I0028418

READINGS IN MEDICAL CARE

READINGS IN MEDICAL CARE

Edited by the

Committee on Medical Care Teaching

of the Association of Teachers
of Preventive Medicine

Chapel Hill

THE UNIVERSITY OF NORTH CAROLINA PRESS

Copyright, 1958, by

THE UNIVERSITY OF NORTH CAROLINA PRESS

FOREWORD

THE crucial resource in the complex industrial society that is the United States today is the capacity of the individual to achieve. Health is vital to achievement, whether for the individual or the Nation. Only a healthier America can become more productive.

To meet his expanding responsibilities, the physician must have a broad understanding of health and disease and of the many forces that are introducing change at an accelerating rate. The doctor does not treat his patients in a vacuum. His ability to make the correct diagnosis and to recommend, administer, and supervise treatment is increasingly dependent upon the availability to him and to his patient of many facilities and assistance from other professional, technical, and lay people. This requires a financial base and an administrative structure adequate to provide modern medical care. Doctors alone cannot mobilize the indispensable resources. This takes organized effort—the effort of doctors, their patients and families, and their community: local, state and national.

The objectives of the physician at mid-century far exceed the cure and alleviation of disease. More important are its prevention and early recognition. Beyond that, the obligation has been accepted by the doctor to strive for the maximal physical, mental, and social efficiency of the individual, his family, and community. To move toward this ideal requires that the physician have a realistic appreciation of the organization of medical care. But that is far from enough! The physician must also understand the deeper forces at play in the Nation. By 1980—less than 25 years from now—it is reliably estimated that the population of the United States will have grown from 173 to 240 million. Medicine must prepare at once for the largest increase in population in our history. Other social changes may have even greater impact. Suburban living is becoming the American mode of life. Families are becoming more mobile. The numbers and proportions of older citizens will steadily rise. Progress in such areas as health management and the care of chronic and mental illnesses will probably call for more intensive medical service per unit of population. The upgrading of our people in terms of education, occupation, and income betokens increased demands for medical services. *Indeed, many of our people now regard the opportunity for good health as their basic human right.* The challenge to society and medicine is already tremendous to expand and redirect our facilities and opportunities for medical education.

It is implicit that the physician as a citizen must bring to bear on social problems his special education, proficiency, and responsibility. He is expected to advise his community, his state, his nation—expected to play a role of leadership as our democratic society endeavors to extend the benefits of expanding scientific knowledge to the service of mankind.

The medical schools are the wellsprings whence will flow the better health of tomorrow. They must constantly adjust their educational offerings for future doctors to the changing conditions and needs of society. Medical students must obviously continue to have an opportunity to build their professional educations on a solid foundation of the natural sciences. The behavioral sciences, particularly psychology, sociology, and cultural anthropology, must receive greater emphasis. Although these disciplines are in their infancy in comparison to physics, chemistry, and biology, they are beginning to make an important impact on medical thinking. Furthermore, an adequate understanding of the setting of medical care is essential for the future physician. Thus, students must learn about the factors that affect the availability and quality of medical care. They need to learn also how to evaluate their experiences and those of others in a number of developing programs such as, for example, health insurance and group practice. Good medicine cannot be practiced independently of the intricate framework in which other health personnel function. The clinical medicine of the future will be indissolubly a part of the future organization of medical service with all the relevant professional activities, facilities, and financing.

At Harvard, interest in the field under discussion started to develop several decades ago. The earliest reported organized teaching program concerned with the structure of medical care in any medical school in the United States took shape in 1945 as a series of special lectures for Harvard medical students. Experts recognized nationally were brought to Boston to present their divergent points of view. These lectures were published in the *New England Journal of Medicine* (January 3 to February 28, 1945) and have also been republished as a booklet entitled, "Medical Sociology." The practice of presenting to medical students all points of view on sociological problems as they relate to medical care has been continued at Harvard by the Department of Preventive Medicine. This is as it should be in a democracy.

The Association of Teachers of Preventive Medicine sponsored with the Association of American Medical Colleges, at Colorado Springs in November of 1952, the Conference on Preventive Medicine in Medical Schools. The *Report* of this Conference was published as Part Two of the October, 1953, number of the *Journal of Medical Education*. Subsequent to that searching exploration of the growing importance of Preventive Medicine in medical education, the Committee on Medical Care Teaching of the Association of Teachers of Preventive Medicine have devoted their efforts to understanding, evaluating, and recording changes in the patterns of organization of medical care and health service. During the past few decades there has grown up in this field an extensive literature consisting of documentation of fact, analysis, postulation of theory, and exposition of philosophy. From this literature the Committee on Medical Care Teaching has selected for the present volume, READINGS IN MEDICAL CARE, a balanced and representative collection. For the first time in a single textbook the background material is available to students in a form to help them appreciate their future roles and responsibilities as physicians and citizens. This worthwhile enterprise has obviously filled an important gap. Medical students can now equip themselves to form balanced judgments of their own concerning many controversial questions.

The rapid changes in our industrial society and the equally rapid changes in medical science mean that the framework and content of medical care and health service will inevitably have to change. The Committee has now equipped all of us in medical education to assist our medical students more effectively as they seek to understand the interaction of social forces to the end that they, when they have become physicians, can mold and guide the resulting interaction in a way to provide at the least expense the finest type of medical care for the greatest number of people.

GEORGE PACKER BERRY, M.D.
Dean, Faculty of Medicine
Harvard University

Boston, Massachusetts
May 1, 1958

PREFACE

THE Committee on Medical Care Teaching of the Association of Teachers of Preventive Medicine has prepared this volume in response to a widely felt and frequently expressed need for teaching material on the organization of medical care. The many and varied documents essential for an understanding of current problems in this field—problems of providing the necessary resources, of payment for services, and of administration of medical care programs—include basic studies dating back to the 1920's as well as important recent publications. Scattered in numerous books, journals, and monographs, these documents are often difficult to obtain; a number of them are no longer in print. Inability to consult them conveniently has been a serious hindrance to students of medical care organization.

Programs of medical care under public and voluntary auspices have grown rapidly in recent years. Paralleling this development, a body of knowledge concerning principles and techniques of medical care organization has accumulated as a result of both research and practical experience in administration of medical care programs. Increasingly this knowledge has become systematized through the joint efforts of persons representing many disciplines.

At a few universities, specialists in medical care organization have established introductory and advanced courses in the subject, relying for supporting material on personal and institutional collections of the relevant documents. But they have been handicapped in their teaching because their students have hitherto lacked a source-book of basic information about the field which is logically organized, inclusive, and readily obtainable. The lack of such a volume has been even more keenly felt by the large number of teachers of medical care organization who are not specialists in the subject, including professors of preventive medicine in medical schools; professors of public health administration in schools of public health; teachers of public health in schools of dentistry, nursing and pharmacy; teachers of community health organization in schools of social work; and faculty members of schools of hospital administration. These instructors and their students have had to depend, in general, on slender and fragmentary collections of documents.

It was primarily in order to provide teachers and students with easier access to sources of medical care data that the Committee on Medical Care Teaching compiled this volume of readings. The book is also intended, however, for members of the health professions—physicians, nurses, medical social workers, hospital administrators, and others—and for those who organize and operate medical care programs under both voluntary and public auspices, whether such programs are financed through insurance, general taxation, or other means. It will contribute, it is hoped, to sound and realistic solutions of medical care questions of the future by making knowledge about past and present problems more conveniently accessible.

Responsibility for organizing the volume and selecting text material, for writing introductory statements for each chapter, and for preparing the lists of additional readings has rested with an editorial subcommittee of the Committee on Medical Care Teaching. The editors have endeavored to choose the most useful and informative writings available and to include items representing differing points of view on controversial questions. The opinions expressed in individual selections are naturally those of the authors rather than those of the editors.

The Committee on Medical Care Teaching has advised the editors on the scope and general orientation of the volume, but not on the choice of specific material for inclusion. The Association of Teachers of Preventive Medicine, while it has taken no active part in either development of the format for the book or determination of its content, has encouraged the undertaking as a useful addition to the literature. Neither organization, of course, is responsible for the viewpoints presented in the various selections.

The book is divided into thirteen chapters, each of which covers a major aspect of the organization and administration of medical care in the United States. The editors had originally hoped to include a chapter describing the experiences of several other countries in organizing medical care services. But, much to their regret, they were forced to eliminate this section of the manuscript owing to space limitations. For the same reason, they also had to omit a number of selections describing American experience that otherwise merited publication in a work of this kind, and to delete extensive passages from some of the selections retained.

Except for the brief introductions to each chapter and a few scattered editorial footnotes, the continuity of the text has not been interrupted by explanatory material. The editors believe that this approach not only makes the book more readable, but also enhances its flexibility as a teaching device, since it permits each teacher to establish his own framework for relating the selections to one another.

Although the editors have attempted, in the arrangement of the book's chapters, to treat sequentially the various facets of medical care organization, they consider that each chapter can stand, in a sense, by itself. Students and other readers interested only in special aspects of the field may profitably explore them by concentrating on specific chapters; and instructors may assign individual chapters for study in order to underscore particular points emphasized in the classroom.

As a guide to more intensive investigation of the different segments of the medical care field, a selected bibliography has been provided at the end of each chapter. Only books, monographs, and pamphlets are included in these lists. While articles in professional journals represent a rich source of data on medical care organization, it would have been impossible within the brief compass of these reading lists for the editors to strike an appropriate balance among the numerous articles that have been published on each topic. Furthermore, since some time must necessarily elapse before the permanently valuable books and monographs issued yearly in the medical care field can be identified, no work published later than 1956 has been included among the recommended readings. Works from which excerpts have been reprinted have not been listed in the bibliographies; the entire book, monograph, or article from which an excerpt has been taken, however, may be considered by the reader as recommended for further reading.

The manner in which statistical material is treated in the volume warrants brief comment. Tables and other numerical data have an important place in certain selections. When they appear in selections dating back several years or more, such data should be viewed by the reader as links in the author's chain of argument rather than as accurate statements of the current facts about the problem under discussion. In certain cases, of course, statistical information which is several years old will still be the best available on a particular subject. In others, it will be obvious that the specific figures presented in the text are definitely out-dated. Where this is true in connection with a few key points discussed in the volume, the editors have used footnotes to refer the reader to sources of more recent information— either in other selections in the book or elsewhere; occasionally, some of the newer data have actually been included in these notes. But in the belief that "old" statistics alone do not impair whatever inherent validity there may be in a given author's ideas on medical care organization, the editors have not, for the most part, attempted to bring such material up to date.

*   *   *

Many individuals and organizations played a part in helping this volume to reach publication. The Committee on Medical Care Teaching wishes to take this opportunity to acknowledge the contribution of those whose role was a particularly significant one.

The Committee appreciates deeply the cooperation it received from the many authors and publishers of selections represented in the volume who very graciously granted permission for the reprinting of excerpts from their works. In most cases publishers gave such permission—in view of the educational purpose of the book— without requesting payment of a fee. The Commonwealth Fund and Harvard University Press were especially generous in permitting the Committee to republish an extensive amount of material from works originally issued under their joint imprint; and several other publishers—including the American Public Health Association, the American Medical Association, Harper and Brothers, the Massachusetts Medical Society, and the American Academy of Political and Social Science—were most cooperative in granting permission for the reprinting of a number of selections from their copyrighted publications.

The Committee wishes also to thank, for the use of excerpts from their writings, the authors of selections reproduced from government publications, as well as those whose publishers granted reprint permission on their behalf. Special thanks are likewise extended to each of the authors who permitted the Committee to reprint excerpts from several of his works, and to each of those who consented to deletions from his material in order that the over-all length of the book might be kept within manageable limits.

The Committee desires, lastly, to emphasize its considerable debt to the persevering members of its editorial subcommittee: S. J. Axelrod, M.D., Franz Goldmann, M.D., Jonas N. Muller, M.D., Cecil G. Sheps, M.D., and Milton Terris, M.D.; to Edward B. Kovar, whose devoted work as the subcommittee's editorial associate made completion of the book possible; to the Association of Teachers of Preventive Medicine and the Subcommittee on Medical Care of the American Public Health Association, for their encouragement and assistance; to individual members and friends of the Committee on Medical Care Teaching, for their financial contributions and advice, which were most helpful in the accomplishment of a difficult editorial and production task; to the University of North Carolina Press, for its continued interest, patience, and understanding; and to the Josiah Macy, Jr., Foundation, for its generous grant of funds which made publication of the volume possible at a price within reach of students preparing for the health professions.

Committee on Medical Care Teaching
of the
Association of Teachers of Preventive Medicine

February, 1958

EDITORS' NOTE

MOST authors' footnotes have been omitted from the present volume; in general, however, original footnotes that either clarify narrative statements, explain tables, or identify sources of direct quotations have been retained. These footnotes are numbered serially within each selection, except for footnotes to tables, which are identified by upper-case letters.

Editors' notes are designated by either asterisks or daggers. The first page of each selection carries an acknowledgment note containing the author's name and most recently reported official position; an indication—when appropriate—that special reprint rights have been granted to the editors; and a reference to the original publication from which the selection has been taken.

Omission of tables, graphic material, or one or more initial paragraphs from the text of a selection as originally published is also mentioned in the acknowledgment note. Otherwise, the usual ellipsis symbol is used throughout the book to indicate that portions of the original text have been deleted by the editors. Ellipses at the end of a paragraph may denote omission of the remainder of that paragraph or of one or more following paragraphs.

Contents

Readings in Medical Care

CHAPTER I

Problems in Medical Care:
The General Background

THROUGHOUT KNOWN HISTORY, men living in communities have had to reckon with the fact that man is a biological organism. As an organism, he has manifested many variations of disorganization owing to interaction of his essential nature with the physical, chemical, biological and social forces of his environment. As we have recognized them, we have called these evidences of disorganization, disease or ill health. Man has attempted to cope with the problems of health and disease in many ways. The provision of medical care, under one title or another, has long been prominent among those ways.

Medical care, as a social device, has constantly developed and changed in response to the movement and pressures of the community in which it has functioned. The degree of change, and the relative emphasis upon the problems of medical care, has varied quite directly with the intensity of general social and economic ferment. It is apparent that we are now in a period of accelerated change.

Knowledge of the significant developments which have led to the present picture of medical care and of the details of that picture will help us to understand what is happening today. With understanding, we can interpret the problems of medical care and help to shape its future through intelligent action. This chapter presents some of the more important facets of the background of modern medicine—in terms of its chief protagonist, the physician; and of its history, social setting and the central socio-economic problems of its existence and distribution. Succeeding chapters will fill in the details of the modern picture.

1. The Physician in Modern Society *

THE RELATIONSHIP of the physician to the patient as an individual and to his immediate family is well understood and has formed the basis of medical practice for centuries. The doctor, in the simpler society of the past, has always been close to the problems, anxieties, and economic situation of his patients. Those contacts were direct and personal. The complexities of present-day living have had a severe impact upon those earlier relationships. . . .

Yet the needs of the individual in matters of health, sickness, and disability are still personal. They are related fundamentally to the same questions as Democracy itself, because the concern of the physician, as it is of Democracy, is for the welfare of the individual.

It is during the same period of rapid change in our economic and social system that we have witnessed the phenomenal development of scientific knowledge. It probably is not an exaggeration to say that the advances in medical knowledge during the last fifty years have exceeded those of the previous five thousand. It is self-evident that no individual can master every phase of medical practice. However, in order to apply that knowledge we must seek new methods which would make available up-to-date medical and health services to the individual, the community, and the country.

It is now evident that in the future an increasing proportion of the population will be in the older age groups. This is an inevitable result of the improvement in public health and in the widespread application of new knowledge in the prevention, control, cure, and treatment of crippling and killing diseases. These changes in the age composition of the population are now having a definite effect on the character of medical care and public health. A large part of the problems in these areas comprises disabilities associated with middle and late life, particularly the chronic and degenerative disorders, physical, emotional, and mental. These disorders often handicap the individual and may limit his ability to work or to live a normal life. The families of many of these persons are not able to take care of them in their own homes because of economic circumstances and conditions of living, particularly in the cities. This presents at once an urgent problem for the hospitals, the medical profession, and community agencies, because proper care requires a wide variety of diagnostic, therapeutic, rehabilitation, re-education, recreational, and psychotherapeutic programs.

Since knowledge regarding the diagnosis, treatment, and prevention of disease is now far in advance of its application, co-operation and teamwork, as represented among other things by some form of group practice, are a necessity. While special-

* From "The Physician in Modern Society," by Willard C. Rappleye, M.D.; *The Diplomate* 22:245-51, Nov. 1950 (No. 7). Reprinted (with omissions, including initial paragraph) · by permission of the author and publishers. The author is dean of the Faculty of Medicine and vice-president in charge of medical affairs at Columbia University, New York.

ization is inevitable and, within limits, desirable, it must be accompanied by a mobilization of skills and talents which will provide every patient, as far as possible, with the highest quality of medical care.

It has long been recognized that illness is unpredictable, but that the economic risks of sickness and incapacity can be distributed on a community-wide basis by spreading these hazards over large numbers and over a long period of time. The voluntary prepayment insurance plans covering different aspects of sickness have been conspicuously successful in recent years. . . . Probably about 75,000,000 people in the country have some degree of financial protection during sickness, most of which protection, however, is partial.*

What must be developed further are provisions for comprehensive medical care for the entire family and emphasis upon preventive medicine, early diagnosis, and competent treatment. Such efforts will focus attention upon preventive rather than purely curative medical practice. There is also a strong trend toward group practice for reasons suggested above and because of such other factors as providing competent medical care at reduced costs. Another consideration is the inclusion of the entire family in any program, together with a sound prepayment insurance coverage.

The rapid growth of prepayment medical care programs sponsored by the leading labor unions in recent months, either independently or jointly with industry, needs special emphasis because it indicates a significant and immediate new development in American medicine and public health. Many of these plans are tied to pension contracts which are actuarially unproved and probably financially unsound. They carry with them the hazard that they will lead ultimately to government supported or aided, voluntary or tax-supported, pension and sickness insurance programs under the sponsorship of labor unions or the government rather than under local community auspices. In our anxieties for security we may well barter away our most precious possession, individual freedom and our American way of life.

Mention need only be made of the increasing emphasis upon ambulatory care of the sick. Early ambulation of hospitalized patients, the development of diagnostic clinics, the modernization of home medical and nursing services, the increasing support of organized public health programs, the improvement in sani-

---

* The Health Information Foundation reported in 1957 that about 112,000,000 persons—almost 70 per cent of the nation's population—were carrying "some form of voluntary health insurance," and that this insurance paid for more than half the costs of all hospital services to insured and uninsured persons, more than 40 per cent of the costs of all surgical operations, and more than 25 per cent of physicians' fees in maternity cases ("Health Insurance Benefits and the American Family," *Progress in Health Services* (a periodical publication of the Foundation), Vol. 6, February 1957; p. 1).

According to the Health Insurance Council (which is sponsored by the insurance companies that offer various forms of protection against hospital and medical expenses), the extent of voluntary protection against hospital, surgical, and "regular" medical expense in the United States, as of December 31, 1956, was as follows: against hospital expense, approximately 116,000,000 persons; against surgical expense, approximately 101,000,000 persons; and against "regular" medical expense (i.e., not including so-called "catastrophic" or "major" medical expense protection), approximately 65,000,000 persons (*The Extent of Voluntary Health Insurance Coverage in the United States*, New York: The Council, 1957; p. 7).

tation, the control of milk and water-borne diseases, the reduction in occupational hazards, and many other efforts may be cited as contributions to the improvement of the health, well-being, and safety of the population. The health of the people is the greatest single asset of any nation and, conversely, illness is probably the most important single cause of economic and social dependency. Adequate medical care may well be America's most essential industry.

It would be quite erroneous for us to assume that these urgent and immediate problems of medical care are new. In varying degrees, the health of the people has always been the concern of society. The very nature of the care of the sick explains why many of the earliest known records dealt with sickness and medical care. Documents show the methods of treatment in the Egyptian dynasties as early as 4,500 B.C. Specialization, in the light of then existing knowledge, was recognized in Egypt about 2,500 B.C.

We hear a great deal these days about specialty boards, qualifying boards, medical licensure, lists of approved institutions, societies, and organizations, but you may be reminded that one of the earliest codes of medical practice was that of Hammurabi, promulgated in 2,250 B.C. That code prescribed the conditions of practice and defined the fees which a physician might charge. . . . It was in ancient Rome that numerous mutual aid associations were created. To illustrate that human nature has changed but slowly, it was specified in Rome in the fourth century that "where there is a question of fees, the medical officer must take as a standard not what men fearing death will pay, but what men recovered from illness will offer."

The need to provide collective protection against sickness was first formulated in modern times in the French Convention of 1794, when the idea of sharing the economic risks of sickness and disability by spreading those hazards over a large population group was initiated. This was done as a direct result of the Industrial Revolution. After the French Convention of 1794, a large variety of organizations were inaugurated to apply the principles of distributed risks in relation to many of the hazards to which employed persons in an industrial society are liable, including unemployment, old age, sickness and survivor benefits, funeral payments, and numerous other financial considerations. In his imperial message to the Reichstag in 1881, Bismarck outlined the first proposal of a nation-wide sickness insurance plan. The program went into effect in Germany in 1883. . . .

Practically every leading country in Europe, however, adopted one or another modification of the original sickness insurance plan of Germany. Much is being said these days in criticism of the National Health Service of Great Britain, but please keep in mind that the antecedents of that service date back at least one hundred years. Great Britain has had national health insurance since 1913. . . .

Increasingly, as the years have gone by, medical-care plans have been linked with other aspects of social security, particularly tying in with such questions as unemployment, cash benefits during periods of illness, hospitalization, rehabilitation, maternity benefits, retirement allowances, and disability assistance. Inevitably, in countries where regulation of the whole economy came into practice, problems of sickness were linked with such matters as the rationing of food, rent controls, allocation of scarce commodities, job assignments, price controls, and various forms of insurance against industrial and occupational hazards. Anyone who to-day disregards the relationship of medicine to current social, economic, and the political conditions must be literally unwilling to face the facts.

The American people are convinced of the value of adequate medical services and are determined that in some way the benefits of modern medicine must be made available to all. It is important for the public as well as for the doctors, dentists, nurses, public health officers, hospitals, and others concerned with community health matters to realize that medical care is for the people and not for the benefit of the professions. The latter have been granted special privileges and recognition by virtue of their ability, knowledge, and skill in rendering the services that must always be, in the last analysis, in the public interest.

The organization and administration of health and medical services must of necessity avoid the proposals of extremists who, on the one hand, advocate complete governmental control and management or, on the other, hold vigorously to defense of vested interests and the status quo. It is often difficult to steer a course in the middle of the road, particularly because that requires a high order of judgment and courage. Our progress must be by evolution, but it also must be progress.

Medical security in this country is coming and it is up to our professions to formulate ways and means by which sound, progressive plans can be drafted. It would be short-sighted and, in the long run, futile to ignore the broad implications of medicine, which must be recognized as much a social as it is a biological science. It is our responsibility to propose and to help in the creation of an environment for medical and health services which will provide opportunities for the very expression of individual freedom which has made medicine and its allied health sciences so conspicuous in the improvement of the welfare of man.

It would not be possible in these brief comments even to mention the many different methods that must be, and are being, employed to meet many facets of this vital responsibility. It is an axiom, however, that any sound program can be only as good as the personnel who operate it. Any plan of organization of professional services, whether developed from within the profession or imposed upon it from without, which lessens the responsibility of the trained professional worker or denies him the rewards of superior ability and character will, in the long run, be detrimental to the public welfare. Since the success of any health and medical program depends upon its personnel and since in our American system that personnel is produced almost entirely in our universities, may we just take a glance at what that may imply. Society in one way or another has contributed substantially to the rapidly developing and expanding areas of basic and medical sciences and to the maintenance of the institutions and organizations which have been created to apply that knowledge to the needs of the individual and the community.

It can be emphasized again that such institutions as universities, medical schools, hospitals, clinics, and professional organizations which enter into this great American effort justify their existence only to the extent that they serve the public interest. Conversely, those functions carry with them an obligation upon the part of the public, through governmental, private, philanthropic, voluntary plans, or other devices, to insure that an adequate supply of well-trained and competent physicians, nurses, dentists, and public health officers are recruited, educated, and placed satisfactorily in our social scheme and that they are properly financed.

Much has been said about the alleged shortage of physicians. It is true that there is a shortage in some areas, particularly certain rural communities. The distribution is faulty but, as facilities and inducements are developed in smaller and rural communities and in certain undermanned specialty fields, there will be a redistribution of professional manpower into these areas.

It is unsound to assume that physicians and expensive hospital facilities need to be distributed into every small community. Modern transportation and communication have made available to many areas a higher quality of medical, hospital, and health services than they have ever had. There is plenty of evidence that the building and equipping of new hospitals where they are not really needed may be more of a professional than even a financial liability. It would be uneconomical and short-sighted to advocate that we train larger numbers of physicians unless we first work out some method of absorbing and distributing the well-trained personnel which we now have where they are actually needed. Inducing doctors to move from those congested areas where there is already an oversupply of physicians would be the quickest and most satisfactory way to meet many of the needs of the regions now short of physicians. Merely producing a surplus of doctors who will congregate in the cities cannot possibly solve the problem of medical care in the smaller and rural communities.

It is disappointing indeed to hear those who should be informed advocate that we return to the mass production of professional personnel that existed forty or fifty years ago when medical education was still in the pioneering stage in this country. If that were done, it could easily result in a return to the relative standards of the diploma-mill era.

Some propose a large increase in the output of medical graduates of the country without safeguards for the maintenance of proper standards of training and competence, on the general theory that over-production of physicians would force the surplus doctors into the areas where physicians are actually needed. The idea is fallacious that economic competition would result in the maintenance of high standards of medical care, because laymen cannot be expected to have a basis for judgment or selection of professional competence.

The training of professional students must be supplemented by continuing education throughout their careers if they are to keep abreast of rapidly developing new knowledge and methods. Hence, graduate and postgraduate education are essential features of any comprehensive health program for the nation. . . . It is highly important to recognize that true education is largely self-education. The responsibility of the universities and the medical schools is to provide an environment in which a student can learn the methods and acquire habits of self-education which are indispensable to the proper discharge of his professional obligations later.

In view of the enormous value of understanding the economic and social factors in the maintenance and extension of proper medical and health services, it is of paramount importance that undergraduate medical instruction and graduate training be permeated with emphasis upon those very elements which will so largely determine many phases of medical and health services of the future. This cannot be brought about so much by adding new courses in sociology and economics to the medical school curriculum as by presenting forcibly to students and faculty alike the importance of these features and trends in modern medicine.

The first step in this process is to awaken a wider social consciousness in the faculties of our own institutions and to introduce that flexibility of medical instruction which will permit a freer interpretation of the obligations of the doctor. Of equal importance is the selection of students who are motivated not to be technicians but to be citizens and leaders in medical thinking, because medical practice is not a private enterprise but a public responsibility. It is unfortunately true that many students have a better social motivation when they enter medical school than when they graduate. Please be assured that all of the leading medical schools are fully aware of these questions and are studying the ways and means by which this point of view can be presented to medical students. They are making every effort to move, perhaps conservatively—and that is wise—in the direction of finding a solution without destroying or undermining the high quality of medical care which has been the cherished tradition of American medicine.

Mention has been made of the selection of students, and here again important contributions can be made to this over-all problem if we will look upon the college period as offering as broad a humanistic and cultural education as the college can provide, including a grounding in the principles of the natural sciences. This critical period in the development of the physician, even before he has come to medical school, should be a preparation not for medicine but for life itself and should not be regarded as "pre" anything. This means a wider concept of the functions of the American colleges. Perhaps we would make immediate gains if we abolished so-called "premedical" education and encouraged students who desire to go into any of the professional fields to prepare themselves for real citizenship. Emphasis should be placed not alone upon better subject matter but upon the functions of learning by the student as distinguished from teaching by the faculty. What we need to-day are more educated men and women who are self-starting and self-propelling and whose interests are not narrow concepts of technical skills but rather a broad grasp of humanistic and social understanding.

The hope of Democracy lies in trained leadership. The medical and allied professions are the trustees of the essential knowledge which will contribute substantially to a solution of the problems of individual and national well-being, happiness, and vigor. Possessing that knowledge, the professions are in a position to make, and are challenged with the responsibility of making, a vital contribution to the public welfare. Our profession will occupy its proper place in modern society to the extent that it provides that leadership and that educated personnel who will be equipped to meet the responsibilities of the future. . . .

2. The Social Framework of Medical Care *

THE PROVISION of medical care has always been linked with the social and economic conditions of specific groups of people, and its quantity and quality form an index to their civilization. Medicine is deeply rooted in the general civilization of a period, and like general culture is a product of material conditions. The position of medicine in society, the tasks assigned to it, and the conduct expected of its practitioners change from one historical period to another. These are determined primarily by the social and economic structure of society, and by the technical and scientific means available to medicine at the time. Seen in historical perspective, it is clear that the provision of medical care is not something eternally fixed and eternally envisaged by all good doctors of whatever age and country, but is rather a problem more or less constantly changing whose solution is changing with it.

Like other arts and crafts, medicine in ancient Greece was an itinerant vocation. The number of physicians was small, and like other craftsmen, such as the shoemaker or the artist, the Hippocratic physician practised his craft while wandering. In smaller towns medical service was provided exclusively by these itinerant physicians. When a doctor came to town, he would knock at the doors offering his services like other craftsmen, and where he found sufficient work, he opened a shop, the *iaterion,* and settled down for a while. Larger communities had permanent municipal physicians. About 600 B.C. individual cities began to appoint such physicians. When a community wanted a doctor to settle down, it offered him an annual salary which was raised through a special tax. This arrangement became general throughout the Greek cities by the end of the 5th century. The physician was not prevented from accepting fees, but he was guaranteed an income even when there was not much work. To a large extent, the community doctor served the need. During the Hellenistic period this practice was to be found wherever Greek culture prevailed.

During the early days of the Roman Republic, medicine was chiefly in the hands of priests. It was then practiced by slaves, and later by freedmen. Greek physicians began to migrate to Rome in the third century B.C., and were soon much sought after. From 91 B.C. on, physicians were always to be found there. Under the Republic and the early Empire, however, all medical knowledge and technique benefited only the wealthy class. No one cared for the poor, no official authority ordered anyone to help them, and no physician thought of treating such unfortunates free of charge.

By the second century A.D., however, municipal physicians, known as *archiatri populares,* had been instituted. Antoninus Pius (131-161 A.D.) decreed that large

* From "Society and Medical Care: An Historical Analysis," by George Rosen, M.D.; *McGill Medical Journal* 18:410-25, Dec. 1948 (No. 4). Reprinted (with omissions) by permission of the publishers. The author is professor of public health education at the School of Public Health and Administrative Medicine, Columbia University, New York.

cities should have no more than 10 municipal physicians, while the middle-sized cities and small towns should have but seven and five respectively. The principal business of these doctors was to give medical attention to the citizens, especially the poor. They were apparently allowed to take fees, but were expected to provide free care for those who could not pay.

In addition to the municipal physicians, medical care in Imperial Rome was provided also in several other ways. Most doctors were in private competitive practice. There were a number of other groups of salaried doctors. Some were attached to the imperial court, others to gladiatorial schools, or to baths. In some cases we find an arrangement whereby physicians were attached to a few families who paid them an annual sum for all attendance throughout the year.

With the downfall of the Roman Empire and rise of the medieval world, the conditions under which medical care was provided also changed. Medieval society was dominated in all its aspects by the Church. It was relatively static, with well demarcated social ranks. Each group was organized and its sphere of action rigidly delineated. During the early Middle Ages, physicians were generally clerics for whom the Church provided living so that they could practice medicine as a charitable service. They were permitted to accept gifts, but were not supposed to ask for any payment. In fact, throughout the Middle Ages, many physicians, because of their clerical status, did not have to take account of economic considerations. From the eleventh century on, however, laymen began to enter the medical profession in increasing numbers. As they were not supported by the Church, they had to earn a livelihood in some other way. This they did by accepting a salaried post, either as body-physician to some lord or as municipal doctor in a town. In either case, the duties as well as the remuneration of the physician were specifically stipulated. Municipal physicians were required to treat the sick poor, investigate the occurrence of unusual or epidemic disease, and to supervise pharmacies. Most salaried physicians also carried on private practice. When doctors treated private patients they had to follow rigid codes, and fees were charged according to strict and binding fee schedules.

During the Middle Ages, a sharp separation developed between physicians and surgeons. The surgeon who worked with his hands remained a craftsman, and learned his art from a master, frequently his father. Each group occupied a different status in the social hierarchy, the surgeons being relegated to a lower position, and organized in the barber-surgeon guilds. During this period, the learned physicians and recognized surgeons neglected almost completely diseases that could not be treated except by dangerous surgical manipulations, with the result that alongside the recognized settled medical personnel there developed a class of travelling empirics who performed such difficult and serious operations as couching cataracts and cutting for the stone. But while itinerant oculists, lithotomists, and hernia operators did not rate highly in social status, yet their services were needed. As a result, various arrangements were made whereby their skill could be utilized. In addition to the itinerant practitioners there were already during the Middle Ages some who settled down in one place. An oculist is mentioned in 1366 at Speyer, and another in 1372 at Esslingen in Germany. In cities where there were no resident specialists the authorities endeavoured to engage the services of such persons, even if only for a certain time during the year. By and large, these conditions continued to persist up to and during the seventeenth and eighteenth centuries.

The conception of the necessity for social assistance in case of sickness was highly developed during the Middle Ages. The guilds had funds for the relief of their sick and disabled members. Wealthy guilds built their own hospitals. Others paid regular fees to a cloister hospital, which was made responsible for the accommodation and care of sick guild members. Among the oldest of these funds in Germany were those of the miners which remained in existence (*Knappschafts-kassen*) until the latter part of the 19th century. When Bismarck introduced his sickness insurance legislation in 1883, it was based in part upon the existing miner's benefit funds. The political power of the guilds was lost following the rise of the absolutist state, but their social insurance functions remained intact.

From the sixteenth century on, with the decay of medieval society and the development of the new economic and social order, that we know as capitalism, medicine in the Western World underwent a gradual but radical change. Attitudes and traditions originated by the medical profession in the precapitalistic era were not easily given up. For a long time the medical profession remained organized as a status hierarchy with the physicians at the top, and below them, in descending order of prestige, the surgeons, apothecaries, cutters for the stone, and itinerant oculists. For the most part, the physicians during the seventeenth and eighteenth centuries were established in the upper ranks of society, and generally their services were not available to the mass of the people. In Germany, many physicians were in the service of the numerous princes, while in England and France they were associated with the world of wealth and fashion. To a lesser degree, the same may be said of the surgeons. In England, physicians and surgeons were generally well enough trained in the diagnosis and treatment of the recognized diseases, but their number was so low that some type of practitioner, by the mere logic of the situation, was found to fill the gap. This was the apothecary, whom Adam Smith described as "the physician of the poor in all cases, and of the rich when the distress or danger is not very great."

Concurrently, forces outside the medical profession were inexorably altering the social and economic framework within which it performed its functions. Under feudalism life for the laborer was generally stable. His economy was undisturbed except for the direct impact of famine or the forays of war. With the distintegration of the old system came the separation of men from the land and the beginning of a mobile labor force. Wages came into wide use. Thereby men escaped feudal bondage, but at the price of their security. The growth of an urban civilization, of commerce, and of manufacture went hand in hand with the creation of new social relationships, the balance and functioning of which were susceptible of acute disturbance. . . .

The problem of the laboring poor, concretely symbolized in the figure of the pauper, occupied a strategic position in the social logic of the eighteenth century. It was in relation to the question of property that various social pioneers began to explore the problem of provision against sickness, inclusive of medical care.

One of these was Daniel Defoe. In 1697, there appeared his *Essay Upon Projects,* in which he pours out suggestion after suggestion for the common good. Among these is "The Proposal for a Pension Office" which Defoe offers "as an attempt for the relief of the poor". With strong faith in business-like methods, he proposed the application to the poor of the principle of collective self-help, the insurance principle. As part of this scheme, Defoe included the provision of medical care.

In 1714, John Bellers, a Quaker cloth merchant of London, published a treatise in which he set forth a plan for a national health service. Bellers proposed the establishment of hospitals to be used as teaching and research centers, the erection of a national health institute, and a plan for the provision of medical care to the sick poor.

Neither problems nor plans, however, were a British monopoly, for in 1754, Piarron de Chamousset, a Frenchman who dedicated his life to reforms in public welfare, proposed a plan for hospital insurance.

The projects of Defoe, Bellers, and Chamousset never materialized, but several plans for the relief of the unemployed, which also provided medical care, did come into operation at Bristol, Hamburg and Munich. . . .

For the most part, medical care for the sick poor in England was provided on a parochial basis. During the eighteenth century parish after parish began to make its medical arrangements by contract. These contracts varied from parish to parish. Sometimes the doctor contracted to attend all cases, and supply medicine as well. In others it was agreed that certain illnesses should be left out of the contract. A typical example of a vestry contract for medical attention to the poor is the following: At Cardington, in 1777: "It was agreed that Mr. Edw. Jackson of Bedford, surgeon, bonesetter, and apothecary and man-midwife (if a woman can't do) attend the poor in illness (the small pox excepted) for the sum of £10. 10 s. to Easter 1778, the overseer sending an order." . . .

Similarly, in the American colonies, practically the only means of providing medical aid to the sick poor was to contract with some private physician for attendance on a salary or visits basis. At an early date the services of a salaried municipal physician were made available to the needy in New York City. Dr. Johannes Kerfyle took office in 1689 and served at least two years. . . . Municipal medical care, however, was not limited to the services of the city physician. Direct and indirect medical aid to needy individuals was often administered through other sources at city expense. In 1729, for instance, the city treasurer was ordered to pay Dr. Jacob Moene three pounds "for setting and Curing the broken Leg of A poor Saylor Named John who was an Object of Charity." The custom of appointing midwives for the service of the poor seems to have been practiced in larger towns throughout the colonial period. . . .

Finally, in considering the provision of medical care in the eighteenth century, note should be taken of efforts by employed laborers and artisans to protect themselves against the exigencies of illness. Urban trade clubs, or friendly societies as they were called, contracted with surgeons to attend their members when sick, at a small annual or quarterly sum per head. By the latter part of the eighteenth century, these societies had become numerous enough in England to arouse at least two legislative efforts to put them on a sound actuarial and financial basis. Bills embodying plans for enabling the laboring poor to provide for themselves in sickness and old age were approved by the Commons in 1773 and 1789, but were rejected by the House of Lords.

The French revolutionary struggles and the reaction to them pushed problems of health into the background, but as the Age of Enlightenment became the Age of Economic Man a welter of new and unsolved problems appeared. Western Europe, and particularly England, came under the domination of iron and coal. Industrial capitalism brought into focus a new social class, the industrial workers and with them the social question of the nineteenth century.

The need for new methods of distributing medical services has been felt since the beginning of the industrial era. Throughout the nineteenth century attempts were made to bring medical care to increasingly large groups of the population. Beginning with the Poor Law Amendment Act of 1834, the medical relief of the sick poor in England was taken over by the Poor Law authorities. After a few ineffectual attempts to reduce the provision of medical relief, steps were taken to provide medical care through Poor Law doctors who received fixed salaries plus an additional payment per case. Various critics of this system pointed out, however, that the provision of medical care should be separated from poor relief. It was pointed out that medical care was beyond the means of half the English population. . . .

The realization that medical care could not be provided for the majority of the population on a commercial basis led to the proposal of various solutions. One English suggestion was to have "a set of public officers distributed through the country, having no private practice, but attending entirely to the sick poor and matters of public health." This awareness of the importance of the people's health was not primarily a humanitarian view-point, but one that was based on very practical considerations. It was recognized that a sick labor force was a health menace. Thus, while economic liberalism was still the dominant social philosophy the establishment of a system of free medical advice to all wage-earners in England and Wales was seriously under consideration in 1870 by the Poor Law Board.

Similarly, provision of medical care for the indigent was a problem of great urgency in Germany. The medical reform movement that developed in Germany during the revolution of 1848 took cognizance of this problem, and its leaders among them Rudolf Virchow, put forth proposals for public medical services for the poor, including free choice of physicians. As in England and other countries wage earners were organized in mutual benefit societies that provided sickness benefits including medical care. From 1869 on, communities in Bavaria, Baden and Wuerttemberg were authorized to establish public sickness insurance funds membership in which could be made compulsory for all unmarried wage earners no living with their parents. In short, the idea of compulsory sickness insurance was accepted long before Bismarck, although its application was quite limited. In 1883 Germany inaugurated compulsory sickness insurance as a part of a comprehensive system of social insurance; and one country after another in Europe adopted a similar solution. In 1911, Great Britain adopted a plan for sickness insurance based on the friendly societies and existing governmental facilities.

In Russia, as in the countries of Western Europe, the situation at the middle of the nineteenth century was such that medical service could not be provided on a private basis for the majority of the people, that is, the rural population. To cope with this problem, Russia in 1864 established a system of public medical service. This was the so-called Zemstvo system, which after the 1917 Revolution provided the basis for the present Soviet medical organization.

In the United States, some recognition of special and limited problems in the provision of medical care can be traced to the colonial period. Mention has already been made of the provision of medical care for the sick poor through municipal physicians and midwives. The need for providing medical care for sick and disabled seamen led to the establishment of a sickness insurance system for this group in 1798. (Parenthetically, it may be recalled that it was out of this scheme that the U.S. Public Health Service eventually developed). Some awareness of a special rural health problem can be traced at least to the Civil War period when, in the report of the first Commissioner of Agriculture to President Lincoln, a chapter was devoted to the health problems of farm families.

It was not, however, until the present century that the problem of medical care began to intrude itself into public consciousness. The social and economic environment within which this development occurred is that of American industrialization, with its accompanying urbanization. American society during the past century shifted from a locally subsisting agricultural economy with handicraft production to an urban mechanized industrial economy, with wide income variation, in which men no longer made their living but worked for wages. These changes in working and living conditions created significant health problems in both urban and rural communities, and have decisively influenced the provision of medical care.

Simultaneously, the advance of medical science led to the use of new diagnostic and curative procedures and instruments. Urbanization and industrialization also contributed to the centralization of medicine in the hospital. These developments facilitated access to medical care through concentration of population, but at the same time, the costs of medical care increased and complicated the problems of its distribution. The fact is that the cost of medical care increased more rapidly than purchasing power, and it was realized by some that to serve the new industrialized American society, medicine required new forms of service.

The first extensive movement for a comprehensive system of compulsory health insurance in the United States appeared in 1916, as a natural and logical sequence to the great success of the campaign for workmen's compensation during the preceding five years. The movement operated through the American Association for Labor Legislation. The methods were of a traditional character—propaganda, publicity, research and legislative drafting. Although bills were introduced in many state legislatures, the health insurance project failed. Its advocates had neglected to take into consideration the class and group interests involved. Various groups united against such legislation and so completely silenced the movement that even agitation ceased for several years.

... It was at this time also that the first discussions of sickness insurance appeared in Canada.

From 1920 to 1932, when the reports of the Committee on the Costs of Medical Care began to appear, all public interest in health insurance seems to have disappeared. The earlier movement for health insurance had developed in the atmosphere of the Wilsonian New Freedom, and declined with it. The period between World War I and the depression of the thirties witnessed an intensification of the social ideology of individualism, and a strengthening of the feeling against so-called paternalistic action.

It was not until the crisis of 1929 and the subsequent depression, that a resurgent movement for the better provision of medical care made its appearance.

The economic conditions that prevailed in the early thirties accentuated the necessity of securing adequate medical care for people of limited incomes. These conditions included as a basic element the depression of 1929-1933, and as subsidiary elements the financial plight of hospitals and the irregular incomes of physicians. It was on the basis of these conditions that various studies in the field of medical care were carried out. . . . It was recognized that large numbers of the population could not finance their medical needs. The National Health Survey of 1935-1936 showed that the frequency of illness was much higher among the poor families than among the well-to-do or rich groups. Disabling illness occurred 57 per cent more frequently among families on relief than among families with an annual income of $3,000 or over. Chronic illnesses were 87 per cent higher for relief families. Non-relief families with an income of less than $1,000 had twice as much illness disability as families with an annual income of more than $1,000. Other surveys substantiated the fact that the amount and quality of medical care received was closely correlated with the family's income. . . .

Out of this realization of the disparity existing between the receipt and costs of medical care and the ability of many people in the lower income brackets to pay for such care, there developed the various efforts to achieve a more equitable distribution of medical care and its costs. These efforts have taken a variety of forms. . . . There are numerous private prepayment medical care programs in the United States at present. . . . These programs vary in type of sponsor, membership, coverage, facilities, services, and charges. The sponsors may be industrial groups, medical societies, private group clinics, consumer groups and governmental units. . . . The second important effort has been the remarkable development of group hospitalization, especially since 1937. And thirdly, there are the efforts to bring about governmental action in the field of medical care, and the increasing tendency of the Government to undertake some form of action. . . .

What the future organization of medical care will be no one can predict with absolute accuracy. But I believe we can agree with the remarks that George E. Vincent * made in 1926: "It looks," he said, "as if society means to insist upon a more effective organization of medical service for all groups of people, upon distribution of the costs of sickness over large numbers of families and individuals,

* President, Rockefeller Foundation, 1917-1929.

and upon making prevention of disease a controlling purpose. Just how these ends will be gained only a very wise or a very foolish man would venture to predict. One thing seems fairly certain: in the end society will have its way."

3. CHANGING PATTERNS OF AMERICAN LIFE *

DURING THE LAST CENTURY in the United States, social changes have occurred which are more far-reaching than any in the previous history of mankind. These changes have embraced all aspects of human relationships. They have stemmed largely from transformations that have occurred in economic life, and in the social relations involved in the production and distribution of commodities, but there is no phase of human behavior that has remained unaffected.

Changes in the economic life of the United States from a locally self-subsistent agricultural economy with handicraft production to a modern industrial economy had commenced about 1800 when machine methods were introduced into the New England cotton textile industry. In the same period, commercial agriculture had begun to expand based on trade between states and regions. The extensive building of railroads between 1830 and 1860 accelerated these developments.

The Civil War had a marked effect in stimulating the mass production industries. The large-scale manufacture of standardized commodities, particularly clothing for the soldiers, and the mass production of guns with interchangeable parts encouraged the development and utilization of the new industrial technology. The accumulation of fortunes from war profits afforded the basis for capital expansion, as did the increasing use of the corporate form of business organization which utilized the capital of small investors. The growth of industrial capitalism both provoked and was benefited by the higher tariffs of the post-war period, the immigration of unskilled workers, and the increase and urbanization of population. Because of these developments, the United States, after the Civil War, became increasingly an industrial country in which production was mechanized and concentrated in large factories. Workers could no longer own the machines which required large amounts of capital, but were obliged to sell their labor power for wages. These changes occurred slowly. The net value of manufactured products did not exceed that of agricultural production until about 1890, while people employed in manufacturing did not exceed those employed in agriculture until 1920.

The need for access to raw materials and for markets for the standardized products of industrial production led to the development of a vast network of transportation facilities that accelerated the breakdown of the insularity characteristic

* Reprinted by permission of the publishers and the Commonwealth Fund from Bernhard J. Stern, *American Medical Practice in the Perspectives of a Century;* Cambridge, Mass.: Harvard University Press, 1945. (The excerpt reprinted, with omissions including one table, is from Chap. I, "Social and Economic Changes in American Life," pp. 1-18). The author was, from 1931 until his death in 1957, a lecturer in sociology at Columbia University, New York.

of earlier periods. The small communities, previously well-nigh self-sufficient in the satisfaction of their own demands for consumers' goods and able to market their products locally, now became webbed with, and dependent upon, the commerce of the world. The turnpike and stage-coach, waterways, the railroads, and then later the automobile and the airplane shortened distances by making comfortable and rapid travel cheaper and more convenient. The changes that have occurred in this regard are well illustrated in the experience of two physicians. Dr. N. S. Davis, prominent in the founding of the American Medical Association, who discussed his journey from Chicago to the session of the Illinois State Medical Society in 1852 at Jacksonville, Illinois, wrote: "I had a journey by stage of one day and a good part of a night, then a ride on the Illinois River, then another piece of a ride on the construction train of a railroad on top of a load of ties, part way to Jacksonville, and I think we came into this city on a stage coach." In 1943, the President of the New York Academy of Medicine, Dr. Arthur F. Chace, as the personal physician of former Ambassador Joseph E. Davies, returned from Moscow to Seattle by air, in the traveling time of 30 hours. The movement of population and materials made possible by these improved means of travel has created problems in the control of communicable diseases beyond the power of local communities to solve. On the other hand, among the effects of the advent of the automobile is the reduction of the number of horses stabled in or near cities, with the result that the population of house flies, the carriers of gastrointestinal infections and especially the summer diarrhea of young children, has been greatly reduced. Better transportation has also widened the service area of the rural physician and hospital.

Industrial production accelerated urbanization. In 1840 the population of the United States was 10.8 per cent urban and 89.2 per cent rural. In each successive decade it became increasingly urban, and in 1940 it was 56.5 per cent urban and 43.5 per cent rural. The rate of urban growth declined markedly between 1930 and 1940, but the industrial concentration associated with World War II has again accelerated the urban trend.

The urbanization process was from the beginning marked by the development of unsanitary, disease-ridden cities, and congested tenements are still a feature of urban life. . . . In general, the objectives of the humanitarian movements organized to achieve fundamental changes in the living conditions of urban residents have not been attained, although certain grave abuses have been partially eliminated.

Some technological changes have, however, improved urban living. Increase in commerce brought demands for wider and better paved streets, and provided the capital required for these improvements. The substitution of brick for timber in building material permitted the erection of more hygienic buildings which offered fewer breeding places for rats and vermin. The manufacture of cheap glass increased the number of windows in homes and factories and made living and working conditions healthier. Improved mining methods and transport increased the fuel supply which, along with better heating techniques, permitted better warmed houses and facilitated the cooking of food. As long as the water mains and service pipes were made of wood, the water supplies passing through them were frequently contaminated by seepage from polluted soil through cracks and joints. When iron, lead, and later terra-cotta mains were utilized, a serious hazard to the lives of city dwellers was eliminated.

Congested housing and unhealthy living conditions are still prevalent and are a detriment to the health of the American people. A comprehensive survey of housing in 1934 revealed that about four-fifths of the 1,500,000 residential dwelling units in the 64 cities studied were still made of wood, about one-third were more than thirty years old, one-sixth were substandard—a large proportion being in a serious state of obsolescence and disrepair. It was found that even by moderate housing standards, 16 per cent of the houses were overcrowded. The National Health Survey also concluded, after a door-to-door study, that contrary to the popular impression, overcrowding is a problem of the small as well as of the large cities. . . .

Sanitary engineering has made great strides during the last hundred years, and this has prevented cities from devouring their inhabitants as was once threatened. . . . A serious lag in the application of present knowledge of sanitation persists. This is true not only in the war centers where the war emergency and material and labor shortages have impeded the establishment of sanitary systems. Before the war, it was estimated, after extensive surveys, that approximately four million urban American families and eight million rural families were without what are still called "modern improvements," that is, running water, private indoor water closets, and bathing facilities.

The health of the inhabitants of cities has been promoted by the purification of urban water supplies. Although large sections of the United States are still without filtered water, great progress has been made in this regard. . . . It is because of advances in sanitary engineering and in public health measures and their administration, as well as the concentration of medical resources in the cities, that the death rate in the cities has declined more rapidly than the death rate of the rural areas, so that the differences between urban and rural mortality rates are diminishing.

In spite of the real distress they have engendered, industrialization and urbanization have been, in the long view, favorable to the social welfare and the health of the masses. Urban living has made possible contact with variant cultures of diverse groups, and so has broadened horizons. It has decreased the coercive pressures of intimate groups, giving freer play to the development of individual personality. It has furnished fruitful soil for the growth of secularism and has helped to dissipate the fatalism hostile to medical progress. Above all, the prodigious scientific and technological changes accompanying industrialization during the last hundred years have made possible a marked improvement in the standards of living of the American people, although these benefits have by no means been equally shared by all sections of the population.

Technological changes have taken place in three major areas: in sources of power, in manufacturing processes, and in types of materials. There has been an increasing shift from manpower to machine power, and machine power has expanded to include not only water, wind, and steam, but electricity and internal combustion engines. Each type has developed in efficiency in recent decades, thereby further multiplying power resources. Because of changes in the sources of power, human service associated with the machine is no longer labor power in the old sense.

The function of labor is no longer primarily to provide power, but to regulate its degree and direction and to manipulate it for productive ends.

The new forms of power have accelerated concentration of population in cities. In the days of water power, mills and factories had to be built where water was available. Steam engines required that factories be built around them. But the electrical transformer and the high-voltage transmission line make it possible to decentralize industry and to locate factories and machines planfully in relation to raw materials, labor supply, and markets.

The importance of machine tools has increased in the process of manufacturing. It was not until the 1850's that the invention of the turret lathe permitted self-controlled tools to perform their successive jobs automatically without the intervention of a human operator. Since that time, there has been a vast extension of automatic machine manufacture, most dramatically illustrated by the continuous strip mill in the steel industry and by developments in automobile and aircraft production. Mechanization has involved a standardization of products and processes, specialization of parts, the conveyor or belt system, and time-motion studies which divide the work processes of the individual laborer into component motions and eliminate unnecessary movements and waste in energy. Management methods and labor-saving industrial instruments, like the photo-electric cell or "electric eye," have greatly multiplied the output per man-hour. These changes are significant from the point of view of medicine, for the health problems of the man who works on an electrically operated conveyor belt or operates a power-driven machine or tractor are not the same as those of the man who uses a hand-operated tool, a pick, or a plow.

The new materials used have also had important consequences. The large-scale manufacture of cotton garments has brought about a higher standard of bodily cleanliness. Cheap artificial fibre materials, such as rayon and nylon, have supplemented and have been combined with the natural fibres to make clothing and other consumer fabrics more numerous, more comfortable, more durable, and more attractive. In construction and production, wood has given way successively and increasingly to iron, to steel and lighter metals, to cement, and to plastics. As a result, metal bedsteads, china or plastic dishes, and aluminum and enamel cooking utensils have facilitated cleanliness, and the use of materials with greater tensile strength in the construction of houses and machines has lessened the rate of accidents.

In general, the living conditions of the American people have been improved by the innovations of goods and services since the Civil War. Motion pictures, automobiles, telephones, electric lights, phonographs, radios, refrigeration and air-cooling, wireless, and airplanes are a few of the hundreds of inventions that have raised the standard of living in the United States during the last century, creating a different psychological milieu as well as a different material environment. Technological inventions have, moreover, made possible a marked decrease in hours of work and a corresponding increase in leisure time and recreation, changes which are all conducive to good health.

Technological advances have also contributed to a considerable growth in national income. It has been estimated that during the period 1849 to 1938 the income received by individuals in the United States increased from under $2.5 billion to $62 billion in terms of constant purchasing power. When account is taken of the increase in population arising both from natural increase and from immigration, and also of changing price levels, the average per capita real income, or income in terms of goods and services purchasable with the dollars received, is estimated to have increased from under $250 in 1849 to $531 in 1938.

The increase in the national income, consumers' goods and services, and leisure time has tended to obscure a simultaneous development in the social structure of the United States which has had a crucial effect upon the well-being of the American people, namely, the trend toward concentration of economic power. Concentration of ownership and vertical as well as horizontal control of production and markets by large integrated corporations have become fundamental features of the economy of the United States since the Civil War.

The ramifications of corporate power have modified considerably the nature of capitalist competition in the United States. In 1904 when corporations engaged in manufacturing comprised 23.6 per cent of the number of establishments, they employed 70.6 per cent of the wage earners, and produced 73.7 per cent of the total value of products. By 1929 they comprised 48.3 per cent of the manufacturing establishments, employed 89.9 per cent of the wage earners, and produced 92.1 per cent of the total value of products. . . .

Corporate ownership is concentrated in a comparatively small number of large corporations. The three hundred and ninety four largest corporations, comprising about 0.09 per cent of the total number, owned in 1937 about 45 per cent of the total corporate assets. On the other hand, the 228,721 corporations with average total assets of less than $50,000, or 55 per cent of the total, owned only 1.4 per cent of the total assets of reporting corporations. The proportionate holdings of the 200 largest non-financial corporations increased from approximately 33 per cent of the total corporate assets in 1909 to over 54 per cent in 1933. . . .

The ownership of the assets of corporations is highly concentrated, so that few persons receive the profits from these undertakings. A study by the Securities and Exchange Commission revealed that in 1937 the 10,000 persons with the highest dividend incomes owned about one-fourth of all stock of American corporations. Less than 75,000 persons, or less than one per cent of all stockholders, and less than one-fifth of one per cent of all income recipients, owned fully one-half of all corporate stock owned by individuals.

While the ownership of farm land and equipment remains less concentrated than that of other economic resources in America, there have been drastic changes in its pattern since the frontier period of settlement. This can be seen in the increase in tenancy in almost all farm areas and the appearance of large quasi-industrial farm enterprises. In 1880 tenants operated 25.6 per cent of all farms, while in 1910 the figure had risen to 37 per cent, and in 1935 to 42 per cent. In recent years the increase in the use of farm machinery has tended to increase the number of large land holdings at the expense of other farm owners and tenants. This mechanization has tended to force displaced farm owners from the better lands to areas where the soils are poorer. Those who are dispossessed altogether have become agricultural laborers or have joined the migration to the cities.

In spite of the vast increase in national income and in consumers' goods derived from technological progress, the ownership structure of American economy has engendered a situation in which a large segment of the American people have incomes which do not permit them to share fully in the social gains that have been made. The distribution of incomes of American families has fluctuated in periods of depression and prosperity. In 1942, according to the findings of the Division of Research of the Office of Price Administration, 10.1 per cent of the 32,650,000 families in the United States had incomes less than $750, 17.7 per cent less than $1,000, 34 per cent less than $1,500, 65.7 per cent less than $2,500. In the higher income groups, 26.3 per cent had incomes between $2,500 and $5,000, 8 per cent had incomes over $5,000, and 2.8 per cent had incomes over $10,000.* The families comprising the lowest third, that is, the group with incomes below $1,480, received only 11 per cent of the aggregate consumer income, while the highest third with incomes above $2,545 received 66.4 per cent. . . .

Concentration of production and ownership has had far-reaching effects not only on income distribution but on all aspects of American life. It curtails the movement of individuals from class to class. It places in the hands of a few men the power to control, through patents and other means, the utilization of scientific and technological innovations, to establish international cartel arrangements with foreign corporations, to regulate plant expansion, to determine the character of the competitive market by fixing the quality, amount, and prices of consumer goods, and to decide working conditions as well as wages. By affecting the basic aspects of the life of the people, it influences profoundly the health of the nation.

These economic developments within the political framework of a democracy have been accompanied by the efforts of workers to organize themselves to protect and advance their interests in the face of the extension of monopoly power. . . . As long as the frontier was open, and the movement of workers out of their class was relatively frequent, trade unions made slow progress, but they grew in strength at the end of the nineteenth century. . . . The Congress of Industrial Organizations began the successful organization of mass production industries in 1935. Both the C.I.O. and the A.F. of L. are now not concerned exclusively with collective bargaining in relation to wages and conditions on the job. They have extended their functions to represent the interests of their members and their families as consumers and as citizens, including their medical care.†

* For purposes of comparison with these 1942 data on income distribution, the following figures regarding 1955 distribution of money income among American families, as reported by the Federal Reserve System on the basis of its 1956 survey of consumer finances, may be noted: of the estimated number of 49,200,000 "family units" contained in the population of the continental United States in 1955, 33 per cent had incomes under $3,000; 26 per cent, from $3,000 through $4,999; 24 per cent, from $5,000 through $7,499; and 17 per cent, $7,500 and over. (Source: Table entitled "Distribution of 1955 Money Income," Vital Statistics Charts Section (unpaged) of *Facts on the Major Killing and Crippling Diseases in the United States Today,* New York: The National Health Education Committee, Inc., 1957).

† Organized labor in the United States has continued to maintain its interest in the status of its members as consumers and citizens, and in procurement of certain "fringe benefits" (such as

As the United States has developed from a loosely knit agrarian economy to an extremely complex and closely knit industrial nation in which corporate control predominates, a considerable expansion has occurred in the functions of government. In the early stages of this country's growth, most social, educational, and economic services were supplied by local governments, or by private institutions and philanthropies. Gradually, however, some of these functions have been assumed first by the states and then by the federal government. Federal activities and finances have tended to expand greatly during wars, natural catastrophes, and economic depressions, when state and local treasuries are incapable of meeting emergencies, and to contract during succeeding years. The long-time trend, however, has been toward an increase in federal services.

The enlarged scope of the government's operations on all levels was in response to the new economic situation, to increased wealth which gave a social surplus on which to operate, to the growth of humanitarianism, and to the influence of organized labor. The growth of population and the expansion of industry obliged city governments to offer a vast array of social services for the welfare of the community, and to impose higher taxes. With the growth of business activity, state governments had to extend considerably their regulatory functions to protect their citizens and to expand their social services.

The federal government likewise found it necessary to expand its regulatory functions in order to meet the situation arising out of interstate business, which could no longer be regulated successfully by individual states. At the same time it extended both direct and indirect aids to business and agriculture in the form of high protective duties for the benefit of domestic manufacturers, grants of land and loans of money for the benefit of railroads, purchases of silver for the benefit of the western mining population, and improvements of rivers and harbors for the benefit of business interests in various parts of the country.

Only at the turn of the twentieth century did the federal government begin to broaden its activities, beyond aids to business, to improve social conditions. Reforms were initiated which ran counter to prevailing laissez faire philosophy. Measures were enacted to protect consumers against harmful foods and drugs. Tariffs were reduced and simultaneously progressive income taxes were established. Machinery for the mediation of labor disputes in the railway industry was set up and control of working conditions of employees on American ships was instituted. The federal Department of Labor was organized and the Children's Bureau was established. The conservation of natural resources, which had been threatened with depletion through reckless exploitation for profit, was undertaken, and provision was made for the reclamation and irrigation of desert areas, the control of national forests, and the preservation of valuable mineral lands. Anti-trust legislation was tightened in an effort to check evasion, the powers of the Interstate Commerce Commission were strengthened, and the Federal Reserve System was established to

medical care) for them, since the A.F. of L. and the C.I.O. merged in 1955 to become the A.F.L.-C.I.O.

provide greater governmental control of banking in the public interest and more adequate credit facilities in different parts of the country.

The economic crisis beginning in 1929 accelerated the expansion of the functions of the federal government. . . . When economic conditions failed to improve and state and local governments, with treasuries depleted and taxes delinquent, proved unable to cope with the problems of relief of the unemployed, the federal government, in unprecedented action, furnished direct aid to the unemployed and to the distressed farmers. In an effort to prevent some of the abuses partly responsible for the economic crisis, it then increased its control over financial and business practices by the passage of such laws as the Securities and Exchange Act. It sought, further, to protect the workers, the middle class, and the farmers by establishing facilities to extend low cost credit to home-owners and small farmers, by passing the National Labor Relations Act, by instituting an extensive system of old-age and unemployment insurance benefits through the Social Security Board, and by extending maternity and child care services. Current controversy over federal responsibility to cope with problems of health must be understood in the setting of these developments. The war has necessitated further extension of federal authority covering all phases of production and the utilization of goods and services as well as of social welfare.

In a brief review, we have traced how the United States has changed from an agricultural to an industrial economy, from a small-scale handicraft to a large-scale machine technology, from a rural to a predominantly urban society. The shift from manpower to machine power, the increase in the use of machine tools which make manufacturing processes automatic, the changes in types of materials used, all have bettered the quantity and quality of consumers' goods and improved the working and living conditions of the American people. Concurrently, there has been a change in the structure of American economy involving the concentration of ownership and the vertical as well as horizontal control of production and of markets by large integrated corporations. In the face of the vast increase in national income and of consumers' goods, a situation has developed in which a large segment of the people of the United States have incomes that do not permit them to share fully in these social gains.

These changes in the social and economic structure of American life had decisive influence upon the functioning of the medical profession. . . .

4. The Impact of New Medical Techniques *

Only during the past generation has any question about our system of medical care arisen. The reason for the comparatively recent origin of the arguments on the

* From: *Private Enterprise or Government in Medicine*, by Louis H. Bauer, M.D.; Springfield, Ill.: C. C. Thomas, 1948 (Chap. I, "The Background of the Problem"). Reprinted (with omissions) by permission of the author and publishers. The author is a practicing cardiologist in New York City.

subject can be seen easily if we review all the developments of medicine in the United States.

Medical Education

SEVENTY-FIVE YEARS ago the ordinary medical school course was one or two years; it consisted largely of lectures. There was little clinical teaching. The medical student apprenticed himself to another doctor to learn the clinical side of medicine. It was quite possible for one man to know all there was to know about medicine. Oliver Wendell Holmes, the senior, was at that time a professor of both anatomy and physiology at the Harvard Medical School and did clinical teaching as well. He is said to have remarked, when asked what chair he held in the medical school, that he did not hold a chair, but a settee.

When Mr. Hyde became president of Bowdoin College, he found that the course at Bowdoin Medical School consisted of two years, the second exactly like the first; the idea being, apparently, that if a student were exposed to the same subjects twice, he would absorb more. Medicine was purely an art and was not a science.

The discoveries of Pasteur became practical, and they affected the whole course of medicine. The antiseptic era of surgery was followed by the aseptic, and surgery made great strides. Bacteriology helped develop medicine into a science. Immunology and biological chemistry gave it another boost, and medicine developed then as rapidly as surgery had previously. Medicine was no longer just an art, but became a science as well. All this affected medical education. Medical courses were gradually extended to cover four years, and clinical teaching became more and more important.

In order to understand the medical sciences properly, it became necessary for the prospective medical students to be trained in physics, chemistry, mathematics and biology. So college credits became necessary for entrance to medical school. More and more specialties evolved, and it became impossible for one man to cover the field of medicine. Post-graduate training then became a necessity. Hence, instead of one or two years of training, now, anywhere from seven to thirteen years are required for the training of a physician *after he graduates from a high school*. This has resulted in medical education becoming much more expensive, and the medical graduate has become much older before he is qualified to take up the practice of medicine. He is often thirty or more years of age before he earns a living and, hence, his professional life is comparatively short. Besides being short, a large part is given to the public. The public has usually realized that the services of physicians are on a higher plane than services based purely on a monetary reward. Recently, there has been an attempt to undermine the confidence of the public in the doctor.

Diagnosis

As MEDICINE became more complicated, so did diagnosis. It was no longer possible for a doctor to carry his armamentarium around with him. The development of the x-ray in the early part of the century resulted in more careful diagnosis in many conditions. No doctor would now think of caring for a fracture without the benefit of x-ray. The x-ray has also entered the diagnostic field in diseases of the gastro-intestinal tract. Diagnosis of ulcers, cancer and colitis are confirmed by the x-ray. Diseases of the lungs are followed closely by the x-ray, as much more detailed information is available from x-ray of the lungs than is possible by physical examination. The x-ray, the fluoroscope and the electrocardiograph have added a great deal to our knowledge of heart disease. As a result, both our accuracy of diagnosis and our prognostic ability have made great progress. Basal metabolism is a necessary adjunct of thyroid diseases. Blood chemistry has not only increased our knowledge, but has facilitated diagnosis and therapy of diseases of the kidney, of the liver, and metabolic diseases. Bacteriology and immunology have made possible modern therapy of infectious diseases. All these new methods are not only essential to modern medicine, but neglect of them would leave the physician open to severe criticism. They have, however, increased the expense of medical care.

Hospitals

THESE CHANGES have also closely affected the hospitals. Usually, it is not remembered in these days of de luxe hospitals that hospitals were originally established for the sick poor. No one of independent means ever thought of going to the hospital. However, as surgery developed, the surgeon was no longer willing to operate on the kitchen table. He wanted and needed proper surroundings and equipment which he found only in the hospitals. So private wings were added to public hospitals and these were followed by exclusively private hospitals.

Just as surgery needed the hospitals, so medicine also needed them. The complicated procedures of diagnosis and treatment in many diseases can be carried on more effectively in the hospital. The public attitude toward the hospital has also changed materially. People used to have a horror of them, whereas, now more and more people prefer to go to one when they are ill. This again results in an increased expense in medical care. The maintenance cost of hospitals has increased greatly. The overhead of a hospital for administration, laboratory facilities, x-ray, operating suites, and many diagnostic facilities which must be available, to say nothing of equipment for the patients, laundry, and food, have made hospitalization more and more expensive.

Nursing

THERE HAS DEVELOPED a greater demand for nursing care, and this is more expensive. Nursing in the early days was pretty much of a trade, and a rather poor trade at that. The new demands of medicine have called for increased education and training of nurses and this has made it more expensive. An increasing number of patients desire, and, in many cases, need private nurses, and the cost of this special nursing care has increased over the years.

Specialization

ALL THESE FACTORS of increased medical education, hospitalization, diagnostic procedures, and nursing care have not only raised medicine from the status of an art to one of both art and science, but have called for increased specialization and, hence, greater expense. Not only is it no longer possible for one individual to know all there is to know about medicine, but it is difficult for him even to know all there is to know in one restricted field. Years of training and experience are necessary to train a competent specialist.

Fees

THE INCREASE in medical fees has been mostly in the diagnostic procedures and in the fees of specialists. The general practitioner receives little more today than he did a generation ago. In fact, if one compares the value of the dollar today with the value of the dollar a generation ago, he receives practically no more.

Therapeutic Agents

ANOTHER INCREASE in the cost of medical care is in therapy. Many of the new drugs and biologicals are expensive. The same is true of oxygen, which is being used more and more. Some states provide various vaccines, serums and other biologicals free of charge to those unable to pay. The time has long since passed when the patient was treated with pills out of the doctor's bag or by a "shot-gun" prescription filled at the local drug store. . . .

5. MEDICAL CARE ECONOMICS: A PROBLEM AREA *

PRACTICALLY ALL of [the problems that have arisen in the economics of medical care] have come from the fact that medical care has increased in quality so rapidly within our own lifetime—within our professional generation almost—and this

* From: "Socio-Economic Problems Confronting Medicine," by Paul R. Hawley, M.D.; *Cincinnati Journal of Medicine* 30:181-86, April 1949 (No. 4). Reprinted (with omissions, including initial paragraphs) by permission of the author and publishers. The author is the director of the American College of Surgeons, Chicago.

great improvement in the quality of medical care has brought with it new and weighty problems in the economics of medical care.

The first of these problems is the increased cost of medical care. To the public medical care comes in one package. The public will not separate the cost of a serious illness into the cost of hospitals, the cost of doctors, the cost of drugs or prosthetic devices. It is the cost of illness insofar as the public is concerned.

In considering the increase in cost of medical care, we must consider all of the factors which have gone into this cost. The cost of operating hospitals is reflected in the cost of everything hospitals must buy. The cost of operating hospitals, like the cost of operating a home, has increased, but with the addition of the greatly increased cost of labor within the hospitals. Twenty-five or thirty years ago the administrative overhead in hospitals was very low. The increasing requirements for records, for good business administration, and for countless other things that have improved the quality of hospital operation, have added greatly to the number of people employed in hospitals. Furthermore, the new and precise technics in diagnosis have greatly increased the proportion of skilled people required for the operation of hospitals. When I was an interne, nurses were practically the only skilled people other than the medical components of the staff of the hospital. Dietitians were just being added at that time. A few people were being trained in the laboratory technics. But other help in hospitals was largely unskilled. Now we have all sorts of medical technicians that are necessary to these precise technics of diagnosis and treatment. When I was an interne, some hospital personnel worked about 76-78 hours a week; all of the personnel worked well over 60 hours a week. Now, most of the hospitals are reduced to 44 hours, and some to a 40-hour week. All those things have added very greatly to the cost of hospital care.

So far as the patient is concerned there is another addition to the cost of medical care, because more and more people must now go to a hospital in order to get treatment that is possible only in hospitals. Much of modern treatment and diagnosis is not possible in the home. Increased costs of the hospital operation, therefore, have added much to the over-all medical bill of the people.

In the treatment part of the doctor's services, there has been relatively little increase in cost—surprisingly little considering the general increase in prices and the devaluation of the dollar. The fees charged by physicians today, by and large, are not much greater than they were when I was a medical student and interne. . . .

On the other hand, the cost of diagnosis has increased very, very much. Thirty years ago there were very few diagnostic technics to apply to a patient, other than those the doctor applied himself with his hands, eyes and ears. Perhaps a blood count was done or a broken bone x-rayed. X-ray was just coming into its own and was not very widely used. There were few precise technics. Very little thorough clinical laboratory work was done. The cost of diagnosis thirty years ago was low and added very little to the cost of medical care of the patient.

The next problem that has arisen in the economics of medical care is a shortage of hospital beds. There is an over-all shortage of beds in this country but no one knows now exactly how great this shortage is. The American Hospital Association realizes full well that the surveys completed only 2 or 3 years ago are now highly inaccurate. The principal reason for this is the decreasing duration of treatment of patients in hospitals—due to many things, principally to early ambulation in surgery and certain medical and neurological conditions. There is, however, some shortage of beds but it is more a question of bad distribution of hospital beds throughout the country. This must be corrected if we are to give to all of the people of the country the benefits of modern medical knowledge. This shortage of hospital beds is one that is rather difficult to meet at the present time because of the high cost of construction. . . .

Another thing, when income and other taxes were lower it was not too difficult to get philanthropists to contribute hundreds of thousands of dollars toward the building of hospitals. The growth of our own medical center here, for example, was due in large part to the philanthropy of a few citizens of Cincinnati. That would not be possible today. There is just not that much loose money after the government gets through with the taxpayer. . . .

A third problem to be met in this changing economy of medical care is the increasing cost of medical education. It is very difficult to determine the average cost of medical education in the United States because bookkeeping in various schools varies. Some charge the entire research program to the cost of teaching medical students, for the very defensible reason that they could not operate a medical school without research. Other schools separate the cost of research from the cost of actual teaching. The schools with which I have been in contact during the last year or so estimate the cost of educating one student for one year to be between $3,800 and $6,000. The high figure I have given is from a school which charges all of its research program to teaching. The tuition charged medical students ranges only from about $600 to $750 a year; so students are paying not much more than 20 per cent of the cost of their medical education. Someone else has to pay the rest. This fact, coupled with greatly decreased returns on endowments, has placed the endowed schools of the nation in a bad financial position. It was the endowed schools in my time that were the wealthier schools. That position is now reversed, and today it is the State-supported schools of medicine that are in the better financial condition; and the endowed schools are in serious financial condition.

The fourth problem in this changing economy of medical care is the shortage of personnel in the entire health field. I realize fully that there are people in medicine in this country who say we have enough doctors but that they are badly distributed. I think the answer is that, if we had more doctors and more competition, the matter of distribution might solve itself; but whether or not there are too many doctors in clinical medicine, it is an indisputable fact that there are too few doctors in the field of public health. There are many areas in this country who have no organized and well directed health departments. There are numerous communities that would like to establish a public health department now and have the funds to do so, but are unable to get trained personnel. Again, whether or not there is an actual shortage of physicians in medicine, there certainly is a shortage of general practitioners of medicine, especially in the rural areas. There are millions of people living in this country today who never see a doctor of medicine year in and year out. There are millions, literally millions, perhaps 15 or 20 millions of people in this country, who are forced to depend on osteopaths and chiropractors for the medical care they get because there are no doctors of medicine in their part of the country. This shortage also extends to the other people in the health field—dentists, nurses, medical technicians of all categories. This is a problem which must be met if we are to extend good medical care to all of the people in the country.

Now to explore a little farther for the moment this problem of increased cost— the increased cost of medical care has made the prepayment of medical care an absolute necessity for a large segment of the population. It is insurance like any other insurance.

I like to illustrate the necessity for medical care insurance with a rather homely example. My forefathers came down the Ohio River on a flatboat, about the turn of the 19th century; and they debarked at the mouth of the Little Miami and took out "soldier land" in Clermont County. They felled the trees on that land and from them built a log cabin. They made all their own furniture and many of the utensils that went into the cabin. The actual capital needed for such a home was very small indeed. If the home burned down the loss was not great. It was no catastrophe, no disaster, at best only an inconvenience, because the home would be replaced with the same work and materials that went into the original. Often, when a home was built, there was a "log rolling" which everyone attended, and the home was under roof by nightfall. The risk from a fire of a home like that was so little that no one would think of carrying insurance. Compare that to the modern home, built of expensively processed materials, by skilled workmen commanding high wages, furnished with expensive furniture and equipped with all modern appliances, fine draperies and perhaps even a television set. There are very few people in this country who can afford to carry the risk from fire to a home like this, even if they have capital in the bank to replace it. So everyone carries insurance against such a loss.

Now take the practice of medicine. When I was a small boy, and even when I started to practice medicine, what happened in the case of illness? There were two doctors in our own household, my grandfather and my father. My mother never thought of consulting them if I became ill until she had exhausted her own pharmacopoeia, which consisted of a dose of castor oil, a liquid diet, and if there were respiratory symptoms, a concoction of turpentine and lard rubbed on the chest. If these didn't work, my father or grandfather was consulted. So it was in every family. The doctor was not called until the illness had gotten out of hand and all home treatment had failed. The doctor came into the house with his little black bag. In it he had a clinical thermometer, a stethoscope (although often when my father did detect something with the stethoscope, he would ask for a towel and put his ear to the chest to verify what he heard. He had learned in school to auscultate the chest directly). There was no tongue depressors because the family always furnished a spoon. That was the complete diagnostic equipment of the family doctor, in addition to his eyes, ears and hands. About all the clinical laboratory work he could get done was a urinalysis—and many of those were done by exposure on the window sill. That was not a costly kind of medical care. Death frequently stepped in to limit a medical bill in those days. So most of the people could afford to pay for the medical care of that time. There were no nurses—the family or neighbors served. There were not those refinements that are now an accepted part of medical treatment. . . . No one thought of insuring against the cost of medical care.

Compare that with the medical care of today and you have the comparison of the modern home and the log cabin. Medical care today is very fine, very luxurious, very efficient, but very costly. . . .

FURTHER READINGS

Cabot, Hugh. *The Patient's Dilemma.* New York: Reynal and Hitchcock, 1940. 284 pages.

Clapesattle, Helen. *The Doctors Mayo.* Minneapolis: University of Minnesota Press, 1941. 822 pages. (Includes references).

Flexner, Simon and James T. *William Henry Welch and the Heroic Age of American Medicine.* New York: Viking Press, 1941. 539 pages. (Includes references).

Galdston, Iago (ed.). *Social Medicine: Its Derivations and Objectives.* New York: Commonwealth Fund, 1949. 294 pages. (Includes references).

Riesman, David. *Medicine in Modern Society.* Princeton, N. J.: Princeton University Press, 1938. 226 pages.

Sand, René. *The Advance to Social Medicine.* New York: Staples Press, 1952. 655 pages. (Includes references).

Shryock, Richard H. *The Development of Modern Medicine.* (2nd ed.). New York: Knopf, 1947. 457 pages. (Includes references).

Sigerist, Henry E. *Civilization and Disease.* Ithaca, N. Y.: Cornell University Press, 1943. 255 pages.

Stern, Bernhard J. *Society and Medical Progress.* Princeton, N. J.: Princeton University Press, 1941. 264 pages. (Includes references).

CHAPTER II

The National Health Picture

KNOWLEDGE OF THE STATUS of the nation's health is fundamental to any consideration of the needs of the people in regard to medical care and its future. The definition of health varies with the knowledge and understanding of its content and with the culture of those who offer the definition. In practice, our definition is usually in the negative terms of the extent or absence of disease or defect. It is in essentially such terms that this chapter offers a description of the health of our people.

The appraisal has been made in terms of mortality rates, the average expectation of life at birth, and the incidence and prevalence of disease and disability as determined by sample surveys of the population. Ample evidence has been accumulated to indicate that our people are subject to an enormous volume of both acute and chronic illness, with the latter accounting for an ever-increasing proportion of the burden. Considerable progress toward better health is indicated by the increases in the average expectation of life at birth and the marked reductions in infant and maternal mortality over the past few decades. However, the average obscures the sharp contrasts that exist among the various regions of our country and the many segments of our population. Continued study of the detail is essential if further progress is to be made.

The extent of that progress will depend also upon the acceptance of the new and positive concept of health as "a state of complete physical, mental and social well-being and not merely the absence of disease." We have been primarily concerned, to date, with sickness and death. Modern medicine and the society in which it functions would seem to be ready for an increasing concern with health and life.

We will need to know more of the manifestations of health, of its incidence,

30

and of the extent and nature of associations between specific factors in the individual and social environment and a state of well-being. The best planning for health requires such knowledge. The current picture of relationships between environmental factors and illness offers us leads for future studies, and for the application of current knowledge as well.

6. A DEFINITION OF HEALTH *

BY "HEALTH" IS MEANT something more than vitality or even actual survival. An individual may possess a physical impairment that handicaps him or presages death within a few years, may be frequently or constantly ill from a disease, may be mentally abnormal or even insane, and still be counted as a survivor. Health is marked by vigor, but not by vitality in the sense of inherited longevity. Nor is the health of a people characterized by fertility, since to survive beyond the age of reproduction and to be fertile are two distinct biological capacities and, as far as we know, are not even associated, although both may vary in similar or opposite ways because of common environmental conditions. Nor does health necessarily imply painless adjustment to an environment, for the reason that the individual and his environment are constantly changing ad the process of continuous readjustment may entail normal reactions without ill health or harm. A healthy state is difficult to define precisely; it may be described as freedom from physical and mental impairments (except those that are the natural concomitants of the aging process, the wearing out of the human machine), from disease, and from illness. This is the commonly understood interpretation of the word, and it is sufficiently precise for our purpose without putting too fine a point upon it.

. . . Since resistance to disease, quality of vigor, and capacity to cope with environment vary with age, we ought as far as practicable to have [the morbidity and mortality] picture [for the American people] at each state of life. And since defects, impairments, illness, and death differ in kind and cause, it will be well to have some idea of the nature of ill health and of the ways in which failure to survive occurs at different ages.

The necessity for all this factual detail would not exist if it were feasible to discover or construct some single index of health. Various indices have been proposed, such as the "index of physical fitness" suggested by Dreyer, or the height-weight tables for children of either sex, or the "index of robustness" proposed by Pignet. The trouble with all these statistical devices is that they do not take into account *all* of the salient symptoms of ill health and *all* of the structural and func-

* By permission from *Health and Environment,* by Edgar Sydenstricker. Copyright, 1933. McGraw-Hill Book Company, Inc. (The excerpt reprinted, with omissions including initial paragraph, is from Chap. II, "The Nature and Extent of Ill Health," pp. 18-20). The author was, from 1928 until his death in 1936, director of research for the Milbank Memorial Fund, New York.

tional differences among individuals. Each type of impairment, each disease, is characterized by a syndrome of symptoms. Furthermore, the biological diversity of individuals is enormous. The best that any index so far invented can do is to select out from the mass those persons who are so far away from "normality" that their divergence is perfectly apparent to anyone; the statistical index thus is likely to be merely an interesting device with which one may divine the obvious. On the other hand the details of the evidence, unsatisfactory as the data often are from the viewpoints of accuracy, precision, and completeness, afford an insight into the situation that no index, however ingenious or sensitive, can possibly give. . . .

7. The Decline in American Mortality *

THE ENTIRE POPULATION of the United States doubled during the first half of the twentieth century and the number of persons 65 years of age and over quadrupled. Reductions in mortality have been only one factor in aging our population; the other two factors were changes in birth rates and in immigration. These three factors are interdependent and not mutually exclusive causes of change. For example, reduction in deaths of children from birth to age 18 or 21—that is, until the age at which they would normally leave their homes—has undoubtedly been an important part of the story of the downward trend in birth rates prior to the last half dozen years. Parents now can get a house full of children without the nineteenth century level of birth rates. We economize on the lives of children. The interrelationship between mortality reductions and the low level of immigration for almost thirty years would be too tedious to develop at this point. . . .

The crude death rate has declined from 17.2 per 1,000 population in 1900 to 9.6 in 1950. Infant deaths probably accounted for one-fifth of all deaths in 1900 but only for one-twelfth in 1950. The infant death rate was probably at least 15 per cent whereas it is now 3 per cent; the death rate among the children of one to four years of age has declined from about 2 per cent to one-seventh of 1 per cent. In 1900 probably about 750 of 1,000 babies born were scheduled to reach their twenty-first birthdays under the mortality conditions of 1900, whereas about 940 of 1,000 babies born today are scheduled to reach their twenty-first birthdays. I say "scheduled" to allow for the fact that all survivorship probabilities derived from a life table of a particular calendar year are forecasts which are based solely on the mortality conditions of that calendar year.

I am always intrigued by the great improvements in maternal mortality because there is no better place to start telling the story of longer life than with the story of the mother's chances of surviving pregnancy, childbirth and confinement. This

* From "Significance of the Half-Century Decline in Population Mortality," by Frank G. Dickinson; *Proceedings of the Fraternal Actuarial Association* 23:25-36, 1950-51 (published in Rock Island, Ill.). Reprinted (with omissions) by permission of the author and publishers. The author is the director of the Bureau of Medical Economic Research of the American Medical Association, Chicago.

probability is slightly above 999 in 1,000. This is a great social gain and a source of comfort to our own wives and daughters. The improvement in maternal mortality has been quite general throughout the nation. The *highest* state maternal mortality rate in 1949 was only slightly more than half the *lowest* state rate in 1933, the year when all the states were first included in the registration area.

The increase in life expectancy at birth from 49 to approximately 69 years is the purest and most general measure of mortality reductions. This is a pure figure in the sense that the base is not influenced by immigration, emigration and fluctuations in the birth rates.

I wish I could take time to discuss the evidence that longer life means healthier life, age for age. The question is worthy of an entire paper, for the evidence is conflicting. For example, as physicians gained increasing control over the progress of diabetes the patients were enabled to live on in comparative comfort as useful citizens though with shorter average future lifetimes. The death rate from diabetes in the age group from 65 to 74 has more than doubled while the general death rate for this age group has declined more than one-fifth. This increase for diabetes suggests that medical progress can produce a rising age-specific death rate from one cause of death simply because more young people suffering from this disease are enabled to live on to the higher ages of life. Age-specific fatality rates for diabetes, based upon 100,000 persons with the disease in an age group, would be superior in some respects to age-specific rates based upon all persons in that age group.

If we were to consider diabetes alone we would conclude that longer life does not mean healthier life. But a full discussion would require an appraisal of the great reductions in the impairments of later life which have resulted from the increasing control over some of the causative diseases, such as pneumonia, scarlet fever, measles. And before a balance could be struck in determining whether longer life means healthier life, a student would want to go into the field of genetics to see if longer life for laboratory animals produced a higher or lower percentage of well days, age for age. Unfortunately, our data on morbidity are too inaccurate to serve as a measuring rod. But I must leave this topic with the observation that the medical progress which enables modern society to maintain the life of an individual who would have died under the medical knowledge of several decades ago or several years ago is a force which has tended to make the healthy, unimpaired person even healthier. It seems very unlikely that longer life could mean a less healthy life for the average person. But longer life, whether a healthier or a less healthy existence, is a basic gain for mortals.

Now for a few more general statistics of an historical rather than an actuarial nature. The mean age at death has risen from 34 to 59 years. One-third of the funerals in 1900 were for persons who had lived for at least 50 years; now three-fourths of the funerals are for such persons. The median age at death has jumped from 30 to 66 years. One-fourth of the people dying in 1900 had lived 62 years or more; now 76 years or more. Three-fourths of the people dying in 1900 had lived two years or more; now 49 years or more. Since the distribution of deaths by age is a U-shaped curve and since the mode is age zero to one year, it is necessary to use several measures of central tendency instead of relying on one alone to explain the changes since 1900. That the mortality reductions have not been the sole cause of altering the values of the mean, the quartiles and the median ages at death need not concern us too much today. My purpose today is to choose data which point out the social significance of dying later. I do regard mortality reductions as the major cause, although the causes can scarcely be evaluated separately because they are interrelated. . . .

8. THE NATION'S HEALTH STATUS *

THERE APPEARS TO BE a wide divergence of opinion as to the status of the nation's health; some contend that we are the healthiest nation in the world, others cite comparative mortality rates to prove that the United States ranks seventh among the nations with the lowest death rates.

Close scrutiny, however, promptly reveals that neither of these contentions is meaningful. The six countries that boast of lower death rates (the Netherlands, Uruguay, Canada, Denmark, Sweden, and Norway) cannot really be compared with the United States, first because they are so different from this country, and second, because there are so many variations within the United States in conditions affecting health indices that any figure for the country as a whole is meaningless. . . . Climatic variations, cultural homogeneity of the population, variations in degree of industrialization, in standards of living, in age and sex composition, in health literacy, in record-keeping, are important factors which render the comparison of the health indices of different groups, either inter- or intra-nationally, rather fruitless. In none of the above-listed respects is the United States as a whole comparable with other countries; the comparison of its death rate with that of any other country cannot serve as an index of its health.

Indeed, the death rate itself does not afford a clear picture of the health conditions of any country. Our current national death rate is compounded of a high rate of maternal mortality in some states and a low rate in others; it takes in the rich and the poor, the babies lost in early infancy, the adults killed in traffic and in home and industrial accidents. Being an average figure, the death rate swallows up and thus conceals all the particular and meaningful items by which the state of the nation's health might be judged approximately.

General Problems of Medical Care

THERE ARE BOTH LIGHT and dark spots in the American picture, and some of the dark spots are very dark indeed. These deficiencies are not revealed in the gross

* From: *Medicine in the Changing Order,* by the Committee on Medicine and the Changing Order, New York Academy of Medicine; New York: Commonwealth Fund, 1947 (Chap. III, "The Health of the Nation," pp. 37-40). Reprinted (with omissions) by permission of the publishers.

fact that life expectancy at birth rose from 49.24 years in 1900-02 to 64.5 in 1943,* but they begin to emerge when detailed comparisons are made between one state and another and between one economic level of the population and another. Although there is ample ground for satisfaction with the progress already made, there is also much evidence that many persons are in sore need of more and better health services.

It is in the contrast between the good and the bad that one perceives the most disturbing aspects of the American health situation. In 1942, for example, the infant mortality rate for the nation as a whole was 47 per 1,000 live births, while that for New Mexico was 99.6. But in Connecticut the rate was only 34.1.† Had the Connecticut rate obtained throughout the country, thousands of infants would have been saved in that year alone. To take another comparison, if the 1945 death rate for tuberculosis had been as low for the entire country as it was for the state with the best record, many more thousands of lives would have been spared. Whatever the reasons for these variations, it is not to be denied that if better health facilities were in some way made available to all sections of the population, our gross mortality would certainly be reduced.

But mortality statistics tell only part of the story. There is a vast amount of illness which, while it does not lead directly to death, has far-reaching and immeasurable effects on individuals, families, and social groups. No one can gauge the suffering and anxiety caused by sickness. A number of attempts have been made to establish just how much and what kinds of illnesses and physical disabilities prevail among the population of the United States at any given time. Much of the data yielded by these efforts is of uncertain value. The induction examinations during World War II did reveal, however, that close to a third of those examined were unfit for military service because of physical and mental deficiency and disease. Even granting that the examination standards were high, and that some of those unfit for military service may yet be fit for civil life, the residual facts still constitute a serious charge against our national well-being. There are evidently many among our people who are below par and whose condition would be improved by raising their standard of living and by making available to them more and better medical services.

* For 1954, provisional figures on life expectancy for the American people, as reported by the National Office of Vital Statistics, were as follows: entire population, 69.6 years; white males, 67.4 years; nonwhite males, 61.0 years; white females, 73.6 years; nonwhite females, 65.8 years. (Fetal deaths and deaths among members of the American armed forces overseas were excluded from the calculations on which these figures are based.) (Source: Table entitled "Total Deaths and Death Rates, Deaths Under 60 Years of Age, Median Age at Death, and Life Expectancy by Race and Sex: Death-Registration States, 1927-1955," in Vital Statistics Charts Section (unpaged) of *Facts on the Major Killing and Crippling Diseases in the United States Today*, New York: The National Health Education Committee, Inc., 1957). (Note: All 48 states and the District of Columbia are now included in the "death-registration area").

† Cf. these rates with those listed for 1946 in Selection No. 10A, below (pp. 40-42), and with the provisional national rate for 1955 given in the footnote on p. 40.

Means to Health Improvement

THE PROVISION OF better living conditions involves economic complexities which cannot be entered into here. But an increase in real income among the poorer elements of our population would doubtless lead to a substantial improvement in health even in the absence of a change in the medical services available to them. There is no question, for example, that there are a great number of Americans whose food is inadequate, and that if these people had larger incomes and were better instructed their diet and therefore their health would be improved.

But the elimination of poverty, involving as it does the whole economic system, is of necessity a slow process. It is no argument against immediate steps for extending medical care to say that complete solutions will have to wait upon long-range economic changes. Furthermore, it is evident that in some instances adequate medical care is a more pressing need than economic advancement. The contrasts in infant mortality rates cited above for Connecticut and New Mexico may serve as an illustration. Many of the people in Connecticut are quite poor, yet in that state only 34 babies died per 1,000 live births; while in New Mexico the infant mortality rate was nearly 100, about one in ten. The most striking difference in the two states appears when the medical services available in each are examined. In Connecticut in 1943 virtually all births were attended by a physician and took place in a hospital; in New Mexico nearly a fourth were not attended by a doctor and about half occurred outside of hospitals. Even if we assume what is surely questionable, that the *quality* of these services was as good in New Mexico as in Connecticut, the difference in *quantity* is obvious. In a situation of this sort, medical care improvements could be effected more promptly than could a general improvement in economic status. . . .

9. EXTENT OF DISABLING ILLNESS *

NEW ESTIMATES of the prevalence of disabling illness among persons aged 14 to 64 years in the United States have recently been compiled from the results of two sample surveys, identical in plan, undertaken in February 1949 and September 1950. The findings of the first of these surveys have been available for some time, but users of the data were cautioned to take into account the fact that the amount of illness in the country is usually at or near the top of the seasonal cycle in February. The statistics presented for February 1949, therefore, over-estimated the amount of disabling illness that one would find in the United States on an average day. On the basis of that survey it was estimated that 4.6 million persons between

* From: "Two Surveys of Disabling Illness," by Theodore D. Woolsey; *Public Health Reports* 67:807-10, Aug. 1952 (No. 8). Reprinted with omissions. The author is assistant program director of The National Health Survey, Division of Public Health Methods, Public Health Service, Washington, D.C.

the ages of 14 and 64 years, inclusive, were unable to carry on their usual activities because of some illness or other medical condition.

TABLE 1. *Estimated number* A *of persons with a disabling illness or condition in the civilian noninstitutional population, 14 to 64 years of age, by age and sex, United States, February 1949 and September 1950*

Sex and date	Numbers of persons (in thousands)						
	14-64 years	14-19 years	20-24 years	25-34 years	35-44 years	45-54 years	55-64 years
	All disabled persons						
Both sexes:							
February 1949	4,569	387	364	650	797	1,044	1,330
September 1950	3,605	225	259	534	618	804	1,167
Male:							
February 1949	2,341	196	150	274	366	566	791
September 1950	2,005	124	118	243	306	426	789
Female:							
February 1949	2,228	191	214	376	431	478	539
September 1950	1,600	101	141	291	312	378	378
	Persons disabled over 3 months at the time of the survey						
Both sexes:							
February 1949	2,300	120	121	260	343	562	893
September 1950	2,206	75	103	266	338	517	909
Male:							
February 1949	1,412	71	73	160	190	338	580
September 1950	1,378	46	61	158	205	293	616
Female:							
February 1949	888	49	48	100	153	224	313
September 1950	828	29	42	108	133	224	293

A All figures in this and other tables are estimates from a sample survey and are, therefore, subject to sampling variability which may be relatively large for the smaller figures and the small differences between figures. Each cell of this table was rounded separately; hence, the detail figures do not always add to give the exact total shown.

As had been expected, the second survey revealed a lower prevalence (table 1). In September 1950, the estimate indicated that slightly more than 3.6 million persons aged 14 to 64 were disabled, using the same criteria of inability to carry on usual activities. Most of the difference between the two figures was in the cases of illness of short duration, that is, the cases for which disability had lasted a month or less. Many of these illnesses were probabaly the minor respiratory infections which are responsible for the greater part of the seasonal differences.

On the other hand, the number of persons who, at the time of the survey, had been disabled for more than 3 months was not greatly different in September 1950 from the corresponding number in February 1949. The estimate from the earlier survey was 2.3 million and from the later survey, 2.2 million. These must have been chiefly chronic disabling cases, and the stability of the number is in accordance with expectation.

A comparison of the numbers of persons disabled for more than 3 months (lower half of table 1) and the numbers of all persons found to be disabled (upper half) indicates that the cases of longer duration form a proportion of the total that (*a*) increases steadily with age; (*b*) is higher in September than in February; and (*c*) is higher for males than for females.

The surveys did not cover the population of resident institutions, such as hospitals for mental disease, tuberculosis sanatoriums, homes for the aged, and orphanages. The number of disabled persons 14 to 64 years of age in these institutions is estimated at roughly 750,000. Most of these have undoubtedly been disabled for more than 3 months, and, hence, would have appeared in the lower part of table 1, as well as in the upper part, if they had been included in the survey.

In addition to supplying national estimates of the numbers of disabled persons, the two surveys also afford an opportunity to make comparisons of the prevalence of disabling illness in the main age and sex groups of the population aged 14 to 64 years and in urban, rural, and employment status categories.*. . .

TABLE 2. *Estimated percentage ᴬ of persons with a disabling illness or condition in the civilian noninstitutional population, 14 to 64 years of age; by age, sex, race, and marital status for females, United States, February 1949 and September 1950 combined*

Sex, race, and marital status for females	Average percentage of persons with a disabling illness or condition, by age						
	14-64 years	14-19 years	20-24 years	25-34 years	35-44 years	45-54 years	55-64 years
Both sexes	4.19	2.46	2.78	2.58	3.45	5.40	9.38
Male	4.59	2.62	2.50	2.37	3.37	5.89	11.96
Female	3.82	2.31	3.02	2.78	3.52	4.93	6.84
Married	3.45	2.46	3.18	2.33	2.92	4.34	6.16
Not married	4.70	2.28	2.70	5.35	6.85	6.97	8.18
Both sexes:							
White	4.03	2.39	2.66	2.46	3.29	5.17	8.97
Nonwhite	5.77	3.01	3.80	3.93	4.91	7.87	15.00
Male:							
White	4.51	2.55	2.52	2.34	3.30	5.78	11.59
Nonwhite	5.42	3.33	2.28	2.71	4.06	6.92	16.88
Female:							
White	3.58	2.25	2.78	2.56	3.28	4.56	6.41
Nonwhite	6.07	2.70	4.94	4.87	5.63	8.77	12.96

ᴬ See footnote A, table 1.

The data in table 2 reveal three points which are worthy of particular attention. First, there is the high prevalence of disabling illness among males at ages 45 years

* These comparisons are made in Public Health Monograph No. 4, which is a more extensive analysis of the two surveys discussed in this selection. See list of further readings at end of chapter for the appropriate reference.

and over. A higher rate for males than for females has been observed in previous surveys but not for males as young as 45 to 54 years. Second, there is a rather striking excess of disabling illness among unmarried women in all age groups from 25 years on compared with rates for married women in the same age groups. This, too, is a relationship that has been observed before, although no completely convincing explanation has been given for it. Finally, a consistent and not unexpected disadvantage of the nonwhite population with respect to disabling illness shows up clearly in the prevalence rates.

The rates in table 2 are based on cases of disabling illness of all prior durations. This means the rates include cases in which the disability had lasted as short a time as one day and other cases in which the person had been continuously unable to work for as long as 10 years, or had even been completely disabled since birth. The rates in table 3, on the other hand, are averages for the two surveys of the percentages of persons aged 14 to 64 who had been disabled for more than 3 months.

TABLE 3. *Estimated percentage* A *of persons in the civilian noninstitutional population disabled for over 3 months at the time of the survey, by age, sex, and race, United States, February 1949 and September 1950 combined*

Sex and race	14-64 years	14-19 years	20-24 years	25-34 years	35-44 years	45-54 years	55-64 years
Both sexes	2.31	0.79	1.01	1.16	1.67	3.16	6.78
Male	2.95	.97	1.26	1.46	1.99	3.75	9.06
Female	1.71	.62	.78	.88	1.37	2.59	4.53
Both sexes:							
White	2.23	.79	1.01	1.09	1.56	3.04	6.43
Nonwhite	3.15	.82	1.01	1.83	2.69	4.37	11.37
Male:							
White	2.91	.98	1.31	1.42	1.94	3.71	8.74
Nonwhite	3.40	.87	.69	1.96	2.46	4.15	13.23
Female:							
White	1.59	.61	.72	.79	1.19	2.39	4.18
Nonwhite	2.94	.78	1.25	1.73	2.89	4.58	9.36

A See footnote A, table 1.

For these chronic disabling cases it is apparent that the rates for males are higher than those for females at all ages included in the survey. The ratio of male to female prevalence ranges between 1.45 and 2.00 in the six age groups shown. In these same six age groups the ratio of male to female mortality from all causes of death ranges from 1.47 to 1.74. In general, there is a noticeable similarity of pattern between the distribution of the disabling illness of longer duration by age, sex, and race and that of mortality in the same groups. . . .

10. HEALTH TRENDS IN THREE POPULATION GROUPS

A. HEALTH TRENDS: CHILDREN *

THE UNITED STATES may feel justly proud of the gains which have been made in protecting the health of its children. Mortality in infancy and childhood has decreased; certain diseases which accounted for a high proportion of deaths twenty-five or even ten years ago have become less frequent or have largely disappeared. The death rate among preschool children (ages one to five) has shown a decline from 20 deaths per 1,000 population in 1900, to 10 in 1920, to 2 in 1945. Among school-age children (ages five to fifteen) the rate has declined from 4 in 1900, to 3 in 1920, to 1 in 1945.[1]

The phenomenal record of improvement for the preschool ages is due mainly to the control of communicable diseases. It is a striking fact that among preschool children the death rate from all causes in 1945 was less than the combined death rate from pneumonia, influenza, and the other communicable diseases in 1935. The reduction in mortality from diarrheal diseases, scarlet fever, whooping cough, and measles has been particularly noteworthy. During the last fifteen years the death rate in this age group from diarrheal diseases, although still important, has been cut to one tenth of its former level.

The rapidly changing mortality picture has brought about major shifts in the relative importance of the various causes of death and, consequently, new concepts regarding the chief problems and objectives in child health today. Accidents are now responsible for about 1 in every 4 deaths among children beyond the age of one year, outranking every other cause of death in this age group. Among children of school age chronic illnesses are increasing in importance as morbidity and mortality from acute diseases diminish. Today rheumatic heart disease is at the top of the list of causes of death from disease. A rather surprising finding is the entrance of cancer, including leukemia, into the picture as one of the leading causes of death among children.

Where children receive the best that modern medical science offers, health records are outstanding. But if we look within the averages, there is little room for complacency.

Infant mortality serves as one useful index of general health conditions. The national average in 1946 was 34 deaths under one year for every 1,000 live births,†

---

* Reprinted by permission of the publishers and the Commonwealth Fund from the American Academy of Pediatrics (Committee for the Study of Child Health Services), *Child Health Services and Pediatric Education;* Cambridge, Mass.: Harvard University Press, 1949. (The excerpt reprinted, with omissions including initial paragraphs, is from Chap. I, "The Study of Child Health Services," pp. 16-20.)

1. Figures are for states in the death registration area for the years specified.

† The National Office of Vital Statistics reported for 1955 a provisional national infant mortality rate (i.e., deaths of children under one year, exclusive of fetal deaths) of 26.5 per

FIGURE 1. Death rates have decreased steadily among infants . . .

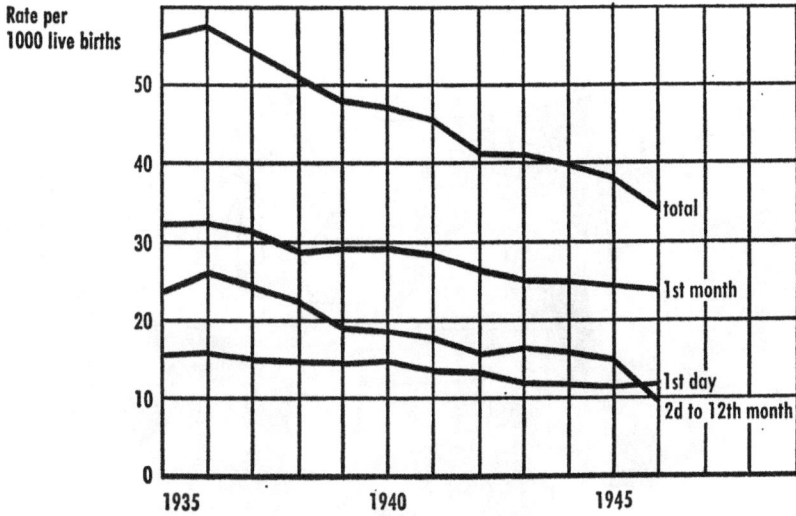

Rate per 1000 live births

50

40

30 — total

20 — 1st month

10 — 1st day / 2d to 12th month

0

1935   1940   1945

. . . and among children.

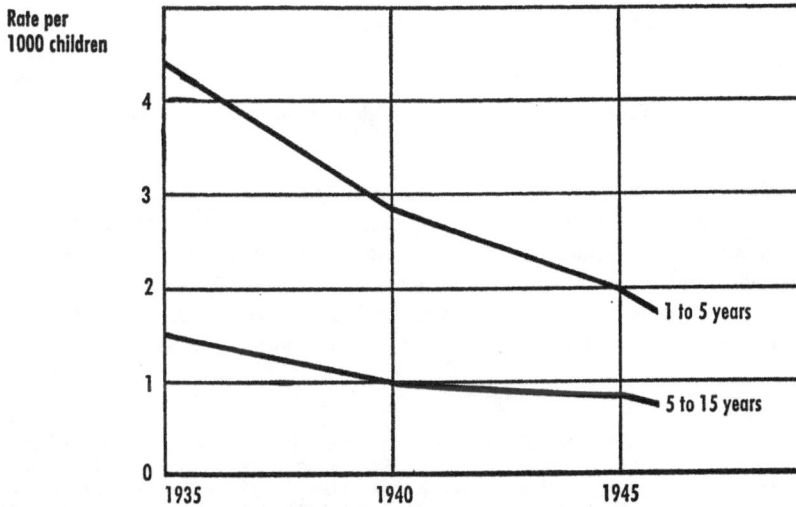

Rate per 1000 children

4

3

2 — 1 to 5 years

1 — 5 to 15 years

0

1935   1940   1945

the lowest ever attained up to that date. Utah, Oregon, and Connecticut succeeded
in bringing their death rates below 28. On the other hand, in New Mexico the rate
was 78, three times the rate in the best states and the same as the national average
of twenty-five years ago.

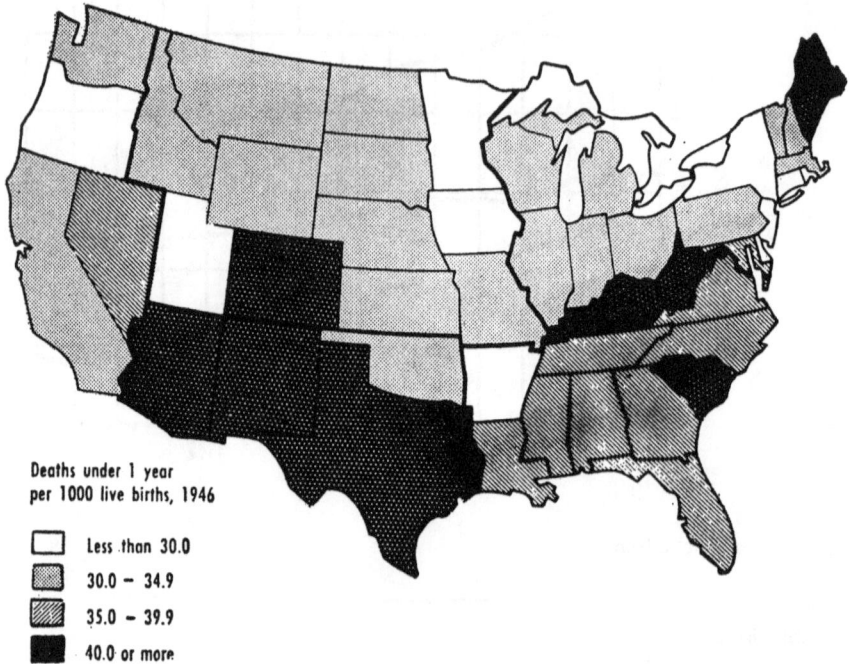

Deaths under 1 year
per 1000 live births, 1946

☐ Less than 30.0
▨ 30.0 – 34.9
▧ 35.0 – 39.9
■ 40.0 or more

FIGURE 2. Yet infant mortality is still high in some states (New Mexico 78).

Variation in infant mortality among county groups has been determined for the
five-year period, 1941-1945, in order to obtain sufficient data, particularly in those
counties where the annual numbers of births are relatively small. The rate in the
isolated counties was about a third higher than in the greater metropolitan counties.
A striking contrast often exists between the infant mortality rate of greater metropolitan counties and that of the isolated rural counties in the same state. For ex-

1,000 live births for the birth-registration area (currently the entire continental United States).
The provisional maternity mortality rate for 1955 reported by the National Office of Vital
Statistics for the birth-registration area was 0.48 per 1,000 live births (estimated on the basis of
a 10-per cent sampling study). (Source: Table entitled "Maternal Mortality Rates and Infant
Mortality Rates: Birth-Registration States, 1927-1955," in Vital Statistics Charts Section (un-
paged) of *Facts on the Major Killing and Crippling Diseases in the United States Today,* New
York: The National Health Education Committee, Inc., 1957).

ample, in Arlington County, Virginia, which is a greater metropolitan county, the infant mortality rate was 25, but in the isolated rural counties of Virginia the rate was 59, almost two and a half times as high.

There are many factors other than geographic location which influence the level of child health. Where there are poor sanitary conditions, families crowded together, ignorance of proper hygiene, babies born at home with no help at all, or at best the help of a midwife, infant mortality is high. This situation is illustrated forcefully in the nonwhite population, as for example, Negro and Indian families. The national infant mortality rate in 1946 for nonwhite infants was 50 as compared with 32 for white infants. In New Mexico the rate for nonwhite was still at the startling height of 152, a condition due essentially to the notoriously poor health conditions among Indians.

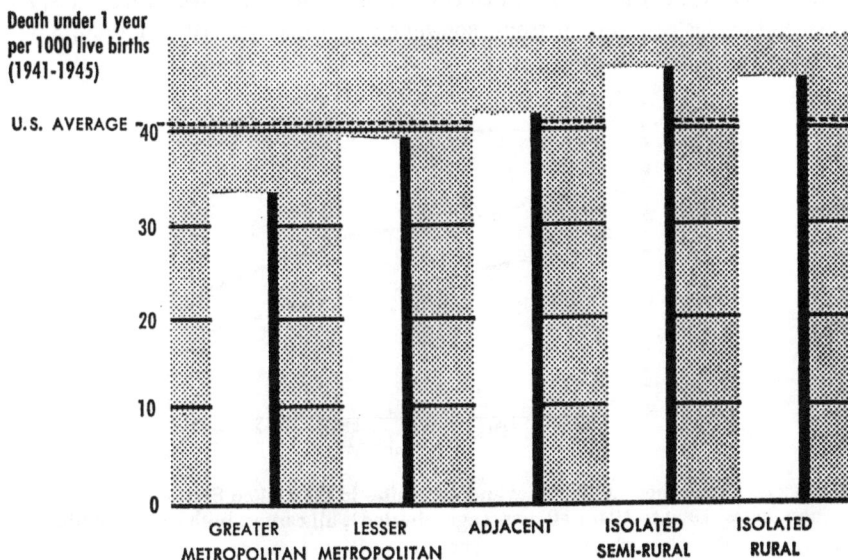

Figure 3. And infant mortality increases as we go from metropolitan to isolated counties.

In respect to death from premature birth, progress has also been made, but the fact remains that a large number of premature babies die needlessly. There has been a gradual decline from 15.4 per 1,000 live births in 1935 to 12.1 in 1946. However, premature birth still ranks as the leading cause of infant death in the United States. If all ages are considered together, it is one of the ten leading causes of death. In 1946 premature birth was recorded as the cause of death of nearly 40,000 infants, more than one third of all deaths during the first year of life.

The cost to the nation from infant deaths is demonstrated vividly by a comparison with the experience of World War II. From Pearl Harbor to V-J Day 281,000 Americans were killed in action. During the same period 430,000 babies died in the United States before they were a year old—3 babies dead for every 2 soldiers. . . .

B. HEALTH TRENDS: THE NEGRO *

MORTALITY

Total White and Nonwhite Mortality.—Remarkable progress has been made in the last half century in reducing the rate of mortality in both the white and non-white groups. Thus the rate of 8.4 deaths per 1,000 whites and of 12.6 deaths per 1,000 nonwhites in 1949 was in each instance less than half their respective rates of 17.6 and 27.8 in 1900.[1] The relative differences between the mortality rates of whites and nonwhites has remained much the same over the years (fig. 4: 58 per cent in 1900; 70 per cent in 1925; 50 per cent in 1949). In terms of absolute rates, however, the gap has narrowed considerably, especially since 1925; thus, the excess of deaths per 1,000 persons, nonwhite over white, was 10.2 in 1900, 8.6 in 1925, and 4.2 in 1949.

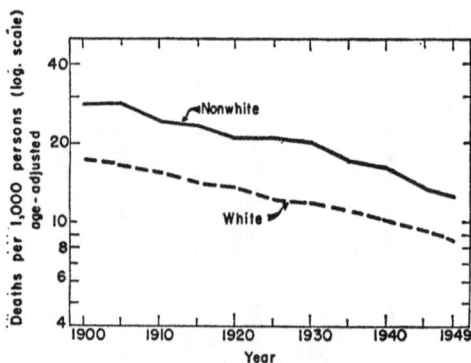

FIGURE 4. Deaths per 1,000 whites and nonwhites in the United States, Death Registration States, 1900 to 1949: all ages (age-adjusted), all causes, both sexes combined.

Taking the period 1925 to 1949, a reduction in mortality rate occurred at all age levels during this interval among both nonwhites and whites (fig. 5). The differential between the two groups, measured by the ratio of nonwhite to white rates, diminished during this period between ages 1 and 25, but did not change or had become even slightly wider for infants under one year and at ages 25 to 74.

As far back as 1916, an Assistant Surgeon General of the Public Health Service questioned whether "color and race" (apparently used in a biological sense) were

* From: "Longevity and Health Status of Whites and Nonwhites in the United States," by Marcus S. Goldstein; *Journal of the National Medical Association* 46:83-104, March 1954 (No. 2). Reprinted (with omissions, including initial paragraphs and some tables and figures) by permission of the author and publishers. The author is a public health research analyst for the Division of Public Health Methods, Public Health Service, Washington, D.C.

1. Rates are age-adjusted and refer to all causes and both sexes combined.

the most important factors in the high rate of mortality among nonwhites in the United States. Bearing on this question are the recent available data on mortality in various countries: the mortality rate of the American nonwhite population in 1949, for example, was lower than that of Ireland, Mexico, and Egypt at this time.[2] Indeed, a high correlation between income level and mortality, as well as between food consumption and mortality, was found to be a world-wide phenomenon in 1930. . . .

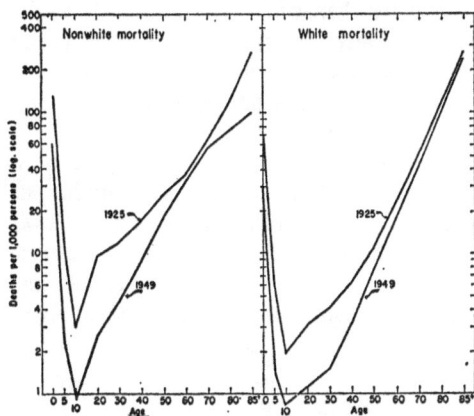

FIGURE 5. Death rates per 1,000 whites and nonwhites in the United States, by age, both sexes combined: 1925 and 1949.

Medical Care and Mortality.—That availability of adequate medical, hospital, and public health services is essential to the maintenance of health and life is attested by an abundance of published evidence. It is also common knowledge that there are substantial differences between the white and nonwhite population in the availability and utilization of medical and hospital services. Several examples of these differences in medical care between the two groups may be cited.

At latest report (1948), there were in the United States 3,681 Negroes per Negro physician compared with 755 persons per physician in the general population. White physicians, to be sure, also provide medical care for Negro patients, yet it seems more likely that Negro physicians would settle and serve regions preponderantly populated by Negroes; other things being equal, therefore, a more ample supply of Negro physicians would be of especial benefit to the nonwhite population.

In regard to hospital beds, the lower number available for nonwhites than whites (1.9 compared with 2.6, per 1,000 population) found in four States (Virginia, North Carolina, Georgia, and Mississippi) in 1950 is probably the pattern in the country at large. In the case of hospital insurance, the proportion of older people

2. Crude death rates are not of course strictly comparable on an international scale, since they are influenced by such factors as age composition, under-registration of deaths, and the like. Yet the crude death rates give some measure of relative position of the various populations in regard to mortality.

possessing such protection has recently been found to be lower by nearly two-thirds among nonwhites than whites, a differential that probably also holds for the population as a whole. In regard to hospital admissions, a criterion of availability and use of hospitals, the American Academy of Pediatrics has provided data on admissions of children under age 15 in six States in 1946-47.... The disparity between the white and nonwhite group was and no doubt still is substantial.

Medical care in terms of fewer births attended by a physician and delivered in a hospital among nonwhites than whites ... also attests to the much lower level of care available to the former, and is especially relevant since the incidence of births delivered in a hospital is inversely related to the rate of infant mortality. Immunization of children, an index of preventive medical care, has been less common among nonwhite than white children.

The disadvantageous position of the nonwhite population in the United States with regard to availability and utilization of medical and hospital care undoubtedly has been the end result of a complex of interacting causes: low occupational status, low income, concentration in rural areas, educational deficiencies, historical mores, and the like.... However, there has been substantial improvement in these cultural factors affecting the health status of the nonwhite population. ...

MORBIDITY

GOOD HEALTH while alive undoubtedly contributes to a long, as well as, indeed, a happy life, and hence some data on morbidity that appear to be relevant to the present problem will be discussed briefly....

The prevalence of disabling illness in the civilian United States population aged 14-64 years, based upon sample surveys in 1949 and 1950, has been estimated for nonwhites as 5.8 per cent and for whites as 4.0 per cent.[3] As shown in this report, the differential between whites and nonwhites in disabling illness prevalence increased with age, and was particularly marked between white and nonwhite females. Disabling illness prevalence in relation to employment is also considered, although no breakdown by white and nonwhite group is given. However, it is of relevant interest that a statistically significant excess of disabling illness was found among the unemployed males.

It may be well to recall at this juncture [Myrdal's point] that "resistance to disease is a function not only of heredity and environment at a certain time, but also of environmental conditions throughout the life history of the individual under observation."

The various elements making up the standard of living have long been recognized as having a considerable if varying influence on both morbidity and mortality, as a number of previously cited references have made plain. Rarely, however, has an attempt been made to adjust rates for living standards. One such effort is that of Perrott and Griffin, as shown in table 4. In the words of these authors:

3. A person was considered to have a disabling illness or condition if it prevented him from doing his regular work on the day of interview or if, as a result of a disability, the person had been able to work only occasionally.

... making an adjustment for differences in the incomes of relief and nonrelief families cuts the difference between the relief and nonrelief disability rates from an excess in the relief population of 250 per cent to an excess of only 33 per cent for whites, and for Negroes from an excess of 97 per cent to a deficiency of 13 per cent.

TABLE 4. *Per cent of the population aged 16-64 of Dayton, Ohio, reporting disabilities as of July, 1934, by relief status, race, and sex*

Sex and Relief Status	Adjusted Rates ᴬ		Crude Rates	
	Nonwhite	White	Nonwhite	White
Both sexes:				
Relief	7.1	8.0	14.4	16.2
Nonrelief	8.0	6.0	7.3	4.6
Males:				
Relief	6.9	9.3	14.1	18.9
Nonrelief	8.2	7.7	7.8	5.7
Females:				
Relief	7.3	6.8	14.8	13.4
Nonrelief	7.9	4.4	6.9	3.6

ᴬ Adjusted for age and for family income.

The findings of the National Health Survey in 1935-36 corroborated the results cited above. In [the Survey] report by Holland and Perrott, the results of a health survey of several cities in 1933 are also given. The most unique aspect of this particular study is that the nonwhite population was reasonably comparable to the white groups in terms of economic status. . . . When economic status was held fairly constant, the prevalence of disabling illness in nonwhite females became about the same as in white females, and considerably lower in nonwhite males than in white males. Comparison of these same data on the basis of per capita income indicates again the influence of environmental factors in the health status of both whites and Negroes, and the tendency of differences between the two groups to level off when reasonable comparability is attained in regard to age distribution, sex, place of residence (urban and rural), occupation, economic status, and like considerations.

C. HEALTH TRENDS: THE AGED *

THE AGING OF OUR population has many and fundamental implications for the Nation. Persons aged 65 and over are rapidly increasing both in absolute numbers and in relation to the total population (an estimated 20 million and 10.8 percent of

* From: "Health Status and Health Requirements of an Aging Population," by George S. Perrott, Marcus S. Goldstein, and Selwyn D. Collins; in *Illness and Health Services in an Aging Population* (Public Health Service Publication No. 170), Washington: U.S. Government Printing Office, 1952. Reprinted from pages 1-11, 21-23 with omissions, including some tables and figures. The authors are, respectively, chief of the Division of Public Health Methods; public health research analyst for the Division; and chief of the Division's Morbidity and Health Statistics Branch; Public Health Service, Washington, D.C.

the population by 1975 compared with some 3 million and 4 percent in 1900). The health status of this old-age group measured by prevalence of illness and the receipt of medical care, and estimates of future national trends in volume of illness and medical care in the light of an aging population, are pertinent to geriatics and to the public health aspects of the problem.

The most recent illness records of Nation-wide scope are still those obtained in the National Health Survey of 1935-36, a house-to-house canvass conducted by the Public Health Service. The data of this survey, supplemented by the morbidity studies of the Eastern Health District of Baltimore of 1938-43, probably the most comprehensive household canvass of its kind, provide in large measure the statistical basis for the present discussion. . . .

THE OLD-AGE GROUP AND THE TOTAL POPULATION

Frequency and duration of disabling illness.—The annual frequency of all disabling illnesses among persons 65 years of age and over, compared with that in the total sample population as found in the National Health Survey and in the Baltimore study, is shown in figure 6.[1] The Baltimore data in this instance also refer to

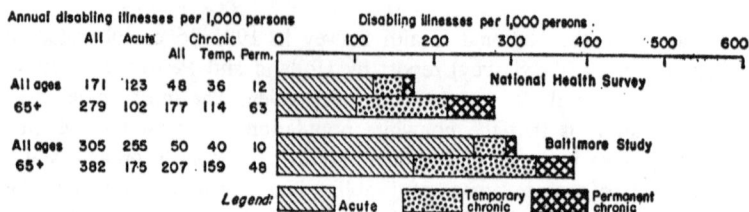

FIGURE 6. Annual frequency of acute and chronic illness disabling for seven consecutive days or more, all ages and 65 years and over.

illnesses lasting 7 or more consecutive days and are comparable in this regard with the National Health Survey material. A similar pattern of disability frequency is discerned in the results of both surveys. All disabling illnesses, including both acute and chronic conditions, occurred relatively more often in the group aged 65 and over than in the population as a whole: the number of illnesses per 1,000 persons was 63 percent greater in the old-age group than in the total sample population according to the National Health Survey, and was 25 percent greater in the Baltimore study.

In both surveys, the ratio of chronic to all illnesses was much higher in the old-age group than in the total sample population (63 percent as compared with

1. The total population, that is, all ages, rather than the population under 65 years, seems to us a more useful measure of comparison with the old-age group in the present instance. Findings for the total population will, of course, be weighted by conditions in the old-age group, although scarcely to the extent of masking any substantial differences between the latter and the population under 65 years of age in view of the much smaller number in the old-age group.

28 percent according to the National Health Survey; and 54 percent as compared with 16 percent in the Baltimore study). The chronic cases were further divided according to temporary or permanent disability, and it is significant that even in the old-age group most of the chronic cases were temporarily disabling (64 percent in the National Health Survey, 77 percent in the Baltimore study).[2] This finding agrees with the fact that many of the serious chronic diseases, such as those of the heart and arteries, may cause disability of relatively short duration even though they may end in a sudden and fatal attack.

. . . A note of caution may be interpolated here, namely, that the number of chronic cases, in contrast with the rates, is much greater in the middle years than in the old-age group: of all chronic cases found in the National Health Survey, 39 percent occurred at ages 35-54, 53 percent at ages 35-64; and only 16 percent of the total number were at 65 years or older. As much as 35 percent of all invalidism (persons disabled for the entire 12 months immediately preceding the visit) occurred at ages 45-64, compared with 30 percent at 65 years of age and over.

The differences between the rates of disability in the National Health Survey and in the Baltimore study, it may be mentioned, are probably due in part to the fact that visits were made each month to families in the latter study and over a 5-year period of time, while families were visited only once in the National Health Survey. Accordingly, many more illnesses of short duration were undoubtedly picked up in the Baltimore study.

[When] frequency of illnesses other than that of seven or more days' duration in the Baltimore study is [considered], the rate of disabling illnesses of 1 day or longer is less in the old-age group than for the entire population, primarily because of the larger number, and rate, of short-term acute illnesses in the population under 65 years of age. . . . Cases of disabling illness lasting 30 days or longer, on the contrary, occurred more than twice as often in the old-age group as in the total population sampled.

In the aggregate, the relatively large incidence of disabling illness of short duration (less than 7 days) is probably of considerable importance: in time lost from productive work, in demands on medical facilities, and in receipt of medical and other health services.

The duration of illness, measured by total days of disability per person per year, was over three times greater in the group 65 years old and over than in the general population, almost entirely ascribable to the higher rates of chronic diseases in the former (fig. 7). Indeed, in both the total population sample and in the old-age group, the chronic diseases exact the greatest toll of days disabled—two-thirds or

2. The term chronic in the National Health Survey referred to illness the symptoms of which had been observed for at least 3 months before the day of visit to the household. Chronic permanent disability represented that of persons who were disabled when the family entered the study and throughout the time of observation in the Baltimore study; in the National Health Survey, chronic permanent disability represented disability of 12 months' duration immediately preceding the visit. Chronic temporary disability pertains to chronic patients who were well enough to be about their work or other usual activities for a part of the period of observation.

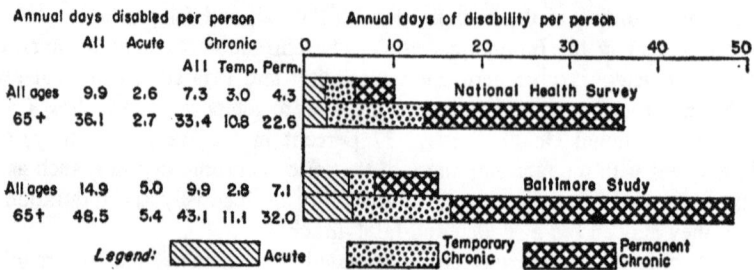

Annual days disabled per person   Annual days of disability per person

	All	Acute	Chronic		
			All	Temp.	Perm.
All ages	9.9	2.6	7.3	3.0	4.3
65+	36.1	2.7	33.4	10.8	22.6
All ages	14.9	5.0	9.9	2.8	7.1
65+	48.5	5.4	43.1	11.1	32.0

Legend: Acute — Temporary Chronic — Permanent Chronic

FIGURE 7. Annual days of disability from illness disabling for seven consecutive days or more, all ages and 65 years and over.

more of all days disabled in the former group and about 90 percent in the latter. These observations on duration of disabling illness are derived from the data in both the National Health Survey of 1935-36 and the Baltimore study of 1938-43. . . .

TABLE 5. *Illnesses, all ages and 65 years and over, confining to house, bed, and hospital, respectively, per year, as found in the Eastern Health District of Baltimore, 1938-43*

[All causes; both sexes: A disabling illness represents a disability lasting 1 day or longer]

Item	All ages	65 years and over
Illness confining to house:		
House cases per 1,000 persons observed	595	482
Days confined to house per person observed	9.4	29.9
House days per house case	15.7	62.0
Percent of disabling cases confined to house	91.5	88.3
Bed illness (includes hospitalized illnesses):		
Bed cases per 1,000 persons observed	365	321
Days in bed per person observed	4.95	8.52
Days in bed per bed case	13.5	26.6
Percent of disabling cases in bed	56.2	58.7
Hospitalized illness: A		
Hospital cases per 1,000 persons observed	70.6	57.4
Hospital days per person observed	2.60	2.45
Hospital days per hospitalized case	36.9	42.7
Percent of disabling cases hospitalized	10.9	10.5
Chronic diseases:		
Individuals with 1 or more chronic illnesses per 1,000 persons observed:		
All chronic illnesses	68.7	211.3
Disabling chronic illnesses B	41.6	157.1
Nondisabling chronic illnesses	27.1	54.2
Percent of hospitalized cases that were chronic	23.8	70.8

A All types of hospitalization are included, regardless of duration.
B These rates, referring to individuals regardless of number of attacks, differ from those given in figures 6 in that the latter refers to cases in the sense of disabling attacks of chronic disease.

The annual number of illnesses confining to house, bed, and hospital, respectively, as well as additional data on the extent of chronic illness, in the old-age group and in the total sample population of Baltimore, are shown in table 5. It may be observed here that (*a*) the relative frequency of cases confining to house, bed, or hospital was lower in the old-age group than in the population as a whole, and concomitantly (*b*) the proportions of all disabled cases confined to house, bed, or hospital were about the same in the old-age group as in the total population; (*c*) the duration of an illness confining to house or bed, per person or per case, was considerably greater in the old-age group (e. g., persons 65 years of age and over who were bed cases remained about twice as long in bed as did bed cases in general); (*d*) the relative number of individuals having a chronic disease was three times greater among persons aged 65 or over than in the total population; and (*e*) chronic disease was the cause for hospitalization three times more often in the old-age group than in the population as a whole.

Kinds of illnesses.—[When] the frequency of various kinds of disabling illness found in the National Health Survey, in old age and for all ages combined [is analyzed], the most common group of diseases in the old-age population is the group described as "degenerative" (30 percent of all cases), although diseases of the respiratory system, excluding pneumonia, are also a considerable portion of the total in the old-age group as well as in the whole population sample. It is of interest that the illness rate is considerably higher in the old-age group than in the population as a whole in each of the major diagnostic categories listed, except the communicable diseases.

[With regard to] the 10 most frequent causes of disability (1 day or longer) ascertained in the Baltimore study, among persons 65 years of age and older and for all ages combined, both chronic and acute illnesses, about equally divided, were among the leading 10 in the old-age group, whereas almost all were acute diseases in the total population sample. Heart diseases in the old-age group were by far the most severe in number of days disabled, representing nearly three times the disability rate found for the second most severe disability, arthritis.

Medical care.—The number of physicians' services per person per year is a useful yardstick of the receipt of medical care. Available data from several sources on utilization of medical services by older people and by the total population observed are given in table 6. The very low figure of the National Health Survey is undoubtedly the result of counting only illnesses that disabled for seven or more consecutive days; physicians of course often attend illnesses of shorter duration.

Perhaps of greatest import is the question whether the old-age group per person utilizes a significantly greater volume of medical services than that received by the population as a whole. According to the experience of the Health Insurance Plan of Greater New York, as indicated in table 6, older persons do not receive appreciably more than the usual amount of medical care. The HIP population, it will be recalled, is enrolled in a prepaid, comprehensive medical care program. The Swift Current medical care program in Saskatchewan, Canada, which also provides comprehensive physicians' services on a prepayment basis, shows much higher rates for the older age group.

The experience of HIP is only partly borne out by the Baltimore study. The group aged 65 and over in Baltimore received more physicians' calls (*a*) for disabling cases per person observed, especially chronic cases, and (*b*) per attended disabled case.... There was little difference, however, between the old-age group and the total population in number of calls by physicians on nondisabling cases or in the percent of cases attended by a physician. Indeed, except for chronic cases, fewer were attended by a physician per 1,000 persons observed among the older people than in the whole population. And, although relatively many more people in the old-age group were attended by a physician for chronic illnesses, the number of physicians' calls per attended chronic case was about the same in both the old-age group and the population as a whole.

TABLE 6. *Physicians' services per person per year, all ages and 65 years and over, according to different surveys*

Source of information	All ages	65 and over
Committee on the Costs of Medical Care (1928-31)[A]...................	2.37	4.95
National Health Survey (1935-36)[B].....................................	.85	2.15
Eastern Health District of Baltimore (1938-43).........................	2.60	3.72
Health Insurance Plan of Greater New York (1948)[C]...................	4.4	4.7
Swift Current (Saskatchewan) Medical Care Program (1949).............	3.84	10.59

[A] Includes nondisabling illness and illness disabling for 1 day or longer; all causes, exclusive of confinements terminating in live births.

[B] Refers to disabling illnesses of 7 or more consecutive days; confinements, fatal cases, and hospital cases are included without reference to duration of disability.

[C] All attended cases plus calls for all preventive services.

In brief, in the Baltimore study the number of physicans' calls per person, for disabling illnesses and especially for chronic illnesses, tended to be definitely greater among the older people than in the total population. Cases of illness attended by a physician, however, were about the same or even lower in the old-age group.

Of pertinent interest is the question of hospital utilization, in the old-age group and in the general population.... The rate of hospitalized cases is somewhat higher in the old-age group than in the total population, according to both the study of the Committee on the Costs of Medical Care and the National Health Survey; in Saskatchewan the rate was 1.5 times greater among those aged 65 or over than for all ages combined. Apparently contrary results were obtained in the Baltimore study; namely, a lower rate of hospitalization among the older people than in the total sample population. The reason for this difference in the results of the several studies is not clear. All surveys cited, however, agree that the average number of days of hospitalization per person is definitely greater in the old-age group than in the general population—as much as three times greater in Saskatchewan. Indeed, the differences between hospital utilization in Saskatchewan and the rates found in the several surveys in the United States are striking, both in cases hospitalized and length of stay in the hospital.

It should be noted at this point that the Saskatchewan Hospital Service Plan is a form of governmental compulsory hospital insurance which in 1950 covered about 92 percent of the people of the Province; it imposes no limits on duration of needed hospitalization or on type of illness that may be hospitalized, except that the general hospital accepts tuberculous and mental patients for diagnosis only, after which they are transferred to special hospitals.

FUTURE VOLUME OF ILLNESS

THE FULL IMPORT of the increasing number of older people in the population with respect to disabling illnesses may perhaps be better sensed in terms of the volume of people affected.

The old-age and total populations of the United States at the specified dates referred to subsequently are given in table 7. Here is also indicated the relatively much greater future increase of the old-age group than of the total population—an increase of 45 percent in the total population compared with 156 percent in the old-age group between 1935 and 1975. The ratios in the table also indicate an increasing proportion of females in the population, especially in the old-age group. . . .

TABLE 7. *Population of continental United States at the specified dates: For all ages and for group 65 years and over, by sex (estimated for 1935, 1960, 1975)*

Age and sex	1935	1940 ▲	1950	1960 ▲	1975 ▲
	Population (thousands)				
All ages:					
Both sexes	127,250	131,669	150,698	162,012	185,072
Male	64,110	66,062	74,633	80,670	92,572
Female	63,140	65,607	76,065	81,342	92,500
65 years and over:					
Both sexes	7,803	8,964	12,324	14,675	19,935
Male	3,858	4,378	5,712	6,838	9,028
Female	3,945	4,586	6,612	7,837	10,907
	Ratio (1935 = 100)				
All ages:					
Both sexes	100.0	103.5	118.4	127.3	145.4
Male	100.0	103.0	116.4	125.8	144.4
Female	100.0	103.9	120.5	128.8	146.5
65 years and over:					
Both sexes	100.0	114.9	157.9	188.1	255.5
Male	100.0	113.5	148.1	177.2	234.0
Female	100.0	116.2	167.6	198.7	276.5

▲ Estimates for 1960 and 1975 assume high fertility, low mortality, and net immigration of 1,000,000. The 1940 population is the Census enumeration of April 1940.

The health status of persons in the United States aged 65 and over and the medical and other health services received by this age group have been considered in some detail. By 1975, the group aged 65 or over will represent one-tenth or more of the total population. Aging of the population will materially affect the extent and types of disabling illness in the population and will also increase the volume of services furnished by physicians, nurses, hospitals, and other health personnel and facilities. The latter observations are based on conspicuous differences between the old-age group and the population as a whole as found in surveys of illness and receipt of medical and other health services. . . .

Projecting the findings of the National Health Survey of 1935-36 and of the Baltimore study of 1938-43 to future years, it is estimated that the number of disabling illnesses in the United States lasting seven consecutive days or longer will be 25 to 30 percent higher in 1960 and 40 to 50 percent greater by 1975. Total annual days lost from disability are expected to rise 30 to 40 percent by 1960 and even more by 1975. These anticipated increases in disability will not only result from the larger size of the population, but will also reflect the future rise in number and proportion of older people in the population—in age groups that show the highest rates of chronic illness. Similar findings in medical care, assuming that rates in 1960 and 1975 will remain essentially like those found in the National Health Survey of 1935-36, indicate increasing demands for the services of physicians, hospital care, and nurses' services.

The number of cases of cardiovascular-renal diseases in the United States population aged 65 and over may reach 3.8 million by 1975 as compared with an estimated 1.5 million cases in 1935. Of the total number of cardiovascular-renal cases in the all-ages group, some 1.7 million are expected to be disabled for seven or more consecutive days in 1975, about 2.5 times the number in 1935. By 1975 cardiovascular-renal diseases in the old-age group alone may result in an annual total of 628,000 years of disability, including 214,000 years in bed, and 21,000 in the hospital. An estimated total of 7.3 million physicians' calls (office, home, and clinic) were made on the old-age population having cardiovascular-renal diseases in 1935. If the same rate of physicians' calls on older people with cardiovascular-renal diseases prevails in 1975, the annual total may reach 18.7 million by that time. On the basis of hospital beds used for cardiovascular-renal conditions in 1935, it is estimated that more than 25,000 hospital beds will be required by 1975 for persons aged 65 and over suffering from these diseases.

Advances in medical knowledge and techniques, changes in the incidence, prevalence, and severity of illnesses, as well as economic factors that may alter patterns of utilization of medical and other health services, may well require later modifications in these forecasts of future disability and medical care in the old-age and total populations. Yet a few conclusions appear inescapable. Larger numbers of people, especially women, will live to old age in the years to come. The health status of these older people will require expanded resources to meet increased demands for physicians' services, hospital care, and nursing services. An increasing proportion of all medical, hospital, and nursing services will be concentrated on the chronic diseases as a result of aging of the population. Control of the chronic diseases—perhaps by early detection in the middle years or before—and prevention or amelioration of their consequences would greatly reduce not only the time lost from disability but also the patient load on hospitals, nurses, and physicians.

11. SOCIAL AND ENVIRONMENTAL ASPECTS

A. INCOME, EMPLOYMENT STATUS AND ILLNESS *

ILLNESS IS GREATEST in the population group least able to bear the economic burden involved. Although this fact is well known, the National Health Survey data are of value as corroborative evidence and also contribute information on certain novel aspects. No attempt will be made to assess the proportion of the total excess which is due to factors connected with low income, or the proportion in which low income has resulted from chronic sickness. The point to be made is that, regardless of cause, the groups in poor economic circumstances have excessive illness rates.[1]

Distribution of persons surveyed by family income and relief status.[2]—Persons in families with annual incomes under $1,000 comprised about 40 percent of the surveyed group; about 65 percent were in families with annual incomes under $1,500, and 80 percent in families with incomes under $2,000. Almost one half of the lowest income group had received relief during the year 1935.

Frequency of serious illness at different income levels.—In table 8 is given the frequency of illness disabling for a week or more according to the income and relief status of the family. The excess in the relief group over the rate in the group with incomes of $5,000 or more is 59 percent for all causes, 49 percent for acute diseases and 85 percent for chronic diseases. There is also a definite excess for the nonrelief group with incomes below $1,000, and some excess in the next higher group. However, above the $1,500 level there is no excess.[3]

* From: "The National Health Survey: Some General Findings as to Disease, Accidents, and Impairments in Urban Areas," by Rollo H. Britten, Selwyn D. Collins, and James S. Fitzgerald; *Public Health Reports* 55:444-70, March 15, 1940 (No. 11). Reprinted with omissions, including initial paragraphs and some tables and figures. Mr. Britten was, until his retirement in 1946, chief of the Health Economics Section, Division of Public Health Methods, Public Health Service, Washington, D.C.; Dr. Collins is chief of the Morbidity and Health Statistics Branch of the Division of Public Health Methods; and Mr. Fitzgerald was a research analyst in the Division of Public Health Methods at the time of the National Health Survey (1936).

1. In the Health Survey, families were classified by income received during the 12 months preceding the interview and also according to whether or not relief had been received during that time. Information on employment status of the individual was obtained as of the day of the canvass.

2. For the purpose of this comparison, all persons living in a household are classified according to the total income of related members of that household.

3. There is some difference in the age composition of the various groups, which explains the slight rise in the rate for chronic diseases at the higher income levels.

TABLE 8. *Annual frequency of acute and chronic illnesses disabling for 1 week or longer (per 1,000 persons) as related to economic status*

Annual family income and relief status	All illnesses	Acute	Chronic
All incomes	171	123	48
Relief	232	160	72
Nonrelief:			
Under $1,000	176	120	56
$1,000 to $1,500	155	117	38
$1,500 to $2,000	146	111	35
$2,000 to $3,000	145	110	36
$3,000 to $5,000	145	109	36
$5,000 and over	146	107	39
Relief and nonrelief under $1,000	*200*	*138*	*63*

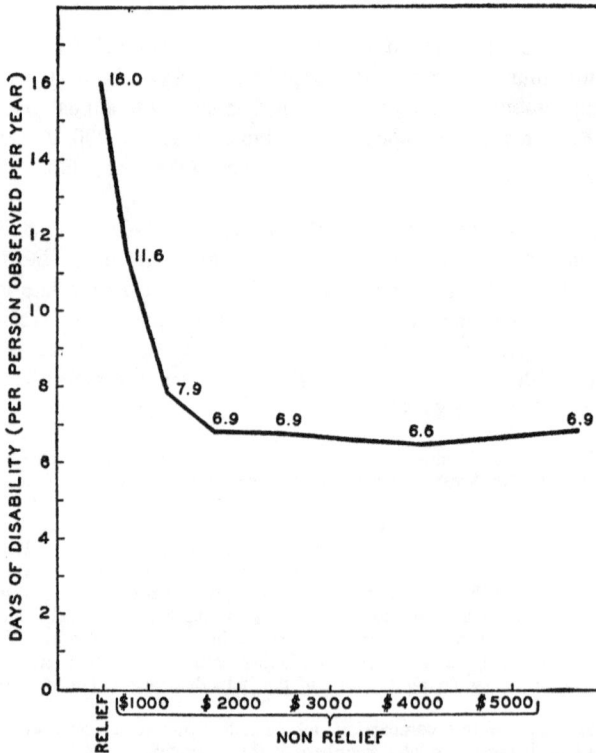

FIGURE 8. Disability rate according to annual family income and relief status.

Amount of disability at different income levels.—The excess in the low income groups is greater in terms of days of disability per person per year than in terms of frequency, because of a longer average duration of cases in the low income groups. The relief group shows an excess of 132 percent over the $5,000 class, and the nonrelief group under $1,000 an excess of 68 percent. Above $1,500 there is no excess. The rates are presented in figure 8, which gives a vivid portrayal of the problem of illness in the low income groups.[4]

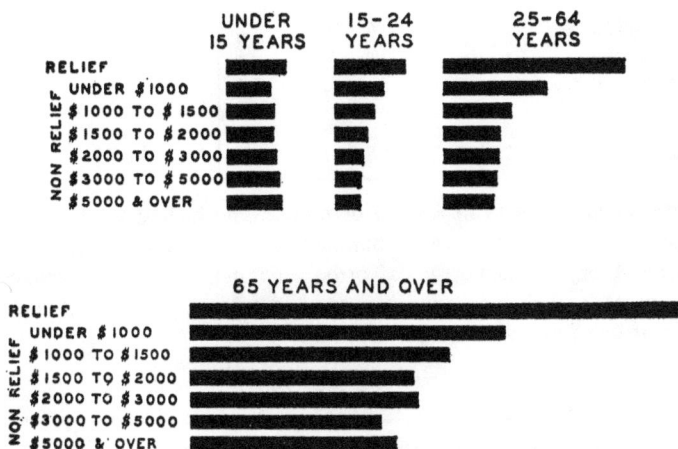

FIGURE 9. Disability rate according to age and annual family income and relief status.

Differences by age.—The greatest relative excess of illness in the lower income groups over the higher is found in the productive ages, as shown in figure 9 and table 9. The excess in the relief group over the $5,000 class is as follows for the different ages:

Age	Percentage excess
Under 15	8
15-24	177
25-64	263
65 and over	139

Diagnoses chiefly responsible for excess amount of disability in low-income groups. —Further light is thrown on the problem of excessive illness rates in the lower income groups by consideration of the degree of excess for specific diagnoses. . . . For simplicity, the data given . . . (table 10) will be limited to the ratios of the annual per capita volume of disability for different income groups to that in the

4. The income for the relief group is placed at $500 in the chart, which figure was taken as a rough estimate of the average annual income of urban relief families.

TABLE 9. *Days of disability (per person observed per year) for persons of different ages, according to economic status*

Annual family income and relief status	All ages	Under 15	15-24	25-64	65 and over
All incomes	9.9	5.7	5.4	10.5	36.1
Relief	16.0	6.8	8.6	21.8	58.8
Nonrelief:					
Under $1,000	11.6	5.0	5.9	12.4	37.6
$1,000 to $1,500	7.9	5.4	4.7	8.0	30.7
$1,500 to $2,000	6.9	5.3	4.2	6.8	26.7
$2,000 to $3,000	6.9	5.7	3.6	6.6	27.0
$3,000 to $5,000	6.6	5.8	3.4	6.4	22.8
$5,000 and over	6.9	6.3	3.1	6.0	24.6
Relief and nonrelief under $1,000	*13.5*	*6.0*	*7.1*	*16.0*	*44.4*

group with annual incomes of $3,000 or more.[5] The highest ratios are found for hernia, tuberculosis, varicose veins, blindness and deafness, diabetes, diseases of female genital organs, hemorrhoids, orthopedic impairments, miscellaneous digestive diseases, and rheumatism. In general, diagnoses of an acute nature show much less association than chronic diagnoses.

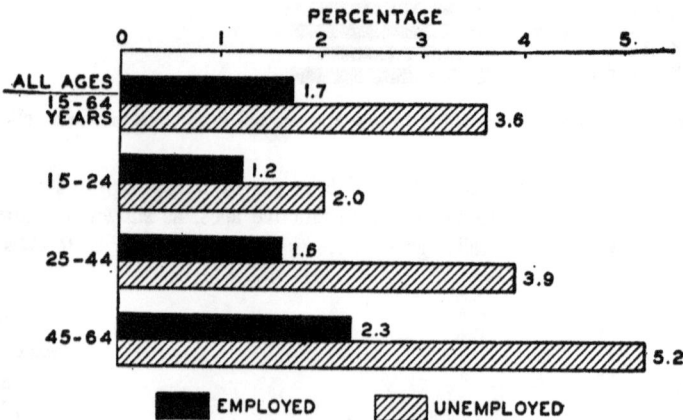

FIGURE 10. Percentage of employed and unemployed workers disabled on the day of the canvass, in different age groups.

Proportion of employed and unemployed workers disabled on the day of the visit. —Intertwined with the problem of illness in the low-income groups is that of illness among the unemployed. Since employment status was recorded in the survey as of the day of the visit, the most appropriate illness measure is the percentage of persons unable to work on that day. The comparison in figure 10 excludes persons who had

5. Persons in institutions for the care of disease for the entire 12 months immediately preceding the visit are excluded from these comparisons.

TABLE 10. *Ratio* [A] *of annual per capita volume of disability for different income groups to that in the highest income group, according to diagnosis*

Diagnosis	Relief	Annual family income and relief status					
		Nonrelief					
		Under $1,000	$1,000 to $1,500	$1,500 to $2,000	$2,000 to $3,000	$3,000 and over
Hernia	1,261	435	304	191	200	100
Tuberculosis (including nonrespiratory)	886	392	253	177	139	100
Varicose veins	714	329	171	193	136	100
Blindness and deafness	562	312	171	146	150	100
Diabetes mellitus	423	231	154	141	128	100
Diseases of female genital organs and complications of pregnancy	420	230	160	150	150	100
Hemorrhoids	371	182	153	129	135	100
Orthopedic impairments	367	251	153	123	112	100
Diseases of digestive system other than appendicitis, hernia, and diseases of teeth, mouth, and gums	361	191	121	97	100	100
Rheumatism and allied diseases	351	202	132	105	110	100
Anemia	310	198	133	110	124	100
Diseases of bladder, urethra, urinary passages, and male genital organs	304	174	110	101	88	100
Nervous and mental diseases	298	212	140	120	112	100
Confinements	289	200	205	168	142	100
Diseases of skin and cellular tissue	279	176	137	101	97	100
Diseases not elsewhere classified	276	168	118	105	103	100
Cardiovascular-renal diseases	272	158	112	101	101	100
All diagnoses	266	167	121	107	106	100
Cancer and other tumors	248	148	114	114	100	100
Accidents	213	167	124	109	107	100
Pneumonia (all forms)	193	120	100	93	107	100
Diseases of respiratory system other than tuberculosis, pneumonia, and tonsillitis	192	125	92	90	95	100
Communicable diseases other than those common to childhood	183	125	83	73	78	100
Diseases of teeth, mouth, and gums	147	147	100	100	87	100
Tonsillitis (including tonsillectomies)	138	108	100	100	108	100
Diseases of ear and mastoid process	132	101	93	87	101	100
Diseases of thyroid gland	122	94	61	68	69	100
Common communicable diseases of childhood	110	86	93	95	100	100
Appendicitis (including appendectomies)	104	83	87	83	87	100

[A] Based on rates adjusted to the age composition of the total population.

been removed from the labor market by reason of chronic disease or impairment—the "unemployables."... Had they been included the contrast between the illness rates for the employed and the unemployed would have been far greater. Also many of the disabled persons in the unemployed group presented in figure 10 are potential "unemployables." However, the data bring out the great excess of illness among unemployed persons who have not yet abandoned the hope of working.... The rates for all groups are higher than they would have been had the visits not been confined largely to winter months.

A more intensive study, to be published later in this series, will show that the illness rate among the unemployed is related to the relief status of the families and of the worker. The rate is higher in relief than in nonrelief families, and among relief families it is higher for workers who were not on work relief than for those who were.

Proportion of "unemployables" in different income groups.— A still further aspect of the problem of illness and income is the concentration of persons reported to be "unemployable" by reason of disability in the low-income groups and especially in the relief group. . . . The base for these calculations is the number of workers plus the unemployables themselves. . . . In proportion to the number of persons, there were 13 times as many unemployables in the relief group as in the group with incomes of $5,000 and over. The relative excess is greatest in the age group 35-44. . . .

B. INCOME AND MORTALITY *

THE GREAT VARIATION in health status from one individual and from one population group to another constitutes a continuous challenge to all those concerned with improving the health and well-being of the population. If an understanding of the causes of this variation could be achieved, a more rational basis for action to raise the general level of health would be available.

The causes of variation are generally classified into two main groups, hereditary and environmental. Many published studies point to the influence of one or the other of the two groups. Since environmental factors are more amenable to modification, major emphasis is placed upon investigations of the association between disease and income, nutrition, education, occupation and other conditions susceptible to improvement.

It has been shown from studies in this and other countries that variations in infant mortality are related to economic conditions and all that these imply in terms of hygiene, nutrition, etc. For mortality in general, a study based on deaths among 1,300,000 life insurance policyholders shows that there is an association of relatively higher mortality with low occupational class.

When the relationship between sickness and environment is studied, similar results are obtained. . . .

In appraising the many studies reported, two facts stand out:

1. Only in the case of infant mortality has there been shown a clear-cut relationship with socio-economic conditions.

2. There is little quantitative information on the relationship between the

* From: "Relationship between Per Capita Income and Mortality in the Cities of 100,000 or More Population," by Marion E. Altenderfer; *Public Health Reports* 62:1681-91, Nov. 28, 1947 (No. 48). Reprinted with omissions, including one figure. The author is supervisory statistician in the Division of Public Health Methods, Public Health Service, Washington, D.C.

individual elements of the environment, in terms of socio-economic status, and disease.

There are two exceptions. First, the supplements to the annual reports of the Registrar General of England and Wales, published decennially, contain extensive material on male mortality by occupation. Second, Hirshfeld and Strow have used data for the 48 States and the District of Columbia to study the relation between health status and such environmental factors as percent urban, sanitation facilities, medical facilities, health insurance, economic resources and degree of culture. Hirshfeld and Strow used as measures of health status infant mortality, mortality from heart disease, tuberculosis and infectious diseases, and draft rejections.

The information furnished in this study is valuable though limited by the size of the unit chosen. . . .

. . . In the present study of the relation between health status and environmental factors, it has been decided to use all the counties in the United States and the cities with 10,000 or more population in 1940 as units. These political divisions more nearly meet the requirement of internal uniformity than do larger units. Mortality rather than morbidity data will be used as the measure of health status because that is all that is available on a national scale. The relation between mortality from selected specific causes, maternal mortality and infant mortality and percent urban, per capita income, medical facilities, occupational class and degree of culture will be systematically investigated. The results will be presented in a series of reports. In this first report, the results based on the 92 cities which had 100,000 or more population in 1940 are presented. The questions asked are—What is the relation between the per capita buying income of the community and mortality from several causes? What is the influence of the color composition of the population on this relationship? . . .

TABLE 11. *Relationship between per capita buying income and total mortality, infant mortality and maternal mortality, 1939 and 1940*

Income group of cities	Number of cities	Average per capita buying income	Total deaths per 100,000 population (age adjusted)	Infant deaths per 1,000 live births	Maternal deaths per 1,000 live births
Total cities, 100,000 or more. .	92	$792	1,134.1	42.2	3.6
Lowest	31	668	1,211.5	47.9	4.3
Middle	30	789	1,097.4	41.1	3.1
Highest	31	918	1,092.2	37.5	3.2

Relation between income and mortality.—The 92 cities were divided into 3 approximately equal groups on the basis of per capita income, and an unweighted average for each mortality rate was computed for each group of cities. Table 11 shows the results for total deaths and for infant and maternal mortality. The table also includes the average per capita income for each of the three groups of cities.

The average total death rate decreases sharply between the group of cities with an average income of $668 and the group with an average income of $789.

There is a slight additional decrease between this middle group and the group with average income of $918. The infant mortality rate shows the same pattern of association with income. The trend in the maternal mortality rate is similar except that the rate in the highest income group is slightly higher than that in the middle income group. There is considerable variation in the mortality rates from city to city in each income group. . . .

TABLE 12.   *Relationship between per capita income and mortality from a selected list of broad diagnosis groups, 1939 and 1940*

[Deaths per 100,000 population (age adjusted)]

Income group of cities	Diagnosis group								
	Infec-tious A	Tuber-culosis B	Syph-ilis	Cancer	Diabetes	Exoph. goiter	Pella-gra	Chronic C	ENT D
Total cities, 100,000 or more..	4.6	49.4	15.9	133.4	29.5	3.0	0.9	493.9	5.5
Lowest	5.6	56.7	18.2	132.8	29.5	2.8	2.0	514.9	6.2
Middle	4.1	44.9	15.2	130.5	30.1	3.1	0.4	487.0	5.1
Highest....	4.2	46.4	14.2	136.9	28.9	3.1	0.5	479.7	5.2

	Infl., pneu.	Ulcer of stom.	Appen-dicitis	Hernia E	Cirr. of liver	Dis. of gall-blad.	Accidents	
							Motor vehicle	Other
Total cities, 100,000 or more..	73.3	8.1	10.7	10.3	10.7	6.9	24.7	46.0
Lowest	86.8	8.3	11.7	11.2	10.4	6.7	23.9	48.6
Middle	68.2	7.9	10.4	10.1	9.8	7.1	25.1	44.2
Highest....	64.9	8.2	10.0	9.5	11.9	7.0	25.2	45.0

A Includes typhoid and paratyphoid fever, meningitis, scarlet fever, whooping cough, diphtheria and poliomyelitis.
B Includes respiratory and nonrespiratory forms.
C Includes intra-cranial lesions of vascular origin, all forms of heart disease, diseases of the coronary arteries and nephritis.
D Includes diseases of the ear, nose and throat.
E Includes hernia and intestinal obstruction.

Certain of the diagnoses included in the basic data were combined into broad groups and the average mortality rates computed for each of the three income groups of cities (table 12). . . . It will be seen that some of the average rates decrease with increased income, some increase and others seem to show little or no association with income.

The following facts are shown in the table:

1. The average mortality rates for syphilis, chronic diseases, influenza and pneumonia, appendicitis and hernia decrease consistently from the lowest to the highest

income group. As was true for the total death rate, the decrease between the lowest and middle groups is much greater than that between the middle and highest groups.

2. For the infectious diseases, for tuberculosis, pellagra, diseases of the ear, nose and throat and "other" accidents the average rates decrease between the lowest and middle groups but show a slight increase between the middle and highest groups.

3. The rates for exophthalmic goiter and motor vehicle accidents increase slightly with increased income.

4. The rates for cancer, cirrhosis of the liver and diseases of the gall-bladder increase irregularly with increased income.

5. There seems to be no association with income for diabetes and ulcer of the stomach. . . .

Relation between color composition and mortality.—The income level of the communities in the United States is roughly related to geographic area and this in turn requires consideration of the color composition of the population. The 92 cities differ in color composition from 58.5 percent white for Memphis, Tenn., to 99.9 percent for Lowell, Mass. Since nonwhites experience higher total mortality, infant mortality and maternal mortality than white persons, it is to be expected that cities with lower proportions of white persons will have higher mortality rates than cities with high proportions of white persons.

It is not possible to investigate the relationship between color and mortality directly for the 92 cities because the basic data are shown by color only for cities with 10 percent or more nonwhite populations. Therefore the following indirect method was used. The percent of white persons in the population was calculated for each city. The cities were then divided into three groups on the basis of this percent and the average rates computed for each group for total, infant and maternal deaths. It will be seen from table 13 that there is a marked inverse relation between the mortality rates and percent of white persons in the population.

TABLE 13. *Relationship between the color composition of the population and total mortality, infant mortality and maternal mortality, 1939 and 1940*

Percent of white persons in the population	Number of cities	Total deaths per 100,000 population (age adjusted)	Infant deaths per 1,000 live births	Maternal deaths per 1,000 live births
Total cities, 100,000 or more..	92	1134.1	42.2	3.6
Less than 90.0.............	31	1260.3	48.6	4.2
90.0-96.9	33	1097.1	40.6	3.5
97.0 or more	28	1038.0	36.8	2.9

For nine of the diagnosis groups of table 12 the mortality rates for the total United States differ considerably for white and nonwhite persons. The average rates for each of these causes were calculated for the cities in the three color composition groups. Table 14 shows that for the five diagnosis groups for which the nonwhite rates are higher than the white rates for the United States, the mortality, as expected, is higher in the cities with more nonwhite persons than in those with less. The reverse is true for those four diagnosis groups for which the nonwhite rates are considerably lower than the white rates.

TABLE 14. *Relationship between the color composition of the population and mortality from selected causes, 1939 and 1940*

[Deaths per 100,000 population (age adjusted)]

Diagnosis group ᐃ	Percent of white persons in the population		
	Less than 90.0	90.0-96.9	97.0 or more
Diagnoses for which nonwhite rates are higher than white rates:			
Infectious	6.2	4.1	3.6
Tuberculosis	64.6	49.3	32.6
Syphilis	23.1	13.3	10.8
Pellagra	2.2	0.4	0.2
Influenza, pneumonia·	93.3	68.6	56.9
Diagnoses for which nonwhite rates are lower than white rates:			
Cancer	125.8	137.7	136.9
Diabetes	27.8	30.1	30.7
Exophthalmic goiter	2.9	3.0	3.2
Diseases of the gall-bladder	6.2	7.0	7.8

ᐃ See the footnotes to table 12 for the diagnosis titles included in each broad diagnosis group.

Effect of color composition on the association between income and mortality.— In order to examine the effect of the observed association between color composition and mortality upon the relationship between income and mortality, each of the three income groups of cities was divided into the three color composition groups. For the nine groups of cities thus formed the average total, infant and maternal mortality rates were calculated. The results are presented graphically in figure 11.

For the total death rate, the average rates decrease with increased income in the cities with the lowest and highest percent white populations. For the infant mortality rate, there is a consistent decrease with increased income in all color composition groups. There are two exceptions to the general trend for the maternal mortality rates—the minimum rate is in the middle income group for both groups of cities with less than 97 percent white populations.

A careful examination of figure 11 will reveal that, at each income level, the higher the proportion of white persons in the population, the lower the mortality rates. This might be the result of an association between income and color composition within an income group. However when the average per capita income is computed for the nine groups of cities, no marked association is found between income and color composition within an income group. In the lowest income group, there is a difference of $38 between the groups with lowest and highest percent white; in the middle income group, this difference is $18; in the highest income group it is only $7. These differences are small in comparison with the differences between income groups (table 11). Therefore the association between mortality and color composition shown in figure 11 is apparently not the result of income variation alone.

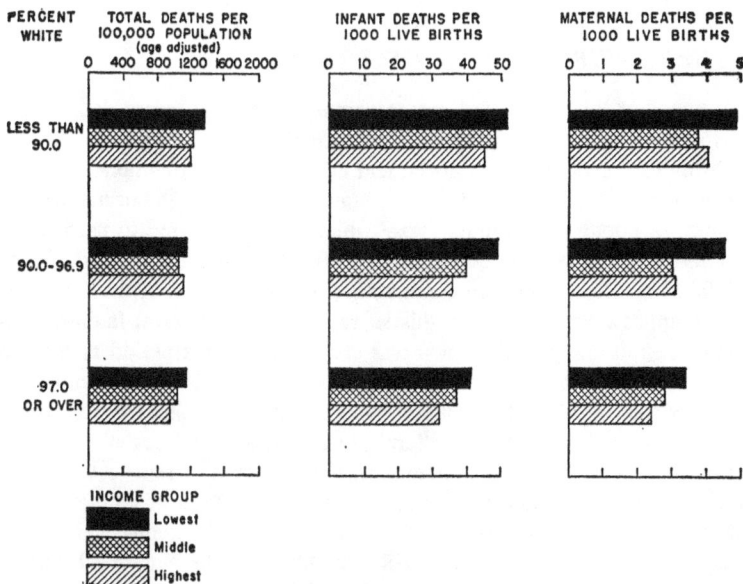

FIGURE 11. Relationship between the per capita income and color composition of the population and total, infant and maternal mortality in the 92 cities of 100,000 or more population, 1939 and 1940.

The average rates for each diagnosis category of table 14 were computed for the nine groups of cities, [making it] possible to examine what effect the color composition of the population has upon the association between income and mortality from selected causes.

Only nine of the diagnosis groups of table 12 are [considered here]. The rates for the remaining diagnoses show only a small color differential. For six diagnoses— infectious diseases, tuberculosis, syphilis, influenza, pneumonia, pellagra and cancer —the pattern of association between mortality and income shown in table 12 is also present in two or more of the color composition groups. The exceptions to the general trend are slight. The rates for exophthalmic goiter and diseases of the gall bladder show a more irregular pattern in the color composition groups than in table 12. For diabetes, the pattern of association between income and mortality is differ- ent in each color composition group.

Therefore, on the basis of the above analysis it would seem that in the largest cities in the country, economic status as measured by per capita buying income is inversely related to the frequency of death from all causes, of infant and maternal deaths, and of deaths from infectious diseases, tuberculosis, syphilis, pellagra, diseases of the ear, nose and throat, influenza, pneumonia, chronic diseases, appendicitis, hernia and "other accidents." This association is independent of the age composition of the population and is affected only slightly by variations in color composition. . . .

C. OTHER ENVIRONMENTAL FACTORS *

THE PURPOSE of this paper is to present some of the most recent data drawn from various sources which illustrate the breadth or the limits of our knowledge of the relationship of illness to various social and environmental conditions.

Data of total morbidity have been obtained only through special investigation of samples of population groups. Those which will be referred to particularly are: the National Health Survey of 1935-36 of slightly more than 2,000,000 persons in 917,000 households in urban communities in various parts of the United States [1] (Negro families were included in this survey); a study of farm families in Michigan; and the morbidity study which was conducted over a period of five years in some 2,000 white families living in the Eastern Health District of Baltimore.

In all of these studies of morbidity, information was obtained concerning certain aspects of the environment of the family, such as age and sex of the population under consideration, size of community, income, amount of rent or value of owned homes, certain data on housing conditions, and occupation of employed members of the family. In addition to these, educational level of the family members was included in the Eastern Health District Study. Also, for the National Health Survey population, information was obtained as to whether the head of the household had moved to the city from a farm during the ten years preceding the survey. Thus it is possible to consider morbidity in relation to some of these factors. . . .

Illness by Age.—Statistics of illness at adult ages portray conditions and disease as manifestations of impaired vitality. The frequency of all illness is highest in childhood, due chiefly to respiratory diseases and the acute communicable diseases, lowest in the ages 15-24, and increases gradually after age 25.

That the increase of illness with age is a manifestation of impaired vitality may be illustrated by a study of the prevalence of the more serious chronic diseases among some 1,200 husbands and their wives in the Eastern Health District of Baltimore. As shown in figure 12, at ages 20-34, about 4 per cent had chronic disease; in each of the next two age groups the rate more than doubled; and at ages 65 and over, 43 per cent had chronic disease. Chronic disease here includes conditions which are leading causes of death: cardiovascular disease, hypertensive vascular disease, cancer, and diabetes, as well as conditions such as the psycho-

* From: "Social and Environmental Factors in Illness," by Jean Downes; *Milbank Memorial Fund Quarterly* 26:366-85, Oct. 1948 (No. 3). Reprinted (with omissions, including initial paragraphs and some figures) by permission of the author and publishers. The author is a member of the technical staff of the Milbank Memorial Fund, New York.

1. The urban surveyed population was so distributed as to give a sample which was, in general, representative of cities in the United States, according to size and region.

neuroses and arthritis, which cause a great amount of disability.[2] It is a significant fact that at ages 45-64, which should be a most productive period of life, slightly more than one-fourth of these husbands and wives had chronic illness. The fact that the prevalence of the chronic diseases increases rapidly as age increases and that such conditions occur most frequently within well-defined age limits might be taken to constitute presumptive evidence that some environmental condition, either external or internal, peculiar to middle and old age is necessary for their development. The usual explanation is that the "aging process" is common to those specific ages and that chronic disease is associated with the "aging process." This explanation is not entirely satisfactory and is cited only to emphasize the complexity of the problem of studying environment and disease.

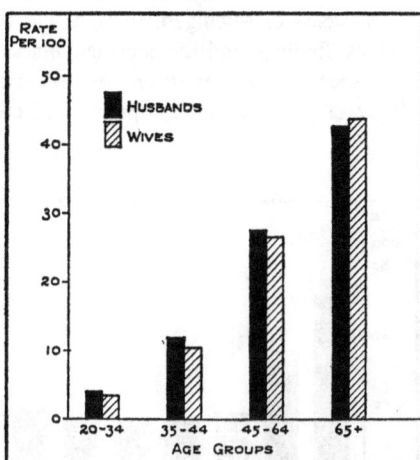

FIGURE 12. Prevalence of chronic disease among 1,289 husbands and their wives.

Chronic disease is not a result of age *per se* inasmuch as it occurs at relatively young ages in some people and not all persons at advanced ages develop the same chronic condition. Thus it would seem that a particular setting or background is involved. The study of the 1,200 spouses offers some suggestive evidence on this point.

The association of chronic disease without respect to cause was studied for husbands and their wives in four different age groups. In each age group the observed number of instances where both the husband and his wife had a chronic disease was considerably greater than the number expected to occur concurrently if such conditions occurred at random among husbands and wives. These differences were statistically significant. Chronic disease by specific cause was considered only

2. The diseases or affections which are included are as follows: tuberculosis, malignant neoplasms, diabetes, psychoses, psychoneuroses, heart disease, hypertensive vascular disease, varicose veins, peptic ulcer, gall-bladder disease, chronic nephritis, arthritis, hernia, and asthma. *Only cases diagnosed by a private physician, clinic, or hospital are included.*

for the married pairs 45 years of age and over. A significant association of illness in both husband and wife was found for all circulatory diseases combined, for hypertensive vascular disease and for arthritis. These spouses had shared the same environment over a period of years and the results suggest that the immediate domestic environment may be a factor of some importance in the occurrence of certain chronic diseases.

A study of significant symptoms and complaints among 1,219 persons in a carefully selected sample composed of 308 farm families in rural Michigan showed that the proportion having such symptoms increased markedly with age. These data are not comparable with the usual statistics of morbidity since they include some impairments and complaints without overt illness. Approximately every sixth family was asked to have a clinic examination made by a physician from the Medical School of the University of Michigan. In eight out of ten cases there was agreement in the physicians' findings and the reported illness or complaint. These data are significant with respect to the proportion affected at different ages and it is evident that the prevalence of persons with symptoms and complaints increases as age increases. . . .

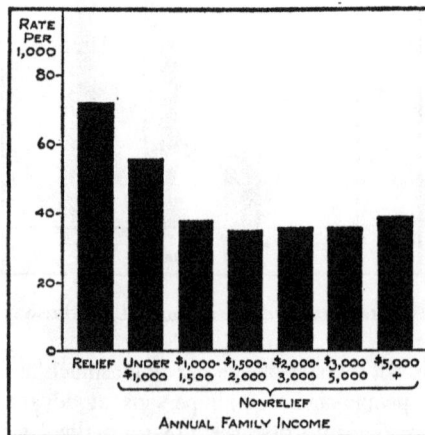

FIGURE 13. Annual frequency of chronic illness—disabling one week or longer.

Illness by Income Groups.—Figure 13 shows the occurrence of disabling illness (three months or longer) from chronic disease among the National Health Survey urban population classified according to income. Here again the highest rate of illness was found to be among persons in the lowest income classes. In the classes where income was $1,000 and above there was little variation in the rate of chronic illness. Except for the lowest income groups there seems to be little association between all chronic illness and family income. This is not surprising since chronic disease is common to so many of the older adults.

Certain specific illnesses, however, do show a more marked association with family income. Illness from pneumonia illustrates this fact. The lower the income the higher was the frequency of this disease.

Rheumatic fever which is considered a chronic disease also shows a marked association with income. . . .

Both the morbidity from pneumonia and rheumatic fever show a closer association with economic environment than does total disabling chronic disease or all illness as expressed in symptoms and complaints.

Illness and Crowding.—One environmental factor, crowding; that is, the number of persons who occupy a dwelling unit in relation to the number of rooms in the

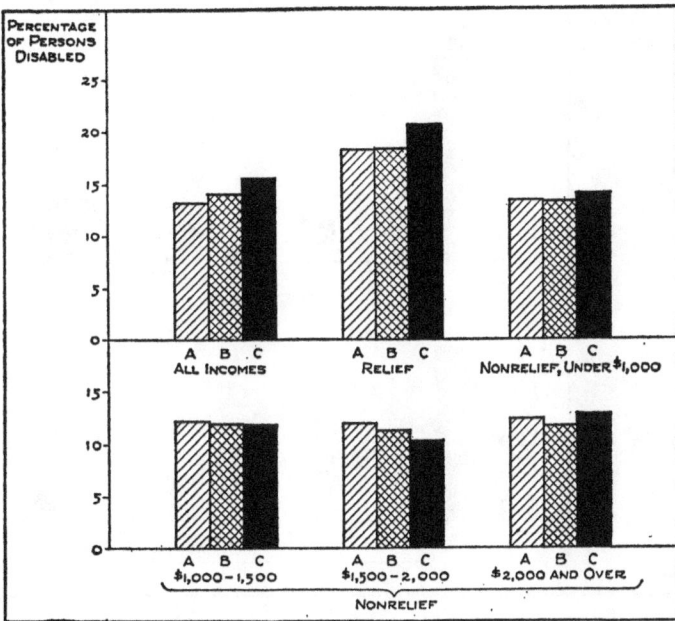

FIGURE 14. Percentage of persons disabled for a week or longer during one year, by degree of crowding and economic status.

unit, has been studied in relation to illness by Britten. The data presented are based upon a population of about 1,700,000 white persons from the National Health Survey. As shown in figure 14, there are three "crowding" classifications: "A", one person or less per room; "B", more than one person but not more than 1.5 persons per room; and "C", more than 1.5 persons per room.[3] Crowding is a crude measure of economic status; the inverse correlation between income and crowding is high. The effect of income is partially eliminated by making comparison

3. The data of illness are adjusted to age and household-size distribution of the total white population studied.

of disabling illness rates within fairly specific income groups. In general, the relative increase in the percentage of persons with disabling illness varied inversely with income. That the ratios of the rates in Category "C" to those in Category "A" were lower for specific income groups than for the population as a whole, according to Britten, is explained by the interaction of two factors: (1) the higher illness rates in the low-income classes, and (2) the greater concentration of these low-income groups in the categories of increased crowding.

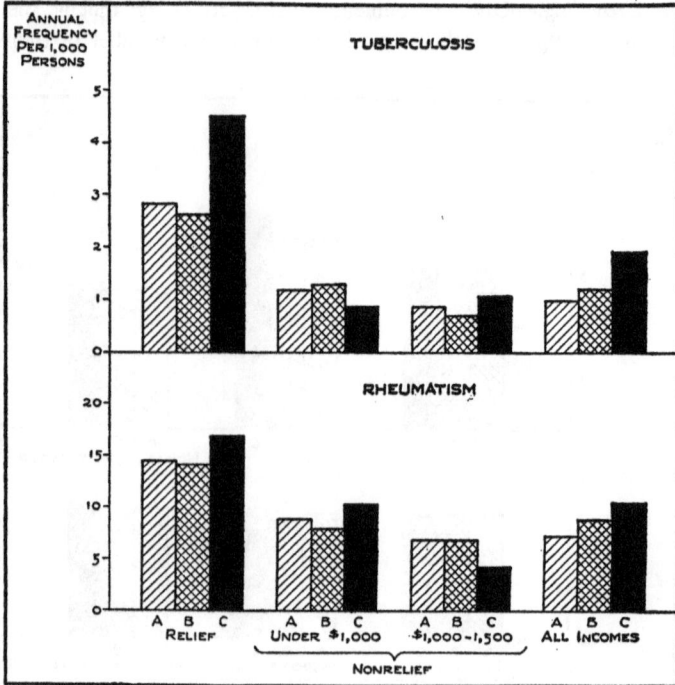

FIGURE 15. Annual frequency among persons of two diagnoses by degree of crowding and economic status.

... Figure 15 shows data for tuberculosis and rheumatism. Here the increase of illness with increase in crowding is more marked for tuberculosis than for rheumatism.

Britten concludes that the data presented in his report, of which only a small part has been shown here, has established an important broad association between housing and health. ...

Chronic Disease as an Environmental Factor.—A study of illness among school-age children may be used to illustrate the possible influence of social factors other than age, income, or crowding which may affect the rate of morbidity. The data presented are based upon a sample which includes 214 families in the Eastern Health District of Baltimore observed for illness over a period of from three to five years. In each of these families there was one or more children of school age, and a school-age child formed the basis of selection of the family for special study. Also, in each family there was one or more cases of chronic disease, usually among the adult members of the family.

It was possible to classify the school-age child who brought the family into the study (the index case) according to his sickness record during a particular twelve-month period. Sixty-three of the 214 children had three or more illnesses; the remaining 151 children either suffered no illness or had less than three illnesses during the year under consideration.[4]

Examination of the illness rates of the school-age siblings of each of these two groups of children revealed a striking difference between them. Siblings in the families selected on the basis of a child who had three or more illnesses had an annual illness rate three times as great as the rate among siblings of the index cases in the other families. This was true for disabling illness as well as for all illness.

Further study indicated that there was a tendency for children to remain at about the same sickness level over a period of five years; that is, sickly children remained sickly. There were sickly families and healthy families as judged by morbidity among the children in them.

This question is pertinent: Were there wide differences between these two groups of families with respect to certain social and environmental conditions which may be related to the differences in the rate of illness of the child population? It was possible to study the following environmental conditions: size of family, degree of crowding, income, educational level of the head of the household, and the type of chronic disease in the family.

There were no important differences between the "sickly" and "nonsickly" families with respect to size or degree of crowding. The median size of family was similar in both groups—5.3 and 5.6, respectively. A relatively high proportion of the families in both groups were graded as crowded; that is, having an unsatisfactory number of rooms in relation to the number, age, and sex constitution of the family members. Thirty-six per cent of the "sickly" families were crowded and 35 per cent of the "nonsickly" were so classified.

There were no important differences between the two groups of families with respect to annual income. Only about one-fourth of the families in each group had an income of $2,000 or more per year.

In about 60 per cent of the families in each group the head of the household had less than an eighth-grade education, very few had any high school education, and there were none who had any college or other advanced schooling.

The head of the household had chronic disease in 44 per cent of the "sickly" families compared with 49 per cent in the "nonsickly" group. Most of this chronic disease was nondisabling. The proportions where the head of the household was disabled were as follows: "sickly" group 5 per cent; "nonsickly" group 3 per cent.

4. Attacks of acute communicable diseases, infectious skin conditions (ring worm, impetigo and scabies) and tonsillectomies are excluded; also chronic disease is excluded.

However, there was a greater concentration of adults with chronic illness in the "sickly" families. The housewife had chronic disease in 80 per cent of the "sickly" compared with 45 per cent of the "nonsickly" group. Both husband and wife were affected in 32 per cent of the former compared with 16 per cent of the latter group.

When type of chronic disease in the family is considered there are striking differences between the two groups. . . . In the "sickly" families there was, [for example], a higher proportion with rheumatic fever, psychoneuroses, and psychoses than was noted for the "nonsickly" group. Fifty-three per cent of the "sickly" families had such cases of illness compared with 20 per cent of the families classed as "nonsickly."

It is not surprising that classification of a family by frequent illness of a child member has selected a relatively large number of "rheumatic fever" families into the "sickly" group. It is recognized that in these families more than one child may be rheumatic and these children are especially susceptible to attacks of respiratory illness and other ailments.

Chronic disease in either the husband or the wife creates an atmosphere in the family which can be detrimental to the other members of the family, especially the children. One can hardly escape the conclusion that a child's reaction to the atmosphere created by a psychoneurotic parent is apt to be frequent illness. Otherwise, we should not expect such a high proportion of these families in the "sickly" group. . . .

Summary.—Economic status as expressed by annual income of the family is an important index of environment because it determines to a considerable extent the paucity or abundance of so many conditions conducive to healthful living: food, housing, medical care, education, and recreation. Yet the relationship of family income to *all illness* is clear-cut only for the very poorest, those with an annual income of less than $1,000. Part of the reason for this is because a relatively high proportion of *all illness* is composed of attacks of the acute respiratory illnesses and the acute infectious diseases, mainly those of childhood. For example, at ages under 15 these illnesses account for 60 to 70 per cent of the total; at ages 15-44, 50 per cent, and at ages 45 and over they account for 30 to 40 per cent of all illness. These illnesses generally do not select only those living under poor environmental conditions. They are fairly common to all population groups irrespective of their level of living.

However, when specific illnesses such as pneumonia, rheumatic fever, or tuberculosis are considered, their relationship to poor environment as defined by annual income is more clear-cut. Undoubtedly, a poor environment tends to lower nonspecific resistance to these and other diseases and thus is an active factor in their production. Yet we do not know precisely the particular factor or factors responsible.

The relationship of family income to *all chronic disease* also is clear-cut only for the very poorest groups in the population. The probable explanation for this is entirely different from that of *all illness* and economic status. It is true that chronic disease affects a relatively high proportion of the middle and old-age population and persons with these conditions are evidently common to all income groups. However, the chronic diseases may be in the process of development over a long period of time and thus their appearance may be one expression of an accumulation of past experience. Information on income as obtained in morbidity studies is related to one particular period of time; that is the present. It is recognized that our population is not static with respect to level of income. Some families with a present income of $2,500 per year may have been in a much lower income class over a period of years; some may have previously been in a higher income class. In a study of social and cultural factors in chronic disease and delayed recovery, Ruesch found that 45 per cent of the cases of delayed recovery were "static"; that is they had remained in the same social class over a period of time; 39 per cent were "climbers"—they had moved from a lower to a higher social class; and the remainder, 16 per cent, were "decliners" or "mixed". To find out whether one type or level of social environment is more productive of the chronic diseases than another type will require either retrospective data on an entire study population or continued observation over a very long period of time.

It seems just to conclude that the study of morbidity in relation to the usual indices of social environmental conditions is of value because such investigation indicates a particular part of the population most in need of public health and medical care. However, if preventive medicine is to function more fully in the control of morbidity, most of which is of unknown etiology, more searching techniques must be employed for evaluating the precise influence of specific environmental conditions in the production of ill health.

FURTHER READINGS

Mortality Trends

Dickinson, Frank G. and Welker, Everett L. *Mortality Trends in the United States 1900-1949*. Bulletin 92, Bureau of Medical Economic Research, American Medical Association. Chicago: The Association, 1952. 32 pages.

Health Status

American Dental Association, Bureau of Economic Research and Statistics. *Survey of Needs for Dental Care*. Chicago: The Association, 1954. 50 pages.

Bureau of Statistics and Department of National Health and Welfare. *Canadian Sickness Survey, 1950-51*. Special compilations, Nos. 5, 6, 7. Ottawa, Canada: The Bureau, 1955.

Collins, Selwyn D., Trantham, Katharine S., and Lehmann, Josephine L. *Sickness Experience in Selected Areas of the United States*. Publication No. 390, Public Health Service. Washington: U. S. Government Printing Office, 1955. 96 pages.

Collins, Selwyn D., Trantham, Katharine S., and Lehmann, Josephine L. *Illness and Mortality Among Infants During the First Year of Life*. Publication No. 449, Public Health Service. Washington: U. S. Government Printing Office, 1955. 20 pages.

Collins, Selwyn D., Lehmann, Josephine L., and Trantham, Katharine S. *Major Causes of Illness of Various Severities and Major Causes of Death in Six Age Periods of*

Life. Publication No. 440, Public Health Service. Washington: U. S. Government Printing Office, 1955. 22 pages. (Includes references).

Falk, I. S., Klem, Margaret C., and Sinai, Nathan. *The Incidence of Illness and the Receipt and Costs of Medical Care Among Representative Families.* Publication 26, Committee on the Costs of Medical Care. Chicago: University of Chicago Press, 1933. 327 pages.

Hoffer, Charles R. and others. *Health Needs and Health Care in Michigan.* East Lansing, Mich.: Michigan State College, 1950. 94 pages.

Milbank Memorial Fund. *Studies of Illness in the Eastern Health District of Baltimore, Maryland.* A collection of papers published between 1940 and 1948. New York: The Fund, no date.

Milbank Memorial Fund. *Backgrounds of Social Medicine.* New York: The Fund, 1949. 202 pages. (Includes references).

The President's Commission on the Health Needs of the Nation. *Building America's Health.* (5 vols.). Vol. 3: *America's Health Status, Needs and Resources: A Statistical Appendix.* Washington: U. S. Government Printing Office, 1953. 299 pages.

United States Department of Health, Education, and Welfare, Public Health Service. *Accident Frequency: Place of Occurrence and Relation to Chronic Disease.* Publication No. 249, Public Health Service. Washington: U. S. Government Printing Office, 1953. 65 pages.

United States Public Health Service. *The National Health Survey, 1935-36.* Publication No. 85. Washington: U. S. Government Printing Office, 1951. 67 pages.

Woolsey, Theodore D. *Estimates of Disabling Illness Prevalence in the United States, Based on the Current Population Survey of February 1949 and September 1950.* Publication No. 181 (Monograph No. 4), Public Health Service. Washington: U.S. Government Printing Office, 1952. 16 pages.

Health Resources

Bachmann, George W. and associates. *Health Resources in the United States: Personnel, Facilities and Services.* Washington: The Brookings Institution, 1952. 344 pages. (Includes references).

Dewhurst, J. Frederic and associates. *America's Needs and Resources: A New Survey.* New York: Twentieth Century Fund, 1955. 1148 pages.

CHAPTER III

Adequacy of Medical Care

WE EXPECT MEDICAL care to make its contribution to the promotion of health and the prevention of disease; its objectives include the cure or mitigation of disease and the rehabilitation of the patient. The achievement of these broad purposes rests, in large measure, on the adequacy of medical care. In turn, the definition of adequacy must be related to these same purposes, and to the more specific criteria established within their framework. As medical science brings new knowledge and skills to bear upon the problems of health and disease, and as social awareness of the ever-new potential of medical care grows, new goals are defined and new criteria may be set. Any concept of adequacy must therefore be a dynamic one.

Adequacy has two dimensions—quantity and quality. Quantitative adequacy implies the provision of all the services required to achieve the stated purposes, in appropriate amounts and effectively timed and balanced. Its essentials include:

1. Enough personnel—all of the members of the medical care team needed to provide the full range of modern scientific care. (See Chapter V.)

2. Enough facilities—from physicians' offices and clinics to health centers and hospitals. (See Chapter VI.)

3. The availability of care in the home, office, clinic, health center, general or special hospital, according to the best interest of the patient.

4. The availability of laboratory and x-ray services, of drugs and appliances.

5. The education of the public in the wise and efficient use of available health resources.

The first half of this chapter is concerned with the quantity of medical care needed and received by various segments of our population.

Quantity not only stands as an independent dimension, but is an inseparable component of the quality of medical care. And the requirements for quantitative adequacy are significantly influenced by the level of quality. Qualitative adequacy depends upon:

1. The competence of the personnel—their education, training and efficiency of function. (See Chapter V.)

2. The standards maintained for equipment and facilities. (See Chapter VI.)

3. The availability of services based on the widest knowledge of modern medical science.

4. The organization and operation of services, whether in independent practice or organized medical care programs, for optimal efficiency and economy, with emphasis on continuity of care and an understanding of the needs of people. (See Chapters VI and VII.)

5. Sound financial arrangements which make possible the timely provision of all indicated services. (See Chapters IV and XII.)

The second half of this chapter provides some meat for these bare bones in a series of discussions of the principles underlying the achievement of medical care of high quality.

A. *Quantitative Adequacy*

12. FACTORS DETERMINING AVAILABILITY OF CARE *

JUST HOW SERIOUS is the lack of proper medical care among the American people? Some idea of prevailing conditions may be gained by a study of the ratio of medical personnel and hospital beds to population. In these respects, and using readily available statistics, the national situation as a whole would appear to be rather good compared to that in the chief European countries. . . .

. . . Despite encouraging national averages, the supply of physicians' services is seriously inadequate in many parts of the nation. Similar contrasts and deficiencies could easily be shown in the supply of other medical personnel and of hospital beds. . . .

Recent studies indicate that three basic circumstances affect the availability of good medical care for any given group. First, there is the economic level of the population; second, the accessibility and the social assets and liabilities of the

* From: *Medicine in the Changing Order,* by the Committee on Medicine and the Changing Order, New York Academy of Medicine; New York: Commonwealth Fund, 1947 (Chap. III, "The Health of the Nation," pp. 41-44). Reprinted (with omissions, including initial paragraphs) by permission of the publishers.

ADEQUACY OF MEDICAL CARE 77

location; and third, the complex of professional institutions (hospitals, clinics, laboratories, specialist and consultation services) to be found in the given community. All are interrelated, but for the sake of clarity each is to be considered separately.

The economic factor is of universal validity. Wherever there is poverty there is a high incidence of illness and, as a rule, less adequate medical service. It is true that certain urban poor have free access to good clinics, but the generalization that "the poor as well as the rich receive good care" is far from accurate. In reality, high-quality care on a charity or low-cost basis is available to the poor in relatively few places.

The factor of location is frequently superimposed upon that of income. The poor, located in rural areas, receive less adequate care than those in urban centers. But even the relatively prosperous may suffer for want of adequate and competent medical care as a result of isolation. Generally the least adequate services are found in villages and in rural areas, and the best in metropolitan environments.

The last factor affecting quality of medical care, namely, "the complex of professional institutions," is in many ways related to the first two factors. The poorer and the rural regions have fallen down in providing medical facilities because the complicated and costly institutions which present-day medicine requires are not easily created or supported where the population is sparse and poor. Yet, though these institutions cannot be created and cannot function without money, money alone will not bring them into being or make them function effectively.

Furthermore, part of this difficulty is to be traced, paradoxical as this may seem, to the very progress of the science and practice of medicine. To term inadequate the medical service available in certain parts of the country, and to some of the people in all parts, is not to say that it is inferior to what was received, say, fifty years ago. In that period of time service has improved even among these groups. But the inadequacy becomes apparent by contrast with the high grade of medical services available to those living on a higher income level and in well-populated centers.

It is evident, therefore, that the inequities in medical services have come into being not because the people were becoming poorer, or more isolated, or more neglected by medical personnel. Actually, the majority are less poor, less isolated, and receive better medical care than did their fathers. We have become conscious of inadequacies in the medical care of some groups chiefly because advances in medical science have out-paced the distribution of its benefits. Yet much of the recent discussion on this subject appears to take as its thesis that poverty and isolation were the starting points in the problem. One result of this has been to place far too much emphasis upon the purely economic aspects of medical care. While no one can doubt that the income factors are very important, exclusive and excessive emphasis on this tends to distort the problem. It certainly is not true that if at a given time and place people had more money to spend they would thereby secure better care, though, of course, in the long run this is most likely to be the result.

The professional factors that initiated recent progress are still much involved in the whole process. Interrelated at many points with financial circumstances, they call for equal consideration. . . .

13. "Effective Demand" versus "Medical Need" *

IT IS PERHAPS unnecessary to point out that the "need" for medical care is not necessarily the same as the "demand." The demand for medical care is conditioned largely by economic factors. It merely represents the medical care actually consumed and is determined by the price and availability of the services, by the relative attractiveness of such substitutes as "irregular" healers and patent medicines, and by popular beliefs concerning health and its maintenance. . . .

The real need for medical care is a medical, not an economic, concept. It can be defined only in terms of the physical conditions of the people and the capacities of the science and art of medicine to deal with them. Thus, it is not always a conscious need, still less an active desire backed by willingness to pay. The ordinary layman lacks the knowledge to define his own medical needs and can rely only on the expert opinion of medical practitioners and public health authorities. But he should be expected to recognize the proper occasion for consulting a physician. Moreover, he must be intelligently able to cooperate with the practitioner in the treatment of illness and in the establishment and maintenance of a regimen of living which will promote the physical and mental health of his family. . . .

14. Variations in Receipt of Medical Services: Three Reports

A. COMMITTEE ON THE COSTS OF MEDICAL CARE †

IN A NATION-WIDE survey of illnesses and costs of medical service among 9,000 white families, the Committee on the Costs of Medical Care found that there was substantially the same incidence of illness per family or per individual in the various

* From: *The Fundamentals of Good Medical Care* (Publication No. 22 of the Committee on the Costs of Medical Care), by Roger I. Lee, M.D., and Lewis W. Jones; Chicago: University of Chicago Press. Copyright 1933, by the University of Chicago. Reprinted (with omissions, including initial paragraphs) by permission of the publishers. (The excerpt reprinted is from the Introduction, pp. 11-12). The authors are, respectively, a consultant in internal medicine in Boston; and president of Rutgers University, New Brunswick, N.J.

† From: *Medical Care for the American People* (Publication No. 28), by the Committee on the Costs of Medical Care; Chicago: University of Chicago Press. Copyright 1932, by the University of Chicago. Reprinted (with omissions, including initial paragraphs and one figure) by permission of the publishers. (The excerpt reprinted is from Chap. I, "The Present Status of Medical Care," pp. 5-13).

broad income groups.[1] Families with incomes under $1,200 or $2,000, however, receive far less medical service than those with incomes of $5,000, or $10,000 and over. This is shown in table 15, which gives the relative amounts of service of various kinds received in a twelve-month period by nearly 9,000 families, at different income levels, in all population groups.

It is evident from table 15 that the two or three lowest income groups receive far less of nearly every service—care from physicians and dentists, hospitalization, eye care, health examinations, immunizations, special nursing, maternity care, and x-ray and laboratory service—than the groups with highest incomes. The group with the lowest amount of service (which was not in every case the group with the lowest income) received only 50 per cent as many days of hospitalization, and 41 per cent as many calls from physicians as the group with the highest amount of service. In every instance the latter is the group with the highest income. Only one-fifth as many persons in the lowest income group receive any dental attention. The families with incomes of $1,200 to $2,000 receive even less hospitalization and preventive services than do the families with incomes under $1,200.

Some persons may object, however, that the higher income groups receive more service than they need, because they enjoy the luxury of being attended by physicians and nurses, or are being kept under treatment to serve the economic interest of the practitioners. While occasional cases of these types are known to everyone, a comparison of the services received by the high-income groups with the standards for good medical care published by the Committee shows that, even among the highest income group, insufficient care is the rule. The only services which this group uses more than appears to be necessary are special nursing of hospital patients and the hospitalization of surgical patients. For all the other services listed, including even prenatal and postnatal calls to maternity patients and immunizations and health examinations, the wealthy families receive less service than these reasonable standards require. The most significant numerical measures of the adequacy of services are the number of home, office, and clinic calls by physicians and the per capita number of days of hospitalization. Of these two items, the well-to-do patients received 84 and 87 per cent, respectively, of the "standard" amounts.

The groups with smaller incomes obtain far less service. In spite of the large volume of free work done by hospitals, health departments, and individual practitioners, and in spite of the sliding scale of charges, it appears that each year nearly one-half of the individuals in the lowest income group receive no professional medical or dental attention of any kind, curative or preventive (table 16).

The figures in tables 15 and 16 give only a partial picture of the lack of medical service. Suitable indices are not available, for example, to show the widespread lack of mental hygiene services. Although the needed data on this point are not available,

1. The incidence of recognized and recorded illness in the Committee's study was lowest in the low income groups and highest in the groups with highest income. It is not known to what extent the higher rate in the upper income classes is due to economic and social factors rather than to strictly physical factors. Data from the U.S. Public Health Service and other sources indicate that when the groups with incomes under $1,500 or $2,000 are further subdivided, a definite relation appears between poverty and illness, the lower income groups having more illness and illness of longer duration.

TABLE 15. *The medical services needed and received*

Units of Medical Service Received per 1,000 Individuals or per 1,000 Illnesses in Families with Specified Incomes Compared with Services Needed to Meet Standards of Good Medical Care. Data on Services Received, Based on 38,668 White Persons in 8,639 Families Surveyed for Twelve Consecutive Months, 1928-1931.

Unit of Service	Under $1,200	$1,200- $2,000	$2,000- $3,000	$3,000- $5,000	$5,000- $10,000	$10,000 and Over	Services Needed to Supply Good Medical Care
	Number per 1,000 Individuals						
Home, office and clinic calls (physicians)[A]	1,931.9	2,045.9	2,296.7	2,741.4	3,621.4	4,734.4	5,649.5
Hospitalized cases[B]	59.4	52.4	59.4	63.1	79.3	98.0	107.0[C]
Days of hospital care[C]	927.9	666.7	757.4	604.2	840.3	1,200.8	1,384.7
Dental care (persons over 3 years of age)	117.9	184.6	247.5	309.4	446.0	622.0	1,000.0
Health examinations[D]	83.2	68.0	69.1	82.2	121.7	234.0	941.9
Immunizations[E]	68.5	49.2	50.9	59.6	84.3	120.2	185.3
Refractions or glasses	24.5	24.6	39.6	53.8	89.6	159.7	175.0
Home and office calls (Secondary practitioners and cultists)	154.6	139.1	230.4	231.1	459.0	569.2	......
	Number per 1,000 Illnesses						
Hospitalized cases[B]	74.0	65.1	71.6	71.6	80.1	88.2	121.2
Surgical cases hospitalized	44.2	42.0	49.6	48.1	58.6	62.6	51.3
Cases having x-ray	23.8	25.2	27.0	31.0	48.5	75.4	186.4
Cases having laboratory service	51.7	61.6	68.8	82.8	120.3	132.3	581.7
Prenatal or postnatal calls[F]	6,939.0	7,230.0	9,551.0	11,386.0	12,382.0	13,000.0	19,360.0[G]
Hospitalized cases having special nursing[H]	67.0	125.0	164.0	251.0	379.0	685.0	578.0[C]

[A] For illness only. Excludes calls for preventive service.
[B] One day or longer in all hospitals.
[C] Excludes care in tuberculosis sanatoria and mental hospitals.
[D] Includes well-baby care.
[E] Includes service whether or not accompanied by illness.
[F] Rates per 1,000 maternity cases. Excludes calls in hospital.
[G] All calls, including those in hospital.
[H] Rates per 1,000 hospitalized cases in all hospitals. Restricted to cases involving 1 day or more of hospital care.

there is agreement of experts in the field that the present service is seriously inadequate. A major objective of the mental hygiene movement, [according to Dr. Frederick H. Allen], is "the development of more real treatment facilities for the early cases found in every community. The thing every mental hospital superintendent faces is the fact that had such facilities existed, a large number of [his] cases would never have developed to the point where hospital care was an emergent necessity." Early detection is fundamental. We have yet to work out methods for such detection, to train specialists in them, and to develop in the medical profession as a whole a knowledge of what can be achieved and how and where assistance can be found.

TABLE 16. *Persons not receiving care*

Percentage of Individuals Receiving No Medical, Dental, or Eye Care—Based on 38,668 White Persons in 8,639 Families with Known Incomes, Surveyed for Twelve Consecutive Months, 1928-1931.

	Percentage of Individuals in Specified Income Classes						
	Under $1,200	$1,200- $2,000	$2,000- $3,000	$3,000- $5,000	$5,000- $10,000	$10,000 and Over	All In- comes[A]
Receiving no medical, dental or eye care[B]	46.6	42.2	37.3	33.4	24.4	13.8	38.2

[A] Weighted for proportions in the several income classes.

[B] The situation is actually even more startling than appears from these data because many of the persons who are counted as having had medical care may have had extremely little.

The Committee's survey does not include data for Negroes. It is well known, however, that the 10 per cent of our population who are colored have health problems which are, on the whole, considerably more serious than those of whites. The Negro is America's principal marginal worker, and he suffers in the North as well as the South from the many disabilities that this entails: poorer housing, less adequate diet, less sanitary surroundings, more employment of married women, and greater economic insecurity. The extensive migrations of Negroes during the last 20 years have added new complications to their problems.* ... In the South, the lack of care for Negroes is only a part of a larger problem. Because of the extreme poverty of large areas, neither Negroes nor whites receive anything but the most deplorably inadequate medical service.

Finally, medical attention may be statistically adequate but of poor quality. Even conceding adequate original education and training, in view of the rapidly increasing body of scientific medical knowledge, it is difficult for a considerable percentage of practitioners under present circumstances to keep up-to-date.

The Situation in Dental Care.—The average annual expenditure for dental care is extremely low among the 90 per cent of families with incomes under $5,000. Thus among families with incomes of $1,200 to $2,000, the average annual expenditure for dental care is $9.01. Families with these incomes or less constitute one-half of the total population. Families with incomes of $2,000 to $3,000, according to the Committee's nation-wide survey of illnesses and costs, spend an average of $16.39.

The significance of these figures is found when we go behind the general averages. If individuals instead of families are considered, only 10.1 per cent of persons in families with incomes under $1,200 received any kind of dental attention during

* See Chapter II (Selection No. 10B) for data on the health status of Negroes.

the year. For those with family incomes of $1,200 to $2,000, the percentage receiving dental care was only 15.5. In the $2,000 to $3,000 income group, the percentage rose only to 21.4, whereas for the $5,000 to $10,000 income group it was 40.6, and for the group with incomes of $10,000 and over it attained a peak of 59.6 per cent. Among the mass of the population, only 21 per cent of individuals secure any dental care during an average year.

Undoubtedly a certain proportion of persons secure care only for the relief of pain or other dental emergency. The proportion of the population who receive systematic and sufficient dental care must be considerably less than 21 per cent. The need for systematic dental care is unquestionable. That there is a latent demand for it is attested by the fact that the great majority of people in the higher income groups purchase a considerable amount of dental service.

. . . The studies of the Committee on Dental Practice of the American Dental Association show that there is unused time among dentists, although not as much as there is among physicians. Undoubtedly, a lack of popular appreciation of the value of systematic dental care is one of the reasons why dental service is not obtained. But the economic deterrent is probably a more important obstacle.

Use of Preventive Medical Services.—Although many practitioners suffer enforced idleness, the American people need far more of the medical services which could be provided on the basis of present knowledge and facilities. This is particularly true of preventive services. For example, in any one year less than seven per cent of the population have a complete or partial physical examination, and less than 5 per cent are immunized against diphtheria or some other disease. In a special survey of pre-school children, the White House Conference learned that only 51 per cent of city children, and only 37 per cent of rural children, have had one or more health examinations prior to their sixth birthday; that only 13 per cent of children in both urban and rural districts have received a dental health examination by their sixth year; that only 21 per cent of city children and only 7 per cent of rural children have been vaccinated by the time they are six; and that only 21 per cent of urban and only 18 per cent of rural children have been immunized against diphtheria.

Several factors cause this limited utilization of preventive medical services. First, most laymen because of habit hesitate to seek medical care except when driven by pain or discomfort. Second, payment on a fee-for-service basis is a greater economic deterrent to the utilization of preventive services than of therapeutic work. Third, in some rural areas, medical practitioners and other facilities are actually unavailable, and, even in cities where there is an ample supply, the training of many practitioners and the avowed scope of many hospitals and clinics cause them to pay little attention to the preventive aspects of service. Finally, the physician who is aware of a patient's needs for preventive work may refrain from urging it because he does not wish to appear to solicit practice.

In view of the potential ability of public health activities to raise the general level of health at relatively low cost, American communities have been pitifully backward in utilizing modern public health procedures. Of the entire $30 per capita spent for the prevention and care of disease, only $1 has been used for public health service, Federal, state, and local. . . .

Niggardly appropriations for public health work not only seriously limit present activities, but also hamper medical schools in their efforts to attract competent students to public health careers, thus weakening the public health work of the future. . . .

B. COMMISSION ON HEALTH NEEDS OF THE NATION *

INFORMATION ABOUT the utilization of health services is most important in planning for the future development of America's health and in pinpointing the areas where health needs are not met. The extent to which physicians' services or hospitals are used, for example, and the change, or lack of change, in utilization over the years can help to indicate the number of physicians and hospital beds we will require. Identifying the population groups who do not use medical services and the reasons for their failure to demand these services makes it easier to determine what kinds of programs should have priority. The use of services made by members of pre-payment plans as compared with utilization rates of the general population is of great importance in evaluating a prepayment system and also in indicating areas and groups of the general population in which too little service is given.

The available data on utilization are limited in scope. There are no compre-hensive current figures on the frequency of physicians', dentists', or other medical and hospital services. Data on utilization of these services are available only from special sample surveys. The only Nation-wide surveys which covered a broad population are the studies of the Committee on the Costs of Medical Care (1928-31) and the National Health Survey (1935-36). More recently two Nation-wide surveys were made of special population groups—one of children (1946-47) and one of the hospital utilization of the aged (1951). In addition, special studies have been made of limited population groups or specific prepayment plans. These special studies are useful but because of the differences in definition of services, scope of services studied or covered, the population and years surveyed, the conclusions drawn must be somewhat limited.

The level of utilization of all kinds of health and medical services is determined by a combination of many factors: income, place of residence, the personnel or facilities available, age, sex, race, membership in a prepayment plan, educational level and probably many others. Although, because of the complex interrelation-ships, it is impossible to identify the exact effect of, for example, income on the demand for medical services, certain broad conclusions are valid. The lower-income families receive far less medical care than families with moderate or high incomes. Rural residents receive less care than urban residents—a function not only of the lesser facilities and health personnel but the generally lower farm incomes

* From: *Building America's Health*, by the President's Commission on the Health Needs of the Nation: Washington: U.S. Government Printing Office, 1953 (Vol. 2, Chap. VII, "Utiliza-tion of Health Services"). Reprinted with omissions, including figures and one table.

84   *READINGS IN MEDICAL CARE*

and the more limited availability of public clinics. The aged receive more physicians' care and more days of hospitalization than the general population, despite their smaller financial resources.

The level of utilization of medical services has generally increased in past years although not significantly for all kinds of medical care. This trend is also the result of the interrelationships of several factors, including the higher standards of living, the greater availability of medical resources, the development of prepayment plans, and improved health education.

UTILIZATION OF PHYSICIANS' SERVICES

DURING THE PERIOD 1928-31, the Committee on the Costs of Medical Care found that the surveyed population had, on the average, 2.4 physicians' visits per year, not including visits in the hospital. Ten years later, in the Eastern Health District of Baltimore, the rate of utilization of physicians' services was the same. More recent studies indicate a somewhat increased use of physicians by the general population. In four rural New York counties in 1948-49, persons in the county with the lowest utilization saw a physician, on the average, 3.5 times during the year and in the county with the highest utilization, the average number of visits was 4.6. . . .

Physicians' services for the indigent, where data are available, indicate a high rate of utilization. Recipients under the Maryland Medical Care Program had 5.7 physicians' visits (including 0.3 in the hospital) and social assistance recipients (age 65 and over) in Saskatchewan had, on the average, 9.7 physicians' visits, including 6.5 in the hospital.

Most group practice prepayment plans show a somewhat higher utilization of physicians' services than the general population. The Health Insurance Plan of Greater New York provided an average of 5.2 visits per member (1950), the Labor Health Institute of St. Louis, 5.6 and Group Health, Inc. (Washington, D. C.), 5.1. The experience of the Health Insurance Plan of Greater New York is perhaps the best guide to the level of utilization of physicians' services to be expected under group practice and prepayment, since it offers all kinds of physicians' service with virtually no limitations and since its experience is based on the broadest base—300,000 members in 1951. . . .

Another measure of the utilization of services is the percent of the population who used any physicians' services during the course of a year. Persons who belong to prepayment plans are more likely to see a physician than those in the general population, but even in those plans where physicians' services are available at small or no extra charge (above the regular premium), a surprising portion fail to see a physician. In the Permanente Health Plan, one-third of all subscribers did not see a physician during a study year and in the Windsor (Ontario) Plan nearly 40 percent did not see a physician. . . . In a Michigan survey (covering a sample of the entire population except in the Detroit area), 63 percent of the population did not see a physician during a 6-month period.

The degree of utilization of specialists is determined by many factors, including family income, residence, and the organization of medical care. In the

Eastern Health District of Baltimore study (1938-43) it was found that about a third of all services were by specialists. In the Health Insurance Plan of Greater New York group practice prepayment plan, utilization of specialists was high—46 percent of all services (excluding those of radiologists and pathologists) were rendered by specialists during 1950. The two surveys are not, however, comparable and neither provides a true reflection of the national pattern. In the Health Insurance Plan of Greater New York specialists are readily available, without extra costs, to any member and the group practice system encourages utilization of specialists. Both studies were made in large cities, in areas with a concentration of specialists.

The Academy of Pediatrics study of children's services provides a Nation-wide picture which is somewhat different. Here the percent of services by specialists is clearly influenced by the family residence. Whereas 25 percent of all physicians' services for children in the United States as a whole were given by specialists, specialists' calls represented only 2 percent of physicians' services in isolated rural areas.

Income and Utilization of Physicians' Services.—Recent data on the variations in utilization of physicians' services among families in different income groups are not available, except for a few areas. The Committee on the Costs of Medical Care Study (1928-31) and the National Health Survey (1935-36) are the only surveys which related utilization of medical services for broad population groups to income. The Committee on the Costs of Medical Care survey found nearly two and one-half times as many physicians' calls per person in the highest income group as in the lowest. Physicians' calls per illness (as reflected in the National Health Survey) increase much less significantly with increases in income, demonstrating that families with higher income have proportionately greater care for minor illnesses and preventive services and that low-income families often find a way of obtaining physicians' services for serious illness.

The more recent data indicate only the proportion of families, by income class, who received no physicians' care during a year. A total lack of physicians' care may be cited for some persons in all income classes, but the percent of persons or families receiving care increases markedly with increases in family income. In 1928-31 the Committee on the Costs of Medical Care found 20 percent of the lowest-income families had no physicians' services during the survey year compared with 7 percent in the highest income group. A more recent survey and one which also covered a diversified population (State of Michigan, 1948), found nearly a quarter of the State's population had unmet medical needs; in the income group under $1,000, 45 percent of the persons saw no physician although they had one or more symptoms which, in the opinion of qualified physicians, should have been the occasion for medical care.

A survey of rural families in New York State revealed that most families received some care during the year; however, the proportion of families receiving no physicians' care was four times as great among the lowest-income class (under $1,000) as among those families with incomes of $3,000 or more.

Age and Utilization of Physicians' Services.—Variations in utilization of all health services with variations in age have a particular significance in view of the rapidly increasing number of aged in the population. Illness occurs more frequently among the aged than among all age groups combined and the incidence of chronic illness is about four times as great among the population age 65 and over. The greater incidence of illness is reflected in the higher utilization rates of persons aged 65 and over. Although the various surveys show wide differences in the utilization rates, the older age groups have consistently high rates. . . .

Today, pediatricians emphasize preventive health services for children. Under such a program children receive a large amount of medical care. In the Health Insurance Plan of Greater New York, for example, infants under one received, on the average, 13.1 physicians' services per year as compared with 4.4 services for all members.

Place of Residence and Utilization of Physicians' Services.—Persons and families in rural areas and small towns generally have fewer physicians' services than persons in metropolitan areas. City size apparently makes little difference in the over-all number of physicians' services; in the National Health Survey which covered only urban families, the differences in utilization between large cities and small ones was insignificant. The lower utilization of rural families is reflected particularly in physicians' calls at home. The study by the American Academy of Pediatrics of health services for children found nearly three times as many home visits per child in greater metropolitan as in isolated rural areas. . . . In the State of Michigan all kinds of medical care were sought less frequently in rural than in urban areas.

UTILIZATION OF HOSPITAL SERVICES

THE WIDESPREAD PURCHASE of hospital insurance and the changing pattern of hospital care in recent years limit the significance of surveys of hospital utilization made more than 5 or 10 years ago. The earlier surveys do serve the purpose, however, of pointing up the changes which have taken place. People are hospitalized twice as frequently as they used to be even 20 years ago and the length of the hospital stay is shorter. The Committee on the Costs of Medical Care found that only 60 persons per 1,000 were hospitalized during a year and that they stayed on the average 12 days. In 1951 more than 1 out of every 10 persons (115 per 1,000) in the United States was admitted to a general or special hospital and the average case lasted 10 days. The pattern of utilization, in 1951, was similar throughout the Nation although persons in the Southeastern States used hospital facilities somewhat less than persons in other regions. Their lower utilization rates probably reflected the higher proportion of Negro people—for whom special problems still exist, the lower incomes and the more limited hospital facilities.

Hospital admissions of the insured do not vary much from the over-all average but the insured have a consistently shorter stay. Hospitalized members of Blue Cross plans stayed 7.4 days as compared with the Nation-wide average stay of 10.1 days in general hospitals and 10.5 in general and allied special hospitals. The average length of stay of the membership of group practice prepayment plans was even shorter; in the Permanente Health Plan, the average hospital case lasted 6.6 days, and members of the St. Louis Labor Health Institute had an average hospital stay of 7.0 days.

Income and Utilization of Hospitals.—Earlier surveys (the Committee on the Costs of Medical Care and the National Health Survey) which related income to hospital utilization are obsolete, primarily because of the rapid growth of hospital insurance. However, even at the time these surveys were made, differences in family income were not clearly reflected in the utilization of hospitals. The lowest-income groups (the medically indigent) apparently received a large amount of free care, and recent studies indicate that they still have higher than average utilization. The Committee on the Costs of Medical Care study found that the lowest-income families and families with incomes of $10,000 or more received nearly twice as much hospital care as did persons in all other income groups.

Hospital admissions per 1,000 population did not vary significantly between States with high and low incomes in 1951, but the average number of days of hospitalization per case is greater in high-income than in low-income States.

TABLE 17. *Hospital utilization in States grouped by per capita income*

State Group	Number of admissions per 1,000 population	Number of hospital days per 1,000 population
All States	115	1,212
Highest income States ᴬ	118	1,361
Upper-middle income States	115	1,248
Lower-middle income States	125	1,146
Lowest income States	103	887

ᴬ Excluding the District of Columbia; if the District of Columbia were included among the high income States, the rate of admissions would be 119 and the number of days per 1,000, 1,380.

Place of Residence, Race, and Utilization of Hospitals.—Rural and farm residents use hospitals to a lesser extent than does the urban population. Although admissions per 1,000 do not vary greatly with residence, the average annual number of days per 1,000 is much higher in urban areas. Among the urban population aged 65 and over the days of hospitalization per 1,000 were twice as great as among the farm aged, and in the 12 most urban States the average number of hospital days was more than one and one-half times the days in the 12 most rural States.

Differences in the rates of hospitalization between the white and Negro population are even more significant. In six surveyed States Negro children were admitted to hospitals less than half as frequently as white children; hospitalization rates for the aged white and Negro showed a similar pattern. Another measure of the differences in medical care for the white and Negro groups is reflected in the percent of live births, for each group, which is attended by a physician in the hospital. In 1947, 92 percent of white births were in the hospital (and attended by a physician) as compared with 55 percent of nonwhite births.

Age and Utilization of Hospitals.—Age differences in the utilization of hospital services are not of great significance except in the age groups 65 and over. Recent data on hospital utilization rates of the aged are available from a special survey conducted in 1951. This survey was made for the Social Security Administration by the Bureau of the Census in conjunction with their monthly population survey. In addition to this survey, experience of prepayment plans and the results of earlier surveys are available. All of these experiences indicate that the aged have more hospitalization than other age groups. This is true in spite of the fact that the aged generally have fewer financial resources. In all surveys it was found that the aged were admitted to hospitals with about the same frequency as other groups but that their longer than average length of stay resulted in nearly twice the number of days of hospitalization per 1,000 persons.

TABLE 18. *Number of hospital admissions and number of days of hospital care per 1,000 persons, all ages and age 65 and over*

	All ages	65 and over
Admissions per 1,000:		
Committee on the Costs of Medical Care (1928-31)	59	61
Eastern Health District of Baltimore (1938-43)	69	56
Saskatchewan Hospital Services Plan (1951)	199	334 ᴬ
General population (1951)	115	93
Permanente members (1950)	104	127
Days per 1,000 population:		
Committee on the Costs of Medical Care (1928-31)	716	1,501
Eastern Health District of Baltimore (1938-43)	1,112	1,682
Saskatchewan Hospital Services Plan (1951)	2,201	7,485 ᴬ
General population (1951)	1,212	2,051
Permanente members (1950)	685	1,040

ᴬ Includes Old Age Assistance recipients. Number of days based on discharged cases and therefore include all days for each case discharged even if that case was admitted as far back as 1947.

UTILIZATION OF DENTAL SERVICES

DATA ON THE utilization of dental services are very limited. The Committee on Costs of Medical Care and the National Health Survey study in Detroit provide the most comprehensive material available. The demand for dental care is probably more closely related to income than the demand for any other kind of health services. Dental care is more frequently regarded as postponable, an attitude which is reflected in the comparative utilization rates of low and high income families and in the rates during prosperity and in a depression.

The previous utilization of dental service by persons seeking dental care during 1928-31 and the reasons for their visits to the dentist are significant. Of all persons in the highest-income group seeking care, 99.9 percent had been to a dentist previously compared with 89.3 percent of the lowest-income families. Seventy percent of the persons in the lowest-income class who visited the dentist did so because of a pain or known cavity while an equal percentage in the highest-income class received care because it was time for a periodic examination. In all income classes combined, only 26 percent of the dental visits were initiated for periodic examination and 60 percent because of a pain or known cavity.

In the Detroit study (1935-36) it was found that nearly 20 percent of all persons had never been to a dentist and that a third of the population had never been to the dentist or had not been for 5 years or more. The same survey found that while 43 percent of persons in families with a professional worker as head had some dental care (exclusive of extractions) during the year, only 16 percent of persons in families where the head was an unskilled worker received care. White persons received care three times as frequently as nonwhite. The variations among the socioeconomic classes may be exaggerated by the fact that this survey was made immediately after a severe depression during which all kinds of medical care were probably postponed, especially by low-income families. A recent study (San Francisco) of moderate-income wage earning families found that about 50 percent had some dental care during the year. This was much higher utilization than was found for similar occupational groups in the National Health Survey where only 31 percent in families with a clerical worker as head and 21 percent of persons in families with a skilled worker as head received any dental services (other than extractions).

Dental care is received less frequently in rural than in urban areas. In Michigan (1948) 19 percent of persons living in the open country and 26 percent of persons in urban areas saw a dentist. . . .

There is almost no dental care for children under 5 and persons age 65 and over see a dentist infrequently. The age groups from about 25 to 40 have the most frequent dental care and at nearly all ages females receive more dental care than males.

UTILIZATION OF OTHER MEDICAL SERVICES

A LARGE VOLUME of nursing services is received free through visiting nurse associations with the result that a high proportion of the families in the lowest income groups receive nursing care. The utilization of private-duty nursing is directly related to income. However, the relatively great amount of visiting nurse services in low-income families does not compensate for the low volume of continuous bedside nursing. The National Health Survey (1935-36) found that a visiting nurse made an average of 5 visits to each person with a disabling illness lasting a week or longer but the days of nursing service for the cases attended by the private-duty nurse averaged 26.

The only recent data on the amount of nursing care are from the experience of the Health Insurance Plan of Greater New York which provides visiting nurse service, but not private-duty nursing, as part of its benefit. In 1951 nurses made 52 visits per 1,000 members. About 1 percent of the membership received an average of 5 visits each. Of all persons receiving any nursing visits, the 5 percent receiving 20 or more nursing services had 40 percent of all the services.

Data on the utilization of other kinds of medical services are almost nonexistent except for the material collected by the Committee on the Costs of Medical Care and very limited data from some of the prepayment plans. Of special interest are the number of health examinations, one measure of the amount of preventive care received. The Committee on the Costs of Medical Care found that only 1 person out of every 4 in the highest-income group had a health examination during the survey year and that in the income groups under $5,000, only 1 person in 10 had this preventive care.

TABLE 19. *Number of services per 1,000 eligible members, selected prepayment plans*

Service	Health Insurance Plan of Greater New York 1950	Labor Health Institute, St. Louis, Mo. 1950	Group Health Association, District of Columbia 1951	Windsor Medical Service, Ontario 1950
Laboratory	A	604	3,164	B
X-ray	255	523	388	141
Physical therapy	A	92	545	B
Nurses visits:				
Clinic or office	A	813	1,663 C	A
Home visits	42	5 D	B	B

A Not available.
B Not included in benefits.
C Injections by nurse.
D Program started during 1951.

The table above shows some of the utilization rates of the members of selected prepayment plans for special services. With the exception of the Windsor Medical Services Plan, all these prepayment plans operate under a group practice system. The several plans cover different kinds of services and even where the same services are included differences may occur in the comprehensiveness of the services offered or in special charges levied. Moreover, not all plans define each service in the same way. These data on utilization, therefore, should be interpreted having in mind that variations exist among the plans. . . .

C. HEALTH INFORMATION FOUNDATION *

THERE HAS BEEN a great increase in the utilization of personal health services in this country since 1940. Some of this increase has been attributed to the rise of

* From: *National Family Survey of Medical Costs and Voluntary Health Insurance: Preliminary Report,* by Odin W. Anderson; New York: Health Information Foundation, 1954 (Part III, "Utilization of Personal Health Services and Voluntary Health Insurance During Survey Year"). Reprinted (with omissions, including tables) by permission of the publishers. The author is the research director of the Health Information Foundation, New York. (A more extensive discussion of this section of the 1953 survey conducted by the Health Information Foundation is provided in pages 55-75 of the volume entitled *Family Medical Costs and Voluntary Health Insurance: A Nationwide Survey,* by Odin W. Anderson, with Jacob J. Feldman;

voluntary health insurance and greater availability of facilities, and some to improved economic conditions for the great bulk of families. Insurance per se is followed by an increase in utilization which is the chief reason why there is still debate as to whether personal health services are "insurable" or not. Fire insurance does not necessarily increase fires nor does life insurance increase the death rate, but health insurance does increase the utilization rate of personal health services, as will be revealed in data to follow, since the need for health services is not as easily determined as the fact of a fire or the finality of death.

Whether or not this increase is good or bad can also be endlessly debated. There are no standards, except very gross ones, of a "normal" hospital rate or a "normal" surgical rate. The rates emerge from the patterns of practice of thousands of physicians in their treatment of hundreds and thousands of patients. What was normal utilization 25 years ago is no longer normal utilization today because so many factors have changed: buying power, new medical discoveries, and people's attitudes towards hospitals and other health services.

A hospital admission rate of 130 per thousand today may be just as normal as a rate of 50 not so many years ago. Both reflect a combination of circumstances the separate elements of which are almost impossible to disentangle. Whatever the utilization rate may be, it can be assumed that the country, individually and collectively, is willing to pay the cost, otherwise insurance would not be so widespread and hospital beds and physicians would not be in such great demand. Thus, it can be said with certainty that the data to follow are a measure of effective demand.

Amount of Hospital Care Received.—On the basis of the national sample of families and individuals interviewed in this survey, the admission rate to general hospitals was 12 per 100 persons per year.[1] Those with some insurance had a rate of 13 and those without insurance a rate of 10. On a national scale the difference between 13 and 10 is a measure of the impact of hospital insurance on hospital admissions today.

Hospital admissions by income group indicates that not until the family income is $7,500 or over does the hospital admission rate for those not insured equal the rate for those insured. In income groups below $7,500 there is an appreciable difference between those with insurance as against those without insurance, generally 25 percent higher for the insured group. On the other hand, among families without insurance there is comparatively little difference between income groups until $7,500 is reached. The high admission rate of 19 in the lowest income group

New York: Blakiston Division, McGraw-Hill Book Company, 1956; 251 pp. This volume—a comprehensive analysis of the survey results—presents essentially the same viewpoint as the preliminary report, but contains additional data as well as minor changes in some of the numerical and tabular material included in the preliminary report).

1. The usual manner in which to present hospital admission rates is by number of admissions per 1000 population. In this survey the number per 100 population is used in order to avoid decimals which imply that there is, for example, a significant difference between a rate of 12.1 per 100 and 12.4 per 100 or 121 per 1000 and 124 per 1000. Instead, both rates are rounded out to 12 per 100.

among the insured can be explained, at least in part, by the fact that this group contains a higher proportion of people 65 years of age and over than other income groups.

The data on the average number of hospital days per person hospitalized by family income and insurance status is difficult to interpret without more detailed knowledge underlying the facts. A high admission rate is usually associated with a short stay as measured by number of days per patient hospitalized. The average length of stay for all persons hospitalized is 9.7 days and there is virtually no over-all difference between those insured and not insured. There are variations between income groups with insurance and those without insurance.

Another method of presenting the amount of hospital service received by people is by calculating the number of hospital days utilized per person or per 100 persons in a year. Throughout the country during the survey year, there were 100 hospital days utilized per 100 persons in all families, and 110 days in families with insurance compared with 80 days in families without insurance. Again, not until the income group $7,500 is reached do the rates for families with insurance and those without insurance begin to equalize. When the volume of hospital care is broken down by rural and urban areas other patterns of hospitalization emerge contrary to usual expectations of the behavior of rural populations, since the rural-farm insured population has a higher admission rate than the urban insured. In fact, the reverse of the pattern would have been predicted, because it has been assumed that rural people have been less inclined to enter a hospital than those living in urban areas. Apparently, times have changed when the rural-farm population with insurance shows an admission rate of 17 per 100 persons as against 12 in urban areas. . . . For people in urban and rural-farm areas with no insurance the rate is the same, but when insurance enters the picture the impact on rural-farm residents is greater than on urban residents. There may be a high selectivity among those insured in rural-farm areas, because relatively few people in those areas are insured.

Further corroboration of the rural-urban pattern is found when there is a hospital utilization breakdown by type of locality as measured by size of city in the area. Again, the more "rural" the area the greater is the hospital admission rate for those who carry hospital insurance, and the shorter is the average length of stay.

Amount of Surgery Performed.—It has been shown that hospital insurance increased the utilization of hospitals. Likewise, it is found that surgical insurance increased the number of surgical procedures. The number of surgical procedures per 100 persons in families with surgical insurance is 7, while in families with no such insurance the rate is 4, a very appreciable difference. The families which have insurance have almost the same amount of surgery, regardless of their incomes. This is also true for families which do not have insurance. Analysis of the two groups reveals, therefore, that the primary factor accounting for the greater amount of surgery is the existence of insurance.

What do these rates mean? Again, it is necessary to know more of the factors underlying the different rates. Very likely there is a higher proportion of so-called "elective" surgery in the insured families, and a higher proportion of "emergency" or "must" surgery in the non-insured families. Is there too little surgery performed in the noninsured group? What is known with certainty is that given a greater accessibility to surgery, the surgical rate is 7 per 100 persons instead of 4.

Dental Services.—To date dental services have not usually been included in insurance against costs of personal health services except for dental surgery. There is a great difference in the amount of dental service received by income group as measured by visits to dentists, contrary to the pattern shown above in hospitalization and surgery. Among all families, 34 percent of the individuals in them sought the services of a dentist during the survey year. In the lowest income group, under $2,000, 17 percent sought service, and in the group $7,500 and over, 56 percent. It can be safely assumed that the lower the income group the higher is the proportion of dental service which is emergency in nature such as relieving pain and extractions, and the lower is the proportion of preventive care and repair work.

15. Medical Care for Children: Prevailing Patterns *

Physicians' Services

IF THIS STUDY had been made fifty or even twenty-five years ago and the medical care of children divided between that given in private practice and that from other sources, the latter would have made up a much smaller proportion than now. Formerly public health officers were concerned almost entirely with sanitation and control of communicable disease. Hospitals had few physicians, other than those concerned with the basic sciences, who were not also in private practice.

Now medical care includes an increasing number of services that do not fall within private practice. Many children in hospitals—and not only the indigent—are under the care of full-time staff members. School health programs, well-child conferences, and many other services are coming into the picture more and more. However, although there are no figures to prove it, it is a fair assumption that the increase in these services outside of private practice was accompanied by a total increase in medical care rather than a decrease in private practice. More children are receiving care who would otherwise have gone without it. Furthermore, it has been demonstrated time and time again that when public health services are brought into a community, there is a concomitant increase in the demand for private care.

* Reprinted by permission of the publishers and the Commonwealth Fund from the American Academy of Pediatrics (Committee for the Study of Child Health Services), *Child Health Services and Pediatric Education;* Cambridge, Mass.: Harvard University Press, 1949. (The excerpts reprinted, with omissions including initial paragraphs, tables, and some figures, are from Chap. III, "Private Practice," pp. 41-44 and 65-66; Chap. IV, "Hospitals," pp. 80-83; and Chap. VII, "Health Services and Per Capita Income," p. 132).

As a community learns the value of diphtheria immunization, more patients request it of their own physicians.

For the country as a whole, approximately 490,000 children were seen by physicians in private practice on an average day. It is obvious that the amount of private care varies widely in direct relation to the number of practicing physicians in a community, state, or region. . . .

There is a wide variation in the rate of private medical service per 1,000 children throughout the country. Comparisons from state to state show the greatest deficiency in the southern states.

It is rather unexpected to find among the states with the highest rate of service, states of such widely differing characteristics as New York and Massachusetts, on the one hand, and Nevada and Wyoming, on the other. In the latter states the average case load is comparatively high . . . General practitioners in Wyoming see more patients per day than practitioners in any other state. . . .

In comparisons of services by county groups, particularly when the five groups * are used, it is important to bear in mind the fact . . . that people do cross county lines for their medical service. Since our data on physicians' visits have been collected from the physicians themselves, the visits were necessarily classified according to the location of the physician rather than the residence of the child. As a result of this factor, the rate of service in metropolitan counties may be exaggerated and that of isolated counties underestimated, particularly for specialists who see patients from far distant areas in their offices or travel into isolated counties on consultation.

The rate of service measured in visits varied from 18 per 1,000 children on one day in greater metropolitan counties to 7 in isolated rural counties. Figure 17 shows the extent to which this difference is attributable to general practitioners in comparison with pediatricians and other specialists. In the metropolitan counties approximately one third of the visits were those of pediatricians and other specialists combined. In the isolated counties, where there were few specialists, practically all of the care from private practice was in the hands of the general practitioner.

The fact that the rate of service given to children by all physicians in isolated

---

* In order to compare the services and facilities available to the child living in or near metropolitan centers with those available to the child living at a distance from such centers, counties were grouped together, for purposes of this study, to form health service areas. These areas were established in terms of two major characteristics: population and proximity to densely populated areas. Consideration was thus given to areas which, although themselves sparsely populated, were relatively close to metropolitan centers and the medical facilities ordinarily available in them. The health service areas were worked out so as not to cross county lines.

In establishing the health service areas for the study, five groups of counties were distinguished: *greater metropolitan counties* (those in or around the twelve major cities of the United States); *lesser metropolitan counties* (the metropolitan districts of all other cities in the country with 50,000 or more population); *adjacent counties* (those geographically contiguous to any of the metropolitan counties); *isolated semi-rural* and *isolated rural* counties (classified as such in terms of the presence or absence within them of an incorporated place of 2,500 or more inhabitants).

According to this classification, two thirds of the 3,076 counties in the United States are "isolated," and relatively few (240) are "metropolitan."

rural counties was less than half of that in greater metropolitan counties does not mean that all of the greater metropolitan children were getting all the care that they needed. It is well known that in the midst of large cities in the very shadow of some of the most prominent medical centers there are children who may be just as isolated from good medical care as the child in an isolated county. Manifestly, to the extent that the attained level of service in metropolitan areas was below the optimum level of service for all children, we have understated the deficiencies in isolated counties.

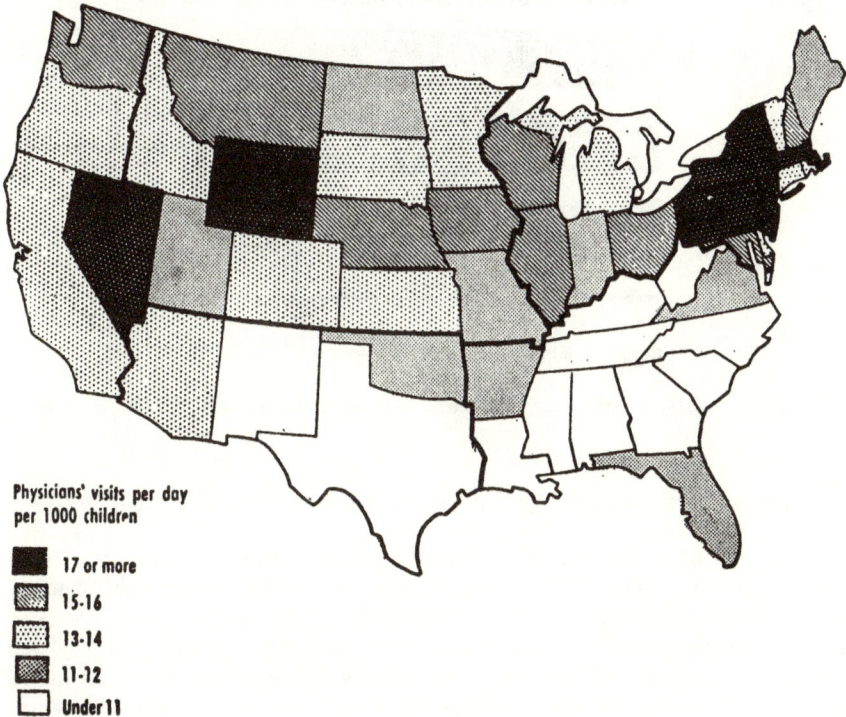

Physicians' visits per day
per 1000 children

■ 17 or more
▨ 15-16
▧ 13-14
▨ 11-12
☐ Under 11

FIGURE 16. Southern children receive far less care from physicians than do children elsewhere.

Regional variations . . . emphasize the relative deficiency of the Southeast and the Southwest regions in comparison with the Northeast, Central, and Pacific regions. In each of the regions the children in the isolated rural counties received much less care from practicing physicians than the children in the other county groups. It follows, therefore, that the children in the isolated counties of the South were the least favored.

It is of interest to note that in all regions the rate of care was less in the adjacent counties than in isolated semi-rural counties. This finding may be attributed to the fact that many of the children living in adjacent counties go to the medical centers of the metropolitan counties to obtain services from private physicians as well as from hospitals and clinics.

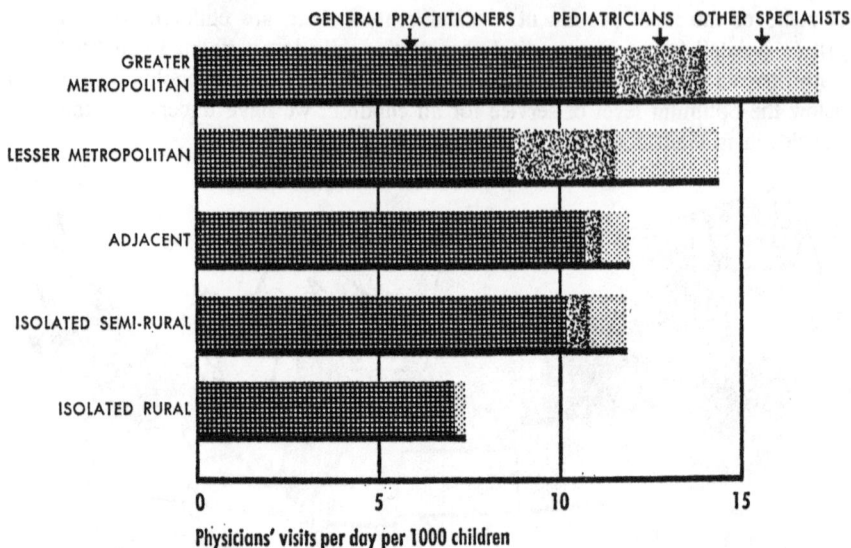

FIGURE 17. The general practitioner carries the load, especially in isolated counties.

Proportion of Care by General Practitioners and Specialists

DESPITE THE GROWING tendency toward specialization and the oft-expressed view that the general practitioner is vanishing from the medical horizon, physicians in general practice still make up the large majority of the medical profession. Two thirds of all physicians in private practice are general practitioners; it is they who take care of most of the children of the country. In fact, they accounted for 75 percent of the children's visits in comparison with 11 percent for pediatricians and 14 percent for other specialists.

In states where pediatricians were relatively few, children were, of course, cared for to a greater degree by general practitioners.... Connecticut's children, [for example], received nearly eight times the rate of pediatric care as the children received from the 4 pediatricians in Idaho....

Dentists' Visits

DENTAL CARIES SHARES with the common cold the unenviable record of being the most common of all diseases.... The years of childhood are particularly susceptible to the irreversible damage caused by caries. If a child is to have and keep healthy teeth, he must not only develop proper habits of oral hygiene, he must also have periodic dental care.

. . . The maldistribution of dentists is extreme, more marked even than in the case of physicians. All children should be able to reach a dentist without traveling long distances. If there is no dentist in the community, children generally go without dental care.

FIGURE 18. The rate of dentists' visits for children . . .

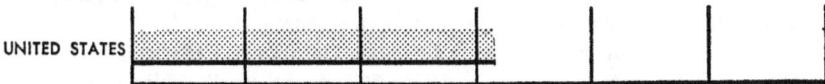

. . . is least in isolated rural counties . . .

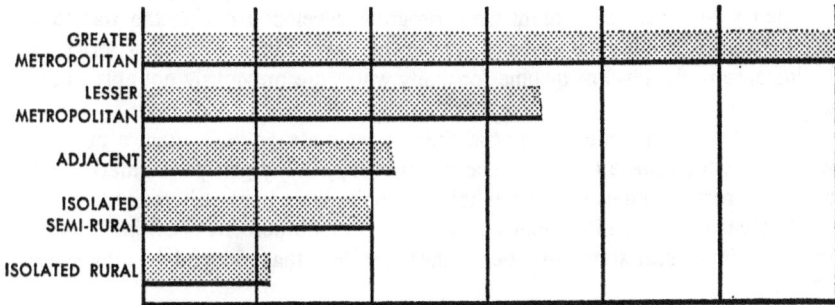

. . . and in the south.

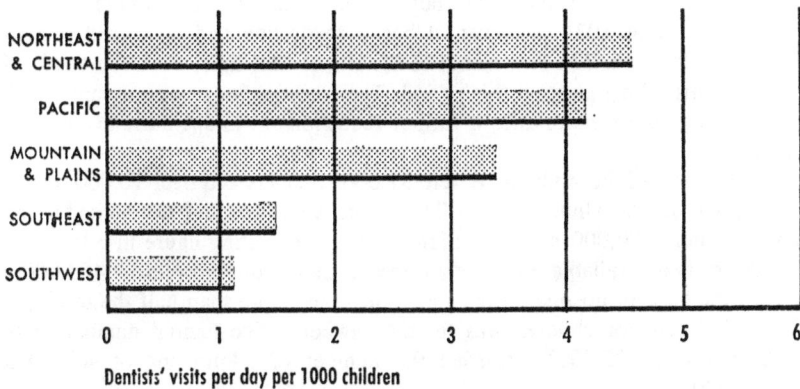

Dentists' visits per day per 1000 children

The rate of visits per day per 1,000 children varied from 6.0 in greater metropolitan counties to 1.1 in isolated rural counties. This striking contrast was noted consistently in the different regions. In view of our knowledge of the insufficiency of dental care in cities, these contrasts are of particular significance and clearly understate the deficiencies in dental care in isolated areas. . . .

Hospital Care for Newborn Infants

THE CHANGE THAT has taken place in the hospital's position in the community is exemplified as forcefully as in any other way by the increase in the percentage of births occurring in hospitals. It is a pretty good guess that few of those who read these pages will themselves have been born in a hospital; it is an equally good guess that few of their children have been born at home.

The percentage of babies born in hospitals has shown a particularly rapid increase during the past ten years. In 1935, 37 percent of all babies were born in hospitals. At the time of this study, the percentage had risen to 82, more than double. Many factors have been associated with this remarkable development prominent among which are: the growth of Blue Cross prepayment plans, the Emergency Maternal and Infant Care program developed during the war to provide maternity care for the wives of men in the lower ranks of military service, and the increase in the level of income for many who were previously not able to afford hospital service.

It is of particular interest that in the greater metropolitan counties only 1 out of 20 births took place at home. The variation by county group was marked, since in isolated rural counties more than half the babies were born at home.

Whereas for the United States as a whole over 80 percent of all births were in hospitals, in several states this percentage was less than 50 and in others nearly 100. . . .

Differences in the percentage of births occurring in hospitals would be expected to be marked as between white and nonwhite babies. For the Southeast states in 1946 the percentage for nonwhite was 25 as against 70 percent for white.

For many years neonatal mortality (deaths under one month) was almost stationary. About 1934, however, it began to decline and decreased one fourth from 1935 to 1946. The first month of life is a critical time, over two thirds of the infant deaths taking place in this period. The facilities for newborn care are therefore of the greatest importance if further reductions in infant mortality are to take place.

At the time of the study there were 91,000 bassinets and over 10,000 incubators in hospitals in the United States. Thus there were hospital accommodations for approximately 100,000 newborn infants, a very interesting figure in relation to the number of beds available for all other ages in these same hospitals—463,000.

On the basis of hospital births and admissions, more than half the total amount of hospital care for children was for the newborn. The annual number of births in hospitals (2,275,000) exceeded the number of admissions of sick children (1,852,000).

From consideration of such data, it is obvious that the pediatrician, along with the obstetrician, stands in a position of major responsibility in hospital planning and the conduct of nurseries for the newborn. . . .

Per capita income, 1944-46

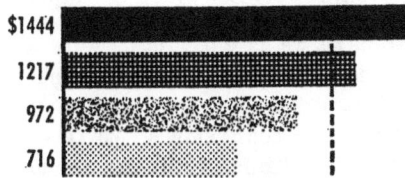

$1444
1217
972
716

Infant mortality rate, 1946

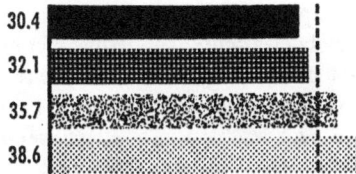

30.4
32.1
35.7
38.6

Total children under medical care per day per 1000

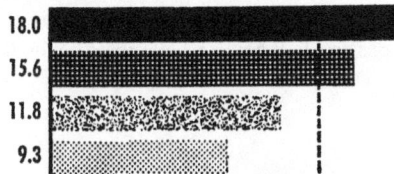

18.0
15.6
11.8
9.3

Preschool children under health supervision per day per 1000

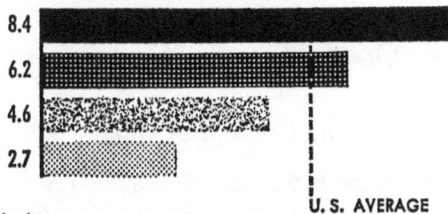

8.4
6.2
4.6
2.7

U. S. AVERAGE

Per capita income

$1350 or more   10 states with 9.4 million children
1100 – 1349   11 states with 9.7 million children
850 – 1099   16 states with 8.3 million children
Under 850   11 states with 8.7 million children

FIGURE 19. Health services for children are directly related to the economic level of the states.

Health Services and Per Capita Income

IN THE FOREGOING pages we have described ... the wide disparities in the amount of health facilities and services for children among differing economic groups and between urban and rural areas in various parts of the country. If there is any one element which seems most consistently to lie behind these differences, it is the economic one. Throughout the report this has appeared as a common factor. The relation is not in the least new with respect to either illness or health care; nor are these areas the only ones which reflect the serious, all-pervasive effects of inadequate income. Perhaps the chief justification for the stress on this element in the report is the relatively clear-cut, quantitative picture which is presented.

The study was not of a type to determine differences in medical needs of individual families on different economic levels. It has been possible, however, to show differences on a broader basis. The classification by county group and by region both primarily reflect economic differences. The clearest contrast lies in state-by-state comparisons. ... Whether with respect to infant mortality, the total volume of medical care, private practice, hospital facilities, or community health agencies, the more wealthy states have rates above the national average and the states with lower per capita income * have rates below the average. The comparisons show a dramatic consistency. ...

B. Qualitative Adequacy

16. GOOD MEDICAL CARE: BASIC PRINCIPLES †

The Concept of Good Medical Care

GOOD MEDICAL CARE is the kind of medicine practiced and taught by the recognized leaders of the medical profession at a given time or period of social, cultural, and professional development in a community or population group. ...

* Per capita income, as used in this report, refers to effective buying income estimates made by Sales Management, Incorporated, on the basis of money actually paid for goods and services, federal allotments, money paid out of savings and surpluses by business and financial institutions, plus the non-money income of farm and village residents. The income is gross income before taxes are paid.

† From: *The Fundamentals of Good Medical Care* (Publication No. 22 of the Committee on the Costs of Medical Care), by Roger I. Lee, M.D., and Lewis W. Jones; Chicago: University of Chicago Press. Copyright 1933, by the University of Chicago. Reprinted (with omissions, including initial paragraphs and some tables) by permission of the publishers. (The excerpts reprinted are from the Introduction, pp. 6-10; Chap. VII, "The Need for Medical Services," pp. 93-96 and 102-9; and Appendix V, "Summary Tables," pp. 296-97). The authors are, respectively, a consultant in internal medicine in Boston; and president of Rutgers University, New Brunswick, N.J.

The concept of good medical care that has been employed in this study is based upon certain "articles of faith" which can be briefly stated.

1. *Good medical care is limited to the practice of rational medicine based on the medical sciences.* There is no place in modern medicine for the quack, the cultist, or the magician: any system of prevention, diagnosis, or therapy which is not founded on rational observation and deduction has a "hit or miss" character incompatible with good medical practice, and it affords an unsound basis for the acquisition of health. . . .

2. *Good medical care emphasizes prevention.* Preventive medicine is by no means confined to "public health" activities. The idea of prevention and the promotion of health must pervade and inspire all branches of medicine. Indeed, in a very real sense all medicine is preventive. There are few specific remedies in the treatment of disease. The purpose of treatment is to assist the body and mind to accomplish restoration of good health, to interfere with the progress of the disease, to prevent complications, and to postpone death. Prevention, diagnosis, and treatment are inseparable aspects of the science and art of medicine. They have a common purpose—the promotion and maintenance of health—and they use a common body of knowledge.

3. *Good medical care requires intelligent cooperation between the lay public and the practitioners of scientific medicine.* Good medical care does not depend on the medical profession alone; often the best of doctors can do little for the patient who does not follow his instructions. The cooperation of patients is quite as important as the efficiency of practitioners and the availability and excellence of the services.

4. *Good medical care treats the individual as a whole.* "Diseases are not individual, but various states of individuals," [according to Sir Clifford Albutt]. Every sick person presents a unique problem, which every physician will attack in his own way. Good practice requires that the patient be considered as a person, a member of a family living in a certain environment. All the factors which concern his health —mental and emotional, as well as physiological—must be weighed in diagnosis, prevention, and treatment. It is the sick or injured person and not merely the pathologic conditions which must be treated. Thus it may happen that while, on purely medical grounds, a woman would be better off in the hospital, her reluctance to leave home and the worry her absence would cause her would far outweigh the benefits of expert hospital care. Good medical care might prescribe that she remain at home.

5. *Good medical care maintains a close and continuing personal relation between physician and patient.* The complex nature of a human being, the intricate relationship between body and mind and between the parts and the whole, establish long familiarity with the patient's personality and habits as the first essential in good medical care. The family physician is the person best qualified to supervise the health of the members of the family, to diagnose their illnesses, and to treat them or to direct their treatment. No amount of technical skill, no combination of mechanical and laboratory devices, is as useful in the diagnosis of many conditions

as a personal knowledge of the patient's medical history, family situation, and general mental and physical idiosyncrasies.

6. *Good medical care is coordinated with social welfare work.* "Where love of man is, there also is love of this art." But love of man must be clarified by an understanding of man and must take note of his social environment and economic needs. The interrelations of sickness and poverty have long been recognized. A low standard of living weakens the bodily resistance to infection, and poor ventilation, overcrowding, and malnutrition are strong allies of disease. The value of medical care among the poorer economic classes is vitiated if the patient is sent back after a course of treatment into the same conditions which gave rise to his ailment. While medicine cannot cure unemployment or abolish slums, much can be done by cooperation with the social agencies to improve the level of health among the poorer members of society.

7. *Good medical care coordinates all types of medical services.* Medicine includes a wide variety of services, ranging from the abatement of sanitary nuisances to the lancing of boils. These services are necessarily furnished by various agencies, and involve various methods and types of organization. Many services can be rendered only on a community basis; examples are the collection of vital statistics and the inspection of food and milk supplies. Others, such as tonsillectomies, can be rendered only to individuals by individuals. Still others could, so far as technical medical requirements are concerned, be rendered individually, but, for social or economic reasons, are ineffective unless they are supplied through some organized public service.

Good medical care requires that a proper balance and coordination exist among all the agencies and institutions through which medical services are provided. The kind of coordination required may be illustrated in the case of diphtheria. Diphtheria immunization, if it is performed by the private physician, should be reported to the health department for purposes of record. Cases of diphtheria are diagnosed by the physician with the help of the public health laboratory; they are isolated by the public health department and treated by the physician with serum probably obtained from the public health laboratory. The investigation of the source of the infection is carried on by the public health department.

8. *Good medical care implies the application of all the necessary services of modern, scientific medicine to the needs of all the people.* Judged from the viewpoint of society as a whole, the qualitative aspects of medical care cannot be dissociated from the quantitative. No matter what the perfection of technique in the treatment of one individual case, medicine does not fulfill its functions adequately until the same perfection is within the reach of all individuals. . . .

The Need for Medical Services

THE NEED FOR PREVENTIVE medicine is shared by all the people, well or ill, from conception to the grave. The extent of the need for diagnosis and treatment depends upon the prevalence of defects and the incidence of disease throughout the population.

The types of medical service necessary for adequate medical care are grouped as follows: community health preservation, preventive services for the individual, diagnosis and treatment of the puerperal state and of diseases and defects, and dentistry. The amount and kinds of service required under each of these heads are set forth in the present chapter.

Preventive Services for the Individual.— ... Preventive services for the individual ... consist in periodic health examinations—with the diagnostic X-ray or laboratory services which they may entail—and immunizations against communicable diseases. ... In table 20 is presented a summary of the physician-hours [1] and visits, the number of immunizations, and the number of X-ray and laboratory services which are required annually by persons of various age groups in the standard population unit of 100,000.

TABLE 20. *Preventive services for the individual required annually per 100,000 of the general population*

Age Group	Per Cent of Population 1930	Physician		X-Ray Services	Immunizations	Laboratory Tests
		Hours	Visits			
Under 1	1.8	5,099	15,300	....	1,800	2,196
1-4	7.5	3,863	7,725	....	5,250	19,050
5-19	29.5	26,255	26,255	1,475	5,900	126,260
20-34	24.4	9,028	9,028	1,220	2,440	44,164
35-64	31.4	26,376	26,376	3,140	3,140	110,842
65 and over	5.4	4,752	9,504	270	....	23,976
All ages	100.0	75,373	94,188	6,105	18,530	326,488

Services in Dentistry.—Periodic dental supervision is an essential part of preventive medicine for every person. Owing to the lack of incidence data on specific dental conditions and the special difficulties of estimating separately the need for prevention, diagnosis, and treatment, the need for all dental service has been combined. ...

Table 21 is a summary of the hours of treatment by general dental practitioner, by exodontist, and by orthodontist, together with the number of X-ray services required annually to give adequate dental care to a population unit of 100,000 persons in the United States. ...

Services For Diagnosis and Treatment.—The quantitative estimates of the services required for the diagnosis and treatment of diseases and physical and mental defects presented in this report are based upon sample opinions and case records of leading practitioners of medicine. The physicians were asked to give their opinions or, if possible, the records of their practice to indicate the amount of service neces-

1. A "physician-hour" is one hour spent by one physician with the patient; it does not include time spent in traveling or in waiting for calls.

sary in each broad disease category (e.g., digestive diseases or respiratory diseases). For each of the representative diseases within the category (e.g., appendicitis or influenza) similar data were requested concerning the amount of service of various kinds required in the treatment of 100 typical cases with such considerations as the average duration of the disease and the normal proportion of severe to mild cases. The physicians' replies were made the basis of arbitrary estimates of the services required.

TABLE 21. *Annual dental services required for 100,000 of the general population*

Age Group	Per Cent of Population, 1930	General Dental Practitioner		Exodontist	Orthodontist		X-Rays	
		Chair Hours	Laboratory Hours		Chair Hours	Laboratory Hours	Number	Hours
3-4	3.7	6,845	.....	....	....	....	1,110	339
5-17	25.7	77,100	.....	1,414	8,995	3,084	29,555	10,280
18-44	42.0	114,379	24,150	9,101	....	....	92,400	32,899
45 and over .	22.9	59,464	10,992	5,496	....	....	34,350	12,881
All ages over 3 ...	94.3	257,788	35,142	16,011	8,995	3,084	157,415	56,399

In general, the services are measured in such units as physician-hours, nursing days, attendant days, and hospital days, which should be applicable to any form of organization through which medical care might be rendered. It is possible, of course, that future developments in medical practice through the training and utilization of nurse-midwives in maternity cases, or the employment of optometrists for refraction and the fitting of glasses, as subsidiary personnel working under a doctor of medicine, might materially reduce the number of physician-hours now requisite for adequate medical care in these two branches of medicine. Further reduction in physician-hours might conceivably be achieved in a highly organized group clinic service. However, the consideration of these problems of efficient organization lies outside the scope of the present discussion. It is hoped that the units of service, as presented in table 22 ... may be sufficiently basic to lend themselves to recalculation of the personnel-hours and facility services under any system of medical practice.

The disease categories are listed in table 22 in the order of expectancy. It is at once apparent that the categories which have the highest incidence are not necessarily the most important from the point of view of the need for medical service. The largest consumer of physician-hours is also highest in order of incidence, but there the correspondence ends. The puerperal state, sixth in order of expectancy, is second in order of physician-hours required. Communicable diseases—third in order of expectancy—required only about 7 per cent of the total number of physician-hours necessary for the diagnosis and treatment of all diseases and defects

TABLE 22. *Annual services required for the diagnosis and treatment of diseases and defects and for the puerperal state per 100,000 of the general population*

Disease Category	Expectancy Rate per 100,000	Physician Hours A	Nursing Days B	Full-time Attendant Days C	Hospital Days D
Respiratory conditions	45,900	60,611	9,859	21,252	57,954
Digestive diseases	11,700	22,600	1,907	1,638	23,000
Acute communicable diseases ...	9,250	13,874	16,686	35,243	35,146
Injuries from external causes	5,400	5,512	2,171	....	4,898
Nervous system E	4,249	11,449 F	7,439	15,759	200,481
The puerperal state	2,356	27,271	5,113	5,395	20,379
Syphilis and gonorrhea	2,300	12,278	1,103	....	5,865
General diseases	2,100	7,561	3,572	4,064	9,152
Diseases of the skin	1,990	2,001	293	....	468
Female genito-urinary diseases ..	1,600	4,964	88	....	3,146
Diseases of the ear and mastoid process	1,500	2,844	667	417	900
Diseases of the muscles, bones and joints	1,300	3,082	328	....	3,765
Diseases of the kidneys and annexa	1,210	7,287	2,562	2,541	5,676
Chronic heart diseases G	1,170	8,180	1,646	....	2,981
Diseases of the eye and annexa ..	850	2,811	126	....	237
Refraction		13,710 H	....	....	....
Diseases of the circulatory system.	680	1,058	381	1,428	142
Male genito-urinary diseases	75	665	229	....	1,056
Total E	93,630	207,758	54,170	87,737	375,246

A A *physician-hour* is one hour spent by one physician (general practitioner, consultant, and specialist) with the patient. It does not include time spent in waiting for patients or in traveling to and from patients.

B A *nursing day* is 24 consecutive hours of the time of one graduate nurse, 12 of which are spent on duty. When both day and night nursing are required, 2 nursing days are counted for every 24 hours. Hospital nursing is not included but is assumed as part of a "hospital day"; but any individual nursing required by hospital patients is counted under "nursing days."

C A *full-time attendant day* is 24 consecutive hours of the time of a partially trained person—not a graduate nurse—who devotes her whole time to the care of the patient, 8 hours being spent on duty.

D A *hospital day* is 24 hours spent by one patient in a hospital. In the general hospitals, all the services of the hospital, including the staff nursing service but *not* including the physician's services, are included in a "hospital day"; in the special hospitals—tuberculosis and mental—the doctor's services are included in a "hospital day."

E Including neuralgia, neuritis, and sciatica, but excepting neuroses and behavior problems.

F This does not include the services of physicians on the staff of mental hospitals and institutions for the epileptic and feeble-minded.

G Diseases of the heart, arteriosclerosis, and high blood pressure.

H Or optometrist hours.

and for the puerperal state. Had a similar table been drawn up years ago, communicable diseases would have headed the list as a consumer of physician-hours; now the group is superseded by three other categories: respiratory diseases, the puerperal state, and digestive diseases.

The need for nursing, full-time attendants, and hospitalization is very unevenly distributed among the various disease categories. Communicable diseases represent by far the largest consumer of nursing days, and they require almost twice as much nursing service as the next highest group, the respiratory diseases. In the need for full-time attendants, communicable diseases also make large demands because patients must be isolated. The outstanding position of nervous and mental diseases in their need for hospitalization is conspicuous. Good medical care requires that more than one-half the total number of hospital days for all diseases and conditions be rendered those suffering from nervous and mental disorders. . . .

The need for service to patients suffering from chronic diseases is enormous, and is increasing absolutely as well as relatively. The great advancements achieved by preventive medicine in reducing infant mortality and in controlling the acute communicable diseases has resulted in a changing age group of the population with a higher proportion of the people surviving into the ages in which the so-called degenerative diseases—organic heart disease, kidney disease, cancer—most commonly occur. Unfortunately, there is no present indication that the incidence of these degenerative disorders is decreasing, even if the effects of the changing age composition of the population be eliminated by considering the higher age groups only. The nervous and mental diseases also appear to be on the increase. . . .

The Total Need for Medical Care.—The need for medical care . . . is compounded of two constantly changing factors: the changing physical condition of the people on the one hand, and on the other, the changing science and art of medicine. The total need for medical services must therefore be considered over a period of years to make allowance for the probable changes in both these factors in any particular community.

The sum of all the services discussed in this chapter would probably exceed even the immediate total need for medical care, and would undoubtedly be an overestimate of future needs. In estimating the need for diagnosis and treatment, the *present* incidence of diseases and defects has been used as a basis for the expectancy rates of conditions requiring medical attention. The provision of adequate preventive services would presumably modify the expectancy of disease, and so reduce the need for diagnosis and treatment.

Some immediate reduction in the need for diagnosis and treatment would result from the application of certain well-known and tried preventive techniques to all the people. So far as the technical powers of medicine are concerned, diphtheria, typhoid fever, and smallpox might very quickly be reduced to negligible factors in the total need for therapeutic medicine. Against this immediate reduction must be set the probable increase in the need for treatment which might be expected to result, through the periodic health examinations, from the discovery of hitherto unsuspected conditions requiring medical service.

Where prevention depends largely upon control of the environment, as in malaria, a gradual but certain improvement is to be anticipated. Other diseases, such as tuberculosis, pellagra, and rickets, to the extent that they are influenced by poor economic and social conditions, are beyond the power of medicine alone to control completely. The need for service arising from the incidence of these diseases will no doubt be reduced by better preventive medical services, but it is likely to remain large until the problems of poverty and congested living have been solved.

There is little immediate prospect of controlling the acute respiratory infections. The common cold and influenza are likely to continue to require a large aggregate amount of service. Though the total social cost of these diseases is large, it is distributed over a very large number of people, and does not as a rule impose a very serious burden upon the individual sufferer.

The problem of the so-called degenerative diseases has already been touched upon. No specific preventive measures have as yet been developed for these conditions. The best hope of combating them appears to lie in the periodic health examination, facilitating early diagnosis and prompt treatment. However, many of these chronic conditions are the sequelae of acute communicable diseases. It is therefore probable that the prevention of the acute disorders and adequate convalescent care of such cases as do occur will eventually reduce the incidence of such diseases as nephritis and organic heart disease. Similar results may be expected from a reduction in the incidence of syphilis and gonorrhea and the institution of a complete course of treatment for every case that occurs.

In short, the provision of adequate medical care would itself alter the need for medical care and would render obsolete and unnecessary certain services which are essential today. The immediate need for physician-hours for annual individual preventive services is estimated to be 75,373 per 100,000 persons, as against a total of 207,758 physician-hours needed for the diagnosis and treatment of all pathologic conditions and the puerperal state. Since the trend is towards a change in emphasis in medical practice from "cure" to prevention, the corrective medical services will assume an ever-smaller place in a reduced total need for medical care. The need for preventive services may be expected to remain at approximately its present level or to expand with discoveries of effective new procedures in preventive medicine.

Thus far, only the changing basis of the need for medicine—due to the decreased incidence of disease or to the changing physical conditions of the population—has been considered. It must be remembered that medical science will itself change, altering the nature of the services required. Whether such technological changes will increase or reduce the volume of services which would be considered adequate, it is impossible to predict. In the past, the tendency has been towards an increase in the services required, as medical knowledge has advanced. Refinements of diagnostic techniques and improved methods of therapy have raised the requirements of adequate care: the more we know how to do, the more service we need. This tendency may continue, so that adequate diagnosis ten years hence may include services which we in our present ignorance neither know nor miss. The total need for service will not, therefore, necessarily decrease as fast as the incidence of disease is reduced by adequate utilization of preventive medicine.

The nervous and mental diseases suggest a possibility of a large future increase in the need for medical care. No data are available on the incidence of neuroses and behavior problems which later develop into complete nervous collapse or insanity. Therefore, these two aspects of nervous and mental disorders could not be included in the estimates of disease expectancy. Even had their expectancy rates been computed, it would have been impossible to obtain any estimate of the amount of service required for the adequate care of these border-line mental disorders. As yet, modern medicine has reached no general agreement concerning the treatment of neuroses and behavior problems. It is conceivable that the next great discovery in medicine will be an explanation of the mind-body relationship and that much of the service for mental disorders which is now merely palliative may be transferred to the functions of preventive medicine. . . .

TABLE 23. *Annual number of home, office, hospital, and operative visits made by general practitioners and specialists for the puerperal state and for the diagnosis and treatment of diseases and defects per 100,000 population*

Disease Category	Total		Home		Office		Hospital		Operative	
	Number	Per Cent	Number	Per Cent	Number	Per Cent	Number	Per Cent	Number	Per Cent
All Physicians										
Puerperal state	47,639	100	5,160	11	30,180	63	12,299	26	....	..
Respiratory conditions	222,927	100	149,442	67	65,417	29	6,439	3	1,629	1
Digestive diseases ...	73,349	100	11,103	15	45,464	62	15,470	21	1,312	2
Acute communicable.	51,503	100	31,483	61	......	..	19,906	39	114	▲
External causes	20,266	100	4,752	23	11,656	58	3,372	17	486	2
Syphilis and gonorrhea	71,161	100	6	▲	66,551	94	4,604	6	....	..
General diseases	29,860	100	8,554	29	11,921	40	8,985	30	400	1
Diseases of the skin .	10,214	100	......	..	9,990	98	179	2	45	▲
Female G. U.	14,833	100	969	6	10,919	74	2,744	19	201	1
Muscles, bones, and joints	10,949	100	146	1	8,278	75	2,465	23	60	1
Diseases of the kidneys	17,770	100	4,305	24	9,005	51	4,299	24	161	1
Chronic heart	27,085	100	16,784	62	9,482	35	819	3	....	..
Circulatory system ..	3,987	100	435	11	3,335	84	122	3	95	2
Diseases of the ear ..	14,687	100	3,307	22	10,297	70	1,000	7	83	1
Diseases of the eye ..	13,167	100	140	1	12,811	97	195	2	21	▲
Male G. U.	2,140	100	20	1	980	46	1,059	49	81	4
Neuralgia, neuritis, and sciatica	5,778	100	......	..	5,699	99	79	1	....	..
Neurasthenia, and N. exhaustion	7,926	100	6,913	87	817	10	196	3	....	..
N. and M. conditions	15,478	100	2,465	16	6,162	40	6,792	44	59	▲
Total	660,719	100	245,984	37	318,964	48	91,024	14	4,747	1

General Practitioner

Puerperal state	43,209	100	4,995	12	29,261	67	8,953	21	....	..
Respiratory conditions	200,716	100	144,594	72	54,470	27	1,652	1	....	..
Digestive diseases ...	48,948	100	10,361	21	36,456	75	2,131	4	....	..
Acute communicable.	49,802	100	30,457	61	......	..	19,345	39	....	..
External causes	16,751	100	4,752	28	9,785	58	2,106	13	108	1
Syphilis and gonorrhea	53,566	100	6	△	50,928	95	2,632	5	....	..
General diseases	17,074	100	8,365	49	8,649	51	60	△	....	..
Diseases of the skin .	8,013	100	......	..	8,013	100	.....	..	....	..
Female G. U.	8,938	100	592	7	8,282	92	64	1	....	..
Muscles, bones, and joints	4,719	100	125	3	4,563	96	31	1	....	..
Diseases of the kidneys	13,659	100	4,232	31	8,469	62	958	7	....	..
Chronic heart	26,834	100	16,784	63	9,231	34	819	3	....	..
Circulatory system ..	2,414	100	435	18	1,979	82	.....	..	....	..
Diseases of the ear ..	4,388	100	2,442	56	1,946	44	.....	..	....	..
Diseases of the eye ..	850	100	......	..	850	100	.....	..	....	..
Male G. U.	177	100	14	8	159	90	4	2	....	..
Neuralgia, neuritis, and sciatica	4,913	100	......	..	4,913	100	.....	..	....	..
Neurasthenia, and N. exhaustion	6,157	100	5,331	87	682	11	144	2	....	..
N. and M. conditions	3,801	100	2,320	61	1,481	39	.....	..	....	..
Total	514,929	100	235,805	46	240,117	47	38,899	7	108	△

Specialist

Puerperal state	4,430	100	165	4	919	21	3,346	75	....	..
Respiratory conditions	22,211	100	4,848	22	10,947	40	4,787	22	1,629	7
Digestive diseases ...	24,401	100	742	3	9,008	37	13,339	55	1,312	5
Acute communicable.	1,701	100	1,026	60	......	..	561	33	114	7
External causes	3,515	100	......	..	1,871	53	1,266	36	378	11
Syphilis and gonorrhea	17,595	100	......	..	15,623	89	1,972	11	....	..
General diseases	12,786	100	189	1	3,272	26	8,925	70	400	3
Diseases of the skin .	2,201	100	......	..	1,977	90	179	8	45	2
Female G. U.	5,895	100	377	6	2,637	45	2,680	45	201	4
Muscles, bones, and joints	6,230	100	21	△	3,715	60	2,434	39	60	1
Diseases of the kidneys	4,111	100	73	2	536	13	3,341	81	161	4
Chronic heart	251	100	......	..	251	100	.....	..	....	..
Circulatory system ..	1,573	100	......	..	1,356	86	122	8	95	6
Diseases of the ear ..	10,299	100	865	8	8,351	81	1,000	10	83	1
Diseases of the eye ..	12,317	100	140	1	11,961	97	195	2	21	..
Male G. U.	1,963	100	6	△	821	42	1,055	54	81	4
Neuralgia, neuritis, and sciatica	865	100	......	..	786	91	79	9	....	..
Neurasthenia, and N. exhaustion	1,769	100	1,582	89	135	8	52	3	....	..
N. and M. conditions	11,677	100	145	1	4,681	40	6,792	58	59	1
Total	145,790	100	10,179	7	78,847	54	52,125	36	4,639	3

△ Less than 1 per cent.

17. THE CONCEPT OF ADEQUACY *

IT IS IMPOSSIBLE to give a precise definition of "adequate medical care." If defined in terms of the best of every type of service now known, it becomes an ideal which is nowhere fully realized. The services rendered in a major medical center and those extended by some solo practitioner "out of a bag" differ widely. Yet even the major medical centers are likely to be deficient in certain respects. They usually provide irregular and insufficient ambulatory services, domiciliary care is frequently non-existent, and no more than lip service is given to the many problems of convalescence and rehabilitation. Nor is adequate medical care always obtained by the well-to-do families and communities. The wealthy individual may receive much attention from able specialists when ill, and yet be quite neglected so far as personal preventive care is concerned. Moreover, excessive attention may have little real value—adequate care is not to be confused with luxury care.

In describing the services and facilities required for adequate medical care there is some advantage in distinguishing between the care of children and that of adults. It would be easier to outline the former, because obstetricians and pediatricians have provided more comprehensive services than most other practitioners. But for this very reason an account of their procedures is relatively unnecessary; these are already well known and approved, if not universally applied. There is more need to emphasize what should be involved in the proper care of adults. Such care should furnish, first, all facilities essential to the recognition and understanding of disease: the complete case history, the thorough and fully recorded physical examination, all of the required laboratory and x-ray examinations. Adequate medical service for adults should provide drugs, surgery, psychotherapy, and physiotherapy—indeed, all therapeutic measures needed for healing and comfort. It should include competent nursing and social service.

Prevention as a part of good medical care involves frequent contacts between physician and patient for supervision and advice, and examinations performed often enough to permit early recognition of physical and psychological abnormalities. Access to the physician should be easy and natural and ought not to depend upon the accident of illness or injury. Much current practice is particularly deficient in early diagnosis and treatment; in this connection, major opportunities exist for rendering really adequate care. Responsibility for early recognition, moreover, is not limited to physical ills. It also embraces the recognition and management in their incipiency of neuroses, anxiety states, and psychoses. Finally, adequate preventive service should include measures against the contraction and spread of infection and infectious disease.

* From: *Medicine in the Changing Order,* by the Committee on Medicine in the Changing Order, New York Academy of Medicine; New York: Commonwealth Fund, 1947 (Chap. VII, "The Quality of Medical Care," pp. 115-18). Reprinted (with omissions, including initial paragraphs) by permission of the publishers.

The concept of adequate medical care also includes fuller consideration than is now generally given to problems of chronic or degenerative disease, particularly common in middle and older age groups, and of convalescence or rehabilitation following illness, injuries, and operations.

In sum, the same degree of concern which has long been displayed for acute conditions should also be devoted to incipient, post-acute, and chronic diseases.

Adequate service requires adequate facilities. For routine examinations, a few simple instruments and elementary laboratory equipment may be sufficient. For diagnostic work, well-equipped chemical and bacteriological laboratories, a fluoroscope, x-ray apparatus, an electrocardiograph, and equipment for the determination of basal metabolic rates represent a standard minimum. This enumeration takes no account of the more elaborate instruments of individual specialists, or the enormously complicated facilities for treatment, or the supplies and instruments involved in physiotherapy, in anesthesia, and in surgical operations. For the maintenance and conduct of these services nurses, laboratory technicians, x-ray technicians, physiotherapists, anesthetists, and others are required to supplement the work of physicians.

It is obvious that the provision of adequate care, as outlined above, calls for many changes in current medical education and practice. In the last analysis, the quality of medical care depends primarily on two factors: first, the caliber of medical personnel, and second, the procedures and facilities through which the latter render services. Much depends on the skill, judgment, and character of physicians and nurses. This is true whether they work as individuals or in group units, in hospitals or in health departments. Without professional competence of the individual worker, the best of institutions or facilities may be more of a menace than a benefit.

In order to complete the circle of professional arrangements here indicated, therefore, simultaneous plans must be made for 1) better selection and training of physicians and auxiliary medical personnel, 2) more effective organization of their methods of practice, and 3) improvement of institutional facilities at their disposal. . . .

18. CRITERIA FOR ASSESSING QUALITY OF CARE *

IN GENERAL, the principles of administration relating to quality of care are equally applicable to any medical care program, whether governmental or nongovernmental, tax supported, or supported by prepayment contributions.

* From: "Improving the Quality of Medical Care: Sound Principles of Administration," by Edwin F. Daily, M.D.; *American Journal of Public Health* 39:337-39, March 1949 (No. 3). Reprinted by permission of the author and publishers. The author is vice-president (medical) of the Health Insurance Plan of Greater New York.

The quality of medical care is primarily of importance to the recipients of services—the patients. It is in their interests I speak, and it is their wishes I am trying to express, rather than considering principles of administration in the abstract.

In order to emphasize the importance of the individuals to be served, I will present some of the principles of administration which I believe most individuals would desire in any medical care program.

The Scope of the Plan

1. I WOULD WANT the plan to provide all professional and auxiliary services, hospital, and convalescent home care that I might need and that could be made available. I would not want anything to do with a plan that is concerned only with assuring payment to surgeons for their operations or providing only fragments of the services required.

The Personnel

1. I WOULD WANT the administrative staff and all professional personnel of my medical care plan to be concerned always with the promotion of positive health, the prevention of illness and disability, as well as the treatment of disease and rehabilitation, for each and every one of us covered by the plan.

2. I would wish to have my medical care plan provide, or pay, for services rendered only by professional personnel recognized as competent in their respective fields. I would hope that my medical care plan would prevent me, if possible, from seeking professional help from individuals who are not competent to provide it.

3. I would wish that those persons who set standards for professional personnel would consider it important that the physicians be as much concerned with environmental and social causes of illness as with their biological and other causes.

4. I would like to have my medical care plan provide physicians and other personnel who are as interested in the long-time treatment of my child with cerebral palsy as they are interested in the dramatic response I made to treatment with a new antibiotic.

5. I would wish the physicians to be selected from among those who would treat me at all times as an individual, giving me as much personal attention as they would wish for a member of their own family. I would not like to be "Case No. 329," and be given a brushoff as one of 50 patients being seen that morning.

6. I would want to see my physician in an attractive office or clinic, where there are comfortable chairs, because I dislike basements of courthouses and hard benches.

7. I would like my office visits to be by appointment, for I dislike waiting for hours on a hard bench *or* in a comfortable chair.

8. I would like to be able to change my physician if I became dissatisfied with him or if he thought I would do better under the care of another physician.

9. I would wish my medical care plan to afford its professional personnel, wherever feasible, opportunities for working in groups—with easily accessible diagnostic equipment they may need—in order that they may easily consult with each other, and in order that I may not need to go from one place to another for a series of consultations or laboratory tests.

10. I would want to know how, when, and where I could get medical care in an emergency, whether such care is required at home, office, or hospital.

11. And, since what is good medical care today may not be good enough a few years from now, I would wish to have the personnel in my medical care plan have regular opportunities for post-graduate training and to be continually considering ways and means of bringing to us—the patients—the most recently acquired knowledge in this great and complex field of human endeavor.

The Facilities

1. I WOULD WISH to have my hospital care only in institutions which meet national standards of performance, and my medical care plan should not provide care in hospitals which do not meet such standards.

The Administrative Machinery

1. I WOULD NOT WANT to be told at any time that I was not eligible for care because of the place of my legal residence, or because my skin was not white, or because my income was up or down during a given year.

2. I would not wish to have red tape, or tape of any other color, delay my obtaining any services I need under my medical care plan.

3. I would want my taxes or prepayment contribution to cover all costs of all services provided, and I would not want the physicians or hospitals to ask me for more money because my case was unusual, or because they did not think the plan paid them enough.

4. I would want the method of payment to physicians and hospitals to be of a type that would prevent the possibility of financial considerations influencing the clinical decisions of the physicians or hospitals.

5. I would want the administrator of the plan and his staff to be fully competent to develop the best medical care plan possible, and to improve it year by year on the basis of experience. I would want this staff to be selected on the basis of merit alone, to serve only the best interests of the community and not the selfish interests of any special group.

6. I would want a group representing those of us served by the plan, and those providing services, to be given ample opportunity, at regular intervals, to confer with the administrator and his staff and to express our viewpoints fully.

7. I would like to have an impartial appeal board established to hear my complaints about the plan, or complaints of the professional staff providing services.

8. And last, I would like to have the amounts of money paid the administrator and his staff, and the professional personnel, high enough to attract and hold in rural or urban areas the best people available, and to have working conditions and other factors conducive to their deriving satisfaction from their work. I would not want bargain counter medical care.

I have stated no new principles. We have all talked about one or more of them on many occasions. It may be new to have them presented together, and from the viewpoint of the patient. At this time, when many public and voluntary medical care programs are developing in this country, it might be of interest to the administrator and the public to evaluate each program on the basis of these principles.

FURTHER READINGS

American Public Health Association, Subcommittee on Medical Care. *The Quality of Medical Care.* Subcommittee Annotated Bibliography No. 9. New York: The Association, 1954. 38 pages (processed).

Josiah Macy, Jr. Foundation. *Administrative Medicine.* Transactions of the Fourth Conference. New York: The Foundation, 1956. 251 pages.

Sheps, Cecil G. and Taylor, Eugene E. *Needed Research in Health and Medical Care: A Bio-Social Approach.* Chapel Hill: University of North Carolina Press, 1954. 216 pages. (Includes references).

See, also, lists of Further Readings for other chapters.

CHAPTER IV

The Costs of Medical Care

SCIENTIFIC PROGRESS has made medical care increasingly effective—also more complex and more costly. But progress has not modified the critical fact that the largest proportion of the costs of medical care are unpredictable for the individual and his family. These two factors—high costs and the uncertainty of their occurrence for the individual—tend to make it difficult for many persons to finance the care they need.

In view of the value of medical care in maintaining life and productivity, we have generally accepted as a socially desirable goal, the ready availability of medical care to all who can benefit from its services. Chapters II and III have given some indication of the extent to which economic factors interfere with the achievement of this goal. Planning to overcome the cost barrier requires knowledge of the size and pattern of expenditures for medical care services. The present chapter will help to provide some of that knowledge.

A. The Changing Pattern of Costs

19. ORIGINS OF THE COST PROBLEM *

PUBLIC CONFIDENCE in physicians was plainly reviving between 1880 and 1910, and state governments reflected this growing confidence in medical science and

* From: *Medicine in the Changing Order,* by the Committee on Medicine and the Changing Order, New York Academy of Medicine; New York: Commonwealth Fund, 1947 (Chap. I, "Origins of Present Problems," pp. 22-26). Reprinted (with omissions, including initial paragraphs) by permission of the publishers.

practice by passing or enforcing laws requiring medical examinations and licensure. Less specific evidence to the same effect was afforded by the behavior of the public at large. The patronage of medical sects declined and many of them practically disappeared. Open attacks on or ridicule of the regular profession largely ceased, and the profession no longer bemoaned its "declining position," as it had in 1850. Leading surgeons and clinicians, and to some extent even laboratory research men, acquired public fame and prestige.

Demands increased in the American Medical Association for a reform of medical education along the lines indicated by new scientific developments. The Johns Hopkins school, founded in 1893, markedly raised standards of admission and training. Finally, in 1910, Abraham Flexner made a general study of American medical schools that revealed the hopeless inadequacy of the proprietary and even of some of the university institutions. Unreserved publicity forced many schools to close and others to raise their standards. A continuous supervision of medical school standards was subsequently established by the American Medical Association.

Similar standardization of hospitals was established by the newly formed American College of Surgeons and by the American Hospital Association. The hospital, long the center of pathologic studies, was revolutionized by the new surgery and therapy. It became a center of elaborate medical facilities—not only for the treatment of the sick but also for diagnostic and research laboratories and other technical services.

Meanwhile the development of professional specialties was on its way. . . .

The newer surgical and therapeutic procedures called for trained nurses as well as for competent physicians, and much of the professional advance of nurses in this era can be credited to these demands in hospital services. The net result was the appearance of trained nurses who impressed the public favorably, and so furthered the growing respect for medical personnel in general.

The growing public confidence in medical science and practice was reflected in a rising demand for medical services. This is to be seen in part in the rapid growth of hospital facilities. In the earliest list of hospitals published in this country, in 1873, about 180 institutions were listed, and these served during that year some 146,000 patients. By 1933 registered hospitals numbered 6,437 and could care for well over a million in-patients at one time. By 1943 the latter figure had mounted to about 1,650,000. This growth was not in proportion to the population growth during the same period. While it resulted from a number of factors, such as the lack of home care facilities among urban families, it clearly would not have occurred unless there had been a growing desire for hospital care.

Here is ample evidence that the medical profession had largely overcome the public's earlier lack of confidence in medical science and practice. But this progress created a new problem. The great developments in medical science which gained and justified the public's confidence added greatly, among other complications, to the costs of medical care.

The lengthened course of medical education increased the investment in both time and money which a young doctor had to make in his career, and necessitated some increase in fees. Modern medical practice involved the use of more elaborate and expensive equipment, such as x-rays and diagnostic laboratory facilities. Such equipment was too expensive for the general practitioner, but hospitals and specialists required it and, of necessity, recovered some of its cost in charges to patients. Even the general practitioner was finding, by the early 1900's, that his essential equipment was greater and more costly than it had been when a bag of drugs, a prescription pad, and a stethoscope were about all he needed.

The development of more complicated diagnostic and therapeutic procedures, carried out by new types of specialists, often required the services of a number of physicians and technicians for each individual patient. In 1875 the family doctor was usually the only attendant even for the seriously ill. A half-century later such patients went to hospitals, and there were tended, directly or indirectly, by a considerable number of specialists, interns, nurses, and technicians. The services received from multiple medical personnel were often greatly superior to those provided by one general practitioner, but the costs to the patient grew in proportion. While this was of no great concern to the well-to-do classes, mounting medical costs created a serious problem for the rest of the population.

The poor had hardly received adequate medical attention in the preceding centuries, yet in the light of the then prevailing standards they had been fairly well tended. The destitute received medical charity, and the self-respecting, low-income families had experienced relatively little difficulty in paying the fees involved in the simple practice available. Moreover, as long as there was no great confidence in professional service no one worried much about the lack of it. Many families depended in large measure on home remedies and patent medicines. Few were conscious of the inadequacy of hospital facilities, and most people were only too glad to stay away from those depressing institutions.

But as medicine and surgery progressed the whole situation changed. The increased cost of care made it difficult for the poor to afford the expert attention now available. The public and the profession became enmeshed in a distressing and paradoxical situation. As the competence of the profession increased, and the public learned to appreciate this and to desire its services, the costs of medical services increased until they were beyond the resources of many.

The mounting costs of medical practice confront the public in the shape of fees charged by physicians, hospitals, laboratories, and the like. But the origins of the costs are essentially those very precise, involved, and expert procedures which make modern medicine so widely desirable and effective. The problem of how to reduce the one and retain the other, how to make medical care widely available without losing its effective qualities, is the core of the current problem in medicine. As this problem emerged after about 1915, the form it assumed and the solutions suggested naturally took their pattern from changing economic situations and social attitudes. To understand the ensuing debate over medical costs and other aspects of medical care, it is necessary to appreciate the changing character of American society during the latter part of the nineteenth century. . . .

20. MEDICAL COSTS: YESTERDAY AND TODAY

A. *FEES IN THE 1870's* *

ONLY A FEW of us here tonight are descendants of medical men, hence the majority of us have little concept of the life and work of our colleagues in this country in the middle of the last century. Wrapped up as we are in our own problems of medical economics, I thought it might be interesting to pause tonight, enlarging our perspective a bit by having a glance backward into the life of a typical successful practitioner of the late sixties.

As we review some of the interesting highlights of this individual, we find that he, too, had his problems related to fee schedules, isolation from medical centers, libraries, and medical journals....

... There was no specialization in practice. The graduate left school to do everything, without internship, without a residency, but starting his chosen profession with a brave heart, and often braver patients. Such a man, in every sense of the word, is the subject of tonight's discussion, Dr. Hiram Buhrman, who was born in Boone Township, Indiana, September 3, 1822....

He had as much education as the young boy of that day could obtain in the Maryland hills [to which his family moved]. He worked hard in physical pursuits and labor. As the years went on, he overcame many obstacles to fulfill his determined ambition to become a doctor of medicine....

... On October 23, 1866, he entered Jefferson Medical College, and on March 7, 1868, eighteen months later, he received the degree of Doctor of Medicine, being one of a hundred and fifty-nine men in the graduating class that year.... He then returned to Maryland to carry on practice during most of his life, practicing in various places.... In those days the horse was the principal means of transportation, and interestingly enough, the doctor was judged by his fellow citizens by the number of horses he was able to maintain. Hence, the less busy practitioner who could afford but one horse, became known as a one-horse doctor, and we still use the term in the same derogatory sense....

... I wish to stress a subject of particular interest to us now, that of fees and the payment of bills owed the physician. [They are recorded in] three daily record books containing the visits, the fees, occasionally the diagnosis, and the manner of payment of the bills through a period in the late sixties and early seventies. They have been remarkably well preserved by Doctor Buhrman's descendants through this period of seventy years since these clear entries were neatly and accurately recorded....

* From: "Leaves from a Doctor's Notebook of Seventy Years Ago," by H. M. F. Behneman, M.D.; *Military Surgeon* 86:547-54, June 1940 (No. 6). Reprinted (with omissions) by permission of the author and publishers. The author has retired from the practice of medicine and has been living in Chicago.

... An office visit was then known as a "call," whereas a "visit" meant a visit by the doctor to the patient's residence. The regulation fee for a call at the doctor's office was twenty-five cents. This included medicine, unless of course expensive medicine was necessary, wherein an extra amount was added to the bill. Owing to the fact that the doctor of the time compounded his own prescriptions, I found little evidence of his therapeutic formulae. One, however, of interest ... is labeled a "tonic mixture". It consists of whiskey, morphine sulphate, tincture of ferric chloride and quinine. Each dose, which a patient is supposed to have taken three times a day, contains two teaspoons of whiskey, one third grain of morphine sulphate, five grains of quinine, and a stout dose of iron chloride. Certainly, after the fifth day on that tonic the patient was either quite restful, or fearless even of his mother-in-law. House visits within the township limits were fifty cents regardless of the time spent in administering to the patient, except in the case of being detained by death, which uniformly was a three dollar fee. At that time, of course, the doctor did most of the work of the present day mortician.

Doctor Buhrman was physician, surgeon, lawyer (as there was none there), and of course, the dentist. All tooth extractions were twenty-five cents, and when a few in a row were removed the fee per tooth was less than that. When chloroform was required for tooth extraction, the total charge for the anesthesia and extraction was two dollars. All obstetrical cases regardless of the length of labor, were five dollars. Abortions were also five dollars, while miscarriages ran a poor third at a dollar and a half. In a careful analysis of these account books of Doctor Buhrman, I can find only two instances wherein he made more than one house visit after delivery, and this was usually the following day. If he did visit thereafter, there is no charge recorded in any of these accounts listed in his books. It appears, therefore, that the women of those days could take it and like it. On the other hand, maternal and infant mortality was high. The fee for setting and caring for a fractured clavicle, including always all material used in the dressing, was five dollars. The reduction of a hernia was the same price. A house visit without medicine was fifty cents, and with medicine seventy-five cents. Setting a fractured arm or a shoulder was five dollars, whereas a fractured thigh brought ten dollars, that being the sum total for proper care. Lancing an abscess or a felon was fifty cents. And thus the fee schedule runs on.

And now, let's look at collections. Frequently, in these volumes I have found the notation: "Patient in hands of the constable." Very often there is a notation: "This bill settled by a note." A careful study also reveals that thirty to fifty per cent of the doctor's bills were paid in merchandise of various sorts....

Some patients poured their money back to him in the form of vinegar at two cents a gallon. There are several turkeys at one dollar each; several tons of coal at six dollars per ton; one hundred and ninety-three pounds of beef at seven cents a pound; many cords of wood at four dollars a cord; one and a half days' plowing, two dollars; and many tons of hay at six dollars a ton. One grateful patient paid with five dozen dill pickles totaling fifty cents. Another patient received credit on her account for a dollar and sixty-three cents for fifteen pounds of pork and four quarters of beef, and twenty-nine pounds of corn meal at one cent a pound....

He sent no bills; when money was needed, he was reminded of it by his good second wife, who also bore him three children. He then would set out in person to his patients, garnering what he could to fill the purse or the larder. He was not rich in worldly goods, but he lived in the biggest house, was a leader in his community, and the family lived simply yet well. . . .

B. A CONTEMPORARY CASE REPORT *

I HAVE WITH ME a few case reports from the hundreds in my files which illustrate how essential coordinated services are for high quality medical care and how difficult or impossible it is for the average person to purchase such services under present methods of payment. Here is one such case:

Mr. C., a teacher, has a wife and two children and earns $70 a week. He came to me on November 10, 1945, complaining that he had been suffering from bad headaches for 2 months and that they were interfering with his work. He had already tried aspirin and a variety of patent headache remedies without success. As a first step, I gave him a thorough physical examination; among other things, I checked his eyes, sinuses, and reflexes; examined his heart and lungs through a fluoroscope, and tested his blood and urine. But I could find no obvious cause for the headaches. I prescribed a medicine for symptomatic relief, gave him general directions about diet and rest; and hoped that the headaches would respond to such a regimen. He failed to obtain any relief, however, and I was compelled to refer him to various specialists who could give him the special tests and services essential to modern medical diagnosis.

I referred him to an otorhinolaryngologist who irrigated his maxillary . . . sinuses but found no infection to account for the headaches. He suggested an X-ray study of all the sinuses to disclose a possible focus of infection. The X-rays were taken by a roentgenologist who reported that they showed no disease anywhere in the sinuses. Having eliminated the sinuses as a cause, and with the headaches as severe as ever, I referred him to an oculist, who, after thorough examination, found no disorder of the eyes to account for the headaches. Since disease of the brain and its surrounding structures is an important cause of headaches, I then referred him to a neurologist who, after a routine neuropsychiatric examination, recommended an X-ray study of the skull and the cervical spine of the neck. He returned to the roentgenologist who found in an X-ray of the spine, changes indicative of an inflammatory process. I recommended application of heat, massage, and exercise of the neck. After 2 weeks of such treatment the headaches were still unrelieved. I then referred Mr. C. to a radiotherapist for a series of X-ray treatments of the spine, a mode of therapy that is frequently successful in relieving headaches due to 'arthritis' of the spine. This treatment finally succeeded in relieving the headaches.

* From: *Hearings before the U. S. Senate Committee on Education and Labor on S. 1606— A Bill to Provide for a National Health Program*, 79th Cong., 2nd Sess.; Washington: U.S. Government Printing Office, 1946 (Part 3, pp. 1255-56). Reprinted with omissions.

The tabulated cost of specialist and X-ray services for Mr. C. was as follows:

Otorhinolaryngologist $15
Oculist 15
Neurologist 25
Roentgenologist:
    Sinuses 15
    Skull and spine 30
Radiotherapist (6 treatments) 60

Mr. C. has spent a total of $160 for these special consultations and services—services that were necessary for the diagnosis and treatment of a single common ailment. His total expenditure during 1945 for medical care for himself and his family amounted to $235. If some member of the family had needed an operation, had been afflicted by a chronic disease or had needed a protracted series of inoculations, such as those for hay fever, the expenditure would have been much greater. . . .

B. Current Expenditures for Medical Care

21. THE NATION'S MEDICAL BILL *

THE NATION'S TOTAL expenditures for civilian health services in 1951 were estimated at nearly $14 billion, a large increase over the $4 billion of 1929. Expressed in uniform dollars, the increase was nearly 130 percent. Health expenditures per capita rose from $32 to $89 or, in terms of constant dollars, nearly doubled.

Two-thirds of the health bill is paid directly by consumers. Almost one-fourth is paid by Federal, State, and local governments for public health services, hospital construction, and other programs, but not including the military. The balance largely represents private hospital construction, industrial health programs and philanthropic activities.

The percent of family income devoted to medical care has risen slightly. Nation-wide surveys, conducted in 1929 and 1935-36 found that on the average, families spent 4.0 percent of their income for medical care. Total consumer expenditures for medical care, relative to disposable income, show a similar pattern. In 1929, 3.6 percent of disposable personal income was spent for medical care; in 1937, 3.8 percent and in 1951, 4.0 percent. Out of each $100 spent on health in 1951, the average consumer paid $28 to physicians and surgeons, $24 to hospitals, nearly

* From: *Building America's Health,* by the President's Commission on the Health Needs of the Nation; Washington: U.S. Government Printing Office, 1953 (Vol. 2, Chap. X, "Financing Personal Health Services," pp. 253-54; and Vol. 4, Part 2, pp. 149-54). Reprinted with omissions.

$18 for drugs and $11 to dentists. Of the remaining $19, $6 went for eyeglasses, crutches or other appliances, $7 for net payments for insurance, and about $7 for nursing and miscellaneous items.

The average consumer health expenditure was about $59 in 1951, roughly $200 a family. The average is misleading because health expenditures vary widely not only because of the uneven incidence of illness but also in proportion to family income.... The proportion of income spent for medical care was more than twice as great in the lowest income group ... as in the highest, ... [according to a survey made in 1941 by the Bureau of Labor Statistics].* Yet it is the low-income group, often suffering from deficiencies in diet and housing and exposed to an unhealthy environment, that has the greatest need for health services....

It is often pointed out that families with incomes of less than $4,000 find money for tobacco, liquor, television, and automobiles. This is undeniably true. Yet it does not necessarily follow that these families could buy complete medical and dental care of good quality, let alone meet extraordinary medical expense. For one thing, a large proportion of the low-income families has not been able to purchase an automobile, a television set, or decent housing. A second factor is that human beings tend to choose the certain and immediate pleasure offered by a car or television instead of laying aside money against the uncertain and wishfully distant expense of medical care. Regular visits to the doctor and dentist, which might help to avoid heavy expense later, are themselves avoided because they require cash that is rarely on hand. These habits may be deplored—but they exist and must be reckoned with. A third factor is the lack of arrangements in most parts of the country for the purchase of comprehensive health services on a periodic prepayment basis....

There is no general agreement on exactly what constitutes complete and insurable medical care. By almost any standard, however, only a small fraction of the population is protected by prepayment for comprehensive health service, the formula that is best designed to cope with the financial and psychological obstacles to a sound program for family health.

What Can We Afford?

TURNING FROM the capacity of the individual family to the capacity of the Nation, how much health care can the United States afford? How much more than the present $14 billion can we spend?

From one standpoint, the expense of an adequate health program is no extra expense at all but simply a matter of bookkeeping. Either we pay to preserve health or we pay to repair it. The choice is the same as with maintenance of a house: either the owner pays to keep a good roof between the elements and the occupants, or he pays for the damages when the roof begins to leak. By this reasoning, we could afford an adequate health program even if there were no further increase in the national income and in per capita income.

* See Table No. 26, page 128.

GOVERNMENTAL EXPENDITURES

TABLE 24. *Expenditures by Federal, State and local governments for civilian health, by type of program, fiscal years 1947-51*

[Millions of dollars]

Type of program	1946-47			1947-48			1948-49		
	Total	Federal	State and local	Total	Federal	State and local	Total	Federal	State and local
Total A	1,717.1	678.4	1,038.7	2,061.5	716.7	1,344.8	2,575.6	828.0	1,747.6
Hospital and medical care B	1,076.0	530.9	545.1	1,324.6	547.2	777.4	1,589.1	603.1	986.0
New hospital construction C	84.8	28.8	56.0	123.1	55.1	68.0	299.4	94.4	205.0
Community and related health services D ...	488.7	63.7	425.0	551.5	66.6	484.4	613.3	74.9	538.4
Maternal and child health care E	51.9	43.7	8.2	34.1	25.1	9.0	30.8	20.5	10.3
Medical rehabilitation F	3.5	1.8	1.7	5.2	2.6	2.6	6.2	3.1	3.1
Medical and public health research G ...	10.1	8.1	2.0	19.8	17.8	2.0	31.3	29.3	2.0
Health personnel, in-service training H ..	2.1	1.4	.7	3.7	2.3	1.4	5.5	2.7	2.8

Type of program	1940-50			1950-51		
	Total	Federal	State and local	Total	Federal	State and local
Total A	2,945.0	1,015.8	1,929.2	3,243.8	1,046.9	2,179.0
Hospital and medical care B ..	1,657.6	644.0	1,013.6	1,763.3	642.7	1,120.6
New hospital construction C ..	521.7	219.7	302.0	571.9	254.9	317.0
Community and related health service D	661.7	65.8	595.9	810.4	61.2	740.2
Maternal and child health care E	28.8	19.1	9.7	34.4	23.1	11.3
Medical rehabilitation F	6.4	3.2	3.2	6.5	3.3	3.3
Medical and public health research G	60.6	58.6	2.0	58.7	56.7	2.0
Health personnel, in-service training H	8.2	5.4	2.8	7.6	5.0	2.6

A Excludes all medical expenditures of the military and the Atomic Energy Commission, medical services under the public aid programs ($225 million in 1951) and medical care provided to Workman's Compensation cases ($210 million in 1951). Further excludes expenditures of State agencies for the School Lunch program.

B Includes hospital and outpatient care in public institutions and expenditures for maintenance and improvement of existing facilities. Excludes expenditures for domiciliary care by the Veterans Administration and institutions for chronic care (other than mental and tuberculosis).

C Federal expenditures include cost of hospital planning and surveys as well as grants for construction; State and local expenditures represent new construction only.

D Federal expenditures represent those made by the U. S. Public Health Service (except for international health activities, the National Institutes of Health, medical and hospital care and hospital construction and professional education and training) and by the Food and Drug Administration; State and local expenditures represent all community health and sanitation expenditures by public agencies except those in connection with schools and public welfare and those classified elsewhere as health and medical services.

E Federal expenditures are for the Maternal and Child Health program, the program for crippled children, and the wartime Emergency Maternity and Infant Care program; State and local expenditures represent required matching of Federal grants under the Maternal and Child Health program and under the program for crippled children.

F Expenditures for medical care and services under the Vocational Rehabilitation Act.

G Represents all expenditures (except for education and training) of the National Institutes of Health, U. S. Public Health Service, and estimated amounts appropriated by State and local governments for medical research.

H Represents in-service training of the Children's Bureau and of the National Institutes of Health, and other units of the U. S. Public Health Service. Excludes professional education and training of nurses, physicians, and other medical personnel and expenditures in State supported medical schools.

TOTAL EXPENDITURES

TABLE 25. *Estimated total civilian expenditures for health and medical services and facilities, by source of funds, selected years, 1929-51*

(Millions of dollars)

Source of Funds	1929	1936	1941	1946	1949	1950	1951
Total expenditures..	3,924	3,299	4,844	9,050	11,654	12,572	13,607
Consumer [A]	3,003	2,523	3,376	6,117	7,774	8,329	8,918
Government (excluding hospital construction) [B] ..	409	442	[C]850	1,938	2,276	2,423	2,672
Philanthropy [D]	82	43	[C]230	300	[C]365	[C]370	[C]400
Industry [D]	[E]225	[E]200	[E]300	[E]525	[E]560	[E]630	[E]700
Hospital construction, total	205	91	88	170	679	820	917
Publicly owned facilities	101	74	42	85	477	476	498
Privately owned facilities [F]	104	17	46	85	202	344	419
				PERCENTAGE DISTRIBUTION			
Total expenditures..	100.0	100.0	100.0	100.0	100.0	100.0	100.0
Consumer	76.5	76.5	69.7	67.6	66.7	66.3	65.5
Government (excluding hospital construction) ..	10.4	13.4	17.5	21.4	19.5	19.3	19.6
Philanthropy	2.1	1.3	4.8	3.3	3.2	2.9	2.9
Industry	5.8	6.1	6.2	5.8	4.8	5.0	5.2
Hospital construction, total	5.2	2.7	1.8	1.9	5.8	6.5	6.8
Publicly owned facilities	2.6	2.2	.9	.9	4.1	3.8	3.7
Privately owned facilities	2.6	.5	.9	.9	1.7	2.7	3.1
Net national product (millions of dollars)	95,012	74,799	117,123	198,947	238,858	262,649	304,606
Percent of net national product devoted to health..	4.1	4.4	4.1	4.5	4.9	4.8	4.4

[A] Based on incomes received by personnel and facilities providing medical services (including hospitals, physicians, dentists and nurses, drug preparations and sundries, net payments for prepayment insurance, etc.); excludes net payments for mutual accident and sick benefit associations. Excludes physicians' income from government and welfare agencies, workmen's compensation cases, life insurance examination and other business organizations. Also excludes private payments to public, hospitals. Includes net payments for accident and health insurance. In recent years as much as half of this item may relate to disability rather than medical care protection; it was a larger proportion in earlier years.... Consumer expenditures in recent years are as follows if these adjustments are taken into account: 1949, $7,627 million; 1950, $8,248 million; and 1951, $8,816 million.

[B] See table 24 for items included.

[C] Estimated.

[D] Expenditure estimates for these items are understatements since some expenditures by philanthropy and industry are included under estimates for consumer and hospital construction expenditures.

[E] Estimated. Includes that part of the total expenditures for workmen's compensation cases that relate to hospital and medical services, in-plant health services, part of employer contributions to prepaid health insurance not included elsewhere and industrial expenditures for medical research.

[F] Part of the cost of constructing the privately owned facilities is met through Federal aid (Hill-Burton Hospital Construction Program); the amount of Federal aid represented would not be in excess of $50 million.

But the steady growth of national and individual income is obviously favorable to expansion of health services. In terms of 1939 dollars, the national income rose from $72 billion in 1929 to $141 billion in 1951 (or $278 billion in current dollars). The average per capita income (in constant dollars) climbed in the same period from $550 to $850.

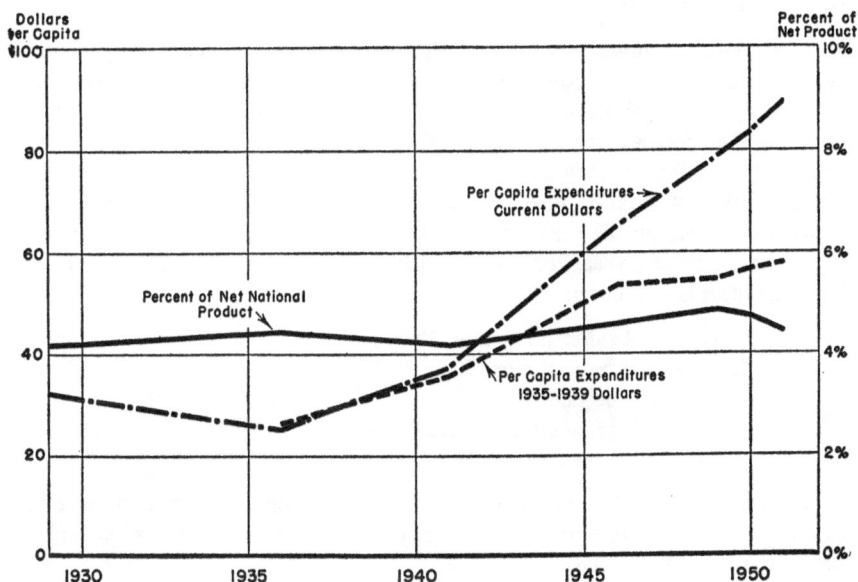

FIGURE 20. Estimated per capita expenditures for civilian health, current dollars and 1939 dollars, and the percent of the net national product devoted to health, 1929-51.

Further increases are ahead, in the opinion of Leon H. Keyserling, chairman of the President's Council of Economic Advisers.* Mr. Keyserling estimates that the expansion of our productive capacity will require an $11 billion increase in consumption of goods and services by 1954 and a level about $100 billion higher by 1962. He points out that additional demand for food, clothing, automobiles, and similar items is limited and that the greatest part of the increase in consumption will derive from new products and expansion of service industries. Much of the added purchasing power would therefore be available to improve the physical well-being of the population through better health services and better housing. . . .

* In the Truman Administration.

22. Trends in Consumer Spending

A. *CONSUMER SPENDING: SOME EARLY STUDIES* *

Unpredictability of illness and costs.—Sickness rates are averages. They conceal the differences between group and individual experience. The average may forecast reliably how much sickness will occur among a thousand or a million persons, but it gives no forecast for the individual. One person may go through the year with no illness; another may have two, three, or more. The illness of one may be mild and brief; of another, severe, long, and incapacitating. For example, studies [of the Committee on the Costs of Medical Care] made some years ago indicated that in the course of a year, in a group of 1,000,000 persons, the approximate incidence of illness is as follows:

> 470,000 will suffer no serious illness.
> 320,000 will be sick once.
> 140,000 will be sick twice.
> 50,000 will be sick three times.
> 20,000 will be sick four or more times.

Variations like these recur year after year; but no one can anticipate whether his family will be the one to go through a year with little or no illness or will be heavily burdened by sickness.

These large variations in the occurrence, duration, and severity of illness among individuals cause similarly large differences in their need for medical services and in medical costs. As medical science advances, there has been great increase in the variety of necessarily costly special skills, laboratory techniques, and hospital services and therefore in the range of medical costs for adequate modern care.

Unlike costs of food, shelter, or other necessities, these costs cannot be budgeted by the individual family because the need for care and the amount required to pay for it cannot be foreseen.

... Household expenses may, for example, be reduced in order to buy a car; the family income will usually determine whether it is a Ford or a Lincoln.

No one, however, can decide in advance what the year's cost of sickness will be or whether the sickness bill will be of Ford or Lincoln magnitude. Unexpected [illness] may require any amount from a month's pay to a year's income or more. Life savings may be exhausted, debts may dog the family for years, plans for buying a home or paying for a college education may be scrapped. The burden

---

* From: *Need for Medical Care Insurance* (Report to the U.S. Senate Committee on Education and Labor Relating to the Bill to Provide for a National Health Program), Senate Committee Print No. 4, 79th Cong., 2nd Sess.; Washington: U.S. Government Printing Office, 1946 (pp. 7-10). Reprinted with omissions, including some tables.

of high medical charges is particularly heavy for low-income families because food, shelter, and clothing take most of what they earn. An expensive illness has wrecked many a family's solvency. The records of charitable and welfare organizations are full of cases in which a long and expensive illness, especially when it strikes the breadwinner, has caused family break-down and dependency.

Uneven distribution of medical costs.—An example or two from the many and detailed studies in this field illustrate the extent of the variation in family bills for sickness.

Among the 8,581 families studied by the Committee on the Costs of Medical Care in 1927-32, 58 percent of the families incurred only 18 percent of the total charges reported in a year, while upon 10 percent of the families fell 41 percent of the total charges (fig. 21)....

SICKNESS COSTS FALL UNEVENLY

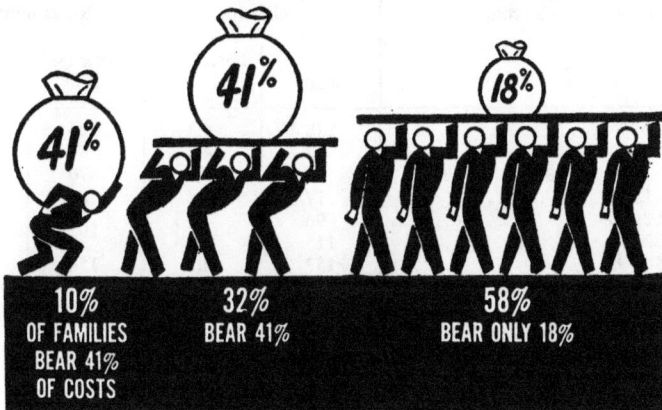

FIGURE 21.

If low-income families were able to pay for all the care they need, the volume of service they receive should exceed that received by the well-to-do since low-income families have more sickness and more serious sickness. Families with low incomes not only receive less care but of course ordinarily spend less for medical services. In over two-thirds of the families with incomes of less than $1,200 studied by the Committee on the Costs of Medical Care, the annual charges amounted to $40 or less, and only a tenth incurred charges of $100 or more. Among families with the highest incomes, on the other hand, barely a tenth fell into the group who incurred charges of $40 or less, and over four-fifths (84.2 percent) had charges of $100 or more.

The relation between income and expenditures is even clearer when the charges per person, rather than per family, are considered. More than twice as much was spent per person in families with $2,000 to $3,000 as in families with incomes below

$1,200. Charges incurred by families with incomes of $10,000 or more were
$115.12 per person, as contrasted with the $10.57 per person incurred by those
in the lowest income groups.

Nevertheless, though spending less in dollar amounts, low-income families
usually spend a greater proportion of their incomes on the costs of sickness than do
the well-to-do and the wealthy. This situation, which was revealed in the Committee on the Costs of Medical Care studies, is also brought out by more recent
inquiries. The following tabulation presents the estimated average medical-care
expenditures during 1941 of all families and single consumers, and the percent of
income spent for medical care, by money-income group and type of community
in the United States: . . .

TABLE 26.

Money income group [A]	Average medical-care expenditures, January to December 1941			
	Urban		Rural nonfarm	
	Average spent	Percent of income	Average spent	Percent of income
Less than $500	$26	8.3	$24	8.2
$500 to $999	32	4.3	51	6.9
$1,000 to $1,499	58	4.7	70	5.7
$1,500 to $1,999	77	4.4	85	5.0
$2,000 to $2,499	96	4.3 ⎱	102	4.3
$2,500 to $2,999	115	4.2 ⎰		
$3,000 to $4,999	153	4.1	154 [B]	4.2 [B]
$5,000 to $9,999	236	3.8	. . .	. . .

[A] Represents annual income for January to December 1941.
[B] Relates to income group of $3,000 or more.

B. CONSUMER SPENDING: A 1951 ANALYSIS *

Personal Consumer Expenditures.—How great is the demand for medical care
in the United States? Medical care is such a vital service that one is tempted to say
"There is no measure of the demand for medical care." While the *need* for medical
service may be incalculable—as indeed is the need for most goods and services—
medical service is an economic good and as such has a *demand* which can be
measured. If medical care were available in unlimited quantities as, for example,
air is, it would be a free and not an economic good. It would have no price, just
as air has no price. The supply of medical care, however, is not unlimited. It
requires the services of people who have livings to earn and requires facilities

* From: *Medical Care Expenditures, Prices, and Quantity, 1930-1950* (Bulletin 87, Bureau
of Medical Economic Research, American Medical Association), by Frank G. Dickinson; Chicago: American Medical Association, 1951. Reprinted (with omissions, including some tables
and figures) by permission of the author and publishers. The author is the director of the Bureau
of Medical Economic Research, American Medical Association, Chicago.

which must be purchased and maintained; and the amount and quality of these personnel and facilities depend to a large degree on the amount of money people are willing to spend for them. Whether the bill is paid by individual consumers, by insurance companies, by government agencies, or by physicians giving "free" services, it must be paid. A complete measure of the demand for medical care would require a vast amount of information on what would be spent if medical care prices were different in addition to data showing the amounts that are being currently spent for medical care at current prices. In this limited sense, the amount spent by consumers for medical care is the measure of their demand for medical care—the "market" demand. Since consumer demand represents the greatest portion of the total demand for medical services, the market demand for medical care is largely reflected in the amounts of personal consumer expenditures for medical care; these exclude expenditures by agencies of local, state and federal government.[1] According to Department of Commerce estimates, Americans spent $8.5 billion on medical care in 1950. (See fig. 22.) At the same time the expenditures for all goods and services were $193.6 billion. Thus expenditures for medical care in 1950 constituted 4.4% of the total amount spent on all goods and services in the consumer's budget; that is, the American people spent roughly 96% of their budgets for items other than medical care. (See fig. 23.) In 1930, expenditures for medical care were $2.9 billion while total consumer expenditures were $70.8 billion; medical care expenditures equalled 4.1% of total consumer expenditures. In 1935-1939, the period commonly used as a base for the purpose of statistical comparisons, average annual expenditures for medical care were $2.6 billion and total consumer expenditures, $63.6 billion; medical expenditures were 4.2% of total consumer expenditures. As a matter of fact, for every year since consumer expenditure data were first compiled, *the proportion of the consumer's budget spent for medical care has fluctuated narrowly around 4%*. The rise from 4.2% to 4.4% between 1945 and 1950 largely reflects wartime conditions in 1945, the tremendous increase in the number of births in the post-war years, the rapid rise in hospital room rates, and the increased use of hospitals.

Of the $8.5 billion spent by consumers on medical care in 1950, $2.4 billion was spent for physicians' services, $2.0 billion for hospitals, $1.4 billion for drugs and sundries, $1.0 billion for dentists' services, and $1.7 billion for "all other medical care." If the total amount of the expenditures for medical care in 1950 is set equal to one dollar, "the medical care dollar," 28.1 cents was spent for physicians' services, 23.1 cents for hospitals, 17.2 cents for drugs and sundries, 11.7 cents for dentists' services, and 19.9 cents for "all other medical care." (See figures 24 and 25.) This compares with 31.8 cents spent for physicians' services in 1930,

1. Personal consumer expenditures as defined in the Department of Commerce estimates include expenditures made by the American people as individuals, but not as taxpayers; that is, these estimates do not cover expenditures made by government. The Department of Commerce personal consumer expenditure series covers 206 items (counting subgroups) which are classified into 12 main groups. The sixth of these groups, "medical care and death expenses," includes physicians' services, hospitals, drugs and sundries, dentists' services, 11 relatively minor medical care items referred to herein as "all other medical care," and three death expense items which will be largely eliminated from this analysis. . . .

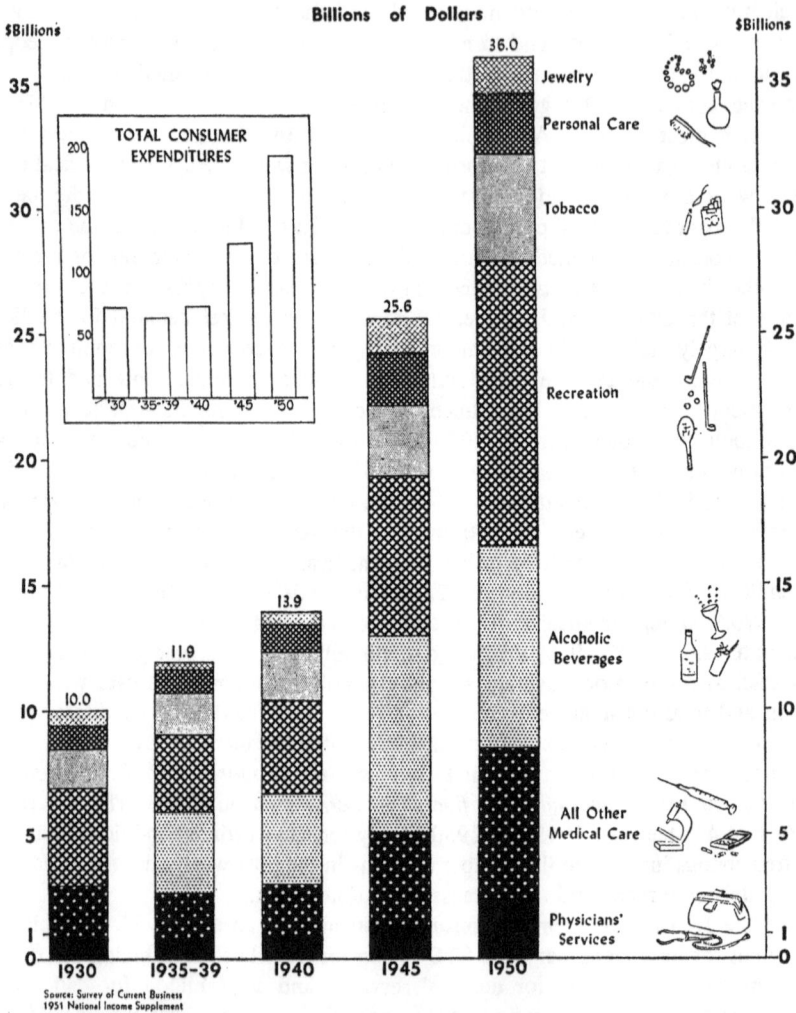

FIGURE 22. Selected consumer expenditures in the United States, 1930-1950.

13.9 cents for hospitals, 19.5 cents for drugs and sundries, 15.9 cents for dentists' services, and 18.9 cents for "all other medical care." * *Thus, over the 20 year*

* This broad category includes the following eleven medical-care items for which expenditures are relatively small, and for most of which the proportions of the medical-care dollar spent have remained relatively constant since 1935-1939: (1) ophthalmic products and orthopedic appliances; (2) osteopathic physicians; (3) chiropractors; (4) chiropodists and podiatrists; (5) private-duty trained nurses; (6) practical nurses and midwives; (7) miscellaneous curative and healing professions; (8) net payments to group hospitalization and health associations; (9) student fees for medical care; (10) accident and health insurance—net payments; and (11) mutual accident and sick benefit associations—net payments.

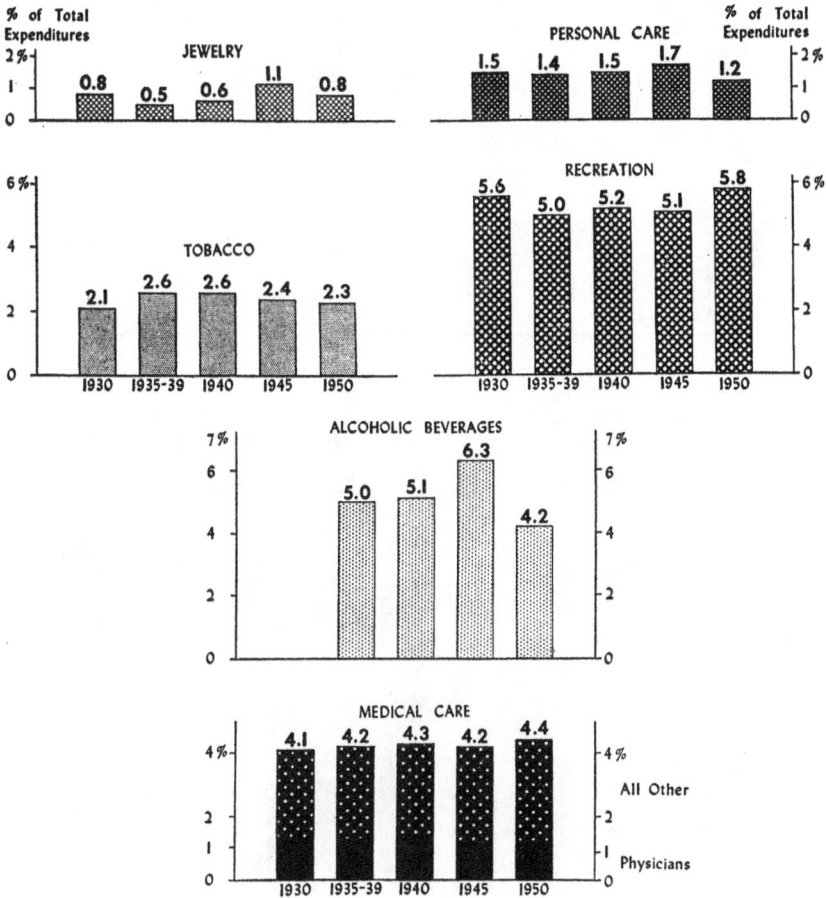

FIGURE 23. Selected consumer expenditures as percentages of total expenditures, 1930-1950.

period, the physicians' average share of the medical care dollar fell 12%, the hospitals' share rose 66%, and the dentists' share fell 26%; the portion spent on drugs and sundries dropped 12% and the portion on "all other medical care" rose 5%. If the base period 1935-1939 is taken as a point of reference, the trend is found to be generally the same. The physicians' share of the medical care dollar fell 10%, the hospitals' share rose 37%, the dentists' share fell 10%, the portion for drugs and sundries fell 17%, and the portion for "all other medical care" rose 9%. Thus, within the medical care group, the portions spent on physicians, dentists,

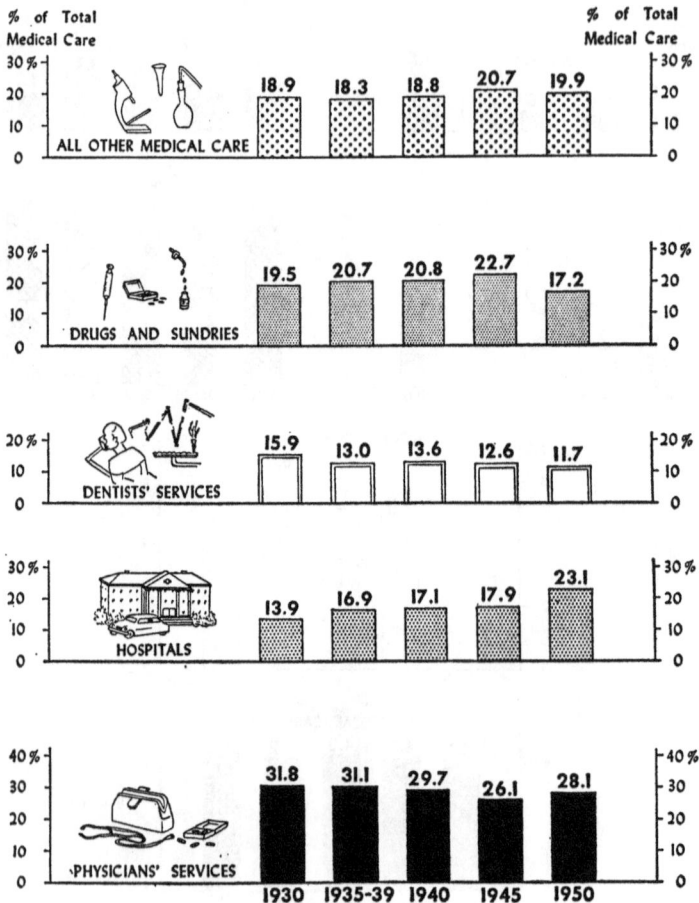

Source: Survey of Current Business
1951 National Income Supplement

FIGURE 24. Percentage distribution of expenditures for medical care, 1930-1950.

and drugs and sundries have shown a continuous decline, while the portion spent on hospitals has been increasing.

Another view of the changes in consumer expenditure patterns is presented in the index numbers (1935-1939 = 100) in table 27. The index for total consumer expenditures was 305 in 1950, for medical care 320, for physicians' services 289, for hospitals 436, for drugs and sundries 266, for dentists' services 287, and for "all other medical care" 348. While the amounts in billions of dollars spent for each of these medical care items have increased, *total consumer expenditures have increased so rapidly that the percentage of total consumer expenditures spent for these medical care items has actually decreased* except for hospitals and some of the minor items included in "all other medical care." The fact that the amount spent for medical care (320) has risen more rapidly than the amount spent for total consumer expenditures (305) is, therefore, due to the extremely sharp rise in the amount spent on hospitals and, to a much smaller extent, on the considerable increase in the amount spent on "all other medical care."

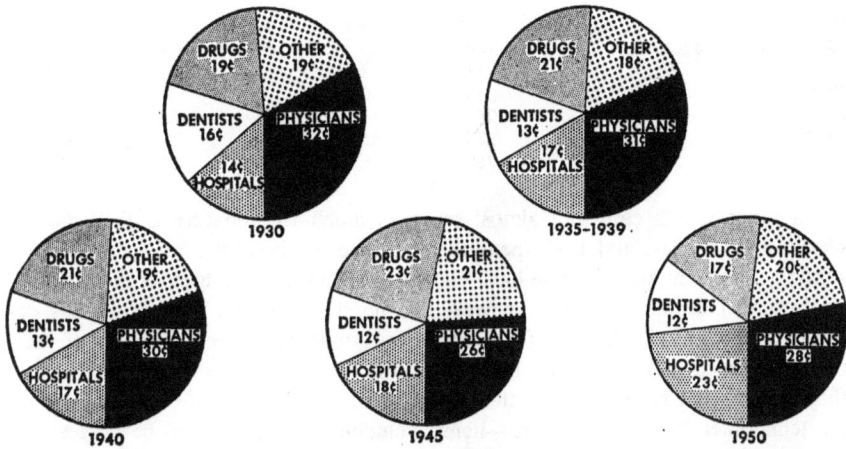

FIGURE 25. The medical care dollar.

How does the demand for medical care compare with the demand for other items in the consumer's budget? The Department of Commerce divides its estimates of personal consumer expenditures into 12 broad groups. Among these, the largest expenditures were for food and tobacco, equalling 33.8% of total consumer expenditures in 1950. The other groups for which expenditures were large were clothing, accessories, and jewelry, constituting 11.8% of the consumer's budget, housing 10.3%, household operation 13.7%, and transportation 11.7%. The lowest expenditures were for private education and research, or 0.9% of total consumer expenditures. Medical care and death expenses constituted 4.9% of the consumer's budget.[2]

Much more meaningful, however, are comparisons of medical care with certain individual items which bear some general resemblance to the medical care items in magnitude of expenditure and frequency of purchase. Of the $193.6 billion spent on all items in 1950, $8.1 billion, or 4.2% of the total, was spent for alcoholic beverages; $11.3 billion, or 5.8%, for recreation; $4.4 billion, or 2.3%, for tobacco; $2.3 billion, or 1.2%, for personal care; and $1.5 billion, or 0.8%, for jewelry. Thus, in 1950 Americans spent about as much for alcohol as for all types and kinds of medical care. They spent over a third more for recreation. They spent as

2. Death expenses (funeral and burial expenses, cemeteries and crematories, monuments and tombstones) counted for $1.1 billion of consumer expenditures in 1950, or 0.6% of total consumer expenditures. In the base period they accounted for 0.8% of total consumer expenditures.

TABLE 27. *Selected consumer expenditures, 1930-1950,*
Medical Care

Year	Total Medical Care	Physi-cians' Services	Hos-pitals	Drugs and Sundries	Dentists' Services	All Other Medical Care
(1)	(2)	(3)	(4)	(5)	(6)	(7)
1930	110%	113%	90%	104%	134%	114%
1935-1939 (average) ...	100	100	100	100	100	100
1940	116	111	118	117	121	119
1945	195	163	206	214	188	220
1948	283	261	354	258	259	301
1949	298	276	385	256	270	322
1950	320	289	436	266	287	348

much for personal care and almost twice as much for tobacco as they did for physicians' services, and they spent slightly more for jewelry than for drugs and sundries. The American people have chosen to spend their budgets in this manner. Each person deciding in his own way how he should spend his income has determined the market demand for every item. Americans spent only 4% of their money for medical care not because they did not have more to spend, but because they thought they could get what they wanted most by spending 96% of their money on items other than medical care—items including jewelry, alcohol beverages, and tobacco. The consumer—the dictator in a free economy—has made his choice. In fact, "personal savings" in 1950, the amount consumers had left over after spending $193.6 billion, was $10.7 billion! The personal savings of 1950 and those accumulated over the years constitute spending ability which consumers can draw upon as they wish. These accumulated savings in 1950 were very large even after allowing for inflated values and the universal failure to consider government bonds as a liability as well as an asset. It is most unfortunate that so many discussions of ability to purchase medical care or other goods and services assume that current income is the sole measure of purchasing power. *An expensive illness is among the rainy days for which people seek to make provision by saving.* As a direct result of ignoring the existence of these accumulated savings—savings which some political leaders point to with great pride—some persons have concluded that the medical and hospital bills not covered by prepayment insurance must be postpaid out of current income. This unrealistic approach to the question of ability to pay the costs of modern medical care deserves more attention that can be given in this bulletin.

Prices and Wages Compared.—While expenditures for medical care and expenditures for all goods and services in the consumer's budget increased at approximately the same rate, medical prices lagged considerably behind prices in general. By 1950, the price of all goods and services, as measured by the U. S. Bureau of Labor Statistics Consumers' Price Index [3] was up 72% since 1935-1939; the price

3. The Consumers' Price Index measures monthly the changes since 1935-1939 in the prices of fixed quantities of goods and services normally purchased by moderate-income families in large cities.

as a percentage of the 1935-1939 average

Alcoholic Beverages (8)	Recreation (9)	Tobacco (10)	Personal Care (11)	Jewelry (12)	Total Columns (3) through (12) (13)	Total Consumer Expenditures (14)
....	127%	89%	113%	170%	84%	111%
100%	100	100	100	100	100	100
114	119	109	121	134	117	113
243	201	180	227	383	215	194
255	320	255	245	421	282	280
248	327	262	242	407	286	283
253	360	271	250	422	303	305

of medical care and drugs had risen only 48%. Physicians' fees were up 40%, general practitioners' fees 40%, and surgeons' and specialists' fees 41%. Of all the medical care items, hospital rates alone rose more rapidly than the price of all goods and services—up 135% in 1950. At the same time, however, that these medical care items underwent a relatively small increase in price, average weekly earnings mounted rapidly. According to the U. S. Bureau of Labor Statistics average weekly earnings of production workers in manufacturing industries increased 165% between 1935-1939 and 1950. With medical care and drug prices rising only 48%, just 56% of a week's wages in 1950 was necessary to purchase the same amount of medical care as a whole week's wages in 1935-1939. Only 53% of a week's wages in 1950 was necessary to purchase the same amount of physicians' services as a whole week's wages in the base period. For the same amount of general practitioners' services or for the same amount of surgeons' and specialists' services a person would have to work only 53% as long in 1950 as in 1935-1939. The hospital services purchased with a week's wages in 1935-1939 would require 89% of a week's wages in 1950. These percentages do not, of course, reflect any changes in the average amount of services or drugs or in the average length of hospital stay required for a given illness.

How do these percentages compare with the percentages of a week's wages necessary to purchase other items in the consumer's budget? For the same amount of food as could be purchased with a week's wages in 1935-1939, 77% of a week's wages would be necessary in 1950; for the same amount of recreation, 62%; personal care, 67%; transportation, 61%; women's housedresses, cotton, 103%; rent, 50%; and for the same amounts of all goods and services, 65%. Since average weekly earnings rose so high in comparison to the Consumers' Price Index, less than a week's wages would be required to purchase most of these other items in the consumer's budget. Except for rent, however, the percentages are greater than those for medical care. This is to be expected since medical prices rose less rapidly than the prices of most items in the consumer's budget. . . .

Over the last 20 years, the American people have spent a constant proportion of their consumer budget, roughly 4%, for medical care. The demand for medical care has been small in comparison to the demand for other consumer items. It has been small, not because people could not afford more, but because they preferred to spend their budgets in this manner. In the past one could say that the irregularity and unpredictability of medical expenses were greater deterrents to the purchase of medical care than the actual amount of the expenses. Today, however, the wide-spread availability of hospital and medical insurance makes medical care a readily marketable item. A family can purchase a typical Blue Cross-Blue Shield membership, which will pay the bulk of hospital and in-hospital medical bills, for roughly 25 cents a day—the price of a package of cigarettes. Insurance helps a particular family to approach the 4% level, the average of all families. With over half the population carrying some form of medical or hospital insurance, the small demand for medical care certainly does not mean that people do not have the money for medical care, but that they are purchasing the amount they desire. And with the index of the prices of medical care, including the high hospital rates, lagging behind the Index of all consumer prices, they are receiving much more medical care for their money. In fact, average weekly earnings have risen so much more rapidly than the cost of medical service, that a production worker today can buy almost twice as much medical care with a week's wages as he could in 1935-1939. And health progress has given him another dividend—more and better years in which to earn. Today, in a period of general inflation, the consumer is getting more and better medical care for the same proportion of his personal consumer expenditures.

C. CONSUMER SPENDING: THE PICTURE FOR 1953 *

IN THE PRESENT survey it has been possible to project the total amount of charges for personal health services incurred by families by a direct examination of family expenditures among a representative national sample of 2,809 families, subdivided by age, sex, income, size of family, rural-urban, occupation and region. At the same time it has been possible to break down family expenditures by income and by type of service such as hospital care, physicians' services, and so on.

National Total Charges for Personal Health Services.—During the survey year families incurred national gross charges for personal health services of $10.2 billion. This figure is exclusive of the amount paid by the government for direct services, workmen's compensation, and private charity. (See table 28.) The medical dollar is divided as follows: physicians, 37 percent; hospitals, 20 percent; prescrip-

* From: *National Family Survey of Medical Costs and Voluntary Health Insurance: Preliminary Report*, by Odin W. Anderson; New York: Health Information Foundation, 1954 (Part 2, "Expenditures for Personal Health Services and Voluntary Health Insurance during Survey Year"). Reprinted (with omissions, including initial paragraphs and some tables) by permission of the publishers. The author is the research director of the Health Information Foundation, New York. (A more extensive discussion of this section of the 1953 survey conducted by the Health Information Foundation is provided in pages 21-29 and 109-13 of the volume entitled *Family Medical Costs and Voluntary Health Insurance: A Nationwide Survey*, cited in the acknowledgment note for Selection No. 14C, in Chap. III).

tions and other medicines, 15 percent; other medical goods and services, 13 percent; and dentists, 16 percent. (Adds up to 101 percent because of rounding of the individual percentages.)

TABLE 28. *Estimated national total gross charges incurred by families for personal health services and goods*

Item	July, 1952 through June, 1953	
	Amount (billions of dollars)	Percent
Total	10.2	100
Physicians A, B	3.8	37
Hospitals	2.0	20
Prescriptions and other medicines C	1.5	15
Other medical goods and services D	1.3	13
Dentists E	1.6	16

A Physicians' charges can be further broken down as follows:

Physicians	3.8	100 percent
Surgery	.8	21
Obstetrics	.4	11
Other physicians	2.6	68

B Includes:

1. Payments to hospital out-patient departments for the services of salaried physicians and other clinical services.

2. Payments by either consumers or insurance for medical services received from salaried physicians in government hospitals.

3. The estimated value (at going rates) of physicians' services received from salaried physicians under some form of prepaid medical care plan.

4. Payments by surgical or medical insurance to independent physicians either directly or through reimbursement of patient.

5. Payments by accident insurance or liability insurance (except employer's liability insurance or Workmen's Compensation) to independent physicians either directly or through reimbursement of patient.

6. Payments for drugs administered by a physician.

7. Payments to independent physicians for services received by persons who were still considered as members of some household in July, 1953 even though they had been institutionalized at some time during the past year and were still in an institution on the date of interview.

8. Payments to independent physicians for services received by people who died during the survey year but who had been living at the time of their death with relatives as members of households still in existence in July, 1953.

(This category thus excludes deceased who had been living in institutions, alone, or only with non-relatives at the time of their death as well as those who lived in households which were broken up after the death.)

9. Bad debts—services by physicians for which patients were actually billed but which will never be paid for.

It is also possible that physicians may sometimes act as collecting agents for the fees for certain services like X-rays, laboratory work, or special tests which they themselves do not perform. The physician may net no income from this and so does not consider these fees as part of his gross income. NORC in general classified all such fees paid to a physician into the physician category.

(*continued on next page*)

Total annual national costs for personal health services paid from all sources are difficult to estimate accurately, but an estimate of $12 billion would seem to be reasonable judging from available data reported by Oscar N. Serbein in *Paying for Medical Care in the United States,* New York, Columbia University Press, 1953. Thus, $1.8 billion should be added to the $10.2 billion charged the families, or approximately 15 percent comes from sources other than individual payments and insurance benefits. The present survey shows that of the $10.2 billion charged families for personal health services, $1.5 billion or 15 percent was covered by insurance benefits. (See table 29.)

It is more meaningful, however, to break the totals down by type of service. One-half of the hospital charges are covered by insurance; also 13 percent of all physicians' charges, 38 percent of charges for surgery, and 25 percent of charges for obstetrics. Insurance benefits to cover other services are negligible, because such benefits are not usually provided through insurance. Thus, as a grand total, it appears that approximately 30 percent of the costs of all personal health services today are from so-called third-party payments, exclusive of disability insurance and life insurance.

B Excludes:

1. Value of services of salaried physician in a government or private hospital or clinic or the services of a company doctor when such services were not paid for by the patient and were not received as part of any form of prepaid medical care plan or insurance.

2. Free care (care for which an independent physician received no re-imbursement and did not bill anyone.)

3. Payments to independent physicians (physicians in private practice) by Workmen's Compensation, employer's liability insurance, or by an employer for a work-incurred injury.

4. Vendor payments to independent physicians under governmental (generally state or local) assistance programs for various categories of indigent families.

5. Vendor payments to independent physicians by foundations and associations like The National Tuberculosis Association, National Foundation for Infantile Paralysis, Crippled Children's Societies, Rotary, Lions, etc.

6. Payments to independent physicians by recipients under governmental assistance programs when these payments were specifically re-imbursed to the recipient by the program.

7. Payments to independent physicians for medical care received by people who were not part of the civilian, non-institutional population of the continental United States as of July, 1953.

C Both estimates are for pharmaceuticals purchased directly by the consumer. The expenditures for pharmaceuticals administered in hospitals or by physicians and dentists are included in the estimated payments to those groups and are excluded from this item.

D The NORC * estimate contains expenditures for medical appliances including ophthalmic products, services of oculists and optometrists, services of paramedical personnel like chiropractors, chiropodists, podiatrists, naturopaths, faith healers, etc., the services of private duty nurses, practical nurses, and midwives, and expenditures for laboratory services like diagnostic tests and X-rays for which the consumer was billed directly by the laboratory.

E It should be noted that the NORC estimate contains expenditures made directly to dental laboratories for X-rays, denture repair, and the manufacture of dentures on the basis of impressions taken by dentists.

* National Opinion Research Center, University of Chicago, which conducted this survey for the Health Information Foundation. For description of the sampling method employed for the survey, see the Introduction to the report from which the present selection is drawn

TABLE 29. *Estimated national percentages of total gross costs incurred covered by total insurance benefits*

Item	NORC Sample—July, 1952 through June, 1953		
	Total gross costs incurred	Total insurance benefits	Percent covered by insurance benefits
Total	$10.2 billions	$1.5 billions	15
Hospitals	2.0	1.0	50 B
Physicians	3.8	.5	13
Surgery	.8	.3	38
Obstetrics	.4	.1	25
Other physicians	2.6	.1	4
Medicines	1.5	A	0
Other medical goods and services.	1.3	A	1
Dentists	1.6	A	0

A Less than $50,000,000.

B Since many patients in non-governmental general and special long-term hospitals, mental and allied hospitals, and tuberculosis sanatoria at the time of the interviewing may not have been considered as members of civilian non-institutional households, the NORC estimate probably does not adequately represent expenditures for this category of care.

Family Charges for Personal Health Services.—After considering over-all national estimates, it is well to come down to the family unit and its experiences with costs of personal health services. Exclusive of insurance premiums and the portions paid by insurance, the average charge incurred by families is $178 per year. (See table 30.) The gross charges including the amounts paid for insurance are $207 per family per year. Families with insurance incurred an average gross charge of $237 and families without insurance an average of $156. The gross hospital charges are approximately $42 per family per year, and physicians' charges would be around $75. Medicines average $31 per year; other medical services and goods, $26; and dentists, $33.

TABLE 30. *Average net costs per family for hospital, medical and dental services and goods*

Item	NORC Sample—July, 1952 through June, 1953	
	Amount	Percent
Total, net A costs	$178	100
Physicians	67	38
Hospitals	21	12
Medicines	31	17
Other	26	15
Dentists	33	18

A The estimates in this table are for incurred "out-of-pocket" charges. Thus, the money paid directly to hospitals and physicians by voluntary health insurance and the payment by consumers for which they received or expect to receive reimbursement by such insurance are both excluded from these estimates. Moreover, insurance premiums are also excluded.

The foregoing discussion was concerned with *average* family charges, but hereafter the *median* charges will be used. The median gross charges for all services is $110 per year, which means that one-half of the families experienced charges of less than $110 and one-half more than that amount. Since the average gross charges exceeded $200, this indicates that there were some extremely high costs experienced by some families which pulled the average up. The median disregards the extremes and is a more meaningful statistical device in some circumstances. Families with insurance incurred greater charges for personal health services than those without insurance; a median of $145 compared with $63 or an average of $237 compared with $156. This is in part due to greater utilization by those with insurance and possibly also utilization of a more expensive type of service, for example, a private room in a hospital instead of semi-private or ward. Obviously, the higher costs incurred by the insured group have great implications for the national costs of personal health services as voluntary health insurance continues to expand.

For all families there are great differences between incurred charges by income groups, ranging from $54 for those under $2,000 to $238 for those over $7,500. Since the dollar-value of free care is undetermined, it is possible that the costs of services received by families under $2,000 would be higher than the gross incurred charges of $54. For example, 27 percent of families had at least one family member hospitalized, but only 26 percent reported gross hospital charges. Similarly, 77 percent of families reported attendance by a physician, but only 75 percent reported gross physicians' charges.

When the net charges incurred by families with and without insurance are calculated—which excludes hospital, surgical, and other medical insurance benefits—there is still a great difference. Families with insurance incur net charges of $117 compared with $63 for families without insurance. (See table 31.) It would seem that the implications of these differences can hardly be overemphasized.

TABLE 31. *Median net charges for hospital, medical and dental services and goods by family income for families with and without insurance*

Family income	Number of families			Median net charges [A]		
	All families	With insurance[B]	With no insurance[B]	All families	Families with insurance	Families with no insurance[C]
Total, all families ...	2,809	1,780	1,029	$ 98	$117	$ 63
0-1,999	560	176	384	53	77	42
2,000-3,499	617	347	270	74	88	54
3,500-4,999	693	514	179	105	112	79
5,000-7,499	577	466	111	144	151	105
7,500 and over	343	272	71	197	198	185
Income unknown	19	5	14	—	—	—

[A] Net charges are gross charges incurred less voluntary health insurance benefits received. That is, net charges are the charges to the family itself. In the case of hospital service plans or comprehensive medical care plans, the cost of service benefits is not included here. In the case

So much for averages or medians by income groups; what is the distribution of charges for personal health services for families within selected income groups? Families experience a full range of charges from nothing to a great deal.

"Catastrophe" as used with reference to costs of personal health services has always been nebulously defined "as an awful lot" depending on family income. . . . It should be possible to arrive at some concept of the area of "catastrophe" depending on what standard is adopted. No standard is proposed, but at what point should so-called major medical or catastrophe insurance begin to pick up the check, and at what point for each income group?

Among all families, 11 percent experienced a cost in excess of $395; 7 percent in excess of $495; and 1 percent in excess of $995. Projected to the entire population this means that approximately 500,000 families in the United States experienced a cost for personal health services in excess of $995. These figures exclude the insurance premium and the portion paid by insurance. Further, in the income group under $2,000, 7 percent incurred a cost in excess of $395; in the income group $2,000 to $3,500 the percentage is also 7, increasing from there on. On the other hand, it is also well to note that almost 39 percent of the families incurred costs under $100 and 9 percent incurred no costs. When families with insurance are compared with families without insurance, it is again borne out that insured families incur greater charges than the uninsured.

These data illustrate again the classic generalization that the costs of personal health services are unpredictable for the individual family but relatively predictable for a group of families. Thus costs, as such, are not an issue in the sense that 10 billion dollars are too much for the country to spend annually for personal health services. The problem is—another classic statement—how to spread this cost equitably so that no one family incurs a heavy cost at any one time.

To make the distribution of the charges for all personal health services more meaningful, a breakdown [has been made] by broad categories of service: hospital care, surgery, and physicians' services, other than surgery and obstetrics, and medicines and dental services. These [figures] are particularly significant because they more or less pin-point the problems of the unpredictability of the cost of personal health services.

---

of indemnity plans or insurance, the amount which the insurance paid either to the hospital, physician, etc., or to the family is excluded.

B These figures are for families with and without insurance at the end of the survey year. Median net charges for families with insurance are, of course, substantially lower than median gross charges. However, median net charges and median gross charges are substantially the same in families with no insurance. Wherever median net charges are lower than median gross charges for families with no insurance at the end of the survey year, it is because at some time during the survey year one or more family members had been covered and received benefits.

C A small part of the difference in median net charges for families with insurance and families with no insurance is accounted for by the fact that the average size of families with insurance (3.26 persons) is somewhat higher than the average size of families with no insurance (2.95 persons). This difference is less marked within each specific income group. In almost all instances this family size difference is too small to account for any substantial proportion of the difference in medians. Later analysis should indicate some of the factors producing these rather substantial differences in net incurred charges.

For all families with and without insurance, 6 percent reported expenditures for hospital service in excess of $195 and 3 percent reported expenditures for surgery in excess of the same amount.

The debate regarding "comprehensive" services is largely concerned with physicians' services such as home and office calls and out-patient diagnostic services, excluding surgery and obstetrics. It is frequently stated that non-surgical and non-obstetric services are not an important unpredictable financial item and families might well finance such services out-of-pocket and not add the administrative cost of an insurance agency.

The distribution of "other" physicians' charges shows that 6 percent of the families incur "other" physicians' charges in excess of $195 per year compared with 3 percent who incur surgeons' charges in excess of the same figure. It is then clear that "other" physicians' charges are a relatively large item for some income groups, even though such charges are incurred in small amounts at a time. Thus, multiples of service incurring small charges at any one time can, during a year, accumulate into a large amount. At this point it would be useful to have a breakdown of the distribution of the costs of home and office calls and costs of out-patient diagnostic services. It may be that the latter services are more difficult to pay for out-of-pocket than home and office calls. At the same time, physicians' calls and diagnostic services are so interrelated that a statistical differentiation of those services is difficult.

The cost of medicines is another item which is usually not included in insurance against costs of personal health services because of difficulty in controlling the range and volume of prescriptions. There is frequent discussion of including high cost drugs, drugs with specific therapeutic effects, and some of the antibiotics. For all families, 9 percent experience costs for medicines in excess of $95 and 2 percent in excess of $195. It is not possible to differentiate between prescribed and unprescribed drugs. In any case, it is apparent that there are families that do incur relatively high charges for medicines, illustrating again that multiples of small cost services can add up to a large annual cost. Comparisons between families insured and those not insured show that the families with insurance generally incur larger costs for medicines, even though medicines received while hospitalized are not included.

Dental costs are also distributed unevenly among families revealing differences within and between income groups. Forty-four percent of all families incurred no dental bills and 4 percent incurred charges in excess of $195. Differences among income groups are sharp, particularly when charges in excess of $45 are included. No expenditures for personal health service appear to be so closely correlated with income as dental service.

The median percent of income paid out for personal health services by all families is 4.1. The range is from 6.1 for families under $2,000 to 3.2 for families over $7,500. When families with insurance and without insurance are compared, the usual pattern is found since the median percent for families with insurance is 4.9 and for those without insurance 2.9. Among insured families, the lowest income group pays out a higher proportion of income for personal health services than the same income group among the uninsured.

When the distribution of total "out-of-pocket" charges for personal health services and insurance premiums as a percentage of incomes of all families are calculated, two percent of the families, or approximately one million families, incurred charges of 50 percent or more of their annual incomes, among whom approximately 500,000 families incurred charges equalling or exceeding 100 percent of their incomes. This [calculation] provides some tangible data for a definition of "catastrophe" wherever one wishes to draw the line.

Proportions of Family Charges for Personal Health Services Paid by Insurance.— A test of the adequacy of health insurance benefits is the degree to which they cover the incurred charges. For all services 21 percent of the families had received some service for which insurance benefits had been paid in whole or in part. For 29 percent of the families who had received insurance benefits, 20 percent or less of their charges for services had been paid by insurance. On the other end, 7 percent of the families had received insurance to cover 80 percent or more of their charges.

These gross figures for all services, however, are more meaningful when they are broken down by specific types of services. The proportion of hospital costs covered by insurance is important, because there is a general opinion that it is desirable to cover all or nearly all services recognized as hospital services. Fifty-nine percent of families experiencing hospital costs and who also carried hospital insurance and received benefits had 80 percent or more of their costs covered. On the other end 18 percent of the families had 60 percent or less of their hospital costs covered by insurance. It is well to remember that these are national figures, and there are undoubtedly regional variations, and variations among hospital insurance plans.

If there is any consensus as to how great a proportion of the surgeons' charges should be covered by insurance, it is accurate to say that families below certain incomes should have all or nearly all of the costs of surgery covered. Thirty-four percent of the families who experience surgical charges have less than 60 percent of their charges covered by insurance, and 45 percent have 80 percent or more of such charges covered.

. . . By and large the payments made by insurance for surgical costs fall far short of equalling the total charges. The difference would seem to involve more than a normal deductible or co-insurance feature. Very useful data at this juncture would be the prevailing surgical fees throughout the country by region and the prevailing surgical insurance benefits in relation to these fees by region. To what extent is the low proportion of costs covered by surgical insurance due to low fee schedules established by insurance in relation to prevailing surgical fees? On the other hand, to what extent does surgical insurance increase the per unit surgical costs?

Even though maternity benefits are very widespread in insurance contracts, many people in the insurance field feel that maternity costs have no logical place in an insurance program. In any case there is a great demand for such benefits, and they appear to have a firm place in health insurance contracts. One-half of the obstetrical cases with insurance and receiving benefits had 60 percent or more of the charges covered by insurance, and one-half had less than 60 percent of charges covered. Maternity benefits, however, are usually not designed to cover the total costs of maternity care. This may account, at least in part, for the relatively low proportion of obstetrical costs covered by maternity benefits.

23. ABILITY TO PAY FOR MEDICAL SERVICES

A. *THE PROBLEM OF MEDICAL INDIGENCY* *

THE COST OF NECESSARY medical attention in a severe, prolonged illness may well amount to more than a family's entire annual income. . . .

. . . To virtually everyone the possibility of heavy expense for medical care is a source of insecurity. The payment of hospital or doctor's bills frequently requires people to draw upon past savings, if they have them, or to go into debt. (Various studies of the small-loan business show that payment of hospital and medical bills is the chief reason why people take out these loans.) Frequently people are unable to pay for service and must either ask for charity care or go without, where they cannot get or will not ask for such care. All of this means that frequently physicians and hospitals are prevented by economic barriers from rendering the necessary services they would like to give and that the economic basis of their services is less broad and stable than it should be. . . .

An important factor in the [medical-expense] situation is the low income of part of the population. We have seen that a large proportion of the population who are not indigent will in serious illness be unable to meet—or will find it difficult to meet—the cost of necessary medical care on an individual payment basis. Moreover, there appears to be a certain part of the population with incomes so low that even on a prepayment or insurance basis they would be unable to pay the full cost of adequate care.

In 1946, 12.8 per cent of all single individuals and families in this country had gross cash incomes of less than $1,000, 15.4 per cent had incomes between $1,000 and $2,000, 19.5 percent had incomes between $2,000 and $3,000, 31.4 per cent had incomes between $3,000 and $5,000, and 20.9 per cent had incomes of $5,000 or more.† These figures relate to cash incomes only and do not include the value of an owned home or of food raised and consumed at home. Although incomes

---

* From: *America's Health: A Report to the Nation by the National Health Assembly;* New York: Harper, 1949 (Chap. VII, "What Is the Nation's Need for Medical Care?" pp. 197-200). Reprinted (with omissions, including initial paragraphs) by permission of the publishers.

† Cf. the figures on distribution of money income among American families in 1955, contained in the footnote to Selection No. 3, Chapter I, p. 20.

have since risen about 10 percent, the cost of living has risen to at least the same extent. . . .

At the present time people spend for medical care about 4 to 5 per cent of their income, on the average, the percentage being somewhat higher than this for those in the lower-income groups and gradually declining as income rises. It might well be that if, through prepayment, medical care were given a firm and established place in the family budget people could be encouraged to spend a larger proportion of their income than at present for medical care. Yet when one reflects that many families with incomes under $2,000 or $3,000 are unable to afford an adequate diet or adequate housing—things which in the long run are as essential to health as medical care—it appears doubtful that families at this income level can appreciably increase their expenditures for medical care. In short, one may conclude that there is a certain proportion of families—over and above the indigent—with incomes so small that they would be unable to afford the full costs of adequate medical care even on a prepayment basis.[1]. . .

B. FAMILY INDEBTEDNESS FOR HEALTH CARE *

BEING IN DEBT is no novelty for the vast majority of American families since they are accustomed to buying a wide range of goods on credit. In fact, "so much down and so much a month" is the mainstay of the automobile, refrigerator, radio and television, and furniture industries. Presumably, going into debt for automobiles, refrigerators, television sets, and many other items is pleasurable because one can "enjoy them while paying for them". There are also the factors of convenience of a payment plan and aggressive salesmanship.

Since being in debt is, so to speak, a normal experience for many American families, is there any cause for concern when one learns that 15 percent of families are in debt to hospitals, physicians, dentists, and other providers of medical goods and services,[2] and that 2 percent are in debt for $195 or more? Translated into absolute numbers this means that approximately 7.5 million families in the United States have some debt and that about one million families owe $195 or more.

If personal health services could be purchased like any other goods or services

1. The U.S. Bureau of Labor Statistics has drawn up a list of the commodities and services considered necessary for a minimum but adequate standard of living for a family of four—man, wife, and two children under 15. It has priced these commodities and services in 34 representative cities and found that the total cost as of March, 1946, ranged from $2,573 to $2,985. In 1945, of urban families with two children, 29.1 per cent had total money incomes of less than $2,500, and 45.3 per cent had total money incomes of less than $3,000.

* From: *National Family Survey of Medical Costs and Voluntary Health Insurance: Preliminary Report*, by Odin W. Anderson; New York: Health Information Foundation, 1954 (Part 4, "Debt among Families Due to Costs of Personal Health Services as of July 1953"). Reprinted (with omissions, including initial paragraphs and some tables) by permission of the publishers. The author is the research director of the Health Information Foundation, New York. (A more extensive discussion of this section of the 1953 survey conducted by the Health Information Foundation is provided in pages 45-47 of the volume entitled *Family Medical Costs and Voluntary Health Insurance: A Nationwide Survey,* cited in the acknowledgment note for Selection No. 14C, in Chap. III).

2. Hereafter referred to as medical indebtedness.

—when desired and in the quantity and of the quality to fit one's purse—perhaps the problem of medical debt could be dismissed as of no more concern than the balance owed by a family on its automobile or television set. The cost of these items is known in advance; the costs of personal health services are not so known and when they are needed the consumer usually has no choice but to seek the necessary services, regardless of the cost, even if it means going into debt. Systematic saving is not a solution since families would not know how much should be saved annually. An effective and accepted mechanism today is an adequate insurance plan to meet the unpredictable costs of personal health services; such a plan is, in effect, a savings program of many people pooling their money and their risks.

In a previous part of this report, the distribution of the costs of personal health services by family income was presented showing that some families incurred no cost during the survey year and some incurred costs equalling or exceeding their annual incomes.* In the data to follow showing the distribution of outstanding medical indebtedness, it will be noted that such indebtedness is considerably less than the incurred charges presented in a previous report.† Apparently, the bills were paid in some way or other—insurance and savings—but a residue of unpaid bills remains. Considering the magnitudes of some of the incurred charges, it is surprising that the residue of unpaid bills is actually as small as indicated in this survey. Given the definition of medical indebtedness in the study, it would seem that such indebtedness excludes minor costs and includes indebtedness which represents some degree of hardship to the families.

Outstanding medical indebtedness includes debts owed to hospitals, physicians, dentists and other suppliers of medical goods and services at the end of the survey year *less* any amount which the family planned to pay on such bills during the month following the interview; that is, the informant was asked how much the family owed (including amounts owed on bills not yet received) and was then asked how much the family planned to pay on these bills during the next month. If the informant reported that the family's only outstanding debt was $10 to the doctor and that the bill would be paid during the next month, the family was recorded as having no outstanding indebtedness for personal health services.

This method of getting at outstanding indebtedness was used to determine the number of families who were not current with respect to debts for personal health services, that is, those families who had owed hospitals, physicians, and others for a period longer than "normal" interim between receiving services or goods and paying for them. The amount of outstanding indebtedness then included all such debts whether incurred prior to the survey year or during the survey year, except that the amount which the family planned to pay in the month following the interview was excluded.

An important point to bear in mind is that medical indebtedness *excludes* debts to financial institutions and individuals which were incurred to pay for personal health services and goods.

---

* See Selection No. 22C, this chapter, pp. 141, 143.
† Average amount of indebtedness reported in this selection is $121, as against the $178 for incurred charges reported in Selection No. 22C, this chapter, p. 139.

All families in this survey showed 85 percent with no medical indebtedness and 15 percent with some debt. The 15 percent with some debt includes 9 percent under $94, 3 percent $95-194, 2 percent $195 and over, and 1 percent where the amount was unknown. The average debt per family with medical indebtedness is $121. In national terms, this means that total indebtedness approximates $900 million.

The percent of all families with some medical indebtedness is quite constant until the income groups $5,000 and over are reached. Thereafter, there is a sharp drop. This is not a surprising fact, of course, since upper-income groups lay out a smaller percentage of their income for personal health services although average family costs are higher. It is also of particular interest to note that having or not having insurance had no real appreciable effect on indebtedness. A final observation is that indebtedness in families with incomes under $2,000 undoubtedly represents a greater burden than indebtedness in income groups with higher incomes. Debts are not necessarily distributed evenly in proportion to incomes. . . .

The lowest income group has the highest percentage of families with medical debt under $95, namely 13 percent; 4 percent of the highest income group has debts of similar magnitude. It would appear that in three of the income groups, those with insurance are more likely to have debts under $95 than those without insurance.

For families with medical debts ranging from $95 to $194 again, the lower the income group the greater is the hardship experienced. The effect of insurance is negligible.

There is an interesting uniformity of percent of families with medical debts exceeding $195, two percent, but the lower the income group the greater is the hardship involved on the part of the families.

. . . By and large the greater the percent of family income paid out for personal health services, the larger is the proportion of families who reported outstanding medical indebtedness. This is also true within income groups as well as between income groups.

Finally, families with children are more likely to report medical indebtedness than families without children. This is another way of saying that increased financial responsibilities are incurred in families with children and that medical indebtedness is distributed unevenly.

FURTHER READINGS

Bradbury, Samuel. *The Cost of Adequate Medical Care.* Chicago: University of Chicago Press, 1937. 86 pages.

Brewster, Agnes W. and McCamman, Dorothy. *Health Costs of the Aged.* Report No. 20, Division of Research and Statistics, Social Security Administration. Washington: U. S. Government Printing Office, 1956. 126 pages. (Includes references).

Bureau of Statistics and Department of National Health and Welfare. *Canadian Sickness Survey 1950-51: Family Expenditures for Health Services.* Special compilations Nos. 1, 2, 3. Ottawa, Canada: The Bureau, 1953.

Dickinson, Frank G. and Raymond, James. *The Economic Position of Medical Care, 1929-1953.* Bulletin 99, Bureau of Medical Economic Research, American Medical Association. Chicago: The Association, 1955. 36 pages.

Dodd, Paul A. and Penrose, E. F. *Economic Aspects of Medical Services.* Washington: Graphic Arts Press, 1939. 521 pages. (Includes references).

Falk, I. S., Rorem, C. Rufus, and Ring, Martha D. *The Costs of Medical Care.* Publication No. 27, Committee on the Costs of Medical Care. Chicago: University of Chicago Press, 1933. 623 pages.

Hollingsworth, Helen, Klem, Margaret C., and Baney, Anna Mae. *Medical Care and Costs in Relation to Family Income: A Statistical Source Book.* Memorandum No. 51 (2nd ed.), Bureau of Research and Statistics, Social Security Administration. Washington: U. S. Government Printing Office, 1947. 349 pages.

Huntington, Emily H. *Cost of Medical Care.* Berkeley, Calif.: University of California Press, 1951. 160 pages.

Serbein, Oscar N., Jr. *Paying for Medical Care in the United States.* New York: Columbia University Press, 1953. 543 pages. (Includes references).

Winslow, C.-E. A. *The Cost of Sickness and the Price of Health.* Monograph Series No. 7. Geneva: World Health Organization, 1951. 106 pages. (Includes references).

CHAPTER V

The Medical Care Team

MODERN MEDICAL CARE of high quality calls for the services of a large number of individuals, most of them professional and technical workers requiring specialized education and training. Many of the supporting members of the medical care team, the non-professional service and clerical workers for example, also require special training and orientation for a maximum contribution to health services. The lone physician, trained through apprenticeship, and assisted by members of the family, or a good neighbor, is no longer the symbol of good medical care.

The physician, however, remains the central figure in the provision of health services. The quality of those services will depend, in large measure, on the standards for the selection of physicians, and for their education and training. It will depend on whether there are enough physicians and where they are. Since physicians, as other health workers, are also people, the quality of the work they do will depend upon the satisfactions received from their work.

The modern physician is assisted, supported and often guided in the care of his patients, well or ill, by a literal host of other health workers, seen and unseen. The proper integration and coordination of the services of these many individuals into the functions of a team is one of the dynamic problems of modern medical care. The highest quality of care depends upon the successful achievement of such team function. Knowledge of the potential contributions of each member of the team, and respect for each member, underlies this achievement. This chapter, although it concentrates on the physician, introduces a few of the other professional members of the medical care team.

A. *The Physician: Education and Qualification*

24. MEDICAL EDUCATION: THE CONTEMPORARY SETTING *

THE PHYSICIAN is educated for responsible professional service to society and for individual achievement and advancement. After he has completed the long process of graduated introduction to the science of medicine, the art of its practice, and the responsibility for the care of patients, the state assumes responsibility for determining whether he shall be licensed to practice medicine. If a physician desires to become an expert in a specialty of medicine, he must pursue further study and training. Under existing state medical practice acts, however, any duly licensed physician has complete freedom of action within his state in the practice of medicine and surgery, and he himself is solely responsible for what he does. . . .

Medical education of the past has been concerned chiefly with education for the practice of curative medicine. Although the importance of preventive medicine and public health has received increasing recognition, it has not been widely appreciated that preventive medicine begins with those basic environmental conditions in the home, school, factory, and office which make for healthful living or its opposite. Doctors will always have ample work to do in repairing the damage of disease and maladjustment, but it is now generally recognized that some of this disability can be prevented through more positive and effective programs of preventive medicine. Medicine long since has moved beyond the problems of public health which have to do with epidemic infectious diseases. Although continued vigilance is necessary to control these diseases, the major problems of preventive medicine of the future lie in the new sphere of occupational disease, malnutrition, maladjustment, psychoneurosis, social deficiencies generally, and health education.

The scope of medicine has extended so greatly that it is no longer possible for the doctor to seek to solve problems of such magnitude single-handed. He cannot be an expert in every field in which the problems of personal maladjustment and social deficiency may arise; but he should be so familiar with the social system that he is keenly alert to detect points of friction which may lead to disability of the individual. This means that a professionally competent physician in the future must be a broadly informed, cultured person who can hold his own with and command the respect of leaders in every phase of human activity. It will not be enough for him to be technically competent as a professional man; he must be so educated as to have the social insight necessary to keep abreast of the changing requirements

* Reprinted by permission of the publishers and the Commonwealth Fund from Raymond B. Allen, M.D., *Medical Education and the Changing Order;* Cambridge, Mass.: Harvard University Press, 1946. (The excerpt reprinted, with omissions, is from Chap. III, "Medical Education and the Contemporary Social Process"). The author is the chancellor of the University of California at Los Angeles.

for healthful living imposed by new technical advances. Physicians of the future must be capable of taking their places as responsible leaders in the community and of viewing the problems of medical service dispassionately. Unless they recognize the right of every person to adequate medical service, the medical profession will degenerate to the level of a trade in which, as tradesmen, physicians will be concerned merely with the techniques of their trade. The medical profession cannot assume full responsibility for supplying complete medical service everywhere; it is no more responsible for the inadequacy of medical service in certain economically depressed regions of the country than teachers are responsible for the high illiteracy rates which are often found in the same places. It *is* under obligation, however, to cooperate fully with voluntary and public agencies so that together they may create the economic and social conditions which make possible an adequate medical service for all.

When economic and social conditions are improved generally, the level of professional services will rise almost automatically. The physician as a highly educated citizen shares responsibility with other community leaders in the endeavor to create the conditions which will improve the general economic and social well-being of the people as a whole. The medical profession should devise the techniques and procedures by which medical service can be distributed; the community as a whole should be responsible for making such plans economically feasible and socially practical and acceptable.

Has the medical profession of this country up to this time shown the necessary social vision to realize its opportunity and obligation to cooperate with the community at large under both voluntary and public auspices in conceiving and carrying out programs for the improved distribution of medical services? The answer is partly yes and partly no. It has cooperated with all levels of government in establishing and developing departments of public health which are concerned chiefly with phases of preventive medicine aiming to control epidemic disease, tuberculosis, venereal disease, nervous and mental disease, cancer, and occupational disease; it has supported the development of government-owned and operated hospitals for the armed forces and veterans and for the care of those civilian patients with nervous and mental diseases, tuberculosis, and contagious and venereal diseases; it has cooperated, although at first reluctantly, with industry, government, and workers in improving health services in industry and in establishing satisfactory workmen's compensation laws. After initial opposition, it did cooperate in establishing prepayment insurance plans for hospital care, and more recently for professional services, which are such a boon to families with modest incomes. The worst that should be said of the profession in respect to some of these socially enlightened and now obviously desirable improvements is that it did not show vigorous, imaginative leadership or social insight in its approach to them. Rather, it tended to hold back until public pressure was such that it had to go along.

The profession as an organization has debated the question of medical services for all beneficiaries of the Federal Social Security Act. A strong position against such an extension has been taken on the grounds that this degree of federal support would mean "state medicine" and the destruction of the independence of the profession. Without going into the pros and cons of this debate, one should point out that at the same time that the organized national profession has opposed proposals from governmental and non-governmental sources to help meet the problem of costs of professional (not hospital) services on a prepayment insurance basis, it has not come forward until recently with concrete plans of its own. On the other hand, some socially-conscious local medical societies, voluntary committees, and a great many progressive individuals in the profession have proposed and carried through plans based on the insurance principle of spreading the cost of professional services widely among many participants and so reducing the cost to the individual patient.

The organized profession has not been enthusiastic about plans to provide medical services on a businesslike basis, such as a clinic where medical services are offered at low cost. This is thought to be unfair competition; and often it is alleged that when a physician is placed on a salary by a clinic and is not personally responsible for charging a fee for services rendered, he loses his initiative and independence. However this may be, and the reader is entitled to his own opinion, the fact is that the organized profession has never interested itself vigorously in the question of establishing expensive specialty and laboratory services on such a basis that their cost to the public could be reduced and the services made readily available to all. It has remained for pioneering individuals to do so without benefit of help from organized medicine.

This is perhaps characteristic of any large group, and leadership is largely a function of individuals. A group tends to be protective in its organizational function and is interested primarily in the security of its vital interests as it understands them. It can be said with emphasis, however, that the organized medical profession has exhibited vigorous concern for the maintenance of high standards of medical education and hospital organization and practice. It has established many councils and committees which endeavor, usually with conspicuous success, to improve the quality of professional and technical services. It is only in the broader sphere of the economics and sociology of medical care, looking toward a wider distribution of high-quality medical service which will ultimately reach everyone in the country, that the profession as it expresses itself through its regular organizations has failed to meet some of its responsibilities to the society from which it derives its right to exist.

The crucial question is: *Does medical education share in the responsibility for the failure of the medical profession to exhibit social insight and aggressive leadership in molding public opinion toward a comprehensive handling of the problem of adequate medical care for all the people?* The answer is undoubtedly yes. The reason is that medical education of the past, which trained the current leaders of the organized profession, concentrated almost exclusively on the science, technology, and art of medicine—this was only natural, after all, because of the phenomenal progress in these fields. Adequate attention was not given to the social implications of medical practice and the social responsibility of the physician. Courses in public health largely concerned questions of epidemiology, water and milk purification, sera and vaccines, and subjects of like character. Such courses were important, to be sure, but they did not explore adequately the larger implications of preventive medicine and public health. There was, in short, little or no attention given to the social problem of how the new and rapidly expanding technology of medicine could be made widely available. This was left to chance. Medicine was not peculiar in this regard, for exactly the same thing occurred in every branch of applied science. It is probably true that this failure to assimilate the new dynamic technology on a socially efficient basis was one of the major causes of the current crisis in western civilization. . . .

Medical education today is increasingly aware that it must educate physicians to meet the problems of the future as well as those of the present in order to close the social gap between medical technology or the "know-how" and medical service or the "doing," for the benefit of all mankind. It is the responsibility of the school and university systems to so educate physicians that they will be as proficient in meeting and solving the social and economic problems of medical service as they are in handling the professional and technical problems of the practice of medicine.

25. Licensure in the United States *

THE IDEA OF MAKING the practice of medicine dependent on a license, a certificate issued by a competent body testifying that the bearer has undergone a training considered adequate, is an idea that originated in the Middle Ages. The European Middle Ages created an institution that was modified in the course of time but survived in its basic idea to the present day. The idea of licensing the medical profession resulted from the general structure of medieval society, which was strictly organized according to status, crafts, trades and professions. Each such vocational group had regulations, standard-setting codes, guaranteeing highly qualified services to society. It was recognized that such standards were particularly important in the case of the medical profession. In no other profession is lack of knowledge so serious in its consequences as in medicine. A wrong legal judgment can be corrected by a higher court. A wrong diagnosis or a wrong treatment may result in the death of the patient. No wonder society tried to protect itself from ignorant physicians. If the profession was to be respected and society was to have confidence in it, standards must be set, and the man living up to these standards had to testify legally that he was a real physician. In this way a clean-cut distinction was established between the physician who had undergone a prescribed training and the pseudophysician or quack. Great credit must be given to medieval society not only for having recognized the importance of these facts but for giving them a legal conformation and for having set an example for all time to come. . . .

* From: "The History of Medical Licensure," by Henry E. Sigerist, M.D.; *Journal of the American Medical Association* 104:1057-60, March 30, 1935 (No. 13). Reprinted (with omissions) by permission of the author and publishers. The author retired in 1947 from his position as director of the Institute of the History of Medicine at Johns Hopkins University in Baltimore to live in Switzerland, where he continued to write on the history of medicine until his death in 1957.

American Medicine

THE FACTS ARE well known concerning the development in this country, so that I can be brief. American medicine went in 300 years through all the periods through which European medicine had gone in more than 2,000 years. In the beginnings, here just as in ancient Greece, medical practice was not controlled. Physicians were badly wanted, and whoever was able and willing to help was therefore welcome. There was some quackery, to be sure, but in the early colonial times the number of quacks was undoubtedly not large. In the small cities, where everybody knew everybody else, it was easy to learn who had real medical knowledge and who had not. Physicians were trained the same as hippocratic doctors, by serving an apprenticeship with a physician, and the only diploma was a certificate issued by the physician, testifying as to how long and how successfully the apprentice had served.

Toward the end of the colonial period, and right after the Revolution, the need for a stricter control of medical practice was felt, and, just as in medieval Europe, so in this country was the doctor's degree of a medical school, foreign as well as American, considered a guaranty for adequate medical knowledge. The universities in this country, however, were not numerous. Their purpose in the beginning was not to replace the system of apprenticeship but rather to complete it. Many students could not afford to go abroad, and many entered practice without having studied at any medical school at home. Who was to confer the license on them? Just as the Royal College of Physicians in London and in Edinburgh became very influential licensing bodies, so the medical societies organized in this country in many states became the agencies controlling medical practice and conferring licenses. This was the case in Massachusetts in 1781 and in New Hampshire in the same year. So far, the development had been very sound and the conditions were very similar to those in England. In addition, several states, New York in 1760 and New Jersey in 1772, attempted a state regulation of medicine by appointing boards of examiners.

The tremendous development in the nineteenth century, the opening up of a continent, created entirely new conditions. Physicians were wanted more than ever before, and endless medical schools were founded, many of them with quite insufficient equipment. The licenses conferred by these schools did not mean much. Besides, an institution developed that had no parallel in Europe—the growth of organized and recognized medical sects that paralyzed the efforts of the medical organizations, as well as those of the state boards. At the time of the Civil War, conditions were chaotic; but after the war the readjustment followed rapidly. As the medical schools could not be trusted, the states, or some agencies representing the states, had to take over the control of medical practice. From 1873 on, beginning in Texas, state boards of medical examiners were established, and by 1895 nearly all the states had such an institution. Every one knows what a fundamental part these boards have played in reorganization of medicine in this country. If America today has a high standard of medical profession and if American medicine is playing an ever-increasing role in world medicine, this is not least due to their activities. They were influential in the reform of medical education and succeeded in raising the standards gradually and constantly. The establishment of the National Board of Medical Examiners in 1915 was a further step in this development.

If the conditions in this country are compared with those in Europe, it will be found that they are similar to those which prevailed in most European countries in the beginning of the nineteenth century. The student has to pass two examinations before two different bodies, one for the degree and one for the license. Just as the medical schools of Europe were reorganized in the beginning of the nineteenth century, so they have been from 1893 on in this country. If the development is to follow the general trend, the next phase would be to reentrust the medical schools with the examination of the candidates, whereby the examinations could be controlled by the representatives of the state boards or national board. I know, of course, that the conditions here are different from those in Europe, that the standard of schools is not yet equally high, and that the different states have different problems to face. . . .

Conclusion

IF I MAY add a personal remark, it is that I do not believe either in tests or in examinations. They are a necessity, as no better method has yet been found, but it is well known that certain students have a special ability to pass examinations while otherwise brilliant students quite often show strong inhibitions in examinations. It is also known that actual knowledge alone does not make a good physician, that the character and the whole personality have to be taken into consideration very strongly. In order to judge whether a man is fit to practice medicine or not, one must first of all know him and must have observed him at the bedside of the patient. The longer one has known him, the more will one be able to pass judgment on him.

The history of medical licensure begins in the Middle Ages. It is a unique feature in the history of medicine, in that the very beginning, the initial solution of the problem, was so perfect that a development of nearly 800 years could not improve it.

B. *The Physician: Manpower and Distribution*

26. IS THERE A SHORTAGE OF PHYSICIANS? *

Increased Rural Medical Service

I WAS BORN and raised in Pike County, a rural section of west-central Illinois. Pike County is bounded on the east by the Illinois River and on the west by the Missis-

* From: *Supply of Physicians' Services* (Bulletin 81, Bureau of Medical Economic Research, American Medical Association), by Frank G. Dickinson; Chicago: American Medical Association, 1951. Reprinted (with omissions, including initial paragraphs) by permission of the author and publishers. The author is the director of the Bureau of Medical Economic Research, American Medical Association, Chicago.

sippi. It is 45 to 70 miles north and slightly west of St. Louis. A county bounded by two rivers is interlaced with creeks and streams and is hilly. On the whole, it would be classed as a poor county because of the land. My home town is Griggsville, whose population has fluctuated around 1,200. The largest town in the county is Pittsfield, the county seat. During my boyhood there were rarely fewer than four physicians in Griggsville. I recall one instance in which there was an emergency need for a physician on a morning when they all were out in the country on calls. The roads were so muddy that not one of them could get back to town within an hour.

I also recall my first contact with the word appendicitis. One of my grade school classmates did not come to school one morning, and the teacher told us that she was very ill with what the doctor called "inflammation of the bowel." We children snickered a little at such frankness on the part of the teacher—that was in 1911. The next day the teacher told us that our classmate had died of appendicitis and wrote "appendicitis" on the blackboard because it was a new word to us. She said that the girl had been brought by her father to the local railroad station, where they had to wait for a train, which was an hour late. The physician accompanied them westward about 32 miles where they were switched onto another railroad line which brought them eventually to Quincy, Ill. The child died soon after she reached the hospital. The teacher told us that the trip from the child's farm to Quincy required six hours. The distance is about 39 or 40 miles.

During many of the years since 1917, there has been no physician in town. Recently I studied the experiences of physicians in Pike County, one of whom practiced in Griggsville from 1923 to 1938. The population of the county declined from 27,000 in 1920 to 22,000 in 1950. There are 16 practicing physicians in the county now; whereas there were 42 in 1923. The number of persons per physician has more than doubled. But the fact that I want to bring out is that these 16 physicians can serve more people now than 42 physicians could 25 to 30 years ago. Why?

This question would be easy for many physicians to answer, especially those who have practiced in rural communities. Being an economist, I went about the matter in what may be considered an odd way. The first step was to consider what other occupational group in Pike County, Ill. might have had a somewhat similar experience during the same period of several decades. I went to the village postmaster, to whom many people in rural towns would go for information. I spoke with an older man who had once served as postmaster in Griggsville. As we discussed the decline in the number of physicians in the county, the postmaster made the observation that improvements in the road system in the county have been tremendously important to the physicians. The most important change in the road system was not the development of the few paved roads in the county but rather in the back roads, where a little grading, a new bridge or culvert, some oil or gravel create an all-weather rural road. . . .

I submit that medical school educators and other students of medical care can learn almost as much about the question of the physician shortage in rural areas in America by studying the whole question of rural mail service as they can by studying the number, the ages and distribution of rural physicians. The practice of medicine can never be isolated from the forces of economic and social evolution. The practice of medicine cannot stand still when the whole way of life of people in other occupations is in the process of changing. Any economic service becomes a part of that social evolution.

But hard roads, automobiles and what happened to another occupational group as a result of these changes do not tell the whole story regarding the doubling of the number of persons per physician in Pike County. I mentioned the death of my classmate whose home, 4½ miles south of Griggsville, was 39 or 40 miles from Quincy. But, instead of being six hours away, it is now about one hour away. Yet that is not the important question in this picture of change. Would another child similarly stricken with appendicitis have to go to Quincy for an operation? She might choose Quincy, or she might go east to Jacksonville which would be somewhat closer (45 minutes away). She might even be taken to St. Louis, with its splendid medical and hospital facilities, in about one and a half to two hours. On the other hand, she might be taken to the 43 bed Illini Community Hospital in Pittsfield, which was erected in 1942—a trip of some 10 to 15 minutes. In fact, if she felt extremely ill, the physician might suggest that she go to the hospital immediately, where there would be better facilities for examination. If her father did not have an automobile or it was in the garage for repairs, there would be many neighbors who could be reached quickly by telephone who could take her to Pittsfield, Quincy, Jacksonville or even St. Louis. A child today would be far closer to a physician than one in 1911 in terms of lifesaving minutes even if there were no physician in Griggsville or Pittsfield and if there were no hospital in Pittsfield.

In our study of "medical service areas," which is based on the trading area principle, the central two-thirds of Pike County has been included in a medical service area (number 394) which has Quincy as its center. This area extends across the Mississippi River into Missouri. I am sorry that there was no similar delineation of medical service areas in 1920. For that reason I have had to make my historical comparisons on the basis of the number of persons per physician in the county—a geographic basis of comparison which I abhor because it is a political, not an economic, area. Little reliance can be placed on physician-population ratios for medical service areas. One of the reasons why fewer physicians are actually needed in Pike County is that trading areas have expanded. Some of the persons in Pike County obtain some of their medical care in Quincy (Adams County), in Jacksonville (Brown County) and in other larger towns.

Technological Progress in Medical Care

SOME OF MY PHYSICIAN friends have been gentle in their criticism of my use of statistical procedures in the studies of the supply and distribution of physicians. I have stated repeatedly that 1,000 physicians in 1950 could (and did) render at least one third more medical service than could 1,000 physicians in 1940. (A rough index of the quantity of medical services delivered by physicians can be obtained by dividing the index of expenditures for physicians' services by its price index.

Using this procedure, I have found that the amount of physicians' services increased at least one third per physician between 1940 and 1950.) I have referred to this as an "increase in output" per physician and as technological progress in the practice of medicine. The increase in the total output also reflects an increase in demand. The increase in demand warrants more consideration than I can give it in this report. The most phenomenal fact of medical economics is the terrific rate of technological progress in the medical care industry in recent years. The tremendous changes in medical practice wrought by the introduction of the wonder drugs, the expanded use of auxiliary personnel by physicians, even the assistance given by other physicians in or not in private practice, and the increase in the percentage of patients treated in the office and in the hospital, rather than in the home, have combined to greatly increase the technological efficiency of physicians. As an economist, I strongly suspect that this rate of increase in output per person exceeds the comparable rate in the manufacture of automobiles, the production of coal, the transportation of commodities, in fact, in practically any industry that could be named. I hope that no one will consider these comparisons as invidious or improper for one in my position to make. I am trying to throw light on a very important question for the medical profession. I am trying to explain why I sincerely believe that as a result of present trends we are more likely to have more physicians than we need in the United States in the 1960's than we are to have fewer. Surely if the tremendous rate of increased productivity is continued throughout the 1950's, those who are concerned with medical education must plan accordingly. No one knows how long the present war emergency will last or can be sure of the type of warfare which may ultimately be our lot. But still physicians must be educated for a working lifetime; they cannot become surplus after a war.

Certain statisticians in the United States Public Health Service have predicted a dire shortage of 17,000 to 47,000 physicians in 1960. These three authors did not prove a shortage, they merely assumed a shortage. In fact, if there had been twice as many physicians in 1940 in each of the 126 "health service areas" which they laid out, the shortage in 1960 would have been twice as great by their methods of computation. Similarly the 1960 shortage would have been one half as great if there had been half as many physicians in each one of these areas in 1940. More generally, these authors have really shown that there was a shortage of about 50,000,000 people in the United States in 1940 if their methods of estimating shortages are applicable to other professions and occupations. . . .

Is There a Shortage of Physicians?

THE INCREASE in the number of medical school graduates from 5,100 in 1949 to a projected 7,000 around 1960 should give pause for reflection. Are we laymen going to say that there is a shortage of physicians until there is one in every block in our cities and one in every community with more than 100 people? Of the approximately 42,000 areas (cities, towns, villages, whether incorporated or unincorporated) in the United States with a 1940 population of 100 or over, between

16,000 and 17,000 places have one or more physicians, counting all physicians; thus more than one-third of all the 42,000 places have a physician. Most studies of distribution ignore the 38,500 towns, villages and hamlets of less than 2,500 population. I doubt that drug stores, hardware stores, electricians or plumbers can be found in that many towns of 100 or more people. Are we laymen going to say that there is a shortage of physicians if one has to spend more than 30 minutes getting to a physician or travel more than 30 miles? Is there a shortage of medical schools unless every qualified candidate can be admitted to medical school? We also need chemists, physicists and elementary and secondary school teachers. The public has an interest in promoting the training of all these professions.

Before one can determine whether a shortage exists in any profession, one must make up one's own mind about the functions of the members of that profession. I deem it to be the function of the medical profession to relieve pain and to increase the length of useful life. This must also mean an increase in the number of persons dying later in life from diseases common in older persons. I observe that excellent progress is being made in the performance of these functions. . . .

. . . We have had enough physicians to enable more and more persons to die later in life. I have no illusions about adequate medical care, for there can be no such thing as adequate medical care to the family of a dying person. The best simply is not good enough, but medical care can and will get better and better.

There is yet another way to indicate how well the physician is performing his function. Although heart disease kills about four and a half times as many people as fatal accidents and although heart disease cuts off about twice as many unrealized remaining life years as fatal accidents, it is nevertheless true that fatal accidents cut off more years from the working lifetimes of the American people (ages 20 to 65) than does heart disease or any other one natural cause of death. Thus the prevention of fatal accidents has become the number one job of preventive medicine in the United States if one is thinking about the productive and military strength of the nation. I appreciate that the number of deaths or the number of years of life cut off by death may be an equally valuable criterion for rating the causes of death.

Let me also examine the function of the physician in a somewhat baleful light. Has medical progress been too rapid during the twentieth century? As for myself and my family the answer is "no." But as a student of the social sciences I might well ask whether it is entirely good to have so many older persons alive. Can medical progress ever be too rapid for our social institutions to digest? If there is anything wrong with medical progress in this century, is it the fact that we have had too much instead of too little? But I think that before anyone can say that there is an alarming shortage of physicians, he must grapple with the problem presented by this simple statistic: Since 1900 the entire population of the United States has doubled, but the population age 65 and over has quadrupled. Does that statistic indicate that the American medical profession is not performing its function and that larger numbers of additional physicians are needed?

There is one curious aspect of this question of shortage which I have heard and read a number of times. The claim is made that the physician has not been responsible for most of the gains in reducing the death rate from the diseases of child-hood, but that the credit should be given to the plumber, the house builder, the sanitary engineer, the immunizer and, of course, to the march of science. Some persons apparently believe that drug stores or even grocery stores should be per-mitted to sell powerful drugs over the counter, which would eliminate the necessity of a physician's diagnosis and prescription. The persons who make this claim get themselves into a terrible position when they add that there is an alarming shortage of physicians. Stated in the very simplest terms, their claim is that physicians are not responsible for health gains, yet there is an alarming shortage of physicians.

About two-fifths of the active physician population of the United States joined the armed services during World War II. On Jan. 1, 1945 there were 60,101 physi-cians in government service according to the estimates of the Directory Department of the American Medical Association. Roughly this meant that 60 percent of the physicians remained at home to take care of the 90 per cent of the population which remained civilian. What happened? The health of the American people continued to improve. I am not saying that I think that fewer physicians are better, but I would like to point out to any student of supply and demand problems that the supply of physicians was stretched during World War II and the results were amazing. This stretching of supply may be thought of as a social experiment in testing the supply. If World War III were to be fought as World War II was fought, I do not believe there is a single person who would contend seriously that several tens of thousands of physicians, for example, 30,000, could not be spared to the armed services. Physicians are professional persons, and the quantity and quality of medical care delivered by them is subject to great flexibility. There would un-doubtedly be differences of opinion as to how long these tens of thousands of physicians could be spared to the armed services without lowering the health of civilians. And, of course, there is speculation about the kinds of auxiliary personnel that would be needed in the event of war in this country.

But the 60,101 physicians in government service on Jan. 1, 1945 are strong evidence of a "surplus" of physicians in the early 1940's. Has that surplus evapo-rated? This brings me to my general thesis: If the present upward trend in output per physician is continued, the number of physicians per 100,000 population need not remain constant but could decline moderately and slowly while health progress is continued. Yet our physician-population ratio has been rising for more than 20 years, and Mountin, Pennell and Berger predict it will be even higher in 1960. At last report our ratio was the highest of any country in the world except for Palestine with its many refugee physicians. More generally, the ratio to population for any occupational group may rise or fall in the process of economic and social evolution. The ratio for rural mail carriers has, of course, declined. Change alone requires that some must rise and some must fall. . . .

Summary and Conclusions

I HAVE TRIED to show that the supply of physicians' services has been expanding at a very rapid rate. I have not intended to say that the geographic distribution of physicians is perfect. I assume that it is imperfect and that there will always be attractive openings for physicians in some cities, towns and villages. The number of physicians writing to the American Medical Association wanting to locate or relocate is now in excess of the number of communities requesting physicians. This reverses the situation of 1946, 1947, 1948 and early 1949. The tide has turned. But in terms of results it seems to me that the general analysis points toward a surplus or a potential surplus of physicians rather than a deficit. The physicians' fees have risen a little more rapidly than half as fast as the cost of living index of all consumer prices. It stands to reason that this index of physicians' fees, as reported by the United States Bureau of Labor Statistics, would have risen much faster if there had been such an alarming shortage of physicians. Average net incomes of physicians have just kept pace with the rise in national income per capita. I conclude that the supply of physicians' services has been increasing at an extremely reasonable rate—favorable to the health of the American people, fast enough to meet the increased demand and sufficient to prevent any unduly sharp general increase in physicians' fees.

I have tried to place the supply of physicians in its proper setting, with only a brief look into the future. I have further narrowed my report to a consideration of physicians as an entity. The demand for physicians could be broken down into the demand for each specialty, but I believe that the direction of physicians into these specialties is a problem for educators rather than for an economist. The results of a study which was recently completed indicate that the free forces of supply and demand in a very disturbed period worked to produce a more even distribution of specialists and of general practitioners (including part-time specialists) in relation to state populations in 1949 than in 1938.

. . . I sometimes think that the only measure of quantity in a profession is quality. High standards of medical education buttress our medical licensure laws and, in turn, assure the people that the physician who holds life in his hands is qualified to assume that awesome responsibility. Whereas a student who wishes to do graduate work in physics or chemistry may go to a class A, class B, class C or even a class D school and receive his degree of doctor of science or doctor of philosophy, a physician must be graduated from a class A medical school to be licensed to practice his profession in all but a few of our states. Thus the contrast between the almost unlimited chances to become a graduate student in chemistry or physics in schools of grades A to D and the limited openings for medical students could be eliminated by repeal of all state medical licensure laws! The demand for quality, to which society has given legal sanction by the state licensure laws, both raises the price of medical education and vastly complicates the task of increasing the number of students quickly.

Finally, our medical schools at present and the other schools that train auxiliary medical personnel have made possible enough medical services to provide the American people with the highest level of health of any large nation and even above that of some of the smaller, traditionally healthiest nations. We have had enough physicians to achieve a truly remarkable record of health progress. Is there any better measure of the supply of physicians' services or of the supply of rural mail carriers' services than performance?

At your meeting three years ago, I discussed the supply of physicians' services and made some references to our study of the distribution of physicians by medical service areas. This study, started in 1947, is nearing completion and should be published in April of this year as Bulletin 94, "Distribution of Physicians by Medical Service Areas." In this paper I will present a brief sketch of the two score conclusions of this study.*

... This morning I shall talk about the supply situation in April, 1950, when the census of population was taken. I shall refrain from any speculations regarding the situation that might exist in 1960. We have spent our time and effort trying to find out what the supply situation was in April, 1950, rather than what it should have been then or what it will be or should be in 1960.

Findings

1. ONE-SIXTH of the land area of the United States was beyond a 25 mile radius from the closest physician in active private practice, but only one-sixth of one per cent of the people resided in these areas beyond the 25 mile radius. Almost 89% of these areas and three-fourths of the population of these areas were in the Mountain and Pacific regions.

2. The circle of fixed radius, the town, or the county are poor areas for indicating the supply of physicians. A fixed radius has implications in the wide open sections of the West different from those in the crowded communities along the eastern seaboard. The town as an area must be rejected as an area because many persons do not live in towns. The county must be rejected as an area because persons cross county boundary lines to do their trading as if those boundaries did not exist.

3. Every place (city, town, or village) over 5,000 population had at least one active practitioner, and 96% of the places with 2,500 to 5,000 population and 88% of the places with 1,000 to 2,500 population had an active practitioner. Slightly more than one-fifth of the places between 100 and 1,000 population had an active practitioner; moreover, three-fifths of the places between 750 and 1,000 population had an active physician, and almost one-half of the small towns under 1,000 population had less than 250 inhabitants. But, as stated above, a town is not an acceptable area.

4. The trading area provides a unit for study of the trading habits of the

---

* From: "How Bad Is the Distribution of Physicians?" by Frank G. Dickinson; *Journal of the American Medical Association* 154:1209-11, April 13, 1954 (No. 14). Reprinted (with omissions) by permission of the author and publishers. The author is the director of the Bureau of Medical Economic Research, American Medical Association, Chicago.

people. It alone can be used for grouping together physicians and the persons whom they serve.

5. Marketing researchers classify goods as convenience, fashion, or service and have delineated areas for many commodities and services within each of the three categories. Since the services of the physician do not fall completely into any one of these categories used in marketing research, it was necessary to describe a completely new set of areas, which we have called medical service areas.

6. A trading area is described by its centers and boundaries. A primary trading center is a town that draws considerable trade from the surrounding territory and loses relatively little trade to other towns. We adapted this definition of the primary center in defining a primary medical service center, as a town which, relative to the surrounding territory, was a primary source of physicians' services.

7. In the literature on trading areas, the United States has been divided into many areas—as few as 13 and as many as 1,461. The type of commodity or service under study influences the number of areas. In our study we found 757 areas. It is a pure coincidence that a study of health districts by the United States Public Health Service in 1945 divided the country into 760 areas, only 3 more than our 757. . . .

9. Actually, there were four distinct steps in the preliminary part of this investigation, which was reported in our bulletins 80 and 80A. First, the 1,051 primary centers were selected. Second, the areas were bounded. Third, those primary centers that offered every type of medical service and surgery were further classified as prime-primary centers; we designated 88 cities as prime-primary centers, although undoubtedly there are more than 88 prime-primary centers today. Fourth, all other places with one or more physicians were designated as secondary centers. These secondary centers should be considered as centers of small "areas" within the larger medical services areas. Of these 14,141 secondary centers 6,109 had only one physician but each of 45 secondary centers had more than 100 physicians. . . .

10. The 14,141 secondary centers were divided into two classes; about 13,000 had at least one active physician, and about 1,000 did not have a general practitioner, part-time specialist, or full-time specialist. Moreover, about 5,300 places had only one active physician; "one-doctor towns," if you please. About 156,000 of the 205,000 physicians in the 48 states and the District of Columbia in April, 1950, were classified as being in active private practice. In other words, three-fourths of all physicians were in active private practice and one-fourth were inactive; roughly, one-half of the inactive were interns or residents and the other half of the inactive were mostly federal physicians or retired and not in practice. . . .

11. Two-thirds of all physicians and 42% of the United States population were located in the 1,051 primary centers. The percentages were 68% of all physicians, 66% of active physicians, and 83% of the full-time specialists. In passing, I might say that these percentages compare rather favorably with the percentage of trade that is done in the primary trading centers selected by marketing researchers, a fact that is not surprising, because the physician is one of many who sells his services.

12. I shall have more to say regarding population-physician ratios for each medical service area, even though such ratios are very inefficient measures of the

supply of physicians' services. At this point note that we found 731 persons per physician in the United States in April, 1950, counting all physicians, and a national ratio of population per active physician of 958.

13. In our study, we examined 33 characteristics of each of the 757 medical service areas. . . . I hardly need to tell this audience that it would be unreasonable to expect uniformity in population-physician ratios or in any other characteristic of these areas. From the standpoint of the statistician, however, the most important result of these computations was a clear indication that the relative variation in population-physician ratios was much smaller than the relative variation in most of our other 31 characteristics of each area. Stated in more general terms, population-physician ratios varied less than most of the other characteristics of the areas. I feel certain that every person here will be very pleased to know that population per active physician was among the most stable characteristics of the 757 medical service areas.

14. In examining the extreme values in the arrays, the medical service areas located in the Mountain states were the most noticeable; for example, their areas were the largest, had the fewest people, and the lowest population density. And, as you would expect, three-fourths of the Mountain areas had no interns.

High and Low Ratio Areas

15. IN BULLETIN 94 we have placed our major analytical emphasis on the 75 areas that had the highest and the 75 areas with the lowest number of persons per physician. In stressing the top 10% and the bottom 10% of the 757 areas, we deliberately avoided stress upon the middle 80% of the areas. We thought that stress on the extreme areas would meet "head on" many questions about the distribution of physicians in the United States, as most such questions do deal with extreme areas.

16. There are two sets of 75 high and 75 low ratio areas, one based on all physicians and one based on only active physicians. Since there is not time to cover both sets of ratios, I shall stress the high-active and low-active areas. Since 63 of the areas were both high-all and high-active, only 87 different high-ratio areas were analyzed in detail; likewise, only 94 different low-ratio areas were similarly analyzed. . . .

18. The more important contrasts between the 75 high-active and 75 low-active areas should be helpful.

(*a*) They were quite similar in size, but the 75 low-active areas had 12 times as many inhabitants and were 13 times as densely populated as the 75 high-active areas.

(*b*) During the 1940's when the population of the United States increased 14%, the population of the high-active areas increased less than 3% as compared with an increase of more than 17% for the low-active areas.

(*c*) Only 2,020 active physicians served the 4,700,000 persons in the high-active areas, or 2,320 persons per active physician, whereas almost 81,000 active physicians served 56,000,000 inhabitants of the low-active areas or only 690 persons per active physician. The ratios range from 5,100 down to 2,020 in the high-active areas and from 900 down to 380 in the low-active areas.

(*d*) Whereas 49% of the active physicians of the United States were general practitioners, 66% in the high-active and only 45% in the low-active areas were in general practice, and, whereas 36% of the active practitioners in the United States were full-time specialists, only 16% in the high-active and 42% in the low-active areas were full-time specialists.

(*e*) Maternal mortality and infant mortality rates were distinctly higher than the national rate in the high-active areas and somewhat below the national rates in the low-active areas. Before jumping to the conclusion that the trouble in the high-active areas was only the fewness of physicians, one should note that in them only 58% of the births were in hospitals compared with 87% for the entire United States and 97% for the low-active areas. The lower percentage of hospital births undoubtedly indicated a large number of factors—among which the general level of health education was unquestionably important.

(*f*) In the high-active areas, there were no medical schools and no prime-primary medical service centers, but in the low-active areas, there were 50 of the 72 four-year medical schools and 42 of the 88 prime-primary medical service centers.

(*g*) The per capita buying power of the high-ratio areas did not present an extreme contrast with the national figure, although the high-ratio areas were below the national figure and low-ratio areas were above it.

(*h*) The total number of centers, including both the primary and the secondary, was less than 700 in the high-active and almost 3,400 in the low-active areas; and the medians were 6 and 31.

(*i*) In general, the physicians in the high-ratio areas were older than those in the low-ratio areas, which is consistent with the sharp difference in population growth.

(*j*) Of the 75 high-active areas, 29 were sparsely settled, 29 were characterized by small-scale farming and small-scale industry, 8 by large-scale farming or cattle raising, 4 by mining, and the remaining 5 might be called urbanized. In contrast, most of the 75 low-active areas were highly urbanized.

(*k*) How many extra physicians would have been required in the high-active areas to have made the maximum ratio 2,000 persons per physician? Only 361! This is less than one-fourth of 1% of the 156,500 United States total! Insofar as this study reveals any possible figure which might remotely be called "a national physician shortage of 1950"—and I do not believe there was a shortage in 1950—it is 361 as a maximum. . . .

(*l*) Some may quarrel with 2,000 as a theoretical maximum ratio for any area as a criterion for judging the excellence of physician distribution. A critic of the attempts of federal bureaucrats to prove a national shortage once told me that if there were no more than 2,000 persons per active physician in a meaningful area, he would consider the distribution excellent and proof of an adequate national supply. Obviously, his standard, like other area standards, inherently assumes a national shortage. His standard is, admittedly, high. Yet it may serve some useful purpose. (The 2,000 maximum ratio is independent of the fact that there were 75 areas that had higher ratios.) Perhaps other critics would claim that a nation is not well supplied with physicians unless no meaningful area has more than 1,500 persons per active physician. Applied to the 262 areas in April, 1950, that had more than 1,500 persons per active physician, an additional 2,530 physicians would have been required under this standard. I daresay that neither 361 nor 2,530 is an alarming national deficit—if any existed—requiring heroic measures. One can, of course, choose any premise he wishes and then prove, at least for himself, that there is, was, or will be a national shortage of physicians. . . .

Summary of Results

1. THE DISTRIBUTION of physicians in the United States in April, 1950, in relation to the persons whom they served, was excellent but not perfect.

2. Physicians and the patients they serve vary so much that population-physician ratios are not good measures of supply. In a phrase, we hope that, by computing them for medical service areas rather than for political areas, we have made population-physician ratios "less worse." The relative variation in population-physician ratios computed for counties was much higher than for ratios computed for the 757 medical service areas—the only "trading" areas ever published for the entire United States that entirely ignore all county and most state boundary lines.

3. Our only speculation on that nebulous subject, "a national physician shortage," is our comment that 361 additional physicians would have been required in April, 1950, in the 75 high-active areas to make our maximum area ratio 2,000 instead of 5,100 persons per active physician. That is intended to be a somewhat pointed comment for the special benefit of those who have predicted a shortage anywhere from 22,000 to 49,000 in 1954 or 1960. One can choose any premise he wishes and then prove, on the basis of that premise, that there is, was, or will be a national shortage or surplus. . . .

27. NEED FOR PHYSICIANS: PRESENT AND FUTURE *

THE UNITED STATES now has the largest number of physicians in relation to the total population in its recent history. Its present position in the quality of medical care reflects the standards of medical education set and maintained by the medical profession through the Council on Medical Education and Hospitals of the American

* From: *America's Health: A Report to the Nation by the National Health Assembly;* New York: Harper, 1949 (Chap. I, "What Is the Nation's Need for Health and Medical Personnel?" pp. 2-7, 24-25). Reprinted (with omissions, including initial paragraphs) by permission of the publishers.

Medical Association, the Association of American Medical Colleges, and the State Boards. These standards require adequate personal supervision by instructors and adequate space, equipment, and material per student in the two years of pre-clinical work in anatomy, physiology, chemistry, pharmacology, pathology, and bacteriology. In the subsequent two years of clinical instruction, each student—working individually in the wards and outpatient departments of well-equipped teaching hospitals—must be responsible for supervised observation and treatment of at least three new ward patients a week, selected for their teaching value, and in outpatient departments must have similar contact with three new patients a day.

Medicine is not a science that can be taught to large classes by didactic methods. Minimum standards—surpassed in the better medical schools—call for at least 1 instructor to each 25 students in preclinical courses and for 1 instructor to each 8 or 10 students in clinical classes. Substandard schools have practically disappeared from the American scene in the last forty years; their return would spell disaster. Any hastily conceived plan to establish new schools or greatly increase the enrollment in already overcrowded existing schools would threaten our major safeguards to the quality of instruction and competence of graduates.

The annual rate of production of physicians has increased materially during the past twenty-five years, partly because of the accelerated medical-school courses that prevailed during the war. With the return to peace-time schedules the production rate will probably reach 5,600 new graduates a year, and as students complete their four-year courses in six new medical schools,* and in others that will doubt-less be established, the supply of physicians will continue to increase. According to estimates of the American Medical Association, we can predict a ratio of one physician for each 707 or 717 persons by 1960, depending on the population estimate used. Of these physicians, possibly about 4 to 6 per cent will be retired or not in active practice.

To avoid overproduction of physicians, as was apparently the case in the depression years in view of the limited demand for their services, long-range needs for additional physicians require careful study of possible fluctuations in the economic cycle and of many economic factors which affect the practice of medicine. Under the stress of war, 60 per cent of the nation's physicians were able to serve 91 per cent of the population. Indications which point to a more efficient use of physicians in the future are improved and expanded hospital facilities, additional

---

* The "new medical schools" referred to in the text are: University of Washington School of Medicine (Seattle); Southwestern Medical College of the University of Texas (Dallas); Bowman Gray School of Medicine of Wake Forest College (Winston-Salem, N.C.); School of Medicine of the University of California at Los Angeles; Medical College of Alabama (Birmingham); and College of Medicine of the University of Utah (Salt Lake City). Four-year medical schools that have been established since the National Health Assembly met in 1948 include: University of Miami School of Medicine (Coral Gables, Fla.); University of North Carolina School of Medicine (Chapel Hill); Seton Hall College of Medicine (Jersey City, N. J.); University of Florida Medical School (Gainesville); Albert Einstein College of Medicine (New York); and University of Puerto Rico School of Medicine (San Juan). In addition, plans have been under way at the following universities since 1955 for conversion of existing two-year basic science programs to four-year medical schools: University of West Virginia (Morgantown); University of Mississippi (Jackson); and University of Missouri (Columbia). A new four-year school is also being organized at the University of Kentucky, in Lexington.

health centers, easier transportation, extension of group practice, expanded public health programs, increased use of auxiliary personnel, and discovery of more highly effective therapeutic agents. On the other hand, the adequacy of the ratio of physicians to the future population must be determined in relation to the higher illness rates among an aging population, the wider use of personnel and facilities with the extension of prepayment plans for medical care and hospitalization, and the probable increased number of physicians in the Federal service, in hospitals and health centers, and in research and teaching positions. The present shortages of physicians in some places and fields of activity stem from social and economic conditions which the medical profession believes need correction on a local basis before any attempts are made to augment greatly the supply of physicians in the United States.

Though opinions * differed on the need for definite and immediate steps to increase the annual number of medical-school graduates, many pleas were made for measures to avoid existing and future shortages of physicians in certain fields of work. Evidence of the lack of public health officers, psychiatrists, physicians for the armed forces and other Federal agencies, and of shortages of physicians in rural areas and among Negroes was presented to the Section [on the Nation's Need for Health and Medical Personnel] in its own discussions and in reports received from representatives of other sections of the [National Health] Assembly. . . .

Much of the difficulty of attracting physicians to the Federal service and to rural areas, it was argued [within the Section] on the one hand, can be ascribed— like the shortage of Negro physicians—more to professional, cultural, and economic conditions than to the insufficient numbers now being graduated from the medical schools; areas and agencies in genuine need of more physicians should therefore attempt to provide conditions—as the Federal service has lately tried to do—which will make practice more attractive. On the other hand, some members of this Section urged that strong statements be made to indicate that the Section on Personnel recognizes the need for (1) more and better training in preventive medicine, psychiatry, and pediatrics, (2) personnel of the highest caliber for teaching and research positions in schools and hospitals, (3) better undergraduate, hospital, and postgraduate training in maternal and child health, (4) opportunities for postgraduate training for rural physicians, (5) externships and residencies for medical students in rural hospitals, (6) formation of a joint committee of medical educators and rural people to improve the orientation of medical education toward the social and technical problems of the rural health services, (7) inclusion of osteopaths in the estimates of the number of physicians available, (8) having medical schools and hospitals recognize and assume a continuing responsibility for keeping their graduates abreast of new developments in medicine, and (9) representation of consumers in studies of the extent to which medical schools are meeting the demand for physicians.

The [Section's] subcommittee on physicians, expressing an unwillingness to modify its report to include specific recommendations on these points, agreed that

* i.e., within the Health Assembly's Section on the Nation's Need for Health and Medical Personnel, whose discussion formed the basis for the chapter (Chapter I) in the published report of the Assembly's proceedings from which this excerpt has been selected.

they were appropriate for inclusion in a separate supplementary report by the Section's chairman.* ...

In a profession like medicine, requiring as it does some five or six years before a student can complete his schooling and internship, preparation to meet any fixed goal of supply for any future year needs advance planning. That goal, moreover, must be carefully established in relation to the probable demand for physicians' services. Estimates of the extent to which people in the United States will seek and receive medical care will depend on the assumptions made concerning the number and distribution of active physicians in relation to the size of the population of the area, employment and purchasing power, health habits, existing health programs and facilities, and the number of physicians serving special groups such as servicemen and veterans. Estimates of future demand therefore require setting some year like 1940 as a base line and some future year like 1960 as an end point, assuming from past experience the probable future rates of graduation, retirement, and death of physicians to derive a reasonable estimate of the available supply, and similarly making certain assumptions from recent trends in fertility, immigration, and mortality to figure the probable size of the population. These assumptions, furthermore, must be revised from time to time to take account of newer and better information. ...

Report of Subcommittee on Physicians

YOUR COMMITTEE finds that the following major forces are creating an increased demand for physicians:

(1) The increasing complexity of medical care.
(2) An increasing health consciousness on the part of the people.
(3) The increasing requirements of government service for physicians.
(4) The increasing number of administrative, teaching, and research positions requiring physicians.

In view of this increase in demand, attention should be devoted to increasing the output of physicians in the years ahead. There are several means by which this may be accomplished. Medical educators should carefully survey existing medical schools to determine how they may best increase the number of their graduates without lowering standards. Additional medical schools are another source of supply. Six new medical schools have been organized in the past six years and the development of several others is being planned.

Your committee recognizes that more Negro physicians should be trained. It also recognizes that this problem is part of the larger problem of improving the opportunities for the education of Negroes in general, in order that there may be a larger supply of Negroes qualified to enter medical schools. The committee [on physicians] recommends that effective action to improve this situation at all levels be initiated.

Your committee calls attention to the fact that good medical education is fundamental to good medical care and that American medical education leads the

* See "Report of Subcommittee on Physicians" in succeeding paragraphs of this selection.

world. Efforts to increase the supply of physicians must assure the continuance of these high standards. Medical education should be available to qualified applicants without discrimination as to race, color, or sex.

A continuing study of the extent to which existing medical schools are meeting the demands of the country for physicians is a responsibility of medical educators. . . .

Intelligent planning with respect to the supply of physicians requires periodic analyses of the demand for physicians, both as to number and special qualifications. To this end studies should be developed which will furnish more precise indices for measuring the magnitude of demand.

The increasing complexity of medical education has markedly increased the cost. As a result, the problem of maintaining the present supply and quality of physicians is definitely a problem of financing.

Possible sources for additional financial support are:

(1) Private contributions

(2) State and community appropriations

(3) Federal appropriations

Your committee recommends that increased efforts be made to secure additional contributions from the public at large as well as from state and community governments. The general public does not fully appreciate their obligations to medical education in return for the benefits that they enjoy. There is evidence to indicate that local support will be insufficient to meet the financial needs of a sound and expanding program of medical education, and that some form of Federal support will be necessary. Federal appropriations should entail no Federal control of the administration, curriculum, and student admissions of the medical schools. Continuity of support should be assured. Funds should be granted in such a way as to increase rather than decrease the stimulus and responsibility for local support of the schools from both private and public sources.

Support will be needed in three areas: for general operation, for capital improvements, and for student support. In allocating funds for capital improvements, consideration should be given to improving the quality of medical education as well as the number of physicians trained.

With respect to student support, funds should be provided in such a way as to widen the opportunity for medical training of qualified individuals throughout the nation. Federal aid to students should carry no obligation to serve in any specified capacity after graduation. . . .

Physicians and other health workers recognize that the United States lacks pediatricians, psychiatrists, specialists in pulmonary medicine and in physical medicine and rehabilitation, pathologists, radiologists, anesthesiologists, physicians in the fields of industrial medicine and public health, and well-trained general physicians.* Medical schools need more faculty members. Many of the people who

* From: *Building America's Health,* by the President's Commission on the Health Needs of the Nation; Washington: U.S. Government Printing Office, 1953 (Vol. 2, Chap. V, "Health Personnel," pp. 183-85). Reprinted with omissions, including initial paragraphs and some tables.

appeared at the Commission's hearings also testified to the shortages of physicians.

Needs have been more precisely estimated in some fields of service than others. It is easier, obviously, to measure demand in salaried fields than in private practice.

In the field of public health, the Public Health Service now requires some 100 additional physicians and expects to need almost a thousand more by 1960. State and local health departments already have almost 500 vacant positions, and it is estimated that almost 1,800 more physicians would be needed to provide adequate local public health services.

For industrial medicine, a subcommittee of the Council on Industrial Health of the American Medical Association has indicated that by 1953 some 1,600 additional full-time (or equivalent) physicians would be needed simply to provide for new workers in defense industry. This estimate was based on the committee's recommendation that a typical defense plant with 10,000 employees and moderate hazard should have four physicians—a ratio of 1 physician to 2,500 workers. Many more physicians would be needed to remedy existing deficiencies throughout industry.

Mental hospitals probably need about three times as many physicians as they now have, or about 4,000 additional doctors. This estimate is based on a staffing standard proposed by the American Psychiatric Association in 1945. The Association suggested that mental hospitals should have 1 physician for each 100 admissions per year, plus 1 physician for each 200 resident patients at the end of the year. Mental hospitals admitted some 300,000 patients last year, and the census of these mental hospitals stands now at about 700,000 persons. In 1949, this Association revised its standards to differentiate between various types of mentally ill patients. But data on types of patients in hospitals are not yet exact enough to allow estimates of total needs on the new basis.

For staffing of tuberculosis hospitals, the American Trudeau Society has recommended as a minimum standard at least 1 full-time physician for the first 100 resident patients and 1 additional full-time physician for each 50 (or portion of 50) additional patients. This standard, which was developed in 1945 on the basis of treatment methods current at that time, would indicate a total need for some 1,500 physicians, or about 500 in addition to the present supply. If levels in the better hospitals are not to be brought down to the minimum standard, the total need is greater than these figures suggest. Also, new methods in treatment of tuberculosis may be adding to physician requirements.

Medical schools have between 200 and 500 unfilled faculty positions, most of them for physicians. About 50 schools, or almost two-thirds of the total, have staffs smaller than the accepted standard of 1 faculty member to 4 preclinical students and 1 member to 3 clinical students. To bring these schools up to standards for clinical departments alone would require the equivalent of 600 full-time physicians. This makes no allowance for clinical faculty in new schools about to be opened; the average-sized school needs about 50 physicians in clinical fields. Further physicians would be needed to help staff preclinical departments.

Data from prepayment plans and other studies indicate that to provide adequate

READINGS IN MEDICAL CARE

medical care to individuals requires on the average about one physician for each 1,000 people.

In the following paragraphs six estimates of total physician requirements are presented. They are projected to 1960, for a population of 171,176,000—the Census Bureau's medium population forecast. These estimates are based on a series of assumptions, ranging from maintaining the status quo to bringing to all areas the proportion of doctors now available only in the most favored areas.

Premise 1.—That in 1960 we should have the same over-all physician-population ratio as in 1940—133 physicians per 100,000.

To maintain this level in 1960 would require 227,000 physicians.

Premise 2.—That in 1960 we should have the same physician-population ratio as 1949—135 per 100,000. This would require a total of 231,000 physicians.

Premise 3.—That in 1960 we should have the same civilian physician-population ratio as 1949 and also meet military needs for somewhat larger Armed Forces, expand personnel in industry, public health, medical school faculties and civil defense so as to meet defense needs.

This is the set of assumptions adopted by the Health Resources Advisory Committee of the Office of Defense Mobilization. Its estimated requirement for 1960 (adjusted to include retired physicians) was for 244,000 physicians.

Premise 4.—That in 1960 we would need enough physicians to:

(1) give direct care to the civilian population at a rate of 1 physician per 1,000 population—which would require about 188,000 physicians; and

(2) maintain present levels of intern and resident training and service in hospitals, meet standards for public health, industrial service, mental and tuberculosis hospitals, and medical schools, and meet the requirements of the Armed Forces at present staffing levels, which would require another 75,000 physicians.

This fragmented approach to medical-care requirements has certain shortcomings of duplication (full-time faculty members and hospital house staffs giving medical care, for example). On the other hand, however, it very much understates needs in certain categories of service (psychiatry, rehabilitation, and industrial medicine, for example).

The total requirements for physicians to provide this standard of service would add to 263,000 in 1960.

Premise 5.—That a reasonable goal in terms of present standards of service would be to bring the lower regions of the country to the 1949 national average ratio of 131 physicians per 100,000 civilian population (including private practice, institutional service, teaching, public health, industry, Veterans Administration, and retired—excluding only physicians in the Armed Forces) and to meet the needs of the Armed Forces at present levels.

The total requirement figure, at that level, would be 255,000 physicians.

Premise 6.—Another approach to estimating need is to assume that the over-all physician-population ratio achieved by a wide area with a long history of a generally high economic and education level and with a relatively good supply of health facilities is a reasonable goal for the rest of the country.

The area of New England and the Central Atlantic States had in 1949 an average ratio of 166 physicians per 100,000 civilian people.

To serve the expected 1960 civilian population at that rate and to meet military needs would bring the total need to 292,000.

These six estimates for physicians are summarized below:

TABLE 32. *Total physician requirements, 1960, 6 premises*

Premise	Total physician requirement
1. Maintaining 1940 gross physician-population ratio	227,000
2. Maintaining 1949 physician-population ratio	231,000
3. Maintaining 1949 civilian population ratio, meeting military and other mobilization needs (based on Health Resources Advisory Committee estimate)	244,000
4. Meeting certain specified standards of service	263,000
5. Bringing low regions and population increase up to 1949 average civilian physician-population ratio, and meeting military needs	255,000
6. Bringing all regions to 1949 civilian physician-population ratio for New England and the Central Atlantic States, and meeting military needs	292,000

The expected number of physicians in 1960 is 233,000. Thus, in 1960, taking into account the expected increase in graduates, the total number of physicians will just about maintain 1949 gross physician-population ratios.

It is apparent that even if there were no other barriers, the shortage of physicians in itself will set a sharp limit to the extent to which better medical service can be provided in the next decade. Increasing the number of physicians to a level at which minimum standards can be met in all parts of the country must be considered as a long-range job. As has been pointed out, increased production of physicians will require more faculty members and more facilities. Even with adequate financing, this will take many years.

For the immediate future, we must not only plan this long-range job, but consider the means of improving utilization of presently available physicians, improving the utilization and increasing the numbers of auxiliary workers, and developing effective methods of bringing physicians into understaffed areas, both geographic and in certain fields of practice.

To accomplish this, it will be necessary to give medical students an understanding of the challenge of opportunities for service, to provide more adequate and attractive facilities and educational opportunities, to make consultant service more generally available, to develop methods of giving some financial security and incentive to physicians in these areas and to increase the use of auxiliary personnel. These needs, in turn, go back to the problem of the organization of medical service and facilities. . . .

28. THE DECLINING SUPPLY OF RURAL DOCTORS *

Background and Trends

THE SEVERE SHORTAGE of rural physicians has not always been a feature of American medicine, nor has it developed overnight. It has been a gradual process developing since the latter part of the nineteenth century. The immediate cause of the growing maldistribution has been the accelerating settlement of physicians, particularly new graduates, in the cities. As early as 1906, when about 56 per cent of the nation's population was regarded as rural, there was a clear disproportion, for only 41 per cent of the available physicians were in rural practice. By 1940 when the nation's rural population had declined relatively by less than one-fourth to 43.5 per cent, the physicians in rural practice fell to about 20 per cent of the nation's total, or half their former proportion. As early as 1914, the increasing settlement of new graduates in the large cities was beginning to be striking. In that year 47 per cent of medical graduates were settling in cities of over 100,000 population, while at the time less than 26 per cent of the national population were located in such cities.

After the First World War there was already a marked discrepancy between the supply of physicians in rural and urban counties. In 1923, when there were 159.5 physicians per 100,000 persons in metropolitan counties (containing a place of 50,000 population), there were only 91.9 per 100,000 in the rural counties that contained no urban place (2,500 or more). By 1940, the proportionate supply in the metropolitan counties had actually increased, while that in the rural counties and even in counties with places up to 50,000 persons had gone severely downhill. . . . Considering settlement by whole states, in 1940-41 urbanized New York State, with about 10 per cent of the nation's population, was getting about 18 per cent of the new physicians, while rural Alabama with over 2 per cent of the national population was getting only 0.3 per cent of them. The wartime drainage of medical personnel to the armed forces, as we shall see, aggravated the situation even further.

An explanation of the accelerated settlement of physicians in the cities and the growing rural shortages is not far to seek. The growing industrialization of the nation has meant the increasing concentration of wealth in the cities. Physicians having a service to sell will naturally choose to sell it where purchasing power is greatest. While this may have always been true, it came to result in serious urban-rural dis-

---

* By permission from *Rural Health and Medical Care*, by Frederick D. Mott, M.D., and Milton I. Roemer, M.D. Copyright 1948, McGraw-Hill Book Company, Inc. (The excerpt reprinted, with omissions including initial paragraphs, tables, and figures, is from Chap. VIII, "Physicians"). The authors are, respectively, the executive director of Community Health Association, Detroit; and the director of research, Sloan Institute of Hospital Administration, Cornell University, Ithaca, N.Y.

crepancies in personnel only as the cities became the concentrated centers of the nation's wealth. Other associated factors, of course, play a part, but economic pressures are at the root of most of them.

At the very time that the cities were beginning to exert a strong "pull" on the available supply of physicians, the total national supply of doctors began to fall. In 1900, counting all licensed physicians, we had a supply of one to every 580 persons in the nation. This was still the period of the "diploma mills" where degrees were virtually sold to any who could pay the price. After the movement to grade medical schools got under way, following Abraham Flexner's monumental report in 1910, the unqualified schools were forced to close down and the supply of new graduates fell off sharply. By 1920 the national physician-population ratio had declined to 1 to 730. After 1922 the output of medical graduates gradually rose again, but at a slower rate than the increase in the population. By 1940, therefore, the total supply of licensed physicians in the nation yielded a ratio of only 1 to 748. It is obvious, then, that the total reservoir from which rural physicians could be drawn was gradually getting lower.

Meanwhile, medical science was advancing rapidly and specialization had to develop. From a mere scattering of specialists at the turn of the century, by 1928 about 26 per cent of the nation's physicians were partially or completely specialized and by 1940 over 50 per cent. Since the specialist under present-day patterns requires a large and relatively prosperous population to provide a "market" for his more expensive services, he tends to settle in the cities. Meanwhile also an increasing proportion of physicians were going into full-time salaried positions—as medical school teachers, hospital administrators, public health officers, research workers— chiefly in the cities. The number of physicians in such full-time positions rose from 13,000 in 1928 to 20,000 in 1942. This clearly made still further drains on the reservoir of physicians from which the private practitioners for rural America could be drawn.

With the dwindling reserve of physicians for rural areas, the economic and other attractions of the cities exerted their effect at an accelerated tempo. . . . It may be noted that in 1923 the highest income counties were attracting not quite twice as high a proportion of physicians as the lowest income counties. Just 15 years later, however, the highest income counties were attracting more nearly three times the proportion of the poorest counties. This increasing "pursuit of wealth" and its associated technical facilities and cultural opportunities is found to apply particularly to the youngest physicians and new graduates.

All the while the costs of a medical education were rising, both in direct outlay and in the indirect withholding of earning power during increasingly long medical school years. This has meant that young men and women from rural families have been less and less able to afford the cost of medical training. Yet it is among country families that one might expect to find the love or appreciation for rural life that is partially necessary to make a medical graduate choose a rural practice. Even for a youth from a rural home, however, modern medical training has become such as to induce him to settle in an urban center. Increasingly the young physician has naturally come to demand the institutions, equipment, and technical assistance in his practice that he has learned to depend on in medical school and internship—and these resources are sparse in rural sections.

The continuous settlement of young graduates in the cities has meant a residue in rural sections of physicians largely in the later years of life. In counties with no urban place, for example, 24.8 per cent of the physicians in 1923 were 58 years of age or over. By 1938 the proportion of these older men in rural counties had risen to 45.1 per cent. Older age levels, moreover, mean higher death rates, so that the over-all loss of rural practitioners through death tends to increase each year. Thus, in 1938 when the general annual death rate for large-city practitioners was 18 per 1,000, in the rural areas it was 29 per 1,000. Between 1923 and 1938, the number of rural physicians dying actually exceeded the number entering rural practice by over 3,400. The rural profession, in other words, is almost acquiring the ominous earmarks of a dying civilization; its members are dying off at increasing rates and they are not being replenished by new blood.

Finally, among the trends leading up to the present crisis in the supply of rural physicians, is the influence of the migration of established practitioners. For even after initial settlement in a rural practice, there has been a growing tendency for physicians to move. The pattern of migration appears to be chiefly to the smaller cities of 2,500 to 50,000 population from the rural districts and, to some very small extent, from metropolitan centers. Thus, between 1923 and 1938 the large cities of the nation lost 643 physicians by out-migration but gained 43,361 by new settlement. In the same period, however, rural areas acquired only 13,654 physicians by new settlement, but lost 4,361, or about one out of three new settlers, by out-migration.

... Between 1923 and 1938 the net supply of physicians in the metropolitan counties increased by 29.2 per cent while the population increased by only 20 per cent. In the counties with small cities of 2,500 to 50,000, the net physician supply increased by 20 percent while the population increased by 25 per cent. In the purely rural counties, however, while the population increased by 10 per cent, the net supply of physicians actually declined by 19.3 per cent.

The Rural Medical Profession Today

WITH THESE TRENDS in the number and distribution of physicians over the last several decades, the present picture of rural medical practice is almost self-evident. No sharp line, of course, can be drawn between the influence of past trends and the pressure of contemporary social forces. All the trends leading to the quantitative disparity between the rural and urban supplies of physicians continue today. The present picture of rural medicine, in effect, is only one "still" in the moving-picture film, stopped at about the prewar year 1940 and thrown on the screen for analysis. . . .

... It may be noted that when the states are arranged by groups in the order of increasing rurality, their per capita income declines regularly and their supply of effective physicians, as measured by physician-population ratios, declines with almost identical regularity. The six most urban states and the District of Columbia, having over twice the per capita wealth of the eight most rural states, likewise have over twice the supply of physicians. One cannot help but be impressed with the fact that the basic factor accounting for the rural-urban distribution of physicians is the economic level of the area in which they practice.

Even among rural counties, of course, per capita income exerts its effect. Thus, in the relatively few rural counties with per capita incomes of $600 or more, the physician-population ratio was 1 to 780 in 1938, while in the more typical rural counties with per capita incomes of under $300, it was 1 to 1,670, or more than twice as poor.

Beyond state or county wealth as a determinant of physician supply, other relationships are found. All things being equal, the county with the greater supply of hospital beds tends to have the better supply of physicians. Which is causal is difficult to say, for while ordinarily one expects hospitals to attract physicians, in many rural communities it is the arrival of the physician that leads to the establishment of the hospital. In general, however, the urban concentration of hospital beds holds definite attractions for the new graduate.

The supply of hospital beds itself tends to be directly related to state per capita wealth. As a result, there tends to be an amazingly constant relationship between physicians and hospital beds in states of all degrees of rurality, regardless of the supply of physicians. When states are grouped by rurality, there are exactly 3.2 general hospital beds per effective physician in five of the six groups of states, with 3.0 beds per doctor in the sixth (the most urban) group.

Other factors, like the mere presence of other physicians with whom to exchange ideas, and the cultural and civic advantages of urban life for the doctor and his family, of course, play a real part in shaping the doctor's decision on where to settle. All these factors, in turn, like hospital beds, tend to be themselves related to local economic levels.

The past and present pressures inducing settlement of younger physicians in the cities, as already suggested, leave a supply of rural practitioners of very different age composition from urban. . . .

In terms of median age levels, the large-city doctor in 1940 was 44 years of age, while the country doctor was 13 years older, 57 years. Actually the median figures, however, overlook the rather numerous octogenarians who are carrying on in the country. In fact, the very survival of some of these venerable and often beloved old country doctors sometimes discourages the young medical graduate from even trying to stake his fortune in certain rural communities.

The age of rural practitioners has implications with reference not only to their "manpower" effectiveness, but also to their knowledge of current developments in medical science. With an obviously greater span of time since the completion of his formal medical training, the average rural practitioner tends naturally to be less responsive to changes in medicine than the younger city doctor. This is obviously aggravated by less exposure in the isolated rural districts to the new medical thinking associated with the urban centers of professional education.

At this particular period in the history of medical education in the United

States, moreover, older age implies a greater residue of graduates from medical schools now regarded as unqualified and, for the most part, out of existence.... National data on this point are not at hand but it has been found in Iowa, for example, that in rural communities of under 1,000 population, 1 out of every 5 physicians is a graduate of a school now out of existence, while in Des Moines (with a 1940 population of 160,000) only 1 out of 14 is a product of such a school. The effect of this situation on the quality of rural medical practice is self-evident.

The rising cost of medical education over the years, already alluded to, has led to a situation in which medical students originate predominantly from urban centers and are naturally predisposed to a city practice. Despite efforts of many medical schools to select candidates from a broad representation of states, the tendency is for students to originate predominantly from the more urban states. Thus, in 1940 the states with 70 per cent or more urban population contributed to the medical schools of the nation students at a rate of 17.1 per 100,000 population; over half of these students, moreover, went to schools in their home states. At the same time the states 70 per cent rural or more contributed medical students at a rate of only 12.9 per 100,000 population, and only about one-third of these went to schools in their native states....

State-wide data, however, fail to express the degree of urban selection, for in neither urban nor rural states do students tend to come from rural districts.... C. Horace Hamilton has, in fact, recently shown that in the period 1938-40, first-year medical students came from urban centers throughout the nation at a rate of 66.4 per million population, compared with 18.6 per million from rural communities. Only 12 out of 6,000 students whose residence was studied gave an address on a rural mail route.

It can hardly be claimed, moreover, that rural youth are not desirous of undertaking professional careers. A study of the occupational preferences of high school students in representative rural counties of Missouri has shown, for example, that medicine or dentistry was the sixth choice of all young men, with 6.2 out of every 100 making this their first choice. Among nonfarm young men in villages and towns up to 5,000 population, a medical or dental career ranked as third choice, with 10.6 per 100 giving this preference. If only the best qualified of all these youth interested in medicine or dentistry were financially enabled to carry through their training, there can be little doubt that the professional schools would be turning out graduates more inclined to elect a rural practice....

With the small supply of rural physicians, one might suppose that the income per physician would be relatively high—higher than in the cities where competition is greater. Because of the wide urban-rural discrepancies in purchasing power, however, the financial advantages of reduced competition are quite lost and the opposite is true. The data on physicians' incomes, in effect, bear out the decision of most practitioners—so far as pecuniary objectives are concerned—to settle in urban communities....

...For years there has been a tendency for physicians to migrate out of rural districts, after a period of trial. Equally significant is the frequent migration within rural sections from one place to another. Turnover among rural physicians is so high that in six rural counties of Wisconsin, between 1912 and 1936, one out of every six or seven local practitioners was lost *each year* through migration, death, or retirement. This turnover tends to be highest, judging by a Virginia study, among the youngest rural physicians. Whatever may have once been true about the perennial family doctor in rural America is manifestly losing its validity.

Migration could hardly be considered objectionable, of course, if only it occurred in the direction of correcting the present maldistribution of doctors. But it is clear that, in general, the very opposite takes place. As a matter of fact, the restrictions of numerous state licensure laws act to prevent the migration or relocation of many physicians into rural states in which they are desperately needed.

29. DISCRIMINATORY PATTERNS *

IT'S EASY TO demonstrate that there is discrimination against racial and religious minorities in medicine. It's not so easy to find and understand the causes of such discrimination. And in some cases it's hardest of all to know what to do about it.

To a large extent, discrimination in medicine is a result of discrimination in society generally. It's important to remember, then, that the doctors and hospitals and medical schools engaging in discriminatory practices are *victims* as well as *culprits*.

Yet it is by no means true, as many claim, that they cannot help to eliminate discrimination in medicine themselves—that they must always wait for community action in other fields and follow, rather than lead, the way to right conduct. We have heartening evidence to the contrary.

First, however, a look at the problem as such.

It's a well-known fact that there is discrimination against Jews in medical schools and hospitals. Many institutions admit Jewish applicants only on a quota basis, and there seems to be a tendency for medical practice to divide into Jewish and non-Jewish groups.

I know a brilliant young Jewish physician, for instance, who has been doing a fine job as administrator of a Jewish hospital. Not long ago, I predicted to his wife that he would one day be chief administrator of some great medical center.

"Act your age," she said sharply. "There aren't half a dozen places in the country that would have him."

She was right, too. But the facts of discrimination against Jews are hard to pin down. Where Negroes are concerned, it's an easier matter. Here are a few simple statistics:

¶ With 10 per cent of the nation's population, the Negro race has only about

* From: "Discrimination and the Doctor," by Robert M. Cunningham, Jr.; *Medical Economics* 29:119-24, Jan. 1952 (No. 1). Reprinted from *Medical Economics* by special permission. Copyright 1952, Medical Economics, Inc., Rutherford, N.J.

2 per cent of the nation's physicians and occupies only 2½ per cent of the nation's hospital beds.

¶ The physician-population ratio for the country as a whole is 1 to 750; while for the Negro population the ratio is 1 to 3,500, or substantially below the 1-to-1,500 minimum standard commonly accepted in the United States.

¶ Of 26,000 students enrolled in medical schools, less than 3 per cent are Negroes; and three-fourths of these are in the two all-Negro institutions, Meharry and Howard.

¶ Negro graduates are eligible for appointment to less than 200 of the country's 10,000 internships; and more than half the 200 are in segregated Negro hospitals.

¶ Of some 12,000 residency appointments on hospital staffs, only about 100 are available to Negro physicians; and three-fourths of these are in segregated hospitals.

It is neither necessary nor desirable that Negroes should look only to Negro physicians for medical care, nor that Negro physicians should limit their practices to Negroes. Yet racial discrimination in hospital staff appointments makes it hard to break this pattern.

"Few Negro physicians have staff appointments at any but all-Negro hospitals," a current report of Provident Medical Associates explains. "Thus they must take their patients to Negro hospitals or turn them over to the care of white physicians in the hospitals to which they themselves do not have access. In all the United States . . . hospital and clinical facilities are segregated or denied. And in most of the South, membership in county medical societies is refused . . . [So] the average Negro physician becomes a general practitioner, isolated professionally and serving a low-income group."

Of course, many of these phenomena are inter-related. For example:

Many hospitals provide that staff appointments shall be made only from among members of the local county medical society. With society membership denied him, the Negro physician is thus effectively barred from hospital practice.

(In fairness, it should be pointed out that the American Medical Association, which has been a convenient target for abuse by liberal groups, is in no way responsible for such exclusions. The A.M.A. is made up of self-governing local and county medical societies. Where Negro doctors are denied admission, it is the local society and not the A.M.A. that is at fault.)

Inevitably, discrimination in the admission of hospital patients results from the discriminatory aspects of medical education and practice. In a hospital where the Negro physician finds it impossible to get a staff appointment, there won't be many Negro patients.

Patient Segregation

IT'S TRUE, of course, that many hospitals today admit Negroes. But even here segregation is the general rule. The colored person is apt to be assigned to a single room or an all-Negro ward. Only in large wards of public hospitals and in a few medical teaching centers is it common to see Negro and white patients in adjacent beds.

Though apologists for such segregation insist that white patients object to sharing hospital accommodations with Negroes, that assumption has often been proved false. A case in point:

For many years, staff members at the University of Chicago Clinics maintained that it would be a mistake to open the doors of the clinics to all races on an equal basis. "In a short time," they protested, "we wouldn't have any more white patients."

At the insistence of former Chancellor Hutchins and others, their objections were finally overcome. The result? Well, in Chancellor Hutchins' own words: "The result has been that there hasn't been any result at all!" Nothing happened when white and colored were assigned to the same rooms.

It's been demonstrated, too, that nothing generally seems to happen when white and Negro nurses work together on hospital floors. Or when Negro nurses care for white patients and white nurses care for Negro patients.

As a matter of fact, discrimination against Negro nurses, technicians, and other hospital personnel is breaking down rapidly. This is an example of arriving at the right answer for the wrong reason: The shortage of hospital personnel has become so severe that many hospitals that used to bar Negroes from all except menial positions have been forced to accept them.

Racial prejudice in medicine is of course only part of the larger social pattern. So it's not surprising that efforts to break the pattern aren't always attended with perfect success. Take, for example, the experience of just one group:

Of 29,000 certified medical specialists listed a couple of years ago by the National Advisory Board for Medical Specialties, only 101 were Negroes. For a long time, Provident Medical Associates of Chicago has been financing graduate medical education for qualified Negro physicians in an effort to improve this situation. But the problem is a perplexing one, since so few Negroes *are* qualified.

Qualification comes from an adequate educational background—and it isn't easy for the average Negro to make the grade. The roots of medical discrimination are buried deep in our educational system—in the segregated grade school, high school, and college.

Steps Forward

BUT LET'S NOT TRY to shift the blame from doctors and hospitals to the rest of society. Though it's obviously true that racial prejudice isn't always the fault of medical and hospital people, it's equally true that we can do something about it if we really want to. There are already signs of a good deal of progress.

Four years ago, a hospital in Gary, Ind., invited applications from qualified Negro physicians in the community. Up to that time, Negro doctors had been limited to a totally inadequate facility in the segregated district. Two of them qualified at once, and five more have since accepted appointments. Today, more than 20 per cent of the hospital's patients are colored. This is roughly equivalent to the proportion of Negroes in the population. And the change has been brought about without a single unpleasant incident!

The number of American hospitals accepting Negro physicians as internes, residents, and attending staff members is steadily growing. In Chicago, Negro doctors are on the staff at Cook County, Children's Memorial, and Michael Reese Hospitals. Elsewhere, colored physicians have been appointed at such representative institutions as Philadelphia General, Newark City in Newark, N.J., Queens General in New York, Allegheny General in Pittsburgh, and Los Angeles County.

Especially heart-warming are developments in the South. The medical school of Emory University at Atlanta has established a post-graduate clinic for Negro physicians; the Johns Hopkins school of medicine at Baltimore now admits Negroes for post-graduate work; community hospitals in Virginia and Arkansas have accepted colored doctors as staff members.

Less important but possibly significant of changing attitudes are several recent events:

The American Medical Association switched its clinical session scheduled for last month from Houston, Tex., to Los Angeles—reportedly because it was learned that the headquarters hotel in Houston would not accept Negro delegates as guests.

At this year's American Hospital Association convention in St. Louis, the association found to its embarrassment that Negro members were kept out of downtown hotels. It immediately announced that no further meetings would be held in St. Louis until all members could expect equal treatment.

A few months ago, several Southern nurses walked out of a Catholic hospital in West Virginia because the Sister Superior refused to discharge three Negro nurses who had been added to the staff. The hospital stood its ground, and—more important—it got the full support of the community, the newspapers, the Mother Superior of the Order running the hospital, and the Bishop of the Diocese.

Rome wasn't built in a day. It's not likely that medicine will eliminate all its discriminatory practices until society stops winking at prejudice and segregation. Until that time comes, though, there's a lot we can do. We can expose the evils of discrimination in medicine whenever we come across them. We can fight with unflagging courage for fair judgments and fair practices.

C. *The Physician: Income and Methods of Payment*

30. AN INCOME SURVEY *

IN APRIL, 1950, the Bureau of Medical Economic Research of the American Medical Association and the Office of Business Economics of the United States

* From: *Survey of Physicians' Incomes* (Bulletin 84, Bureau of Medical Economic Research, American Medical Association), by Frank G. Dickinson and Charles E. Bradley; Chicago:

Department of Commerce jointly initiated a survey of the 1949 incomes of physicians from professional services, excluding incomes from other sources. The first report on this survey was published this week in the July, 1951, issue of the *Survey of Current Business,* United States Department of Commerce.[1] The tabulations and interpretations in that current article are the responsibility of the Department of Commerce although the Bureau of Medical Economic Research was given the opportunity to comment on the manuscript of the article prior to its publication. The designing of the questionnaires, the selection of samples of physicians by name, and the mailing of the questionnaires was a joint responsibility. . . .

We want to thank the more than 55,000 of the 125,000 physicians who received questionnaires for taking the time and trouble to fill out and return the schedules. . . .

Thus [the] article in the current issue of the *Survey of Current Business* has an extremely broad base. On these grounds alone this survey is not in the traditional small sample category; roughly, two out of five physicians responded.

It is very difficult to provide a brief summary of this long article with its 23 tables and three charts. In a word, this study indicates that the average physician has been moving up the inflationary ladder about as rapidly as the average American.

General Averages

THE AVERAGE (mean) 1949 net income from medical practice of the 30,000 physicians whose returned questionnaires were analyzed was $11,058—see row 1, table 33. This was 60.4% of the average (mean) gross income of $18,316. The' median net income reported was $8,835; that is, one-half of the physicians reported net incomes of less than $8,835 and one-half reported higher incomes. These are the two over-all averages to be kept in mind. They are based on all replies, which means that they came from physicians of all classes and types except the excluded classes noted above; * for convenience we shall use the term "all" physicians in referring to data from the 30,000 replies. In this summary we shall stress the means, although many statisticians will consider the medians more representative values in the various distributions of physicians' incomes.

Of the 30,000 physicians reporting, 23,000 were in independent practice (derived more than 50% of their professional income from fees from independent practice); their mean net income in 1949 was $11,858 and their median income, $9,668. The remaining 7,000 of the 30,000 were engaged in salaried practice (received less than 50% of their professional income from fees); their mean net income was $8,272 and their median net income, $7,555.

American Medical Association, 1951. Reprinted (with omissions, including some tables) by permission of the authors and publishers. Dr. Dickinson is the director of the Bureau of Medical Economic Research, American Medical Association, Chicago; Mr. Bradley was an associate in economics for the Bureau at the time this bulletin was written.

1. Weinfeld, William: Income of Physicians, 1929-49.

* i.e., retired and other physicians not in practice; interns, residents, fellows-in-training; military physicians; physicians whose major source of income was from a medical school; and defective replies—or approximately 12,000 returns in all.

The 30,000 replies were also separated into three categories: (1) non-salaried practice (20,000 returns) for which the mean was $11,744 and the median, $9,561; (2) part-salaried practice (5,000 returns) for which the mean was $10,928 and the median, $8,760; and (3) all-salaried practice (5,000 returns) for which the mean was $8,434 and the median, $7,678.

TABLE 33. *Average gross income and net income of physicians by source of income, 1949*

Group of Physicians[A] and Number of Replies Analyzed	Mean Net Income (1)	Median Net Income (2)	Mean Gross Income (3)	Median Gross Income (4)	Percentage of Replies (5)
1. "All" Physicians (29,878)	$11,058	$8,835	$18,316[B]	$14,829[B]	100.0%
2. Independent Physicians (23,213)	11,858	9,668	......	......	77.7
2a. General Practice ...	8,835	7,428	......	......	(32.1)
2b. Partly Specialized ..	11,758	9,902	......	......	(14.1)
2c. Fully Specialized ...	15,014	12,599	......	......	(31.5)
3. Salaried Physicians (6,665)	8,272	7,555	......	......	22.3
3a. General Practice ...	6,281	6,132[B]	......	......	(2.8)
3b. Partly Specialized ..	7,135	6,693	......	......	(2.2)
3c. Fully Specialized ...	8,884	7,953	......	......	(14.4)
3d. Other	8,351	7,890[B]	......	......	(2.9)
4. Non-Salaried Physicians (19,906)	11,744	9,561	19,710	16,108	66.6
5. Part-Salaried Physicians (5,013)	10,928	8,760	12,781	8,993	16.8
6. All-Salaried Physicians (4,959)	8,434	7,678	......	......	16.6

Source: Weinfeld, William: "Income of Physicians, 1929-49," *Survey of Current Business,* July, 1951, U. S. Department of Commerce, Tables 2, 3, 6, 7, and 9.

[A] The group "all" physicians (row 1), including salaried as well as independent practitioners, excludes interns, residents, fellows-in-training, physicians in military service, and medical school personnel. All replies (row 1) were classified into two groups (rows 2 and 3) and then reclassified into three groups (rows 4, 5, and 6). Independent physicians (row 2), that is, physicians in independent practice, are those whose major source (more than 50 per cent) of medical income is fees from independent practice; they include (*a*) all non-salaried physicians (row 4) and (*b*) those of the part-salaried (row 5) whose major source of income is fees from independent practice. Salaried physicians (row 3), that is, physicians in salaried practice, are those whose major source of medical income is from salaried practice; they include (*a*) all of the all-salaried physicians (row 6) and (*b*) those of the part-salaried physicians (row 5) whose major source of income is from salaried practice.

[B] Hitherto unpublished data from the joint Department of Commerce/American Medical Association 1950 income survey of the medical profession. These data were eliminated from the Weinfeld article because of lack of space. We have also quoted a few figures in the text which were deleted from Weinfeld's tables in the final editing.

Before further major breakdowns of the data are presented, several historical comparisons may be useful in providing a general setting. Since more data from the past are available for non-salaried physicians, who in 1949 reported higher average net incomes than did all physicians, the historical comparisons, although limited, can best be made of their incomes. On the basis of Department of Commerce surveys for 1935-1939, Weinfeld concludes that the mean net income of non-salaried physicians was 186% higher in 1949 ($11,744) than in the period 1935-1939 ($4,100), the most frequently used base period in economic reports. Because the incomes of salaried physicians have apparently not risen as rapidly since the base period as the incomes of independent physicians, it follows that the increase in the incomes of all physicians was less than 186%. On the basis of limited data we would estimate that the mean net income of all physicians in 1949 ($11,058) was roughly 150 to 170% above that in 1935-1939 (between $4,100 and $4,400). The national income of the American people was 224% higher in 1949 than in the period 1935-1939; the national income per capita was 179% higher. The increase in the national income when adjusted for the number of persons in the working force—commonly called the number gainfully employed—was 177%. (Some economists might prefer the smaller national aggregate known as personal income as a frame of reference; personal income per capita in 1949 was 159% higher than in 1935-1939.) It appears quite clear that the rise in the incomes of physicians and of the American people—their patients—have kept pace with each other during the 1940's. The average physician has been traveling near the center of the inflationary highway up which the entire American economy has been moving since before World War II. Such is the over-all picture presented by the current survey of physicians' incomes in relation to the general level of income of the American people. Whether physicians' incomes were too high or too low in 1935-1939 has not been determined and, possibly, never will be determined to the complete satisfaction of all people. How much was "too high" or "too low" in 1935-1939? An answer would require almost endless consideration of the alternative economic opportunities of high school graduates of equal talents, the personal and economic sacrifices during 8 to 13 years of premedical and medical education and training, the long work week of practitioners, the economic equivalent of the personal satisfaction of helping restore sick people to health. These considerations are largely beyond the scope of our present interest. . . .

According to the U. S. Bureau of Labor Statistics, the fees of physicians were 38% higher in 1949 than in the base period 1935-1939. This index of physicians' fees is part of the Consumers' Price Index—formerly known as the Cost of Living Index—which is so widely used in making wage adjustments. The entire index for 1949 was 69% above the base period.

Obviously, an increase of 150% or 160% or 170% in the average incomes of physicians since the base period cannot be attributed to a general rise in fees alone. Two other factors, which we believe are probably more important in accounting for this increase in physicians' incomes, are: (1) improved collection—a decrease in the percentage of uncollected bills for medical services rendered and, perhaps, a smaller percentage of charity patients to whom services were given free or at reduced fees; (2) greater "output per physician." These data on the incomes of physicians clearly indicate that 1,000 physicians were doing considerably more medical work in 1949 than 1,000 physicians did a dozen years ago. This increase in "output per physician" resulted from, among other things, changes in therapy and diagnosis, increased use of technical assistants, seeing a higher proportion of patients in the office and in the hospital, and improved transportation.

Reactions of Physicians

DOUBTLESSLY, the reactions of physicians to the average incomes given in this summary and to the many more given in the article in the *Survey of Current Business* will vary considerably. Physicians who were practicing in 1935-1939 and who are now approaching the peak earning period of their lives, around age 50, will probably contend that these reported over-all averages ($11,058 and $8,835) are too low. On the opposite side will be physicians who were in their fifties a dozen years ago and are now well past the peak earning period of life; their incomes have increased, on the average, far less than 150% to 170% since 1935-1939. On the whole, physicians who are now at or near the peak earning period of their lives will regard the averages as too low and older physicians will probably think they are too high. Likewise, many specialists will regard the over-all averages as too low and many general practitioners will consider them too high. Such are the limitations of any over-all average. The averages for each of the various groups of physicians will probably seem more reasonable to most physicians in each group. In thinking about the rise in their own incomes, many physicians will forget that the national income also rose until it was three and one-fourth times as great in 1949 as in 1935-1939. Only by comparing the increase in the incomes of the members of their profession with that of the American people taken all together can physicians get any real perspective on their relative position in a rapidly changing economy.

The concept of the average income of the members of a clearly defined group is useful in making historical comparisons. On the other hand, the concept of the income of the average member of that group is very misleading because no person can remain at the same age as time passes. Two illustrations, based on Weinfeld's table 16, can be used to show that the concept of the average physician must be used very carefully by any physician who seeks to check the changes in his own income during the past 20 years with the averages developed in this and earlier surveys of the incomes of physicians by the U. S. Department of Commerce.

Consider a physician who was just under 30 years of age in 1929 and hence almost 50 years of age in 1949. The average net income of physicians in independent practice in the age group 45-49 in 1949 was somewhat more than twice as great as the average of those in the under-age 30 group. If we assume that this age-earnings relationship has held true since 1929, this physician could have expected his net income for 1949 to have been about twice as great as his net income in 1929 providing he had enjoyed the average gain due to 20 years of experience in the practice of medicine. His income would not have kept pace with the average of his medical school classmates if it had not doubled between 1929 and 1949. In addition to the age-earnings progression of his profession, there is a second factor which should have increased his income—the general increase in the average income of the American people which, on the average, doubled between 1929 and 1949. As already noted the average income of physicians also doubled. (If the average income of all physicians—and of the American people—had remained unchanged, this second factor could, of course, be ignored in our illustration.) On the basis of these two factors combined, the income of this physician should have quadrupled between 1929 and 1949 ($2 \times 2 = 4$).

Now consider a physician who was in his late forties in 1929. In his age-earnings progression Weinfeld groups all physicians 65 and over into one class. On the basis of this age-earnings progression we can assume that the average physician's income at age 67 is about half as high as the average for age 47. This second physician, who at age 47 in 1929 was at or near the peak earning period of his life, should have earned one-half as much in 1949 as he did in 1929 under the assumptions regarding the age-earnings progression already noted above. During those 20 years, however, the average incomes of the American people and of all physicians doubled. Hence, these two factors cancel out, indicating no difference between his 1929 and his 1949 income ($\frac{1}{2} \times 2 = 1$).

These two illustrations were chosen as extreme cases in order to show the differences between physicians who were at their peak earning period of life in 1949 and in 1929. . . .

Average Gross Incomes

THE GROSS INCOME corresponding with $11,058, the average net income of all physicians, was $18,316; thus, the net was 60.4% of the gross. The relationship between the net and gross incomes of non-salaried physicians is probably more significant; the net was $11,744, 59.6% of the gross, $19,710. Weinfeld notes a slight rise in the general cost of conducting a medical practice, from 36.7% of gross in 1945 to 40.4% in 1949. Payroll expense alone rose from 11.1% to 13.2%. The remainder of the 40.4% in 1949 was paid to business firms for drugs and supplies and for such other items as transportation (automobile, train) and rent. More generally, the average physician realizes about three-fifths of the fees paid to him by his patients and the other two-fifths is paid out by him to other income receivers. Hence, our principal interest in this summary, as well as in the article itself, is in net income and not in gross income. Some day we hope to make a survey of the personal consumer expenditure patterns of physicians. We suspect that the percentages spent for homes and automobiles are high and the percentages spent for other items, e. g., tobacco and recreation, are low relative to the expenditure patterns of all families in the same income class. This peculiar pattern may reflect the long work week of the physician.

Incomes of Lawyers and Dentists

THE MEAN NET income of non-salaried lawyers rose from $5,534 in 1929 and $4,363 in 1935-1939 to $8,083 in 1949, increases of 46% and 85%, as compared with the increases of 125% and 186% for non-salaried physicians.[2] The present survey is the first which clearly indicates that the average incomes of physicians are now above those of lawyers. Studies covering the late 1920's and early 1930's placed the lawyers' incomes above the physicians'. The mean net income of non-salaried dentists rose from $4,267 in 1929 and $2,812 in 1935-1939 to $7,146 in 1949, increases of 67% and 154%.[3] Apparently there has been no counterpart in the practice of law or dentistry of the so-called wonder-drug revolution of the last decade and a half in the practice of medicine. Rapid changes in diagnosis and therapy have unquestionably increased very sharply the demand for the services of physicians.

The expected data on the average hours of work per week for physicians, required for the comparisons of income per hour, are not now available. Hence, no comparisons of hours worked and of earnings per hour in these three professions can be presented. The comparisons of these incomes of physicians, lawyers, and dentists are of some significance today but much more significant comparisons of the major professions can be made after future surveys of the incomes of certified public accountants and consulting engineers have been made; these two professional groups outranked physicians and lawyers in earlier studies of the incomes of these five major professional groups.[3]

Our major interest in this summary of the article is the relationship between the trends in the incomes of physicians and of the American people—their patients. For several reasons Weinfeld has a greater interest in comparing the incomes of the different professions; these reasons are closely related to the particular function of his studies for the Office of Business Economics. Although the study has been clarified by the exclusion of interns, residents, and fellows-in-training, we believe that these physicians should be included when comparing the over-all average incomes of physicians with those of lawyers and dentists because the latter two professions do not have any comparable group which could be excluded from surveys. These physicians, under the supervision of senior physicians in hospitals, are providing a very large amount of medical care to the American people. Their monthly salaries are nominal. As noted by Weinfeld, if they had been included in the survey the average net income of all physicians would have been perhaps 10% lower, say about $10,000 instead of $11,000. It is especially necessary to make this allowance in comparing the three professions because young lawyers and young dentists were included in the surveys of incomes of lawyers and dentists. At least the comparisons should have been age for age. We wish to make it clear, however, that for all other purposes we thought that the decision to exclude interns, residents, and fellows-in-training was proper.

2. Weinfeld, William: Income of Lawyers, 1929-1948, Survey of Current Business, (Aug.) 1949, U. S. Department of Commerce.
3. Weinfeld, William: Income of Dentists, 1929-1948, Survey of Current Business, (Jan.) 1950, U. S. Department of Commerce, pp. 8-16. For earlier comparisons of the incomes of these five professions, see Friedman, M., and Kuznets, S.: Income from Independent Professional Practice, New York, National Bureau of Economic Research, 1945.

Income after Taxes

NET INCOMES before and after federal taxes are two quite different amounts. The increase since 1935-1939 in mean net incomes overstates the gain in mean net incomes after federal income taxes. Because physicians, like other citizens, are required to pay federal income taxes, it is proper to mention the peculiar economic pattern of the life of the physician. After spending a long time in training, any professional man starts to earn late in life and his lifetime earnings are bunched into a relatively short period of time. Because income tax rates are steeply progressive he will pay more taxes during his lifetime than another person who earns exactly the same amount of money during his life spread over a longer working lifetime— as much as 10 years longer than the working lifetime of the typical physician. Because of the lack of precise data for the base period, 1935-1939, we can make only general comments about the probable increase in the mean net income after taxes. We have, however, estimated that, assuming a wife and two other dependents, the amount of income taxes on 1949 incomes average about $1,300 per physician as compared with less than $100 of taxes in the base period, 1935-1939. It should be abundantly clear that the increase in the net income after taxes between 1935-1939 (and 1929) and 1949 was far less than the increase reported in the article for mean net income before taxes.

The All-Salaried versus the Non-Salaried

AS PREVIOUSLY NOTED, the mean net income for 1949 of physicians who derived all of their professional income from salaried practice—the all-salaried physicians— was $8,434 as compared with the mean of $11,744 for those in non-salaried practice. The difference of $3,310, uncorrected for age differences, must be examined. The non-salaried physician is roughly comparable to a small retailer; as such, he is a prime risk-bearer in our economy. Accordingly, inflation and prosperity raise his income more sharply than the salary of the all-salaried physician; and vice versa in depression. The excess in the average number of hours worked per week by the non-salaried above the average worked by the all-salaried physicians is not now available. In addition to less exposure to the business cycle, the all-salaried physicians have certain financial advantages which are not reflected in their cash compensation. Among these are various provisions for vacations, sick leave, insurance, and, perhaps most important, pensions. The non-salaried physician, whether he is an individual proprietor or a partner, cannot use any of his gross income to purchase an annuity or pension for himself because he does not qualify under the employer-employee relationship defined in the Federal Income Tax Law. On the other hand, the physician who is employed can have a pension financed in whole or in part by his employer out of his employer's gross receipts. This pension benefit does become taxable to the all-salaried physician when he retires; the extra benefit is merely a tax deferment which will enable him to pay the tax on this benefit during his retired years when, presumably, the income tax rate will be lower for him because his income is lower. It is impossible, however, to assign a specific amount of the $3,310 difference to this pension advantage; our best guess would be one-fourth. Vacation pay and sick leave benefits could account for a similar fraction of this difference of $3,310.

Specialists versus General Practitioners

THE REPORTED MEAN net income of general practitioners in independent practice for 1949 was $8,835, for partly specialized (part-time specialists), $11,758, and for fully specialized (full-time specialists), $15,014. Thus the mean net income of the partly specialized physicians was almost the same as the mean net income of all physicians in independent practice (physicians whose major source of income was fees)—$11,858, as already noted; in that sense, he is an average physician. The spread of about $6,200 between the averages for general practitioners and fully specialized physicians will be of great interest to all members of the medical profession. Weinfeld notes that the spread was considerably smaller percentagewise in 1949 than in 1929 and only $100 more. This important finding is also presented in one of his charts.

Elsewhere we have estimated that the accumulated investment of an intern in his seven or eight years of premedical and medical education and in income sacrificed is well over $30,000. The intern contemplating the three or four years of residency training necessary to become a specialist must reckon with the economic aspects of an additional investment. The income margin between specialists and general practitioners may or may not have a dollar value sufficient to offset the extra financial sacrifice during three or four years of additional training at nominal salary, or the personal sacrifice at a time in life when most young men are starting or have already started to have a family. Furthermore, the tendency of specialists to locate in the larger cities where family living costs are higher may offset some of the extra earnings of specialists. Professional qualifications, interests, and prospects may outweigh these economic considerations in the decision to become or not to become a specialist. We shall defer comment until we know the differences in the age distribution of general practitioners and fully specialized physicians which could account for some of the difference in the mean net incomes. . . .

Which Specialty?

THERE WILL BE considerable interest in the tables showing average net incomes for fully-specialized physicians by specialty. For the full specialists in independent practice, neurological surgery ranked first with a mean net income of $28,628 and a median net income of $24,500. Pathology ranked second with a mean of $22,284 and a median of $20,167. The median incomes are not influenced by the extremely large or the extremely small incomes reported by a few physicians. The rankings of specialty groups by medians is probably more reliable than by means; the two rankings, however, do agree for neurological surgery and pathology. The median ages of the respondents were 42 and 49 years, respectively. We are still in the process of developing age breakdowns which will enable us to make additional tests of the age representativeness of the returns from these specialists; this difference of seven years in the median ages of these two specialty groups seems, on the surface, excessive although pathology is one of the older specialties and neurological surgery is one of the newest. Weinfeld notes that the highest mean and median net incomes are reported for the specialties having very few members. Pathology also ranks second for the salaried full specialists with mean and median net incomes of $11,745 and $10,957, but roentgenology-radiology ranks first with $12,326 and $10,412. Again the author provides only the median age of those reporting, 41 years for pathology and 40 years for roentgenology-radiology. So much detail on the specialties is presented in the article that only this cursory summary of the highlights could be presented here.

Final Comments

OUR APPRECIATION of the indebtedness of physicians and medical economists to the author, William Weinfeld, and to M. Joseph Meehan, Director of the Office of Business Economics, and the difficulties under which they have worked is so keen —among which has been our own inability to furnish them with certain data required for testing the representativeness of their many samples—that we would not at this time care to present many additional analytical comments. For many years to come their tabulations and interpretations of the returns from this survey will stand out as a basic reference point in future studies of physicians' incomes. Frankly, we were surprised that the maximum incomes were reported for ages 40-44 or 45-49 in most of the classifications for we had expected the peak earnings to be found later in life. Higher incomes of partners may be due to specialty, size of city, and age factors; partnerships and group practice are not synonymous terms even for partnerships of three or more members. But, as previously noted, we were unable to furnish the data necessary to eliminate the age factor as a variable. This is the outstanding defect of the study. The large sample (30,000) may actually make this prime defect of lesser importance than it now seems to us. Ideally, data for standardized age blocks should have been developed before the computation of over-all means and medians. Weinfeld also notes the over-response—a higher than expected percentage of replies—from specialists and, in the "Technical Notes," the over-response and under-response from certain states. He has made corrections for the latter, which produced negligible changes in the averages, but none for the former. There are also some indications of an over-response from salaried physicians.

The significance of this survey will probably change as time passes. At the present writing it seems to us that the important implications of this study are as follows:

1. The rise in physicians' incomes of the past dozen or 20 years has been at

about the same rate as the rise in the national income per capita. More generally, the American people have been fair to their physicians in an inflationary era from the standpoint of income; and vice versa.

2. Talented high school graduates will continue to choose medicine for the age-old reasons—a great interest in the natural sciences and a conviction that a medical career will provide an opportunity to serve people. The inflationary 1940's have produced only one new financial reason for choosing medicine, namely, that medicine now pays better, on the average, than law—for the incomes of lawyers have not kept pace with the inflationary trends as have physicians' incomes. The trends for certified public accountants and consulting engineers will doubtlessly be described in future surveys.

3. The highest 1949 average net incomes were not received by physicians in the larger cities where family living costs are high.

4. The differences between the average incomes of the all-salaried and the non-salaried physicians are considerable, but the value of the perquisites of the all-salaried physicians must be weighed.

5. The moderate increase in physicians' fees since 1935-1939, as reported by the U. S. Bureau of Labor Statistics, was only one of the three major factors responsible for the increase in the average incomes of physicians which has enabled physicians' incomes to keep pace with the inflationary trend of the 1940's. The other two major factors were the improved collections of fees and the increased "output per physician."

6. In addition to these three specific factors, the increase in the number of physicians since the base period must be considered. If there had been the nation-wide shortage of physicians in 1949 which some writers have alleged, it is almost certain that physicians' incomes would have been, on the average, far higher and the increases in recent years far greater. This survey of physicians' incomes has revealed no general economic evidence of a national shortage of physicians.

31. PAYMENT FOR PHYSICIANS' SERVICES *

ADEQUATE REMUNERATION of participating physicians is one of the prerequisites for effective operation of a medical care program furnishing direct service and, especially, for maintenance of high standards. Whether such a program is established and administered by a public agency or voluntary organization, whether the funds for its support are raised through general taxation, compulsory insurance, or voluntary insurance, systematic arrangements for payment for physicians' services must be

* From: "Methods of Payment for Physicians' Services in Medical Care Programs," by Franz Goldmann, M.D.; *American Journal of Public Health* 42:134-41, Feb. 1952 (No. 2). Reprinted (with omissions) by permission of the author and publishers. The author is associate professor of medical care at the School of Public Health, Harvard University, Boston, Mass.

made by negotiation and conclusion of more or less formal agreements between the administrative agency and the medical profession. . . .

Basic Methods

THE SEARCH FOR the best method of paying physicians for service under organized programs of medical care has been protracted and intensive in every civilized country. It still continues. Three basic methods have been tried out in the course of centuries: the fee-for-service method, the flat-rate method, and the salary method. All have certain elements in common. They provide for payment for any of the services covered by a program, thereby opening up an important source of income for the physician and reducing the amount of free service and bad debts so often experienced in medical practice. They relate the remuneration of the physician to factors other than the economic conditions of the sick at the time he requests service, in contrast to the sliding scale that makes the *doctor medicinae* a tax collector, taking from his rich patients to give free or low-cost service to the poor. Each of the basic methods possesses distinctive attributes. Each has advantages and disadvantages that must be carefully weighed with due consideration to the circumstances prevailing in a given country, region, or locality.

In evaluating and comparing the financial arrangements, attention must be given to the rate as well as the form of payment, the effect on the type, quality, and quantity of service as well as the time and total professional income of the physician, and to the administrative implications. Comparative studies covering all these points are lacking. Those which have been made have been limited to some factors, particularly the costs. . . .

Fee-for-Service Method

THE FEE-FOR-SERVICE method is characterized by three qualities. Payment is based on the type, number, and value of services actually rendered, standard fees or maximum fees are set for each type of service and published in a special fee schedule for a particular program or a generally valid official fee schedule, and the fees are uniform and binding for all participating physicians practicing in a certain geographic area or rendering service under a given program. In general the fees are somewhat lower than those ordinarily charged in view of the fact that payment is certain, while collections in other practice usually represent only a certain proportion of the charges. The amount of income which the physician receives is influenced by both the number and kinds of service actually rendered and the size of the fees.

Adoption of such a system involves determination of the numerous items of service to be included in the fee schedule, assignment of a price to each item, and formulation of rules and regulations concerning the use and interpretation of the fee schedule, the procedures to be followed in submitting bills, and the control of expenditures. Its effective and economical operation depends on the regular and prompt submission of accurate, itemized bills by the physicians and at least the review and audit of each bill and the regular payment of each account by the administrative agency.

In many countries the fee-for-service method is preferred by the physicians and will be readily accepted by them because it is the very system to which they are accustomed by tradition. In the opinion of its advocates it is better suited to the needs and wishes of all than any other method of payment. It affords not only compensation in proportion to effort—taking at least partial account of the work actually done—but wide opportunity to adjust the fees to the value of the services. Moreover, it provides an incentive to give the best care to the patients and thereby serves to strengthen the bond of sympathy and interest between patients and physicians.

The critics of this method point to a number of disadvantages. The system may have merits if only treatment of selected conditions is included in a program, but it is too difficult to operate and too expensive if the scope of service is comprehensive, including preventive as well as therapeutic services and care by specialists as well as general physicians. The emphasis is placed on "the number of acts done" rather than quality, and upon treatment of disease rather than conservation of health. The highly skilled physician is penalized because the fee schedule is too rigid to offer a reward for work requiring special knowledge and experience. The method hinders early referral of the patient to specialists and encourages excessive treatment, unnecessary service, especially surgical operations, or the use of expensive therapeutic procedures, such as injections, because the physician may be guided by fear of losing his patient to a competitor, by the desire to "hold the good will of the patient," or by financial considerations.

It burdens the physician with much paper work—the very thing he hates—and requires a complicated, cumbersome and costly machinery for its administration. Administrative control by authorization and reauthorization of specific services, reviewing and adjusting of bills, or both is inevitable in order to prevent soaring costs with their detrimental effect on the total budget or other services of the program. It may well happen that the payments to the doctor must be scaled down. What the physician finally receives is a product of two administrative procedures, the approval of his own bill and the reconciliation of all approved bills with the available funds. At best, it is what he has claimed and at the worst it is a fraction of his claim. If different programs in the same locality have fee schedules allowing different charges for the same type of service, dissatisfaction and unrest among the medical profession are inevitable.

Flat-Rate Method

THE GENERIC TERM flat-rate method denotes a variety of specific forms of payment that are alike in two respects: fixed amounts of money are paid regularly and the rates represent average payments that are not related to the number of services actually rendered to the individual patient. The principle of averaging rests on the assumptions that some of the persons covered by a program will require little service and others much and that the total compensation will be in proportion to the total amount of work for all patients.

The basis for determination of flat rates may be (1) the unit of time, taking into account the number of hours, half days or full days actually worked by the physician, regardless of the number of patients seen; (2) the clinic session, taking into account the number of sessions actually held, without regard to the exact number of hours worked or the number of patients examined or treated; (3) the case of sickness or maternity, taking into account the number of cases actually attended, regardless of the type and amount of services rendered; or (4) the number of persons who have chosen the physician for a specified period of time, taking into account the number of persons eligible for service rather than that of the sick, irrespective of the type and volume of services rendered or the amount of time spent. The income of the physician depends on the size of the rate of compensation as well as the extent to which his services are utilized.

In the opinion of its advocates the flat-rate method has advantages outweighing its admitted disadvantages. If amount, scale and range of the compensation are adequate the method stimulates professional competition rather than financial competition. It provides an incentive to prevent illness and treat patients promptly, thoroughly, and economically, as the remuneration remains the same, whether a person is healthy or sick, whether the patient requires much or little service. The physician can rely on a regular and predictable income and is relieved of burdensome paper work, as no itemized bills are necessary. The administrative agency can estimate the probable expenses with a fair degree of accuracy and operate economically, because both computation of amounts payable and control of expenditures involve little in the way of administrative costs. However, the principle of averaging the remuneration is of limited applicability if the system of individual practice of medicine is combined with the method of paying flat rates according to the number of eligible persons or cases of illness.

Under this type of organization the flat-rate method can easily be employed for the compensation of general physicians because of the uniformity and predictability of the basic types of care, but it is not practicable for remuneration of specialists because of the diversity and unpredictability of their services. Quite different is the situation if flat rates are paid to group practice units. Under such an arrangement the organizations receive payment in proportion to the total number of persons who have chosen the group, and the staff members distribute the income according to their own wishes in the form of fees, flat rates, salaries, or a combination of these bases and in amounts determined by more or less formal agreements. This procedure permits recognition of both competence and effort. The potential dangers of relating payment to the number of persons on a physician's list or to the number of cases of sickness attended can be averted by limiting the number of persons or patients to be accepted by a physician or by allowing a higher rate for the first 1,000 persons or cases and progressively declining rates thereafter.

The opponents of the flat-rate method either deny the validity of the arguments advanced by the proponents or question the possibility of making an interesting theory work. Their objections are directed primarily against payment of flat rates according to the number of persons on the individual physician's list or the number of cases of sickness attended by physicians in individual practice. They contend that a limited amount of payment for unlimited service is a temptation to give a little service to many patients hastily and superficially ("rush medicine"), to do indifferent, careless, or inferior work, or to refer as many patients as possible to other physicians, particularly specialists, or to clinics or hospitals for continued treatment. Thus, the quality of medical care will deteriorate, consistency of service will become a mockery, the time and skill of specialists will be requested unnecessarily and excessively, and the total costs of the program may well increase.

The conscientious physician giving freely of his time or the highly experienced physician performing superior service is certain to lose because he will be overworked and underpaid, while the less scrupulous and less skilled is likely to gain. If only the general physicians are paid flat rates and specialists are compensated on the basis of another method, a host of problems is created. The difficulty of defining the two groups may be overcome but profound disagreement over the wisdom of distinguishing between general physicians and specialists rather than between general physician's services and specialist services will prevent a satisfactory solution of the problem. Combination of the flat-rate method for general physician's services with the fee-for-service method for specialist service requires administrative control procedures greatly reducing the possibility of cutting down administrative expenses. Limitation of the work of the physician by placing ceilings on the number of patients or potential patients frequently is considered an infringement on the right to practice.

Salary Method

THE SALARY METHOD is distinguished from the two others by the fact that fixed rates of compensation are paid periodically, usually every month, for performance of certain duties by the physician, regardless of the number of healthy or sick persons seen or the number of services rendered. Salaries are paid for part-time or full-time service and often represent net income. The rates are usually set for a year and their size is determined on the basis of qualification, experience, and age and, often also, of length of service under a given program. The total income of the physician depends on the amount of time he devotes to service under a program, his professional status and skill, the salary scale, and the type and amount of additional provisions known as "fringe benefits."

The proponents of this method argue that a guaranteed annual income commensurate with the duties to be performed frees the physician from the necessity of chasing after the elusive dollar and of the temptation to undertake more than he can master or to accept financial advantages for the referral of patients. The physician can devote his whole energy to professional work rather than spending precious time on financial statements, collaborate with his colleagues without fear of losing patients, and keep abreast of scientific progress without sacrificing income. Price competition is eliminated and quality competition encouraged, with resultant high standards of service. Administratively the method is advantageous because it involves no review, audit, and payment of countless different bills and thereby affords considerable savings.

The full-time salary method is opposed on many grounds that stem from the fear the physician would "sell the soul of his ideals for a mess of financial pottage" and lose his liberty for all time. A monthly salary check would kill the spirit of adventure, initiative, and freedom to act and all incentive to be interested in the patient, with the result of grudging response to calls, indifferent or superficial service, and low quality of care. The personal relationship between patient and physician would be undermined, if not destroyed. Appointments and promotions would be made on political grounds. Instead of being servants of the patients, the physicians would be servants of the program, "regimented units of a system of bureaucratic control," compelled to perform their work at the pleasure of the administration officials and ending up as shabbily treated and underpaid "jobholders."

Supplemental Payments by Patients

REGARDLESS OF THE METHOD employed for the compensation of physicians, a service program may pay for the full cost of the standard services or for a definite proportion only. Full payment by the program implies that the patient is required to pay only for services desired for his special comfort and convenience, that he must not offer "extra" payment for any of the services covered, and that the physician must neither demand nor accept money in addition to the compensation allowed by the program. Under the system of partial payment by the program the patient may be required to make supplemental payments to the attending physician for specified services according to regulations, or the physician may be authorized to make additional charges with or without obligation to observe limits set in official fee schedules.

Full payment by the program, in the opinion of its advocates, enables the patient or potential patient to heed the advice "see your doctor early before he has to see you" and thereby encourages preventive measures, early diagnosis, and prompt and thorough treatment. It protects the sick against unpredictable, annoying, and possibly burdensome additional expenses and removes the temptation for the physician to raise his charges on the grounds that part of the cost will be paid by the program. It preserves the principle of service in contrast to the principle of indemnification for expenses actually incurred.

Those favoring supplemental payments by patients argue that such a policy prevents abuse of the services and excessive demands on the time of the physician. Without "deterrents" patients would "run to the doctor for every sneeze, sniffle, and headache." The obligation to contribute to the cost at the time service is demanded fosters a sense of responsibility and keeps the total cost of the program within reasonable limits.

Between the extremists there is a school of thought advocating full payment by the program for all "necessary" professional services at the office, clinic, and hospital; and partial payment for home visits in general or under particular conditions, for drugs and appliances other than those declared "essential," and for materials needed for certain diagnostic and therapeutic procedures.

Present Patterns

THE EXTENT TO WHICH the three basic methods have been employed in the past and the frequency of their utilization at present vary not only from country to country but from one section of the same country to the other and from one type of program to the other in the same geographic area. . . .

In the United States the majority of all physicians rendering direct service under the various programs of medical care are compensated on the basis of the fee-for-service method, the part-time salary method, or the flat-rate method, in this order of frequency, and the minority hold full-time salaried positions. . . .

. . . The fee-for-service method is generally employed by certain tax-supported programs, such as the Vocational Rehabilitation Service and the "Home Town" program of the Veterans Administration, by the voluntary medical care insurance plans known as Blue Shield plans, and by the Workmen's Compensation programs. It is frequently used by programs of public medical care covering recipients of public assistance and "medically needy" persons and by Crippled Children's programs for the purpose of paying for treatment. Often the fees for the same type of service requiring the same skill and time vary considerably from program to program in the same area.

Payment of flat rates per unit of time or per clinic session is the prevailing method of compensating physicians for service at diagnostic clinics under the Crippled Children's programs and is not uncommon under the other programs of public medical care. Flat rates per eligible persons are paid by some programs of public medical care for the needy, such as that in Baltimore, and by the Health Insurance Plan of Greater New York which makes per capita payments to the group practice units, leaving distribution of the sums to the affiliated physicians.

The part-time salary method is utilized by at least eight state agencies in charge of Crippled Children's programs for the purpose of compensating physicians for a varying combination of diagnostic, consultative, and therapeutic services and by a number of local units of government employing town, city, or county physicians to render home care, office care, or both to needy persons.

Full-time salaries are paid primarily to physicians on the staffs of hospitals operated as centers of medical care programs, such as those of the Veterans Administration and the U. S. Public Health Service, and occasionally to physicians responsible for home, office, clinic, and hospital care, or only some of these types under programs of public medical care for needy persons, as in Buffalo, N. Y., Cincinnati and Cleveland, Ohio, Louisville, Ky., and Sacramento, Calif. Guaranteed annual incomes, comprising a basic salary and additional payments for full-time service, are common under voluntary group-practice prepayment plans.

Comments

IF THE PROBLEM of paying physicians for service in medical care programs is to be discussed fruitfully, the basic conflict arising out of the conception of "medicine as a profession of a cultivated gentleman" (Sir William Osler) must be clearly and fully realized. As R. H. Tawney has said so well, the meaning of the physician's profession, both for himself and the public, "is not that he makes money but that he makes health." Although he enters the professsion for the sake of livelihood, "the measure of his success is the service which he performs, not the gains which he amasses." If the physician lives up to professional ideals and strictly observes the code of ethics embodied in the Hippocratic oath he may well conclude his days in poverty. If he acts like a businessman he can acquire a big bank account and a large estate within a few years but will furnish ample ammunition for complaints about commercialism in the system of private practice. A well organized and efficiently administered system of paying physicians for service in medical care programs can markedly reduce the dilemma confronting the possessor of the most humane of arts.

Experience in the United States with the basic methods of payment permits six broad statements.

1. Missionaries by far outnumber mercenaries among the participating physicians. This very fact testifies to the importance of administrative procedures protecting the honest, conscientious, and careful physicians against those relatively few colleagues who, unintentionally or deliberately, cause serious damage to a medical care program by disregarding established standards of service, ignoring the rules for the operation of the plan, or violating the principles of professional ethics.

2. The payments from both tax-supported and insurance programs to participating physicians have multiplied in the last twenty years. They constitute a steadily growing proportion of the total professional income for a continuously increasing number of physicians in private practice and the sole source of support for more than ten thousand physicians devoting their full time to direct service under public programs. Although some physicians in private practice derive substantial, if not huge, incomes from certain programs, especially insurance plans, the average situation leaves much room for improvement. Fully justified criticism is directed against fee schedules lacking the flexibility so necessary for adjustment of fees to services requiring unusual skill; against flat rates and part-time salaries too low and too limited in range to attract or hold competent physicians; and against full-time salaries insufficient to satisfy specialists or unprotected by tenure.

3. If the countless articles in medical journals reflect opinions correctly, most physicians are concerned more over the rate of payment and the total income than over the form in which they are compensated by a program, provided they are given complete freedom to render service according to their own conviction and to establish and maintain the usual professional relationship with their patients.

Almost all programs have adopted specific provisions establishing the principle of professional independence and protecting the patient-doctor relationship.

4. The dollar buys more service, and administration of a program is simpler and more economical, if payment to physicians is made on the basis of the flat-rate or salary methods rather than the fee-for-service method. However, cheap medical care is always costly.

5. To be satisfactory, a system of payment to physicians must encourage adequate service in health and sickness, provide an income related to ability and effort as well as work load, and be easy and inexpensive to administer.

6. No method of payment possesses the magic power of producing high quality of service. Any systematic arrangement for the compensation of physicians must be an integral part of a service organization designed to attain effective teamwork between general physicians and specialists and highest possible standards of medical care.

D. *General Practice and Specialization*

32. THE GENERAL PRACTITIONER'S FUTURE STATUS *

The Present

THE PRESENT TREND toward specialization and away from general practice began many years ago, but was given impetus during World War II by the great emphasis placed upon specialization in the medical services of our armed forces. Other factors operating to encourage students and house officers to specialize are: (1) the specialty boards, (2) the tendency of hospitals to close their doors to general practitioners, (3) the policy of the Veterans Administration in offering special inducements to certified specialists, (4) the higher fees paid specialists by such organizations as the workmen's compensation commissions, (5) the type of training offered in our medical schools and hospitals, (6) the growing popularity of practice in groups or clinics, and (7) the period of pseudo-prosperity experienced under the artificial stimulus of war.

Inducements to Specialization.—As I see it, the four principal inducements to specialization at present are: (1) greater income, (2) greater prestige, (3) shorter working hours, and (4) easier access to hospitals. Let us consider these separately.

* From: "The Future Status of the General Practitioner," by Wingate M. Johnson, M.D.; *Pennsylvania Medical Journal* 51:265-71, Dec. 1947. Reprinted (with omissions, including initial paragraphs) by permission of the author and publishers. The author is professor of clinical medicine at Bowman Gray School of Medicine, Wake Forest College, Winston-Salem, N.C.

It is doubtful if, year after year, the net income of the average specialist is more than that of the general practitioner—if, indeed, it is as large—when one deducts the greater overhead expense. It is highly probable that some of the young men who have gone out from our recently established Bowman Gray School of Medicine of Wake Forest College are already making more in general practice than some of us who taught them. One of our senior students came to me not long ago for advice. He had been offered a guaranteed income of $1,000 a month to do general practice in a manufacturing community, and was debating whether to accept this offer or to launch upon the long training demanded of a gastro-enterologist. More recently the father of another one of our graduates, who was just getting out of service, wrote me asking that I try to persuade the young man to join him in general practice in a small town in eastern North Carolina. He told me that his income was $18,000 a year. An annual income of $18,000 may not mean much in Pennsylvania, but in North Carolina it "ain't hay."

Still another thought is that the income of the general practitioner is far more stable than that of the specialist, and that he is much more secure. It is quite possible for a man to specialize in some particular branch of medicine, only to have his specialty disappear into thin air. Many years ago a friend of mine made a handsome living in New York by doing nothing but giving transfusions. Nowadays this is done by hospital interns, medical students, and even by well-trained orderlies. There was a time when the treatment of syphilis was a source of much revenue. Now, with rapid treatment centers in operation all over the country, specialists in this field are having to look for other work. Infant feeding was once such an intricate problem that pediatricians could almost limit their work to the first three years of life. Now it has become so standardized and simplified that the Academy of Pediatrics some years ago adopted a resolution to raise the age limit of pediatric practice to 18.

There is grave doubt as to the validity of the second inducement for specialization, namely, greater prestige. Most of the general practitioners I know live in houses just as big as those of their specialist colleagues, and are accorded equal social positions. Furthermore, the prestige as well as the income of the family doctor is more secure than that of the specialist. It may be remembered that during the dark days of the depression many medical men gave up their profession for the less dignified but more lucrative job of operating taxicabs or elevators. So far as I know, none of these were family doctors.

Hollywood and the modern novelists have undoubtedly contributed to the glamour associated with the specialist; but what specialist in movies or fiction has ever touched as many hearts as Ian Maclaren's "Doctor of the Old School"? In real life, the specialist does not have the solid satisfaction that comes with belonging, as a sort of honorary member, to his families. Few specialists are accorded the honor of having babies named for them—except possibly the "Juniors" in their own immediate families.

The third appeal to specialize—shorter working hours—has, it must be admitted, much to commend it. The discrepancy between the working hours of the specialist and the general practitioner is not, however, so great as might be imagined, and it should not be as great as it is. It is only human to see the best side of another man's job, and the worst of one's own. Few specialists, if they are successful, do not put in much overtime work. Certainly the obstetrician cannot—or should not—make all his babies come in the daytime; the surgeon cannot see to it that ulcers perforate or intestines become obstructed between 9 A.M. and 5 P.M.; the nose and throat specialist can never predict when a nose will bleed or a foreign body drop down a bronchus; the pediatrician cannot diagnose over the telephone the cause of a baby's crying; and the cardiologist cannot persuade his patients to have their coronary occlusions in the daytime.

There is no valid reason why a family doctor should not have more spare time than he does, except in such emergencies as influenza epidemics and during changes of the moon, which, I have been told on good authority, encourage the flight of the stork. The general practitioner who will make an honest effort to work by appointments, and will train his secretary to make them, will be surprised and gratified to see how quickly most of his patients learn to appreciate the system. Any doctor—general practitioner as well as specialist—will do better work for taking at least one afternoon a week, exclusive of Sunday, away from his practice. In any community which has more than one general practitioner an exchange of free afternoons should be easily arranged.

Undoubtedly the tendency of hospitals to close their staffs to general practitioners is the touchiest subject in medical practice today. This will be discussed later.

Efforts Being Made to Ensure the Survival of the General Practitioner.—For a long time the plight of the general practitioner was like the weather: everybody talked about it, but nobody did anything about it. Within the past year or two, however, especially within the past year, more and more is being done to restore him to his rightful place as the keystone of the medical profession. Anyone who has kept up with the medical and lay literature must have been impressed with the number of editorials and articles devoted to general practice and the general practitioner. New journals have been established and a number of books have been published especially for the family doctor. All over the country postgraduate courses are being arranged for him. A few medical schools now include courses in general practice in their curriculum, and some of the larger hospitals are offering rotating internships planned especially to train men for general practice.

North Carolina can, I believe, claim credit for having established the first section on general practice within a state society, more than ten years ago. Other states have gradually followed suit, and this year a great number of state societies are taking this step.

For more than two decades I have been attending meetings of the American Medical Association regularly. I can say with assurance that never within its history have the House of Delegates and the officials of our parent organization shown more genuine interest in the welfare of the general practitioner than now. This interest arises, it seems to me, from the realization that the medical profession without the family doctor would be, indeed, like the play of Hamlet with Hamlet omitted. Until recently it has been assumed that we would never have to think of such a contingency, but the multiplication of specialists and would-be specialists has served to shake this complacent attitude. . . .

In the first National Conference of County Medical Society Officers, held in connection with the centennial meeting of the American Medical Association, at least half the time was devoted to discussing the general practitioner and ways and means of building up his prestige.

These evidences of interest, even of concern, over the fate of the general practitioner have been dwelt upon at some length because they augur well for his future. It is to the everlasting credit of the medical profession that it has always cleaned its own house. When reforms in medical education were needed, they were brought about by organized medicine itself, not by outside pressure. When it was evident that too many men were claiming to be specialists without sufficient training, certification boards were set up to protect the public from those who were incompetent or poorly prepared. Now that certification—and specialization—are obviously being overdone, we may be reasonably sure that there are enough able clinicians in our midst to recognize the disease and apply the proper therapeutic measures.

Suggested Remedies.—Among the remedies that have been suggested so far are:

1. The requirement of two to five years in general practice as essential to certification.

2. The establishment of rotating internships or residencies long enough to ensure fairly thorough grounding in the essentials of family practice.

3. A change in the teaching methods of our medical schools, so that the students may be made to realize the importance and the advantages of general practice.

4. The formation of general practitioner sections in hospitals as well as in state societies.

5. A certification board for general practitioners.

6. Scholarships to medical schools for boys who will promise to do general practice in a rural area for a specified number of years.

Until comparatively recent times, it was the usual custom for a physician to become a specialist by a process of evolution—beginning as a general practitioner, and eliminating one branch after another until he was limiting his work to one specialty. Sir James Mackenzie was forced into being a cardiologist—the most famous in the world—after many years of general practice. Renewed interest in this evolutionary process is evidenced by numbers of editorials and articles in medical journals and by the resolutions on the subject which were presented to the House of Delegates in June, [1947]. . . .

The alternate suggestion—that rotating internships or residencies of two to five years be established—has been put into practice in a good many hospitals. The rotating internship, I am glad to say, has always been popular in Pennsylvania.

There is no doubt but that most of our medical schools have, whether intentionally or not, encouraged their students to specialize. Most of the teaching is done by specialists, and the students cannot help being influenced by their example. May I be pardoned for calling attention to the fact that our own school, the Bowman

Gray School of Medicine of Wake Forest College, gives perhaps the only course in the country especially for family doctors? This course may help to explain the fact that half the members of our last graduating class expressed a preference for general practice.

There is no reason why such a course should not be given in every medical school. Certainly in every community capable of supporting a medical school an alert, capable, progressive general practitioner—or an internist with years of family practice to his credit—can be found who is willing to devote an hour or more a week to giving the upperclassmen the benefit of his ripe experience. Another way to interest students in family practice is to let them serve as junior interns for private patients as well as for service patients.

Within the past few years more and more hospitals have been closing their staffs to general practitioners by requiring certification of staff members. That there is now a definite reaction against this policy is shown in many ways. . . .

It is conceivable that exceptions might be made of a few hospitals, especially those connected with teaching institutions. These hospitals are expected to care for the problem cases screened out from the outlying smaller communities. Even in these hospitals, however, the broad experience of a seasoned general practitioner should be of value. Such a man might have prevented the embarrassment of a few eminent internists on the faculty of one of our greatest medical schools some years ago. They were deliberating, in the case of an undergraduate student, between the diagnosis of infectious mononucleosis and acute lymphatic leukemia. When his temperature soared to an alarming height, after a day or two at a low level, they decided to summon his father and mother to his bedside. By the time they arrived, the boy was well broken out with measles—much to the relief of his parents and the humiliation of the professors.

Specialists, no matter how well trained, are prone to forget the favorite maxim of my good friend, the late Dr. Fred Hanes: "Common things are common." On the other hand, the general practitioner is apt to make the opposite mistake of overlooking the occasional rare disease encountered until it is too late to treat it effectively. The lesson is obvious: both the general practitioner and the specialist can learn from each other.

This question of hospital privileges for the general practitioner has been dwelt upon at tiresome length, because it is causing the general practitioner and organized medicine more concern than anything else just now. It is the chief reason for the desire of many family doctors to have a certification board of their own. The more one studies the enormous problem that such a board would create, however, the more he doubts the wisdom of its establishment. Although the House of Delegates of the American Medical Association in December, 1946, authorized the Section on General Practice to create the machinery for such a board, the special committee appointed from the section to consider the matter decided that such a board was not needed—at least, not now. Instead, an Academy of General Practice was organized, which is intended to be to the general practitioner what the College of Surgeons is to the surgeon. One commendable feature of the organization is that membership must be renewed every three years, and that during that time the member must spend a minimum of one hundred and fifty hours in postgraduate work.

Subsidizing young men to go into rural general practice by means of scholarships has been tried in some states but has not yielded the results hoped for. It might be better to try subsidizing the wives or prospective wives of medical students, since they often cast the deciding vote as to location. One of the best talks made before the Second Annual Conference [1947] on Rural Health was by a layman, Mr. Chester J. Starr, of Missouri. In it he made the very sensible observation that in order to attract physicians, a community must offer certain advantages: good roads, good homes and schools, available hospital facilities, and an adequate income. "At the present time," Mr. Starr said, "we believe that subsidization is the last recourse and would prefer, greatly, to correct adverse conditions through voluntary action by all interested groups and persons."

The Future

ON THE BASIS of the past and present developments which have been discussed, an attempt will now be made to forecast the future status of the general practitioner. This will take much less time than the foregoing discussion; the rôle of a prophet is always a dangerous one, and the fewer prophecies made now, the fewer there will be to retract in the future.

The General Practitioner Will Be Restored to His Rightful Status.—I am too optimistic to believe with some that the general practitioner is to become extinct, and that the public will be left to shop around among the specialists without an intelligent guide. Neither am I willing to accept the dictum of that self-appointed adviser to the medical profession, Mr. Waldemar Kaempffert, when he said in the *New York Times* for June 15 * : "If medicine is to be practiced scientifically today, . . . we need something better than the traditional mode of practice. That something would seem to be practice under governmental auspices." I believe firmly that the general practitioner will continue to be the backbone of the medical profession, and that the pendulum is already halting in its swing to the extreme of over-specialization. The concerted action to restore the family doctor to his rightful place of leadership in the community and in his profession is bound to succeed, provided he does not yield to an inferiority complex which, more than anything else, has been threatening his usefulness.

The General Practitioner Will Have More Time.—I believe, too, that the general practitioner of the future will learn to make things easier for himself than he has in the past. By systematizing his work—keeping regular office hours, seeing patients, so far as possible, only by appointment, and training his patients who are not actually bedridden to come to his office—he can conserve much valuable time. Another

* 1947.

way in which the doctor of the future—whether general practitioner or specialist—can conserve time is to have his office in a hospital. I believe that hospitals will come increasingly to be thought of as community health centers, and that it will become the recognized custom for staff members to have their offices in the hospital. It is also probable that doctors will tend to treat all their patients in one hospital, instead of visiting two or more hospitals every day. It is to be hoped that this policy, which does save a tremendous amount of a busy practitioner's time, will not augment the tendency to the formation of medical factions in the larger communities. An active and well-organized county medical society should help to avert this danger.

The General Practitioner Will Be a Family Doctor.—Another prophecy is that the general practitioner of the future will be a family doctor rather than a general practitioner in the literal sense. There is a real distinction between the two terms, even though they are used interchangeably. A family doctor, "although he 'must know the fundamentals of all medical specialties,' may limit his work as much or as little as he chooses. He does assume responsibility for the care of his families, very much as a general contractor would assume responsibility for the construction of a building. Just as a general contractor, however, would sublet contracts for plumbing, heating, lighting and other highly specialized work, so the family doctor will refer cases requiring special skill to those who are trained to handle them. This principle must have been what Hippocrates had in mind when, in his famous oath, he had the prospective practitioner promise not to 'cut for the stone,' but to leave that work for others better qualified."

Two chief criticisms of the general practitioner which have been offered by Drs. S. A. and S. B. Thompson are "failure of the general practitioner, on occasion, to differentiate between the trivial and the serious," and "failure . . . to observe the limitations of his training." Both these criticisms should largely be overcome if more men would aspire to be family doctors rather than general practitioners.

Since the great bulk of the average family's practice is medical, a family doctor is apt to be more of an internist than a surgeon. The law of chances are against a top-notch surgeon's having time to devote to the treatment of measles, influenza, diabetes, and arthritis. I do not believe that it is my personal bias, however, which leads me to say that it is quite possible for an internist to be a family doctor. In our city there are at least half a dozen family doctors who are certified as internists. For a general practitioner desiring certification, the Board of Internal Medicine is the logical one to choose.

The General Practitioner Will Practice Alone or in a Group.—The question of solo or group practice is a matter of individual preference. If, as I have suggested, hospital staff members begin having their offices in the hospitals, they will be doing group practice almost before they know it, whether they form partnerships or not. The general practitioner—or family doctor—is able to take care of himself either as a soloist or as a member of a medical orchestra. Indeed, he is the key man in a group—the best public relations man of all. In spite of vehement denials by those whom H. L. Mencken has referred to as "specialists in other people's duties," it has been proved that a competent general practitioner is capable of caring for 85 per cent of the illnesses for which people consult doctors.

The General Practioner Will Be Better Trained in Psychiatry and Geriatrics.— Another prophecy is that the future family doctor will be better trained in elementary psychiatry, for without it he will often be lost in a diagnostic maze. The newly born term "psychosomatic medicine" is only a rechristening of an old concept. The family doctor has a great advantage over the specialist in his knowledge of a patient's background, his past history, and his temperament. My observation, after having spent more than six years in the intensive study of the problem cases sent to our clinic at Bowman Gray, is that there is no substitute for time in separating the psychic from the somatic elements of a patient's illness. I trust that the general practitioner of the future will recognize that an hour or more spent with a new patient will, in the long run, save time if he is to continue to treat that patient. Furthermore, the patience necesary for eliciting the real cause for a patient's "indigestion" may often be rewarded in many ways: the patient will be saved one, or many, unnecessary operations; the doctor will gain a grateful patient; the quacks and cultists will lose a potential customer, and socialized medicine a potential supporter; and the cause of the general practitioner will be given a boost.

Another branch of medicine hitherto neglected, but becoming of greater and greater importance, is the care of aging and aged patients. The family doctor needs to learn much about the physical ailments of old age, and still more about the psychologic changes that come with advancing years. Geriatrics bids fair to rival pediatrics in importance as a specialty for the general practitioner.

The General Practitioner Will Treat the Patient as a Whole.—Most of what has been said about the general practitioner of the future emphasizes the importance of treating the patient as a whole—and only the family doctor is capable of doing this. What Dr. G. Canby Robinson said some years ago is quite true today: "There is need of placing greater emphasis on the study and treatment of the patient as a whole in these days of advancing specialization, as the development of the general physician is required as a means of improving the quality and breadth of medical care. The task of resurrecting the family physician in a modern form should be a recognized obligation of medical education. He should combine the knowledge and methods of the internist, the psychiatrist, the hygienist, and the medical social worker. The study of the patient as a total individual in relation to his surroundings at home and at work is essential for the education of the general physician."

The General Practitioner and the Specialist Will Work in Harmony.—The final thought I would like to emphasize above all others is that there is no need for rivalry between the specialist and the family doctor. Both are playing on the same team, and both belong to the greatest profession in the world. The patient's welfare should come before all other considerations; and the first thought in the mind of every true physician should be, "What is best for this patient?" The medical profession might well apply to itself the words of one of our naval commanders, spoken when a controversy arose as to who deserved credit for a crucial victory: "There is glory enough for us all." And, we may add, there is work enough as well.

33. GENERAL PRACTICE: AN ANALYSIS *

THE PRIMARY HEALTH need of any nation as socially, technically and scientifically advanced as this is for a health service instrument that will offer an intimate, personal service to which the *individual* can turn for assistance and guidance in time of physical or mental distress; and a sound, *basic* diagnostic and therapeutic service that will assure the *individual* a good, first line of protection against the *common* hazards of illness and injury.

Despite technical progress, hospital development and the use of "screening" devices, culturally, theoretically and to a large degree in practice the family doctor is this instrument.

Any assessment of the health needs of the nation therefore depends basically on an assessment of the success or failure of general practice in discharging these responsibilities.

General practice is here considered against this background and an attempt is made to assess the degree of success attained, to analyze the elements on which this success rests and to set down some principles that might further the growth and development of this and any other related instruments of health service leading to the ends set out above.

In present circumstances it is not possible to talk about general practice as a single, definable entity. It is first necessary to analyze the various elements and patterns of practice.

Types of General Practitioner

BROADLY SPEAKING, there are three categories of general practitioner.

The first consists of the general practitioner who, after graduation, has had one or two years of hospital training (frequently a rotating internship), and has then entered community practice. This doctor at his best should be able to diagnose and treat at least 80 per cent of the illnesses with which he is faced, and should be able to understand his patients as people and to guide and assist them with their personal and family problems.

* From: "General Practice Today and Tomorrow," by Joseph S. Collings, M.B., and Donald M. Clark, M.D.; *New England Journal of Medicine* 248: 141-48, 183-94, Jan. 22 and 29, 1953 (Nos. 4, 5). Reprinted (with omissions, including initial paragraphs and tables) by permission of the authors and publishers. The authors are, respectively, the director of a group-practice medical clinic in Richmond, Australia; and the medical director of Phillips Academy, Andover, Mass.

The second class includes the general practitioner with addtitional training in internal medicine. This doctor has had a year or more of residence in medicine at an approved hospital before going into community practice; he may even have been certified by the American Board of Internal Medicine. He is frequently the technical superior of the physician referred to above, but his field of endeavor is wholly comparable.

The third comprises the general practitioner who is a specialist. He may have reached specialist status by virtue of training (such as qualification by the American Board of Internal Medicine), but more frequently he has developed advanced skills in a particular direction—for example, surgery, obstetrics and anesthesiology— by diligent application, by utilizing postgraduate educational opportunity and by years of hard-won experience. The oustanding and most controversial example of this type is the general practitioner who is also a surgeon. As these doctors advance farther and farther into their specialty field, they can give less and less time and attention to the personal problems of their patients and at some time reach a point where lack of practice combined with interest in a single field makes it impossible for them to fulfill the functions of a general practitioner.

The first mentioned of these types frequently reaches his peak of professional performance by accident and instinct, and many factors prevent him from reaching the level he should attain. The other two categories have the chance to use established channels of medical education. They arrive at the professional level they choose either by the relatively rapid process of formal hospital training or by the slow and arduous path of self-development while actually practicing in a community.

It is possible to elaborate and qualify this classification in many ways, but it provides a good working background against which to consider general practice, although it must be recognized that there are general practitioners who, for a variety of reasons, do not meet the standards—that is, a capacity for sound diagnosis and an ability to cope with the personal problems of people—claimed for the physicians described above.

This unfortunately is by no means a small or insignificant group. For the most part these physicians are victims of cultural and professional forces over which they have little control, or demonstrate little ability to control. They have been cut off from the sources that would normally permit them to develop personally and professionally and are yet forced by public demand to make a showing of abilities and skills they may not possess. These factors and others prevent them from being satisfactory general practitioners in any of the categories described above.

For the most part each of these types of general practitioner falls into reasonably definable social, economic and professional situations, which must be discussed before the problem of general practice can really be understood.

Broadly, there are two patterns of practice—urban and rural. Although they have certain things in common, there are many points of dissimilarity.

Urban Practice

THE URBAN PRACTITIONER, surrounded as he is by readily accessible consultant, laboratory and hospital services, rarely covers the broad scope of work or assumes the high level of responsibility of his rural counterpart.

The scope and nature of the urban general practitioner's activity is in great part determined by the financial, social and educational status of his patients. In the poorer, more densely populated city areas, he frequently works alone without nursing or other assistance, disassociated almost completely from his colleagues (specialist and general practitioner) and often without hospital privileges. A physician in this group usually undertakes the "care" of people from birth to death. Some still assume obstetric responsibilties, but with the rapid development of hospital and specialist obstetrics this is passing from their field.

The very conditions under which these physicians have to work permit only a superficial and unsatisfactory approach to the problems of diagnosis and therapy. Major problems, to be satisfactorily handled, must be referred to the hospitals and clinics in the area.

Some general practitioners in these circumstances, through an inherent or acquired sympathy for the problems of the oppressed, achieve excellent results in the form of guidance and counseling, but contrariwise some of them develop a resistance to the overwhelming appeals for assistance. This type of environment is not attractive to physicians of professional or personal ambition, and like any bad environment it tends to perpetuate itself and to become increasingly worse.

This pattern of practice is common to the large cities of the English-speaking world. There are, of course, individual exceptions to this generalization—such as individual doctors of exceptional talent and zeal, who to some extent overcome their environment; it is doubtful if there are any exceptions to the total pattern.

In urban areas populated by higher-income groups, the picture is modified. Whereas the general practitioner in this area covers much the same scope of work (with an ever-decreasing responsibility for obstetrics and pediatrics but with sometimes the addition of limited surgical responsibility) circumstances permit and frequently demand the exercise of a higher level of diagnostic, if not therapeutic, skills and a somewhat greater attention to the personal problems of people.

This, like the former, is a universal pattern. It is sometimes complicated by an "informed" public demand that the physician possess some of the more expensive and complicated diagnostic machinery. As a consequence, it is not uncommon to find the general practitioner's office equipped with quite elaborate x-ray facilities and to find him undertaking a wide range of radiologic diagnoses.

It is somewhere at this point that the physician of limited training crosses the threshold between the sins of clinical omission and the sins of clinical commission. Here again economic and social circumstances rather than objective professional and human consideration determine the nature of general practice.

Just how much better this situation is than the one previously described is debatable. A section of it undoubtedly is, and the movement toward general-practice specialization seems to have its genesis in this environment.

Rural Practice

RURAL PRACTICE similarly falls into a pattern with two major subdivisions. The general practitioner working in true rural isolation is in many ways a counterpart of the one practicing in poor urban areas. However, here circumstances rather than economy seem to dominate the pattern. Divorced as the truly isolated rural practitioner is from the hospital, laboratory and specialist facilities, he has perforce to be self-reliant. The full weight of responsibility for human safety forces the conscientious physician to be well equipped to diagnose and treat everything short of major surgical and complicated medical problems. He has to be obstetrician and pediatrician to his community and must be able to handle all the minor surgical problems that arise from day to day. Living intimately with his people, he cannot escape being their personal physician in the deepest sense of this term.

The scope of work that this type of practitioner has to undertake is almost self-determined; the quality of his work is nearly completely a function of his own capacity and conscience. The vagaries of human nature, in the form of physician conduct, are best illustrated in this situation.

The second major pattern of rural practice is the small community practice where the physician, frequently of his own initiative, has developed a working environment that permits him to assume clinical responsibilities fully compatible with, or even going beyond, his training and skills. In this situation most general practitioners have open access to the facilities of a small community hospital in which they can usually undertake a reasonably high level of clinical investigation and perform almost any surgical procedure for which they feel themselves competent.

The undeniable fact that in these circumstances the general practitioner sometimes overreaches his capacity (most noticeably, his surgical ability) has brought this pattern of practice under heavy criticism and sometimes virulent attack. Too frequently these criticisms and attacks lack perspective and understanding and on occasion threaten to destroy what would become the pattern for better general practice.

It is here that the general-practitioner specialist flourishes, and this exemplifies the controversial area between specialists and general practitioners. It is regrettable that in this intraprofessional struggle concentration is on the relatively unimportant, if dramatic and tangible, sins of general-practice commission, when it should be on the far more important area of sins of omission.

To complete this analysis the whole scene should be correlated to the large hospital and medical teaching situation. In summary, the great clinical institutions have grown up in the large urban areas, and in the very shadow of these institutions is to be found some of the worst general practice both technical and personal; as one moves away from the large hospitals into the less densely populated and financially better off areas, the level of general practice rises and continues to rise with distance from these medical centers, reaching its peak in small rural communities and then falling off in areas of real rural isolation.

This paradoxical situation can almost be represented graphically. It results in part from a rapid development of hospital and specialist facilities with no concurrent development of general practice, which has merely adapted itself to changing circumstances. Much of this adaptation cannot be called progress. It is almost as though the medical profession had attempted to solve a slum-housing problem by building gigantic skyscrapers, in the midst of the slums, and little attention had been paid to the environment.

Problems of General Practice

THE FOREGOING is a general analysis and requires considerable refinement before the problems of contemporary general practice can really be appreciated. However, before details are presented, it is well to pause and consider such evidence as is available to substantiate what has already been said.

For those who want to look, there is abundant, observable evidence, very little of which has been recorded, to support all that has been said thus far. For those who do not want to look, there is, of course, none. A review of the literature of the last fifty years demonstrates a remarkable absence of objective data and opinion dealing with general practice; most of what has been written fails to descend from the realm of philosophical discourse and emotional claim and counterclaim. For obvious reasons, the available evidence is qualitative rather than quantitative; however, it can serve to establish the various patterns of practice described even if it does not permit more than a general assessment of how widespread these patterns are.

It is equally obvious that in a paper of this nature it is impossible to present a larger amount of evidence, because this must, in present circumstances, depend upon lengthy, detailed and anonymous description. It is not possible simply to cite statistical data dealing with performance in general practice, for very few such data exist. Recommendations given at the conclusion of this paper are designed to rectify this anomalous situation.

However, the serious attention at present being given to general practice after many years of neglect calls in the first place for qualitative rather than quantitative analysis—sound criteria must first be established before any worthwhile quantitative assessments can be made.

No objective observer would attempt to uphold the standards and nature of general practice as it is usually conducted in the poorer, densely populated areas of large cities. Most doctors working in these places have neither the time nor the opportunity to put into effect even the indispensable procedures of history taking, record keeping and basic physical examinations that all of them learned in medical schools and hospital. To earn a satisfactory income from small fees they must do a great volume of work; to do this they must "cut clinical corners," and quickly they become "spot diagnosticians and therapists" not because of, but in spite of, their training and personal desires.

It is almost impossible to get factual data dealing with the diagnostic and therapeutic performance of these men. An example of such data, however, is provided by the experience of the Health Insurance Plan of Greater New York. Before this subject is considered one or two points should be made, to meet criticism of the validity of anything that happens in this huge city and in this particular program.

New York City is often regarded as being "freakish" and representative of nothing else, when actually it presents the quintessence of large-scale urbanization and medical organization designed to meet the demands resulting from its size. The particular program cited, the Health Insurance Plan of Greater New York (H. I. P.), whether one is for or against it as a medical development, does offer to the poor communities under discussion a more comprehensive medical coverage than they can otherwise obtain.

This program uses the services of approximately 400 general practitioners, the vast majority of whom continue to work as they always have, in and from their private offices. However, for their insured patients they can call on (without cost to themselves or their patients) all the radiologic and laboratory diagnostic aids they require.

Even so, it seemed apparent, from a survey conducted by the staff of H. I. P. in 1952, that busy doctors, working alone and divorced from the benefits of hospital and specialist assistance, dependent for a livelihood on small and sometimes uncertain fees, cannot do their work properly or meet the rigid standards required by modern medicine.

The findings of Reed and Failes, in Balitmore, and the experience of the Johns Hopkins Clinic were similar to what has been said above.

Some persons recently reviewing the New York scene regard the general-practitioner situation as beyond "the point of no return" and have seriously suggested that elementary health examinations should be carried out by a specialist team. Impersonal multiphasic screening clinics have their origin in such opinions. For obvious reasons these are neither necessary nor desirable, and such superficial thinking is dangerous and wholly destructive to general practice.

To our knowledge, similar evidence pertaining to other types of practice is not available. Pullen compiled some data on rural practice in Mississippi, but his findings are quantitative rather than qualitative and tell little of how a community is served.

The scope of responsibility assumed by general practitioners in better-class urban and in rural practice varies greatly, as does the manner in which individual doctors practice. Circumstances sometimes permit them to do better work than their less fortunate colleagues in poorer areas and also to assume a greater degree of clinical responsibility. It is generally agreed that many of these doctors take on too great a responsibility for their training and skills—for example, their credentials and experience may not gain them a place on the staff of a large hospital, but they continue to do a level of work for which they have been adjudged unsuitable in their offices and in the smaller, less controlled hospitals.

So far as record keeping is concerned, it can be said, with little fear of contradiction, that the great majority of general practitioners keep poor records. The significance of medical records is more than academic; even if they do not tell all that is to be told about performance as a general practitioner, they are certainly a key index to the quality of medical care. Few general practitioners' records are available as compared to those of specialists in hospitals, and additional means of assessing their performance must therefore be sought.

It is usually assumed that the general practitioner does too much or too little, but his actual functions have not yet been spelled out in any detail; in fact these are usually obscured in the philosophical discourses and homilies about general practice and the general practitioner. In the absence of recorded data a careful analysis of the actual activities of general practitioners working in the various environments described above is the starting point for any serious thinking about contemporary general practice.

What are the functions of the general practitioner in the various environments described above? The following is offered as a breakdown of function based on observations and interrogation of many hundreds of general practitioners over a period of several years.

Functions of Urban General Practitioners in Poor Economic Areas

"Spot diagnosis" in home and office.—This comprises the greater part of the work of these physicians. Most of this work is consequent upon a rapid examination made because of specific signs and symptoms. Time and circumstance do not permit anything like complete history taking or physical examinations.

Advice and guidance based on the limited evidence that can be obtained quickly.— This may be valuable in cases of mild emotional disturbance, but can be dangerous in more serious psychiatric conditions.

Treatment.—Much of this must necessarily be symptomatic and is restricted almost completely to the use of common drugs, medicaments and minor physiotherapeutic equipment.

Radiology (x-ray diagnosis or fluoroscopy, or both).—Many of these men have their own x-ray equipment. The more conservative restrict the scope of their work to the chest and the small bones, doing their own interpretation. Some attempt a wide range of radiologic diagnoses, such as barium series, cholecystography and pyelography.

Laboratory.—Most of these doctors are equipped to do urinalyses, blood counts, hemoglobin estimations and sometimes sedimentation rates. A quite surprising number record and interpret their own electrocardiograms and many take basal metabolic rates. The amount of radiologic and laboratory work most of these men attempt seems to be correlated to their patients' ability to pay them (as distinct from an ability to pay specialists' fees) for these services.

Referrals.—In the poorer areas referrals are usually to clinics and hospital out-patient departments. These physicians seldom have the time or opportunity for person-to-person consultation with specialist colleagues, and their patients can rarely afford private specialist consultations.

Minor surgery.—Probably a majority of these physicians will open a superficial abscess or put in a few sutures.

Obstetrics.—Some of this group still retain a small obstetric practice; 15 to 20 deliveries a year seem to be about the maximum load.

Major surgery.—A small number of this group, with admitting privileges in small proprietary hospitals, attempt major operations such as tonsillectomies, appen-dectomies and gynecologic procedures.

Pediatrics.—This is also approached on the basis of spot diagnosis, elementary therapy and advice and guidance based on such information as can be obtained quickly. Pediatrics frequently forms a major part of this type of practice.

Hospital work.—Few of these men have worthwhile hospital appointments or the desire or opportunity to take seriously such appointments as they have. It is esti-mated that in New York City there are 2500 physicians without any hospital ap-pointment and a majority of these probably fall in this category.

The great bulk of the work done by these physicians is spot diagnosis and elementary therapy. The volume of the other functions set out depends largely on the financial status of their patients.

These physicians continually face the insidious choice of doing too little or doing too much. In such circumstances, good and sometimes even safe medical care (not to mention "health care") is impossible.

Functions of the General Practitioner in Better-Class Urban Areas

THIS PICTURE IMPROVES in degree, but not greatly in kind, in the better-income, urban residential areas. General practitioners in these more stable financial cir-cumstances can sometimes but not always devote more time to individual patients. They frequently do more of their own x-ray and laboratory work, which appears, as stated above, to be primarily conditioned by the patient's ability to buy these services from them. This can be judged as good or bad according to assessment of the individual doctor's abilities. These general practitioners do less obstetrics and pediatrics (sometimes none at all) but, on the whole, more surgery, again largely for economic reasons, but occasionally because they have developed special skills and interest in this field. They may see more of their patients in their homes and for this reason alone probably do a better job of guidance in cases with functional components, but still present the same danger as mentioned above.

The functions of this type of general practitioner are amazingly constant throughout the English-speaking world. In the countries of the British Commonwealth these physicians seldom make x-ray or electrocardiographic examination and so forth, and on the whole do less laboratory work than those in the United States. Otherwise, their functions are wholly comparable.[1]

Functions of the Urban General-Practitioner Specialist

THE PATTERN changes markedly with the urban general-practitioner specialists (usually men eligible for certification by the American Board of Internal Medicine).[2] The clasification of certified internists as general practitioners calls for special comment.[3] Most of these men try to restrict their practice to adult internal medicine (some also do a limited amount of pediatrics). They still make home calls, frequently only because of economic pressure or strong patient demand. They do a considerable amount of hospital work and more frequently have good hospital connections. They usually exclude surgery (even minor) completely and limit radiologic work to fluoroscopic and chest examinations. Many of them do their own electrocardiographic, basal metabolic work and so forth. A better financial return for effort more readily permits the employment of ancillary staff such as nurse secretary, and at this level the "spot-diagnosis" proposition largely comes to an end.[4]

With this improved clinical or technical situation there arises the real problem of the breakdown of intimate personal service. The younger physician, who has struggled for specialist recognition simply does not want to be a general practitioner; in the true sense of the word he has aspired to the status of consultant and wants what he believes to be the benefits of this status.

This is well illustrated by the complaints received against the H. I. P. groups using board-qualified internists as general physicians. Two groups that use almost exclusively qualified men and that undoubtedly deliver an extremely high quality of medical care rate badly (as contrasted with some groups using doctors without such qualifications) so far as patients' complaints about attitudes, human relations and home service are concerned. The same complaint is occasionally made of the general-

1. Descriptive evidence of this type of practice in Great Britain is set out in the report "General Practice in England Today" (*Lancet*, March, 1950) and is supplemented and confirmed by the voluminous correspondence that followed publication of the article.

2. Other general-practitioner specialists eligible for certification in surgery, urology, obstetrics and so forth are not considered here. These physicians are only transitory general practitioners supplementing their incomes until they are established specialists.

3. Within the framework of general practice used here the qualified internist should not really be classified as a general practitioner. The desire on the part of some members of the profession so to classify the specialist internist is unrealistic and more than anything else reflects the latest dissatisfaction with the present standards of general practice.

4. This pattern is the same in British Commonwealth countries for general-physician specialists holding M.R.C.P. and similar qualifications.

practitioner surgeon (usually a rural practitioner) who has compromised his "personal" work for technical achievement in the field of surgery.

This is a natural, human situation and should be studied closely, since it illustrates the balance or imbalance that can be attained between technocracy and humanism in the field of health care. It is closely related to education and social status and is discussed below in relation to education.

Functions of the Rural Practitioner

THE SCOPE OF WORK and responsibilities embraced by the rural physician with access to a community hospital is considerably greater than any mentioned above. The chief additions to the functions described for urban practice are as follows:

Surgery.—Much more major surgery is undertaken by general practitioners in these circumstances. Observation (nonstatistical) indicates that the "average" general-practitioner surgeon in a rural area, like the general-practitioner specialist discussed above, limits his operative procedures to a specific list.

Obstetrics.—This is practiced in greater volume than undertaken by the urban general practitioner and with the inclusion of quite serious abnormalities (frequently requiring cesarean section and very occasionally a Porro section). Except in small cities that will support the services of a specialist obstetrician, the general practitioners undertake all obstetrics, but the most able and conscientious keep in touch with consultants regarding unfamiliar and serious complications that are pending.

Radiology.—This is practiced to the upper limit of that described for the urban practitioner. Those with time, practice and experience place no reliance on their own diagnoses and have nearly all films interpreted by a roentgenologist.

Anesthesia.—The rural physician gives anesthetics as considered necessary for the operative procedures undertaken. These are usually limited to intravenous inductions, open ether, nitrous oxide and oxygen and low-spinal anesthesia.

The functions listed above cover the "average" scope of additional responsibilities assumed by what might be called the "conservative group" of this type of physician. It is based on the interrogation and observation of the work of many hundreds of general practitioners working in comparable rural situations in the United States, Great Britain, Scotland, Canada, Australia and New Zealand. This "conservative group" seems to form the great majority of this type everywhere.

The "radical" minority extend their scope of work considerably farther but still seem to stay within definable limits. These men attempt major bowel operations for even diagnosed malignant conditions, thyroid surgery and much more difficult orthopedic surgery, but this seems to be about the surgical maximum.

Rarely, radiotherapy and even radium therapy are attempted under the conditions described. Some of these men also embark on anesthetic adventures using endotracheal and high-spinal technics, cyclopropane, closed circuits, curare and so forth, which may or may not be successful, depending on the original and postgraduate training.

The studies on which the above description is based also demonstated by observation (without statistical documentation) that the work done by the conservative group of rural practitioners is frequently more thorough and complete, right across the medical board—history taking, record keeping, investigation and diagnosis (quite apart from the therapeutic procedures practiced)—than in the majority of urban situations.

The scope of work that all general practitioners undertake is partly determined by cultural demand and by economics. As personal physicians these doctors are again frequently superior to their urban counterparts; the factors bringing this about are the more intimate nature of rural life and the rapport established in a situation of greater human dependency of patient on doctor.

The additional responsibilities assumed by the rural community doctor force him, unless he is quite unscrupulous, into a much more satisfactory organizational situation in which he may employ nurses, secretaries and technicians.

Just as the unfavorable, densely populated urban environment tends to aggregate physicians content to labor under all the handicaps and limitation described, so "good" rural-community environments attract physicians of professional ambition who want to put into operation the skills in which they have been trained and that they hope to develop.

Limitations of General Practice

WHAT SHOULD or should not be done by the general practitioner? There seems to be unwillingness everywhere to define this categorically. The American Academy of General Practice lays down as one of its objects, "to preserve the right of the general practitioner to engage in medical and surgical procedures for which he is qualified by training and experience," and this broad statement seems to have the endorsement of general practitioners in all countries.

However, the question must be asked, Is this right of self-determination of individual medical function, in relation to training, experience and ability, the correct way to a safe, high level of medical service for everyone? If the residency training program and economic and professional circumstances of general practice were considerably better than they are, the answers to these questions would almost certainly be affirmative. However, circumstances are far from ideal, and as pointed out above, the individual general practitioner is by no means the master of his own professional destiny.

Can American medicine, therefore, afford to go ahead on a laissez-faire policy in relation to general practice, or should professional controls be put into effect at the level of training and community practice, similar to those long since accepted as essential at the level of specialist and hospital practice? Such a laissez-faire policy can no longer be afforded. It is because general practice has drifted for so long, while the various special branches of medicine have followed a charted and controlled course, starting with residency programs, that general practice is today in such an amorphous and frequently indefensible state.

With much right and reason on his side, the radiologist can attack the correctness of the general practitioner's undertaking work in this field. Similarly, the surgeon, the obstetrician, the gynecologist, the pediatrician and the rest of the specialists can attack him for his endeavors in each of these particular fields. Most of these attacks fail to stand up to examination where general practice is properly conducted.

No quantitative or qualitative assessments are available to describe a "properly" conducted general practice. Yet observation shows that there are hundreds (perhaps a few thousand) of physicians whose abilities and conduct might be taken as a pattern for all. These physicians have usually reached this level by accident or chance related to the socioeconomic environment of their practices and postgraduate education. Seldom do they reach early professional maturity through existing residency or specific postgraduate programs.

Never losing sight of the need for a large degree of autonomy and self-determination in general practice, one must define the province and function of the majority of general practitioners of the future, and correlate this with educational and training requirements and the means of establishing and maintaining standards. What follows is offered in an endeavor to do this.

So far there has been no realistic and satisfactory definition of general practice. The great majority of attempts to define this, the largest and considered by some the most important field of medical endeavor, have resulted in broad and often meaningless generalities. This failure of definition has a significance all its own, which will be examined before a practical, working definition is offered.

The main difficulties of defining the work of the general practitioner arise because, in what is loosely called "general practice," there are so many different kinds of physicians doing so many different things. In these circumstances it is greatly to the advantage of many men in the medical profession to leave the work of the general practitioner undefined, or loosely defined, because then the lines of definition can be vaguely drawn to satisfy the prejudices, fears, poses, preconceptions and hopes of different parts of the profession and the public.

General practitioners, themselves uneasy about discrimination in staff appointments, worried about the multiplication of boards of certification and defensive about their rights in certain specialist fields, seem to have avoided attempts to describe and evaluate the exact nature of their work.

Specialists, preoccupied with their own problems and concerned about standards and developments in their own particular fields, have had little time or inclination to think seriously about the man who must perform what are often considered to be the laborious, uninteresting and poorly compensated chores of the profession.

Medical educators also seem to have resisted defining the field of general practice. Faculty members are nearly all specialists, and have little or no opportunity of seeing or working with the general practitioner, in teaching hospitals, medical schools or the community. These teachers, isolated from the actual work of general practice, face the difficult problem of preparing a general practitioner for work that embraces some eighteen specialties, each with a separate board qualification. In these circumstances, it is naturally easier to deal with the problem by going around it than by attempting to define it and meet it head on. As a way out of this confusion, some educators have talked of producing "a new type of general practitioner" who, on close inspection, suggests the product of a *mésalliance* between the public-health officer and the psychiatrist—a product wholly incapable of meeting the practical medical requirements of the people.

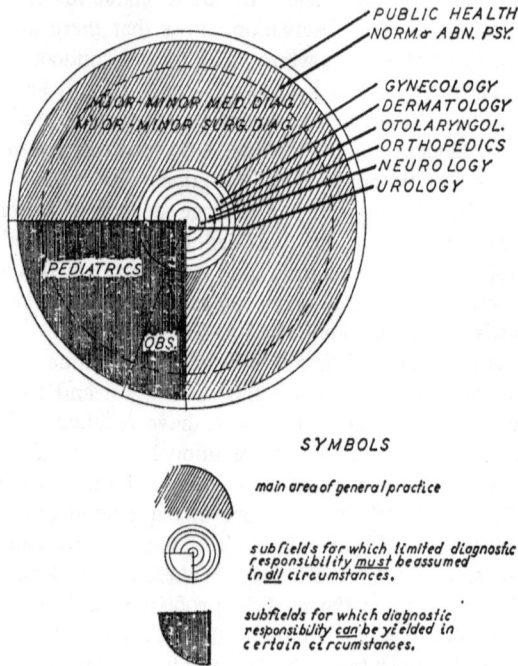

FIGURE 26. Diagnostic responsibilities of the qualified general practitioner.

It is obvious that there are certain specific advantages for a good many groups in the medical profession if the nature of general practice is left undefined. Other, more general circumstances contribute to this failure of definition. Probably the most important of these is the legitimate antipathy of many highly trained and able men for the professionally inadequate who are classed as "general practitioners."

As long as the nature of general practice remains uncertain, it will be impossible for medical authorities, or men in general practice to reach necessary agreement among themselves about what should be the extent of the general practitioner's participation in certain highly specialized fields. It will be equally impossible to establish the exact level of diagnostic and therapeutic responsibility.

Until a specific definition is furnished, it will be difficult to attract men to the field of general practice; it will be difficult to design a sound program for their education, and it will be almost impossible for them to work as general practitioners, with satisfaction to themselves, their profession and their community.

In the first part of this report reference was made to the lack of definition of general practice. Because of this lack, with its resulting ambiguities of status, limitations and responsibilities, many young physicians are unwilling to take up what appears to be an outstandingly thankless form of medical practice. Such a situation

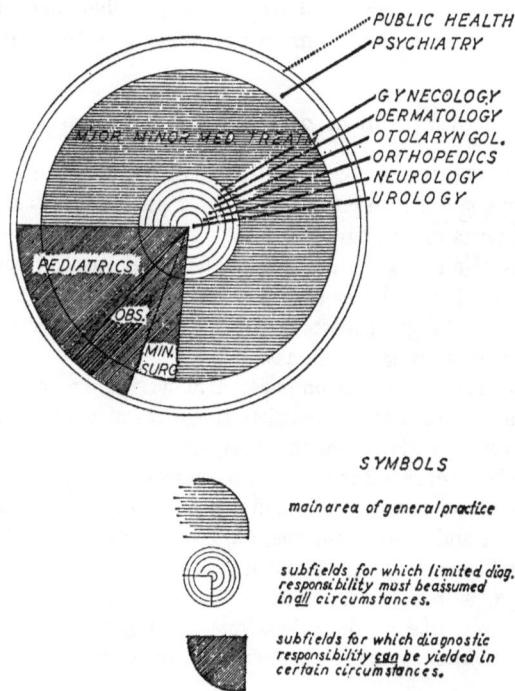

FIGURE 27. Therapeutic responsibilities of the qualified general practitioner.

gives rise to the vicious circle prejudicial alike to the best interests of the medical profession and the public.

Is it, then, possible to define and describe what the general practitioner of the future must *know* and must *do?* This is quite possible, and can best be demonstrated initially by diagrams. Figures 26 and 27 are designed to show the real and practical diagnostic and therapeutic demands of general practice.

In these diagrams, outstanding points to be noted are as follows:

At least 75 per cent of the work in general practice falls into the fields of *major and minor medical and surgical diagnosis* and *major and minor medical treatment,* with undetermined overlapping into the field of psychiatry.

Certain special fields can be, and frequently are, omitted from general practice. (This is important in terms of function and education of the general practitioner.)

Certain special fields—principally psychiatry, dermatology, neurology, gynecology, orthopedics, otolaryngology and urology—cannot be omitted, being an essential part of all general practice.

They are entered on the diagrams in such a way as to suggest their extent in general practice.

Before details of the full implications of all this are considered, a concise and explicit definition of a general practitioner is necessary. The following definition is presented in terms of function and responsibility, rather than in the broad and abstract terms so often used when previous attempts have been made at definition.

Definition of a General Practitioner

A GENERAL PRACTITIONER is a graduate in medicine from an approved medical school who, after a specific hospital training, is capable of assuming responsibility for the following areas of medical care:

The diagnosis of all major and minor medical and surgical conditions (except extremely complicated and rare ones).

The treatment of the great majority of the medical conditions diagnosed (but only the really *minor surgical* conditions).

Obstetrics to the level of uncomplicated deliveries, the early recognition of abnormalities and the necessarily immediate treatment of the few unpredictable but potentially catastrophic emergencies that may arise.

Pediatrics to the level required for medical and surgical diagnosis and treatment.

Psychiatry to a level permitting the differentiation of serious, potentially serious and mild psychoses and psychoneuroses, and permitting the treatment of the last mentioned by intelligent support, clarification and reassurance.

This definition, within broad limits, is specific in terms of function and responsibility. However, like all definitions that attempt to encompass a wide and diffuse range of activities, events or phenomena, it requires considerable explanation and qualification. . . .

Medical Education in Relation to General Practice

MEDICAL CURRICULA and hospital training programs have grown up in a haphazard fashion. Twenty or thirty years ago medical education in the better schools was more or less basic, if for no other reason than at that time the sum total of sound medical knowledge was basic. Since then all sorts of endeavors have been made to superimpose on the basic and essential the almost incredible scientific and technical advances of the last few decades.

The present-day medical student is expected to absorb an immense amount of detailed knowledge, much of which bears little relation to the work he is going to do. He is the victim of rapid technical and scientific progress and the natural enthusiasms of the scientists and educators to embrace and pass on these advances in knowledge.

Medical education has far outstripped the ability of doctors to use and apply widely in a practical way the knowledge and technic at their disposal. A dawning realization of this fact has added to the burdens of medical students. Confusion characterizes present-day thinking in this field.

Endeavors are being made to compensate for the great swing of the academic pendulum to scientific materialism by the addition, to an already overloaded curriculum, of superficial attempts to "humanize" the student, and to teach him "social" and "psychologic" medicine.

The movement toward specialization and the almost total domination of medical faculties by specialists has greatly intensified these trends. Correction can only be brought about with a clear recognition of the real medical needs of the people and the regearing of educational machinery to meet these needs. More than anything else this calls for an objective understanding of the problems of general practice, a functional definition of the essential responsibilities of the general practitioner and the readjustment of educational theory and practice to cope with them.

This paper has endeavored to do the first two of these things; it cannot in any detail attempt the latter. We recognize completely the importance of training and its relations to subsequent medical performance; we appreciate the endeavors of the various specialty groups to establish and promote standards within the confines of the numerous specialties, but we deprecate the over-all trends in relation to the needs of the people, and the needs of the vast majority of doctors who are to serve them.

So far as general practice is concerned theoretical requirements of the present-day medical course go well beyond the requirements of the doctor in practice. This, of itself, would be no crime so long as these theoretical excesses were not carried on at the price of practical essentials, which would promote the general level of medical care in the community. It is suggested that this is the price being paid for some of the great "advances" in medical education.

The enormous developments in hospital practice have elevated the larger of these institutions, particularly the teaching hospitals, to a plane so far above that of community practice that the gap is difficult to bridge, but with great effort (which is far from universal) and by strict adherence to a basic pattern of consultants, physical plant, laboratory facilities and moderate hospital control of qualifications for staff membership (particularly the surgical staff), the present gap could be bridged. To try to eliminate the hiatus by the inclusion of short "orientation" courses in the ways of general practice or by harnessing of the resources of health departments, programs for the medical care of indigents, hospital and outpatient departments, screening clinics and so forth is both inadequate and artificial. The use of such unsatisfactory impersonal substitutes for what should be a personal medical service is no solution, and yet this is the common trend.

We believe that the answer to the educational dilemma lies, first with an understanding of the problems as set out above, and secondly with the harnessing of the huge clinical and teaching resources outside existing teaching hospitals. We do not agree with the readoption of long-discarded technics of preceptorship, which some authorities are again advocating, but suggest rather that tried and tested methods of internship and residency training can be applied in a much more realistic manner and extended to embrace smaller hospitals of satisfactory standard. These hospitals today house the greatest part of the less exotic but absolutely necessary clinical teaching material. To accomplish this, general practitioners and specialists in rural and semirural areas would be expected to give instruction under the auspices of the teaching hospitals after the problem and the method had been carefully studied.

We further believe that it is possible and necessary to develop a new teaching medium outside the hospitals. This should take the form of properly organized group practice, serving community needs to a much higher level than is usually possible for the individual practitioner working alone in his office.

The province of teaching must pass from the monopolistic control of the specialist and make full use of the great contribution that the general practitioners have to offer, when they have shown that, as a group, they are capable and desirous of accepting this great responsibility.

None of these statements in any way imply a turning back of the clock so far as the standards and qualifications of specialists are concerned, but rather a realistic and common-sense turning forward of the clock in terms of standard setting for general practice. This includes, however, an appeal to stop decrying the achievements of general practice in terms of the rightfully exalted, highly particularized requirements for individual specialist fields and to stop trying to set the educational course for the former with the compass of the latter.

It is not possible to discuss in detail the question of curriculum content, but we are firmly of the opinion that a well planned four years of medical education, followed by two years of hospital training, where teaching is properly conducted, will meet the needs of a high level of general practice anywhere. The one exception to this generalization is surgical technic, which calls for a third or fourth year of hospital experience devoted specifically to this end, with perhaps orientation in this direction in the early years of hospital training.[5]

It is emphasized that the financially handicapped make up a large percentage of students who enter this field. The expense of three or four years of internship and residency program may be prohibitive. Direct subsidies in the form of loans, internships during the fourth year of medical school and other suggestions have been made to fit the difficult economic situation to the absolute necessity of longer hospital training for qualified general practitioners and general-practitioner surgeons.

Postgraduate or "continuing" education is a necessity of good general practice. The word "continuing" should forever be replaced by the word "continuous." The key to continuous education is the daily constant and close interaction of doctor with doctor that today is difficult for most men working in individual practice and impossible for those in this position with no hospital appointments. The value of

5. One of us (D.M.C.) believes that three years of hospital training are necessary to qualify a general practitioner and four years of hospital training, with three of these devoted to surgery, are necessary to qualify a doctor as a general-practitioner surgeon.

formally planned postgraduate courses is secondary to that of providing the means for this constant and close interaction.

As a matter of fact, if the residency training for general practice by means of medical journals, hospital meetings and the meetings of county and state medical societies were adequate and young doctors could and would pursue "continuous" education locally, most of the postgraduate courses now offered would be redundant. This is not true of the preparation for part or total specialization (preparing for the American Board of Medicine and so forth), which requires weeks or months of postgraduate work, year after year.

Why is it almost impossible to persuade the majority of general practitioners to use the excellent postgraduate facilities that may be at their disposal? In addition to all the factors mentioned (time, low income and lack of hospital facilities), it is a cold fact that, unlike the specialist, the general practitioner can afford to practice at a substandard level without greatly jeopardizing his hospital appointment, his income or his membership in medical organizations available to him. We do not regard the one-year internship and the program of postgraduate study required by the American College of General Practice as fully meeting the situation. The expulsion from the Academy of General Practice of over 100 physicians in California because they did not meet the required postgraduate study emphasizes the lack of incentive under the present program.

If hospitals demanded qualifications for staff appointments for general practitioners more in line with necessities of practice, if boards of general practice were established to be taken three to six years after completion of residencies, and if admission to the Academy of General Practice required the foregoing qualifications for membership, perhaps the general practitioner of the future would have the same incentive that is common to all the specialist fields and a worldwide pattern.[6] This is mentioned as a partial solution even though some of the less desirable features of the board requirements are appreciated.

Finally, it must be said that educational reform is far from the panacea of all evils in the circumstances of general practice today. Important as it is, it may be secondary to the requirements for social, economic and organizational reform in relation to this field.

34. TRENDS IN SPECIALIZATION *

THE PHYSICIAN specialist is one answer to the problems arising as medicine has become more scientific and complex in character. Where techniques call for great

6. This conception of three-year residency programs and American Board of General Practice qualifications is not countenanced by one of us (J. C.), who believes that for many reasons not more than 5 or 10 per cent of general practioners could or would accept such a program.
* From: *Building America's Health,* by the President's Commission on the Health Needs of the Nation; Washington: U.S. Government Printing Office, 1953 (Vol. 2, Chap. V, "Health Personnel," pp. 152-55). Reprinted with omissions, including initial paragraphs and some tables and figures.

skill, his services are indispensable to high quality medical care. It can hardly be questioned that curative and preventive medicine in the United States owe much of their position of world leadership to the development of specialization. The specialist must be regarded as one of the most important health resources in the Nation.

In 1949 the United States had 62,700 full specialists, 54,900 of them engaged in private practice. A fifth of all full specialists were in the field of internal medicine. Another fifth were surgeons. Fifteen percent specialized in ophthalmology or ear, nose and throat. Together, more than half of all specialists were in these fields.

This pattern of distribution is not the same as it was a quarter of a century ago. While the total number of specialists has grown markedly since 1923, the various types of specialists have increased at different rates. Increases have been relatively gradual, for example, in the fields of ophthalmology and otorhinolaryngology, public health and urology. They have been quite sharp in the fields of anesthesiology, internal medicine, obstetrics and gynecology, orthopedic surgery, and pediatrics.

Between 1923 and 1949 the proportion of all specialists who were in the field of internal medicine increased by more than one-half and the proportion who were obstetricians or gynecologists almost doubled. In contrast, the proportion in the fields of ophthalmology or otorhinolaryngology decreased by more than one-half.

If the present distribution of residents in special fields may be taken as an indication of future trends, the relative numerical importance of the various specialties will probably continue to change. In 1950-51, almost half of the 1949 graduates serving in approved civilian hospital residences were in the fields of general surgery or internal medicine, suggesting that the present predominance of these specialties will grow further. Only about 2 percent were in ophthalmology or otorhinolaryngology.

Certifying Boards

ALTHOUGH NOT ALL specialists in the United States are "certified," such certification is the most readily identifiable mark of specialization. To date, the Council on Medical Education and Hospitals or the American Medical Association has given approval to examining and certifying boards for 18 specialties.

These boards have been established gradually. The first, the American Board of Ophthalmology, was organized in 1917. By 1933, boards had been added for otolaryngology, obstetrics and gynecology, dermatology and syphilology, and pediatrics.

At present the 18 American specialty boards cover the following: anesthesiology, dermatology and syphilology, internal medicine, neurological surgery, obstetrics and gynecology, ophthalmology, orthopedic surgery, otolaryngology, pathology, pediatrics, physical medicine and rehabilitation, plastic surgery, preventive medicine and public health, proctology, psychiatry and neurology, radiology, surgery, and urology.

A nineteenth board, the Board of Thoracic Surgery, is organized as an affiliate to the American Board of Surgery, with prior certification in surgery required for certification in thoracic surgery.

TABLE 34. *Number of specialists and diplomates and percent relationship, 1949*

Specialty	Full Specialists, 1949	Diplomates, 1949	Percent of Full Specialists Who Are Diplomates
Total	62,688	32,714	52
Anesthesiology	1,231	472	38
Dermatology; syphilology	1,609	938	58
Internal medicine	12,490	5,396	43
Obstetrics; gynecology	5,074	2,595	51
Ophthalmology and otorhinolaryngology	9,224	5,362	58
Orthopedic surgery	2,035	1,202	59
Pathology; bacteriology	1,730	1,444	83
Pediatrics	4,315	2,823	65
Psychiatry; neurology	4,720	2,932	62
Radiology; roentgenology	2,866	2,657	93
Surgery	11,127	3,898	35
Urology	2,193	1,194	54
Other	4,074	1,801	44

Sources: 1950 Directory of Medical Specialists. A. N. Marquis & Co. (Chicago, Ill.); 1950 American Medical Directory, pp. 12, 13, table 4. American Medical Association (Chicago, Ill.).

The 1950 edition of the Directory of the American Specialists listed some 32,700 board-certified specialists (or "diplomates of specialty boards"). This means that about half of all specialists in 1949 were certified. The proportion certified was highest in the fields of radiology and roentgenology, pathology and bacteriology, and pediatrics. Surgery had the smallest proportion of diplomates.

Of the 32,700, about a third were divided between the fields of internal medicine, and ophthalmology and otorhinolaryngology. Just under 3,900, or almost an eighth, were surgeons. About 2,900 were psychiatrists or neurologists.

Just as some specialty groups are growing faster than others, so the rate of increase among types of Board-certified specialists has varied. Among the diplomates showing unusually rapid growth since 1940 are those in anesthesiology, dermatology and syphilology, internal medicine, and orthopedic surgery. Members of these groups are also generally younger than average. Diplomates remaining relatively unchanged numerically in the last 10 years include obstetricians and gynecologists, neurological surgeons, otolaryngologists, and plastic surgeons. As a group, these tend to be older than the average.

In addition to the 62,700 full specialists in 1949, there were 23,700 part-specialists, about 23,000 of whom were in private practice. Devoting a portion of their time to general practice, more than three-fifths of these part-specialists were in the fields of surgery, obstetrics, or gynecology. Pediatrics was next in importance, with about 8 percent of the total.

Location of Practice

SPECIALISTS ARE MORE unevenly distributed in the country than are other physicians. In 1949, about a third of the 62,700 full specialists were concentrated in the Central Atlantic States, more than half of them in New York. A sixth were in the East North Central States. This pattern was duplicated almost exactly for the 35,000 diplomates in 1950.

Relative to population, the Central Atlantic and New England States have the most specialists. In 1949, they had 55 and 53 full specialists per 100,000 population, respectively. The Southeastern States had less than 25 and the Southwest, under 30. The range among States was greater, from 72 in New York to 15 in Mississippi. In 1950, the number of diplomates per 100,000 population ranged from 34 (Central Atlantic) to 13 (Southeast) among regions, and from 45 (New York) to 6 (Mississippi) among States.

The ratio of specialists to all physicians varies in different parts of the United States. In the New England, Central Atlantic, and Far West States, between 30 and 33 percent of physicians are specialists. In the West North Central and Southeastern States, the proportion is under 27 percent.

While there are differences of degree among varieties of specialists, the Southeastern States generally tend to have the least relative to population, and the Central Atlantic States, the most. In 17 different full specialties in 1949, the only exceptions were in anesthesiology, industrial practice, orthopedic surgery, public health and urology. In public health the positions were approximately reversed, with the Southeastern States at the top and the Central Atlantic States second to the bottom. In anesthesiology and orthopedic surgery, the top region was New England. In industrial practice, the East North Central States had the most.

More than other physicians, specialists are concentrated in cities. Cities offer them essential hospital and other professional facilities, as well as more favorable living conditions. In all cities of 25,000 population or more in 1949, over half the physicians in civilian private practice were full specialists, while the proportion was as low as 3 percent in communities from 1,000 to 2,500. Part-specialists were proportionately most numerous in medium-sized communities, from 5,000 to 25,000 population.

Organization of Specialist Services

IF SPECIALISTS ARE to serve the needs of the Nation, they must be available to the people. This includes people living outside the immediate area of large medical centers.

It is widely agreed that group practice permits full utilization of the specialist under favorable circumstances and at the same time provides the most medical services for a given amount of money. Group practice is especially advantageous in small and relatively isolated communities. Through organizing the use of their radiologists and pathologists, for example, the Bingham Associates in Massachusetts and the Rochester group in New York have made special services readily available to outlying communities where such services were once unattainable.

In many places local doctors are encouraging specialists to come to their communities. The Wilmington Hospital in North Carolina, for example, has made a practice of calling in outside specialists. Providing consultation for a week at a time, the specialists are enthusiastically received in the community. In some 10 towns within a radius of 70 miles from Cincinnati, general physicians in the Southwestern Ohio Association of General Physicians have similarly obtained specialist services. Throughout the country specialists in travelling orthopedic clinics are being welcomed, with local doctors cooperating wholeheartedly.

The success of plans for utilizing the services of specialists still depends largely on the attitude of local individuals. In some places, unfortunately, eminent specialists continue to be coolly received. Where local cooperation is absent, plans will not work. . . .

E. *The Role of Allied Professions*

35. NURSING *

To ATTEMPT to discuss the progress in nursing during the past 50 years is to face a baffling task. It must be admitted at once that the story is one of confusion—great enough that it might be considered by some critics to exclude altogether the use of the word progress. But before we concede any such decision, much needs to be said, and much can be said.

Let us look, then, at this half-century, namely, the years between 1900 and the present. What has been happening, be it labelled progress or otherwise? What are the boundaries of this service called nursing? What does the word nursing indicate today? Why, as is obvious, has the quantity of service expanded so greatly during this time? Why, in spite of the phenomenal growth in numbers, is there always a shortage of service? Why is there so much discontent with the quality of nursing, and particularly with the quality as given in hospital? Why the extraordinary lack of reasoned argument concerning the conduct of nursing schools? Why are nurses themselves always on the defensive, and almost everyone else on the offensive in regard to nursing? Why must I myself dread the effort to discuss nursing with even my most intelligent friends, when I know that seldom will such discussion get past prejudices based upon ignorance of the real fundamentals of the argument? Why are these fundamentals so elusive? Why am I wondering now how many

* From: "Medicine as a Social Instrument: Nursing," by E. Kathleen Russell; *New England Journal of Medicine* 244: 439-45, March 22, 1951 (No. 12). Reprinted (with omissions) by permission of the author and publishers. The author is the director emeritus of the School of Nursing, University of Toronto, Toronto, Canada.

hospital administrators or medical practitioners—or even what number of nurses —will read this article patiently and with a desire to understand, or with the thought that some new light might appear? It will serve no purpose to open a discussion of nursing unless these questions are recognized at the outset. So much controversy cannot be ignored. Can we find a reasoned and convincing argument to explain the past and give promise for the future? This is my hope in this present writing.

My claim is that the key to an understanding of the whole situation is to be found in a careful study of the social history of the nineteenth century, and especially of the influences that pressed heavily upon the organization of nursing services in that period. If it is conceded that nursing is attempting to serve the mid-twentieth century while living in a strait-jacket fashioned nearly a hundred years ago, much of the fog of misunderstanding may be dispelled, and the way made clear for constructive action. Particularly should we try to discover why the nineteenth-century fetters are still fastened so firmly around nursing—as we believe they are—while other professional groups have escaped these fetters to a large extent.

Glancing back to 1850, we find nursing for the most part a despised domestic service in the relatively few secular hospitals of that period; and it should be noted that neither then, nor at any previous time, did nursing have any real connection with medicine. Apart from the work of the religious orders, where the protection afforded by the order itself maintained discipline and devotion in this service, we find that hospital nursing was an occupation for those women who could earn a living in no other way. The daughters of respectable families did not leave their homes for occupation of any kind unless forced to do so by poverty. There was no thought of even secondary education for girls, and no formal preparation to qualify young women for professional work. Certainly there seemed to be no content in nursing that required either education or training. Furthermore, there was little concern for the miserable condition of the sick poor in the lay hospitals. Finally, the practice of modern preventive medicine was yet to be born, as was also the presumptuous thought that all classes, rich and poor alike, had the same claim to health protection.

Thus came the second half of the nineteenth century: and then appeared in quick succession a trio of influences that have combined to produce the nursing situation of today with all its confused struggles. We see, first, the extraordinary development in the practice of medicine, curative and preventive; secondly, the developing status of women and new provision for their education; and thirdly, a growing sense of social responsibility that forced particular attention upon the social and economic aspects of sickness and health. These three streams of influence should be examined one by one.

First: the growth of medicine. What happened in this field in the nineteenth century that pushed nursing abruptly into an ever-widening range of activity? The reply is found in terse form in Sir George Newman's words, written some twenty-five years ago: "... In the last one hundred years men have witnessed a growth in the science and art of medicine incomparably greater than in any other similar period in the history of mankind"—a growth that has proceeded continuously since Newman wrote these words in 1924. By the end of the nineteenth century the application of this new medical knowledge was bringing much new content into hospital practice with, consequently, an ever-increasing demand for more nurses, and for nurses able to do more nursing of a kind and quality never before dreamed of. At the turn of the century this had started slowly enough, but soon it became a mushroom growth. At last nursing had become directly associated with medicine. Then suddenly came a further complication in the request for nurses to share in the rapid development of public-health practice, though this was not particularly noticeable until the second decade of this century.

Next, we note that the second half of the nineteenth century was bringing a radical change in the position of women as persons, and as active members of society. By the end of the century, through the heroic efforts of devoted leaders, secondary schools and universities were being shared by both sexes. True, there was not yet equal opportunity in education for the woman, but long strides were being taken toward this. At the same time, women began to enter a number of the professions; indeed, the barrier was down from the time that Elizabeth Garrett Anderson qualified in medicine in 1865. . . .

Finally, we trace the effect upon nursing of the movement toward social reform that spread from the late eighteenth century and throughout the nineteenth—reform offered first by the privileged on behalf of the needy and later demanded by all classes on their own behalf. Influences were at work to fix attention upon one after another of the weakest groups in society: the prisoners, the mentally sick, unprotected children, the slaves of the new industrial conditions, and finally the sick poor, particularly the homeless and destitute in hospital. Leaders appeared who campaigned in each field in turn: John Howard, Pinel, Theodore Fliedner, Elizabeth Fry, Lord Shaftesbury, and among others, Florence Nightingale, the powerful but even yet little-understood woman described by Strachey as possessed with a demon. Strachey's description, though slightly sensational, throws more light upon events than the usual representation of the "ministering angel."

At Miss Nightingale's name we must pause and make an effort to assess her contribution to nursing. Other attempts at reform in this field had preceded hers for several years, but the efforts had turned back to old forms—especially the Deaconess Order—and had sought to revive these and make them serve again by adding new patches to the old garment. It took a woman of Florence Nightingale's genius to realize the need for radical change. Sir Edward Cook, her official biographer, says that she may be called "the founder of modern nursing because she made public opinion perceive, and act upon the perception, that nursing was an art and must be raised to the status of a trained profession." What Cook has emphasized is that Miss Nightingale was the chief architect of an institution new in the history of the world: the nursing school. . . . Her work was brilliantly constructive.

Up to this time, the Gamp sisterhood had been the usual source of domestic care (!) for patients in the lay hospitals of both the old world and the new. The almost incredible stories of Bellevue's wards in 1872 provide a good illustration of the miserable conditions in many hospitals at that time. Even so, ridicule and criticism were poured upon Florence Nightingale when she sought to put an end to such conditions; there was the same spate of conflicting argument as is heard at present. The public conscience could soothe itself with remarks such as that quoted by Lord Granville: "Lady Pam . . . thinks the Nightingale Fund great humbug. The nurses are very good now; perhaps they do drink a little, but . . . poor people, it must be so tiresome sitting up all night, and if they do drink a little too much they are turned away and others got." In spite of this kind of irresponsible chatter, the Nightingale school took form in 1860 in connection with St. Thomas's Hospital in London, and soon proved its value to hospital and patients alike.

The next step in the development of nursing—during the last three decades of the century—demands the most careful examination, for here seems to lie the cause of much of the trouble that has followed. Other hospitals sought reform and, gradually, attempts were made, in one place after another, to reproduce the pattern of the school established at St. Thomas's. All over the British Isles, in many countries of the British Empire, in the United States and in the northern countries of Europe, hospitals introduced what was called the Nightingale system of training nurses and of nursing patients. Unfortunately, from the beginning the copy was not exact. The Nightingale school had been organized as an independent institution, self-supporting and distinct from the hospital; apparently the pupils were meant to be supernumeraries, added—at such times and in such places as the school dictated —to a nursing staff already employed to give service to the hospital. But when copied the school lost its essential characteristic of independence and was turned into what is now called a hospital school of nursing—that is, a system of hospital-administered apprenticeship, the "historical accident" of Dr. Esther Brown's comment. Apparently no one had noticed that it was the income from its endowment fund that had made the Nightingale school possible, by giving it independence, and therefore the authority to govern its own procedure. For the succeeding schools there was no endowment, and no other form of income. Lacking this, the school proper was lost: the students became apprentices who were required to work their passage through the training course and consequently were required to service the hospital. Worst accident of all, the Nightingale school itself imperceptibly but surely lost its original form and slipped into the mold of the inexact copy; in place of the distinct one-year training course, the school (?) was found a few years later to be offering three or four years of apprenticeship, and the patients were being nursed to a large extent by the service of pupil nurses. The vestigial remains of the original school exist today in the fact that all student nurses at St. Thomas's live in the residence called the Nightingale Home during their first year of training.

Strange as this story may appear, it is really not difficult to understand how it could happen in the last quarter of the nineteenth century. In the relatively simple conditions of hospital nursing in the 80's and the 90's, the difference between a formal school and an apprenticeship system could, and did, pass unnoticed; indeed, any form of training was bound to give satisfaction as compared with the former unorganized and sordid conditions. But the change from pupil status to apprenticeship gave rise to tragic consequences in a later, more complex period.

The real difficulty lies in the effort to explain the unshakable power that the apprenticeship system has wielded ever since. Unfortunately, by the end of the nineteenth century several influences had been at work to fix this persistent form, in spite of the changing world of both medical and educational practice in which it was expected to serve. Obviously the system had great economic value for the hospital, so hospital authorities welcomed it. Also, the nursing profession itself seemed to accept it without question. It does not appear that thought was given to the growth of educational procedure in other fields, or to the great change that was swiftly taking place in the practice of nursing itself—change that was soon to make the hospital training school more obsolete with every passing decade.

And so we have come to our own period, the first half of this present century. . . . In spite of all the contradictions and controversy, I am quite ready to claim that new foundations have been laid in this present century; it now remains for me to describe the progress that has been made in this time. This progress may be considered under four headings: in the content of nursing; in the personnel of nursing; in the conditions under which nursing is being done; and in the preparation for nursing, that is, in the field of nursing education.

First to be considered is the development in content. . . . By 1900 this content had settled quickly into much domestic work, fairly simple technical skills and even the appearance in district nursing of some social significance when the individual nurse sensed her opportunity to add this, although she had little formal preparation for it. . . . It should also be said that from the end of the past century there were some hospital nurses of high caliber who recognized their opportunity to give their patients something more than technical service: new hope and strength, and healing of mind and spirit as well as of body; while some—also untaught—were using their unique opportunity of contact with patients—much more prolonged than that of the physician—to stimulate or contribute to research. All interpretation of these words must be related to the period.

Today the content of nursing has expanded beyond all possible anticipation of a century ago. Even Florence Nightingale, with her great gift of imagination, could not have foreseen today's nurse, who is often called upon to perform with faultless precision more intricate and responsible treatments than those given by physicians when the Nightingale school was born; she could not have foreseen the great number and size and variety of today's hospitals, with thousands of nursing schools dotted all over the world, and the consequent demand for "lady" superintendents, supervisors, instructors and many, many specialists in nursing services. And, most interesting of all, Florence Nightingale, in spite of her understanding of the service that a nurse might possibly give as a "health missioner," could not have realized the breadth and depth of the health field in which many nurses are now asked to serve, a field where medicine and social work meet, and where the nurse must play the double rôle of medical and social worker.

In summing up the progress in the content of nursing during these 50 years, we see the growth from very small numbers to an enormous army; progress from limited technical service to a wide variety of services, many of professional quality; progress from ancillary status in the sickroom to partnership in the medical services; progress from hospital and sickroom duties alone to participation also in social work that touches the community at many vital points; progress from nursing as a matter of small and somewhat local concern to the 1950 organization of the Expert Nursing

Committee of the World Health Organization. It is little wonder that this rapid growth has caused some confusion.

Secondly, we recognize progress in the type of young woman found in nursing. This is an interesting story, starting from the days of Victorian snobbery and continuing to our own time. Undoubtedly the early Nightingale era brought a sprinkling of recruits from homes of culture, but there is considerable evidence that general opinion, then and all through the intervening years, has tended to relegate nursing to those of mediocre intelligence and limited social background. There is much of this same thought today—especially in the secondary schools from which recruits must come. Often, intelligent and gifted students are directed firmly away from nursing when they show interest in this field. . . . In spite of these indisputable facts, there has been progress in the selection of personnel for nursing. We make no extreme claims, for it is freely admitted that nursing has the same admixture of desirable and undesirable recruits that is found in all professions in today's democracy. Nevertheless, increasingly, young people with first-class ability are found in nursing schools (though not always remaining!); and increasingly, though certainly not always, these students represent the best homes that our countries have to offer in terms of education and culture (in the best sense of this much abused word). Progressing from a decidedly poor social status, the nurse now receives a qualified recognition as a professional worker.

The third aspect of this progress is the material and physical conditions of the work of the nurse, a subject that receives much attention from the public at large. Important as it is, we wish that it would not always be mentioned first in public debate, or even appear to be the only matter for concern. Certain conditions have improved greatly, with the result that many nurses are now leading a much more normal life than has been possible at any other time since secular nursing was first organized. After long delay, this improvement has very recently taken place. I agree that it is important, and a matter for congratulation, that many nurses are working not more than eight hours a day, that many have one free day in seven, that some are receiving an income permitting a modestly comfortable way of life, with protection against unemployment, sickness and old age. It is significant that a few may even leave salaried positions in order to obtain added education to prepare for a special field of service. Another progressive step is found in the correction of mistaken thought on the part of nurses themselves. Earlier in the century we were narrowly exclusive, fearful for our status as "trained" nurses, and afraid of the effect of recognizing an assistant group called at that time "practical nurses" and known today by various names. Indeed, we blocked all such suggestion. Fortunately this attitude has changed, though there is still much progress to be made in establishing wise and happy relations. But these early fears are not going to be soon forgotten or forgiven by our critics; nursing must still live down the unfortunate reputation of having refused to share its services with an auxiliary group.

We are glad to stress all this progress in the conditions of nursing service, but we are bound to bring into the light one other condition, one in which it is not possible to record progress. This bears upon the hospital nurse's work. I refer to the devastating effect felt by good nurses (students and graduate staff alike) when they do not have time to nurse their patients properly. We are forced to conclude that this inability to give adequate time to actual nursing, and thus to afford satisfaction to the nurse herself and to her patients, is the main cause of the constant turnover in staff and consequent lack of stability in the nursing service of many hospitals. It even causes many young graduates to turn quickly away from the hospital as soon as their diplomas are secured. This feeling of frustration and the consequent instability in the service form a vicious circle, which will be broken only when those with power and authority recognize the situation and make a determined attack upon it. The recent world war increased this pressure in hospitals, but the condition was evident long before 1939. Those who have studied the problem most carefully are convinced that the root of the trouble lies in the organization of the nursing school in the hospital and the consequent confusion in a service shared in extraordinary proportions by students and employees. In recent years, the nursing profession itself has unceasingly called attention to the folly and danger of the situation. Year after year, proposals for reorganization have been offered, but with rare exceptions hospitals have been unwilling or unable to take action. A further word is appropriate enough here. Since possibly the nursing profession is now receiving its full quota of the young womanhood of some of our countries, the soundest economy should be practiced in the use of the time of these skilled practitioners.

Finally, in this fourfold recital of progress, comes the topic of nursing education. Paradoxically, our fifty-year span seems to have brought great change, and yet also to have maintained a remarkable sameness. The worst feature of recent years is that while the content of nursing has been developing with great rapidity there has been no corresponding *recognition* of this development. Those who have had much influence in the whole field of nursing education seem to be blind to the fact. Hence, it is folly to hope for logical action on their part. But why this lack of understanding concerning the scope of nursing service? My own conviction is that a curious fixity of thought is obscuring the interpretation of the word "nursing." Through centuries of usage, the word has become chained to a meaning so restricted that it cannot represent anything beyond bedside care; and by most people this bedside care is thought to consist only of domestic service for the patient, plus a few simple treatments, *always under the doctor's immediate direction*. With such a masterpiece of misrepresentation, what is to be done? Again I quote Dr. Esther Brown: surely this same thought was in her mind when she spoke of nursing as "a profession weary from the heavy weight of traditionalism."

. . . Nurses themselves must accept responsibility for many mistakes during these years, for inconsistencies and for grasping often at the shadow rather than the real substance of reform. But the story reflects less credit upon many others who have been in a much better position to understand the educational resources of the community and the appropriate use of these. Hospital authorities, government officials and the senior profession of medicine—all these have been transferring new responsibilities to nursing in steadily increasing quantity ever since the opening of the first world war, but these same groups have done little to support the development of nursing education in corresponding measure. Indeed, there has been considerable sustained neglect, and even definite opposition to progress. The old school-cum-service pattern persists, and is defended with extraordinary zeal. We are grateful to many individuals in these same groups who have given help, but some impression must now be made that will produce a general change of attitude. The present situation is shocking in many respects. Indeed, considering that our educational resources are so limited, some of the increasing demands upon nursing frighten us. The new civilian defence proposals may be in this category.

Certain changes must be made if the nurse's education is to keep pace with these demands. First, the idea must be accepted that all nursing schools should be divorced from hospital administration and re-established as educational institutions. In this case the hospital would have to content itself with its own legitimate responsibility: the employment of a staff to nurse its patients. With this arrangement, it should be easy to fit students into the nursing practice, but also to keep them always under the control of the school authority. As far back as 1923, this change was forecast in a remarkable document, popularly called the Goldmark Report, that was published that year in the United States. Since then, further support for more or less radical change has come from various countries.

It is now quite obvious that schools of nursing of two distinct types are urgently needed. Both have taken form already, but they are very few in number, and even these are fighting for their lives. The one type, perhaps to be called the junior school, is—at its best—taking the form of an exceedingly good technical school that provides the technical training in an atmosphere of science and humanism. This atmosphere can be maintained only by an excellent teaching staff: that is, by nurses who themselves have had the best of technical training combined with broad general education in a university school of nursing. The junior school of which I am speaking may remain on the hospital grounds, as at present, but financially and administratively it should be independent of the hospital. Thus we can prepare the great army of clinical nurses now so necessary to the community's social and medical services.

Secondly, the resources for nursing education must include the university school. The number of nurses to be prepared there will be relatively small, but this school is nonetheless essential. At least three special groups need this educational opportunity: the executive staff for hospitals, the teaching staff for all nursing schools and the medical social workers known as public-health nurses. As there is still much need to defend university education for nursing, let me add some comment. Consider the great and growing number of hospitals. Does the community not understand that nursing provides a very large section of the professional service given in every one of these hospitals? Do we stop to realize that this service does not just happen? Do we not know that nurses must administer this service, and that they cannot administer wisely on the strength of technical skill alone? Only broadly educated citizens can handle today's problems in this vast network of institutions. Look at the woman who is asked to direct the nursing service, with all its complexities, for a hospital containing hundreds of patients whose lives and future happiness may be at stake. Do we see that this nurse-administrator has the opportunity to coordinate all the services so that the work of her professional colleagues may have greatest success? Do we see also that such a person can seriously disrupt this organization if she is inadequate? Is there any more appropriate task for a university than the preparation of this citizen, call her what you will? Consider also the teaching staff being prepared for the junior as well as the university schools of nursing. What teaching have these staff members to do? Just a bit more than the clinician in medicine of not so very long ago, and just as much as the instructor who is developing the professional philosophy of the students in any school of the university. Is there any doubt that some of the young recruits for nursing need general education on the university level?

We should be able to explain and justify what is needed in both content and method from the university school of nursing. The explanation is both simple and profound. The intention is to prepare professional women who, through study of the humanities and social sciences, will grow in understanding and wisdom; with this education in the realm of human values, they may approach with some degree of safety the work that is awaiting them. For these young people, we must "save general education and its values within a system where specialism is necessary." And specialism is necessary, for these same students should have nothing short of excellence in their own technical skills and knowledge. Obviously, this preparation will include a sound scientific basis. We wish to combine the technical with the general subjects throughout the whole university course, believing that the richer result will be obtained by this method.

Amidst a welter of irregular and deplorable arrangements between hospitals and universities, a very few of these fully developed university schools of nursing have taken form. These are organized on the same basis as the other professional schools in the same universities, and offer the regular pattern of degree courses. But let me repeat that they are very few in number, and that for the most part even these are starved, lacking adequate financial support, adequate selection of students and adequate staff. Again the old obstacle interferes: it still seems impossible for the community at large to treat this form of education seriously.

Before closing this discussion of nursing education and nursing schools there is something yet to be said, and all who have followed recent events in this field will understand the reason for adding this. I hope strongly that there will be no class distinction between the graduates of the university school and those from the junior or nonuniversity school. Surely all graduate nurses can be members of the same professional association. Let us put no arbitrary restriction upon the word *professional*. I should add one further word concerning the assistant or auxiliary worker in connection with nursing service. She is important, and her preparation is important, but I shall leave the subject there, for it is quite outside the scope of my present topic. . . .

36. Dentistry *

Surveys reveal that relatively few persons obtain what may be termed complete dental care. To illustrate, a recent national poll indicated that nearly half of the adult population had not visited a dentist within the last two years. Since more than 90 per cent of the American people have dental defects, the conclusion is inevitable that few persons obtain *complete* dental care.

The widely used term "adequate dental treatment" requires interpretation. For the purpose of clarification, the following terminology is suggested: (1) "emergency treatment": service for the relief of pain and removal of acute infections; (2) "expedient treatment": treatment beyond emergency but curtailed by inadequate personnel and limited financial resources, or by indifference to or ignorance of need; (3) "complete dental treatment": *all* dental treatment necessary to establish and maintain dental health. Neither emergency nor expedient dental care will maintain oral health, but complete dental care entails continuity of attention, expenditure of money, and availability of dentists.

Dental Service Requirements

Several estimates have been offered of the number of dentist-hours required to render complete service. Beck estimated that 9.4 dentist-hours would be necessary for initial care for the average person, and 3.6 dentist-hours for annual maintenance care. If all dentists in the United States operated 2,000 hours per year and distributed their services equally among the population, they could give to each person only one hour. Presumably the Nation requires many times the number of dentists currently practicing to meet the present and *potential* dental care needs of all the people.

The following résumé of data on dental care will demonstrate even more convincingly the lags which exist in meeting dental needs: (1) Dental disease affects more than 90 per cent of all persons. (2) Fifty per cent of two-year-old children have one or more carious teeth. (3) At the age of six, children usually have three or more primary teeth which have been attacked by dental caries. (4) Eleven per cent of the children aged 12 to 14 require orthodontic treatment. (5) The average person aged 16 has seven decayed, missing, or filled teeth involving 14 tooth surfaces. (6) It is probable that today's children will lose 50 per cent of their teeth before the age of 40. (7) Persons of low income lose their teeth sooner than do persons of high income.

* From: "Dental Service," by Jacob M. Wisan, D.D.S.; *Annals of the American Academy of Political and Social Science*, Vol. 273 (entitled *Medical Care for Americans*), Jan. 1951, pp. 131-37. Reprinted by permission of the author and publishers. The author is the director of the Division of Dental Health, Department of Public Health of Philadelphia.

One of the complicating factors in meeting dental needs is the uneven distribution of dentists. Some states have approximately four times the relative number of dentists found in sparsely populated states. Within the states, rural areas show relatively fewer dentists than do cities. However, the wider use of automobiles, the improvement of roads, and the establishment of rural bus routes have made it easier for country people to visit city dentists.

One cause for optimism in the field of dental health has been the increased emphasis on research for preventive measures. Topical applications of fluoride and fluoridation of public water supplies have proved their worth, so one may hope for lower incidence and prevalence of dental caries.

Patterns of Dental Practice

IN THE UNITED STATES most of the dental treatment is given by dentists in private practice. The study of child health services conducted by the American Academy of Pediatrics revealed that approximately 96 per cent of the children who obtained dental treatment visited private dentists. In Washington, D. C., where one of the most intensive dental care programs for school age children is conducted, only 12 per cent of the public school population were reported as going to school clinics. Sufficient data are lacking to show the number of adults attending public clinics, but the percentage seems to be low.

About nine out of ten dentists in active practice in the United States are in private practice, though many participate in programs conducted by official and nonofficial agencies. For instance, the United States Veterans Administration has reported that 84 per cent of the service-connected dental defects of veterans were treated in private offices. Similarly, welfare agencies and departments of health defray the cost of authorized dental care rendered by private dentists to persons accepted for treatment at public expense.

The United States Public Health Service provides for the treatment of seamen, coast guard personnel, immigrants at immigrant stations, officers and employees of the Public Health Service, Federal prisoners, lepers, and patients at Federal narcotic hospitals. Demonstrations have been undertaken by the Service with the co-operation of two local communities to treat all school children in order to study needs, costs, and techniques for dental treatment of children. Also, programs have been established in 34 states (1949) to demonstrate topical application of sodium fluoride.

The United States Public Health Service and the United States Children's Bureau administer grants-in-aid to the states for various types of dental care programs or projects related to dental health. The Army and Navy provide dental services for their officers and enlisted men. The Office of Indian Affairs in the United States Department of Interior includes some dental service in the provisions for Indians. An extensive dental care program is maintained by the Veterans Administration. Service-connected defects are corrected in private offices or regional dental clinics. Veterans hospitalized in Veterans Administration hospitals are given routine dental treatment.

Many state health departments, working through local health units or other local groups provide for dental care of preschool and school-age children of low income families. Usually, the care includes prophylaxis, extractions, and fillings. Noteworthy are the provisions for orthodontic service under crippled children's programs, which are operated on the basis of Federal-state co-operation. Welfare departments often are responsible for dental care of patients in certain state hospitals, state institutions, and state prisons. Public assistance agencies in charge of old-age assistance and aid to dependent children assume responsibility for payment for dental service to the persons on their rolls.

Recently several states have organized state-wide dental welfare programs. Maryland has embarked on a program of public medical care for the indigent and medically indigent. About 7 per cent of the total funds are used for dental services. Dentists are paid on a fee-for-service basis and are free to provide whatever treatment their professional judgment indicates. There are restrictions as to prosthesis because of the high cost of dentures and the insufficiency of general funds. As of June 1949, 40 per cent of the practicing dentists provided services for the Maryland program. During 1949, $38,635 was spent for 3,771 dental cases, an average of $10.25 per case. In the state of Washington, recipients of any type of public assistance are eligible for dentists' services when authorized by the county welfare departments.

It is quite difficult to classify local dental treatment programs. The diversity of approaches, policies, and procedures may be due to lack of accepted standards or to variations in needs, resources, or community leadership.

Local tax-supported dental care programs are administered by boards of education, health departments, or welfare departments. In many communities boards of education provide for dental inspections of school children and for treatment of those whose parents cannot afford private dental care. The service given in school clinics is generally limited to prophylaxis, extractions, and fillings. In some instances, only children of the lower grades are included. A number of city or county health departments maintain dental care programs for preschool as well as school-age children. Little service is provided for adults: only a few health department programs include fillings, and even fewer report insertion of dentures. Similarly, city and county welfare departments provide for emergency treatment of needy adults. Dentures where urgently needed are included in a few localities.

One of the most liberal dental programs for the needy is that maintained by the Chicago Welfare Department:

For children "preventive and restorative operative dentistry in all its branches" is made available with the exception of orthodontic procedures and the use of precious metals for filling material. Services for adults include: operative dentistry for relief of pain and elimination of infection; root canal therapy in rare cases; prophylaxis under certain conditions, with cleaning and polishing of teeth for purely aesthetic reasons excluded; fillings (cement, amalgam, synthetic porcelain); repairs of dentures; surgery (simple extractions, removal of impacted teeth when necessary for relief of pain or protection of health, fractures of jaw), roentgenograms if imperative for diagnostic purposes; and subject to special approval, major oral surgery in emergency cases, partial or complete dentures under certain conditions, bridgework in rare instances, and emergency dental service in the home for bed-ridden patients.[1]

As Blackerby has said,

The relatively high cost of dental care programs compelled most administrators to spread their programs thinly over a wide area in order that they might serve as large a part of the population as possible ... the services have been of a strictly emergency nature, encouraging the public to believe that such limited services were adequate for health services.[2]

Among the community dental care programs reviewed, few instances of co-ordination were noted. Where different agencies did collaborate in caring for oral health, facilities were used to better effect, and overlapping was minimized.

Hospitals in many cities maintain dental clinics for outpatients where needy persons may obtain emergency treatment by dentists on the hospital staff. Oral surgeons on hospital staffs treat inpatients with jaw fractures or oral lesions. A few hospitals have comprehensive dental care programs. Examples are the Beth Israel Hospital of Newark, New Jersey, and the Children's Hospital of Boston, Massachusetts.

The Rhode Island Hospital of Providence, Rhode Island, aided by endowments, has established a low-cost dental care program for children of marginal income families in its Joseph Samuels Dental Clinic for Children. Participating dentists are paid either an hourly fee or an annual salary. Dental care is provided for children up to 16 years of age at the rate of $1.00 to $2.00 per visit. Selected cases requiring orthodontic treatment are sent to orthodontists who arrange for special payments by patients.

Endowed institutions such as the Forsyth Dental Infirmary, Boston, Massachusetts, the Zoller Memorial Fund, Chicago, Illinois, the Eastman Dental Clinic, Rochester, New York, the Murray and Leonie Guggenheim Dental Clinic, New York, New York, and the Childrens Fund of Michigan, supplement the services of public agencies by offering dental services to children of low income families. The Zoller Clinic accepts adults as well. These programs, financed by liberal endowments, include research and training of graduate personnel.

Voluntary community agencies not infrequently arrange with private dentists or public clinics to treat persons sent by them. An example of a specialized non-profit voluntary agency supporting a dental clinic for persons unable to pay the fees of private dentists is the Dental Health Service of New York City, organized in 1917. Licensed by the state of New York, it received some philanthropic aid and charged low fees to patients. In 1949 fifteen part-time dentists (nine hours per week) treated 1,903 patients at a five-chair clinic. The total cost of the program

1. Franz Goldmann, *Public Medical Care* (New York: Columbia University Press, 1945), p. 91.
2. P. E. Blackerby, "Treatment in Public Health Dentistry," in Pelton and Wisan, *Dentistry in Public Health* (Philadelphia: Saunders, 1948), pp. 209-10.

was $56,560, or $21 per patient. The majority of dentures cost the patients $65. The 1949 report explains "that a major contribution to the solvency of Dental Health Service remains that made by the dentists and auxiliary personnel constituting the staff of 24. Their compensation still trails well behind that found in comparable employment."

A number of industrial companies provide for dental care as part of the services supported by prepayments or by company resources. Most of these programs furnish X rays, prophylaxis, extractions, and fillings; a few offer dentures and other replacements.

The dental program at the Consolidated Edison System of New York City is one of the oldest dental care projects sponsored by an industrial concern. Employees and the company each contribute seven-ninths of one per cent of the weekly wage of the employee. The company meets any deficits. From these contributions the following dental services are provided to employees earning less than $5,000 annually: pre-employment dental examination; X-ray examination; prophylaxis; silver, amalgam, cement, and silicate fillings; extractions; oral surgery; and alveolectomy. Infected impactions are also treated. Dentures are inserted in specified cases. The treatment is given by private dentists who are paid an hourly fee. Where replacements are inserted, dentists are paid $50 per denture in addition to the hourly fee. Thirty-three thousand, or 99 per cent of the eligible membership are cared for by 49 community dentists.

Most industries having dental programs limit their services to some or all of the following: pre-employment examination, prophylaxis and X-ray diagnosis, emergency treatment, treatment of occupational diseases, and educational programs urging correction of dental defects.

Blue Shield plans cover dental treatment of their subscribers to a limited extent, as the general surgical care provided largely in the hospital is interpreted as meaning "operative and cutting procedures for the treatment of disease or injury and the treatment of fractures and dislocations."

The Group Health Association in Washington, D. C. provides the following dental services: X rays, extractions, fillings, pulp treatment, treatment of gum diseases, bridges, and dentures. Membership is limited to those who pay an initial fee of $10 and who agree to complete dental service. The deposit is applied toward the services, which are paid for on a fee-for-service basis. Because of lack of actuarial data, it has been necessary to postpone the introduction of prepayment until sufficient information on the actuarial basis has been acquired. By July 1, 1950, 2,700 members had been accepted. The staff consists of six dentists (five full-time, one three-quarter-time), two hygienists, six assistants, two laboratory technicians, and one X-ray technician. The director reports the program to be on a paying basis.

The Labor Health Institute in St. Louis, Missouri maintains a department of dentistry staffed by eight part-time dentists. All regular members of the organization received diagnosis and treatment free of charge. Material and drugs are furnished on a cost basis at a standard charge rate.

Schools of dentistry maintain clinics, since they must provide opportunities for teaching and training in all phases of dentistry. They charge comparatively low fees, making dental care accessible to persons of low income.

Proposals for the Future

CONCERNING THE NEED for expanding facilities and enlarging opportunities for dental service, there is virtual agreement. Differences of opinion, however, develop when specific proposals are made for providing more dental care than is presently given to the people in the United States.

The American Dental Association believes that a comprehensive dental program including service, education, and research is needed. The association proposes that dental care should be made available as rapidly as resources will permit to all regardless of income or geographic location. Local communities should determine methods for providing services after consulting representatives of dental societies concerning technical and professional matters. Federal grants-in-aid are considered an acceptable method of supporting state dental programs if precautions are taken to safeguard the right of states to adapt policies to their needs.

Among other recommendations, the association advocates private and community programs which give priority to prevention and control of dental disease in children and to the elimination of pain and infection in adults. Local dental societies are urged to inaugurate experimental voluntary prepayment and postpayment plans for medium and low income groups. Finally, the American Dental Association points out that dental care at the expense of the public should be related to ability to pay.

The Subcommittee on Medical Care of the American Public Health Association issued a statement recommending the following principles for dentists' services:

Dental care should be included in the services provided in a national health program to the extent that available resources of dental personnel make possible. The current severe shortage of dentists and auxiliary dental personnel, however, necessitates a temporarily limited horizon for the provision of dental care to the public. Current emphasis must be directed to preventive and protective dental care for children and to essential therapy for adults. Concurrently, the threefold attack on the overwhelming problem of dental diseases in the nation can be made by: (1) training larger numbers of dentists and other dental personnel; (2) use of multiple chairs by dental practitioners and the performance of subsidiary dental functions by auxiliary personnel under professional supervision in order to increase the number of patients who can be served by a dentist and to achieve reductions in the unit cost of dental service; (3) increased research into the causes and methods of preventing and controlling the major dental disorders.[3]

Congressional bills proposing the introduction of compulsory medical care insurance interpret the term "medical care" broadly, and therefore include dental care, although with qualifications. Payment to dentists would be on a per capita,

3. American Public Health Association, Subcommittee on Medical Care, "The Quality of Medical Care in a National Health Program," *American Journal of Public Health*, July 1949, pp. 904-905.

fee-for-service, or salary basis, as determined by a majority of participating dentists in the various areas. The extent and type of services to be given are not defined.

Voluntary dental insurance has been considered impracticable because of the high cost of correcting accumulated dental defects. Dr. Bissell B. Palmer, secretary of Group Health Dental Insurance, Inc., presented a plan of voluntary dental insurance which attempts to overcome this factor by stipulating that the insurance coverage be instituted in two phases. In the first phase, following examinations, including X rays and prophylaxis, provided by the insurance carrier, the subscriber would pay for the correction of existing defects. In the second, the maintenance phase, all costs would be borne by the carrier.

Since dentists cannot meet the potential need for dental services, it has been suggested that auxiliary personnel fill children's teeth. The advocates of this plan believe that dental hygienists with two years' training could thus increase the quantity of dental services provided for children. Those who oppose contend that personnel with such limited training would provide substandard treatment which would eventually worsen dental conditions.

Admittedly, the dental care problem is a complex social issue. But there is ample agreement among proponents of various plans to warrant the prediction that the oral health of American people will be enhanced when government officials, dental-society leaders, and representatives of the public co-ordinate their talents and resources. The Nation, the various states, and our local units of civil government have within their respective spheres the means to bring about the co-ordination of dentists, officials, and lay persons for more effective dental health programs.

37. MEDICAL SOCIAL WORK *

THE RECOGNITION by physicians of the relationship of the social and environmental factors to the total medical care of the patient has presented to medical social service departments in hospitals and medical care programs an opportunity to integrate social work with medical care. The patient is considered by the physician not only as a sick person but as an individual who has a family, a job and responsibilities in the community. Illness cannot separate him from these and so the factors which affected him in health will also affect him in illness. Furthermore, these same problems are usually exaggerated in illness because of the patient's anxiety and worry. Many patients may have been able before they were sick to face their difficulties with a certain degree of equanimity, but, when ill, become concerned and worried not only over the illness itself but the effect of the illness on

* From: "The Role of the Medical Social Worker in Medicine," by Elizabeth P. Rice; *Bulletin of the Kings County Medical Society* 25: 213-18, Aug. 1946 (No. 8). Reprinted (with omissions) by permission of the author and publishers. The author is associate professor of public health social work at the School of Public Health, Harvard University, Boston, Mass.

themselves, their families and their future. Illness gives to some patients an opportunity to bring to the foreground those problems which may have been lying dormant. Illness also may create new problems for the patient and his family, for it usually presents complications either simple or complex. The patient, whether he is a ward or private patient, has potential problems, therefore, with which he may need some help and guidance. The recognition of these problems is increasing as physicians become more aware of the effect of them on their patients' physical and mental health. More and more private patients are being referred to social service departments and some hospitals have added social workers to their private units.... The idea that illness presents only financial problems to patients is false. Illness creates a situation involving apprehension and anxiety on the part of the patient, problems of relationships with and attitudes toward other members of the family, convalescent and chronic care, as well as work adjustments and financial pressures.

The extent to which the patient is ready to accept advice from the social worker is dependent, I believe, on two points: (1) the degree to which his physician sees the need for advice from the social worker, and (2) the patient's understanding of the services of social workers. We have found that the physician's understanding, not only of the social and emotional factors in relation to the care of a particular individual but also his understanding of the functions and skills of the social worker in being of service to his patient, definitely reflects the degree to which the social service department is used by the physician in the care of his patient. The awareness of the physician of this service is the important criterion in determining the effectiveness of social services. The following situations will illustrate this concept.

In a private room was a 15-year-old boy who had had an amputation following an accident. This boy had been in the hospital for several months and was up and about on crutches, receiving physical therapy. He was occupying a bed needed by patients waiting to come into the hospital. His physician explained to the nurse on the floor that this boy needed to stay in the hospital because his family felt they could not give him the necessary care at home. It was obvious to the medical social worker that the boy was not being taken home by his family not primarily because of the physical handicap of his being on crutches, but because his family was unable to accept his handicap, was disturbed because of the amputation, was rejecting the boy completely, feeling no longer any responsibility for him but trying to press a large settlement by the insurance company. The boy, likewise, was feeling guilty because of the accident, felt pushed aside by his family, realized that they did not want him at home, was apprehensive towards his future, and so was satisfied to remain in the hospital indefinitely. During these months of hospitalization this adolescent had had no interest in working with the school teacher, but was meeting each day as it came, engrossed in the excitement of the hospital. When the administration became concerned that this boy was occupying a bed for so long and was ambulatory with crutches, the needs of the child and family were discussed with the physician, but the physician saw only the fact that this was a liability case and that there were no financial worries and, therefore, no problems for the boy or his parents. We can clearly see the problems which face this boy in the future not only in regard to the emotional adjustment to his handicap but also from the point of view of vocational guidance and training.

In contrast to this illustration of the importance of the awareness of the physician of the social and environmental factors is that one of our senior surgeons who referred a patient to the medical social worker with the request that a study of the patient's social and environmental situation be made to determine whether or not this 56-year-old, unmarried, Scotch lady had potentialities for change in attitude and in social setting which would make it possible to modify her life so that a gastric ulcer could be controlled without surgery. His request was that the social worker, after a complete study, indicate to the surgeon what the chances were for improvement of the patient's total situation and recommend whether or not there could be sufficient change so that operation could be delayed. This referral indicates the extent to which the surgeon was aware of the social and emotional factors as contributing to the patient's physical condition, the physician's recognition of the contribution which the medical social worker could make in the study of the life of the patient, and a real respect for the recommendation which the social worker made regarding the patient's ability to modify her life with help from the social worker. These two extremes of awareness on the part of physicians of the social and emotional factors affect markedly the extent to which a social worker, practicing as a part of medicine, can integrate and contribute her thinking, her analysis of data, and her social treatment to the total medical care of the patient.

In discussing with medical students the contribution of the social and emotional factors to the patient's illness and progress I erred in saying that it was difficult to see any condition which would not be affected by the patient's attitude toward his illness and by his attitude toward his future, unless it were a simple fracture. In a quick response to this statement a medical student disagreed with this and explained clearly to the student group that even in a fracture the degree to which the patient wishes to get well and to leave the hospital has a marked effect on his progress. The students agreed that they could think of no condition where the patient's attitude toward his illness and his social situation might not affect his medical condition and its progress.

On a patient's understanding of the services of the social worker also depends the effectiveness of this service. In hospitals where the medical social worker is closely allied with the medical team, where she has the opportunity to make ward rounds with the staff, where the physician is conscious of his patient's social needs and where the patients are referred to the social worker as they are referred to other consultants, the patient readily accepts the services of the social worker. Unfortunately, many patients, like many physicians, think of the social worker only as a person to give financial assistance. This is an unfortunate heritage. In social work with sick patients a financial problem does not necessarily exist and in many social service departments the department has no money for relief giving. Further interpretation needs to be given to the public as a whole regarding the function of the social worker so that patients who do not have financial problems are aware of the services that can be given.

One can readily think of examples of problems with private patients which exist because of the medical problems and which have no relationship to a financial need. A mother of a new-born baby may be even more disturbed and concerned about a wise plan for her hydrocephalic infant than a ward mother, for this mother on private service has many additional problems to face in regard to social stigma and the attitude of her social group. This problem of a patient with a fractured hip who needs long-time care in a full body cast may be just as much of a problem to a family who does not have financial limitations as he is to the family of a ward patient. The stresses and strains of life which affect men and women occupying important and strenuous positions in the world, who find themselves handicapped because of gastric ulcers or arthritis, may present to these patients even greater complications than these same problems present to ward patients. Recently a private patient operated on for inoperable cancer of the stomach and not knowing his diagnosis was about to make unwise business arrangements which would have complicated the future of his family for many years and he did this because he did not realize the problem which was facing him, nor was he ready or willing to accept the medical facts.

Dr. Francis Peabody's great service to patients in Boston as I worked with him and viewed his relationship with patients was due to his very real concern not only for the illness with which the patient was faced but also for the patient as an individual with problems coincidental to the medical problem. His statement that "the secret of the care of the patient is in caring for the patient" meant that he felt a real concern not only to diagnose the medical problem adequately and treat it skillfully, but that he felt also the importance of treating the whole individual, including his emotional and social problems in order that the individual could be physically, emotionally and socially well. . . .

With the recognition, therefore, that the physician today accepts this point of view, that the patient's social and emotional situation definitely affects not only the extent of the patient's illness but also his progress, many hospitals have added medical social service departments. It was because of Dr. Richard Cabot's early recognition of the effects of social factors on the medical care of his patients that medical social workers were first added to the Massachusetts General Hospital in 1905, and since that day hospitals throughout the country have added or are seeking medical social workers to contribute to the total understanding of the patient and to his total care. Medical care agencies also, such as city, state, and federal health departments, vocational rehabilitation services, private institutions and agencies for the chronically ill and convalescent, have added medical social workers, so that today the demand for this additional service to ill or handicapped people far exceeds the available supply of properly trained medical social workers, and every effort is being made to increase the supply in order that these demands may be filled.

In hospitals we see the medical social worker now being called upon by the physician in charge of the patient for one of three reasons: (1) for consultation, to advise him in regard to the problem which the patient has, and ways of meeting this problem; (2) for social study, to help to determine the facts which cause or complicate the medical condition; and (3) for direct social treatment with the patient. In many hospitals the medical social worker may give advice at the request of the physician to help him to help the patient to meet the problem. Many physicians come to the Social Service Office to ask, for example, for advice as to the best way of meeting the problem of an unmarried mother who does not want to keep her baby, or a man who wishes to overcome his alcoholism and does not know where to start, or a chronically ill patient whose family is not equipped to care for him at home, or for institutional care of children who are physically or mentally handicapped.

In the area of social study physicians refer patients, as did the surgeon in the case of the Scotch maiden lady, to secure supplementary information in regard to the problems which the patient may have which definitely affect his medical care. Situations such as the following have been referred to us: *

A young, married woman on the medical ward was admitted with a history of intestinal distress. Laboratory and x-ray findings were negative, but the patient's complaints persisted. The physician felt that undoubtedly the problem was emotional or social and wanted a social study to determine what factors might be causing this patient's tension. This patient gave to the worker a clear picture of marital friction, followed by desertion by her husband of whom she was very fond, sensitivity to the criticism of her parents and the community because of the desertion, and a very real concern about facing the future without the husband whom she loved.

A 65-year-old Jewish man, born in Russia, who had great difficulty in understanding the ways of an American hospital, had twice refused an operation for carcinoma of the stomach, until the surgeon was exasperated in trying to plan the operative schedule again only to have the patient refuse a third time to go to the operating room. He referred the patient to the social worker with the comment: "He is too sick to leave the hospital but he won't be operated on and you'd better make plans for him in a nursing home," and then added, "unless you can find the reason why he is refusing to be operated and can bring him about to accept this plan." The worker through her social study found that this Jewish man, realizing the seriousness of the operation, could not bring himself to face the possibility of death until he had worked through some of the feelings of guilt towards his past life. An inadequate husband, he separated from his wife and children, throwing the burden of the care of the children and their support on his wife who accepted this responsibility gallantly, and then because of his need for attention he lived in a rooming house with a woman to whom he was not married. Completely cast off by his family and estranged from his church he thought of himself dying in great sin and without the consolation of his family or his church. After a few days the worker was able to help this patient to see the causes for his resistance which were blocking him from getting adequate medical care, to be willing to face his family

* Miss Rice was Director of Medical Social Service, Grace-New Haven Community Hospital, New Haven, Connecticut, at the time this article was written.

and his rabbi, and as best he could make amends for his guilt. Within a short period the patient went to the operating room with a willingness to face what was ahead. . . .

Twin babies were admitted to our isolation pavilion with severe dehydration and pneumonia. An interne felt that the mother seemed bewildered and stupid and he wondered if the condition of the children was due to the incompetency of the mother. The social study proved without a doubt that the cause of the babies' condition was due to the poor care given by a mother with an intelligence quotient of fifty-four. If the babies were to be kept well, care outside the home would be necessary. . . .

Out of the social studies come many problems which need social treatment by the medical social worker, and when this is so treatment is given to the degree to which the patient can be helped to discuss his problems and to have help with them.

Mrs. Jones, a young colored woman, mother of three small children under five years of age, was referred to the medical social worker by the cardiologist with this statement: "This young mother has bacterial endocarditis and if she is to live must remain in the hospital for three months under penicillin therapy. She and her husband refuse to go through this, they have no money, no one to care for the children, and are about to take the patient home against advice. This therapy is the patient's only chance for life. The problem is in your hands." I wish there were time to tell you of the painstaking, lengthy interviews with patient and husband, simple interpretations given over and over and answers to their questions based on fears, prejudices and racial superstitions, of the hours of planning for the care of the children outside the home to the satisfaction of the mother, of the constant encouragement necessary to persuade the husband, highly sexed and dependent on his wife, to leave the patient for these long weeks of care. And then near the time the patient was ready for discharge the help in finding a healthier home, moving them out of the temporary shack with no toilet or running water, and the plans for convalescence and gradual return of the babies. Then the problem of transportation to clinic for supervision and advice. It was a year ago and now this mother is carrying on effectively within her limitations the numerous responsibilities of her household, thus saving a mother for the children and relieving the community of long-time care of three youngsters.

Many times the greatest need of the patient is to have someone with whom he can talk over his problems, verbalize them, and with whom alternative plans can be discussed. Many patients need to be helped to see their problems clearly and then they are often able to go along on their own. Other patients will need more direct help and advice over a longer period of time. Many illnesses present to patients and their families difficult problems of adjustment both for the patient and for the family, and it is with these problems that the medical social worker can be of assistance.

Various methods have been used by physicians in referring patients to the social worker. A patient may be referred by an individual physician, or patients may be referred during ward rounds which the social worker attends, or during weekly conferences with the physicians on a given floor, or in some hospitals patients with certain diagnoses, or in a few hospitals all patients are studied by the social worker. As the physician becomes more and more aware of the problems there is a tendency for him to refer more and more patients. The system of routine study by the social worker of all patients seems to result many times in a delegation of responsibility to the social worker for the discovery of the social factors. This tends to separate the social and the medical rather than integrating the two more closely and it removes from the physician responsibility for the social factors which may be important in his total understanding of the patient. We have found that when the responsibility was placed on the physicians to determine what patients they thought needed the social laboratory, as they determine what patients need the blood chemistry laboratory or the x-ray department, that then the patients were considered as a whole and the integration of the social and the medical became closer to the benefit of the patient.

The extent to which the social worker shares through various means the social material which she has available likewise helps the physician in his understanding of the patient as a whole. Social summaries in medical histories placed along with the physician's notes so that they are readily available to him, social material shared with the staff in ward rounds, material presented in medical staff meetings and in teaching conferences, all help to keep constantly before the physicians the relevant social material which is related to the patient's medical problems. To be most helpful, this social material has to be shared at the point when it will be of greatest help. The relevant material needs to be carefully sifted from the irrelevant and it should be clearly summarized so that the physician can quickly use the pertinent material for his own purposes. Social workers are not always skillful in selecting the pertinent data and in stating the problem clearly and simply.

With the recognition of the importance of the social and environmental factors, physicians have also requested some assistance in teaching the social aspects of medicine to medical students. The American Association of Medical Colleges and the American Association of Medical Social Workers have a joint committee studying this at present. That committee finds that in an increasing number of medical schools the teaching of the social and environmental factors is receiving a greater emphasis than five years ago. In many of these schools the social workers are contributing to the teaching. Some of us, however, have discovered that this teaching has greater validity and acceptance by the student when the student himself observes that his instructor is aware of the social factors and recognizes the importance of these in the care of the patient. It is interesting to note that more and more in all medical schools this subject is now being integrated into the total curriculum and that in some medical schools this emphasis appears as early as the pre-clinical years so that the student will early recognize the integration of the social and the medical. Social Service Departments are being asked to contribute from their own work, the social laboratory, the material which has been used and tested. The opportunities to share with the medical students the social material are numerous within a teaching hospital. Perhaps the best experience comes when the student himself is working with a patient in the clinic or on the wards and when the student himself recognizes and is concerned about the problems which the patient presents. With this experience the student can then apply the gneralized concepts of the social factors which then have for him a clearer and more related meaning.

Medicine of the present day which stresses the understanding of a patient as a person in relation to his total situation presents to medical social workers in programs of medical care, both in hospitals and in the community, a challenge to serve as a scientific laboratory whether this laboratory be used by physicians in charge of the patient or by the medical students who are learning to practice both the art and science of medicine. For this responsibility the field of medical social work needs well prepared and experienced medical social workers who are equipped to meet the challenge presented to them by medicine. . . .

38. OTHER DISCIPLINES *

AN INEVITABLE CONSEQUENCE of specialization and the growing complexity of medicine has been the rapid expansion of medical services. Scarcely more than a century ago medical practice revolved around the general physician working entirely by himself. But today few physicians rely entirely upon their own resources. Besides elaborate hospital facilities and technical equipment, physicians have available a wide variety of specialized assistants. Thousands of individuals are cooperating with the physician in the medical and health fields. This large corps of skilled technicians and specialists who help provide health services are referred to as paramedical personnel.

The word "paramedical" is derived from the Greek "para," meaning beside, or alongside of, and "medical." It is a good choice of words, for the paramedical personnel are working at the side of the physicians and today are making vital contributions to the medical team.

New groups of paramedical workers emerge with each major advance in medical knowledge. Therefore, definition of paramedical workers must not only encompass the existing heterogeneous groups, but also be broad enough to include specialties not yet fully developed.

The following definition is one which approximately fits these needs: Paramedical workers are persons, other than physicians, dentists, and nurses, who are engaged in the investigation, treatment and prevention of disease and disability, and in the promotion of health, by virtue of some special skill. Such skill may be obtained through a recognized course of training or as a result of experience, the required amount and type being determined by professional organizations in the particular fields.

Specifically, the definition is designed to include such diverse groups as the following: Medical laboratory technicians, X-ray technicians, dietitians and nutri-

* From: *Building America's Health,* by the President's Commission on the Health Needs of the Nation; Washington: U.S. Government Printing Office, 1953 (Vol. 2, Chap. V, "Health Personnel," pp. 173-74). Reprinted with omissions.

tionists, physical therapists, occupational therapists, speech therapists, social workers, clinical psychologists, midwives, pharmacists, sanitarians, engineers, hospital administrators, medical record librarians, health educators, operating room technicians, nurses' aides, practical nurses, dental technicians and hygienists, veterinarians, housekeepers and homemakers. It does not include clerical, fiscal, custodial, and other nonprofessional or nontechnical workers.

Of the present groups of paramedical personnel, some work under the close and immediate supervision of physicians. Others, including dietitians, social workers, pharmacists and hospital administrators, have a relatively independent status. Some work as technical specialists and have little contact with patients. Others work directly with the patients. But each specialty plays an important role in the practice of medicine and the promotion of health.

Perhaps because the concept of paramedical personnel is so new, the potential role of these persons is not always appreciated and they are not always adequately utilized.

In general, physicians do not yet know how to use effectively many types of paramedical workers. Medical students have little first-hand contact with the many varieties of auxiliary medical workers. They know little about the functions of dietitians or social workers, not to mention the rest of the long list of paramedical personnel.

This situation may be corrected as the "team approach" to medicine is more thoroughly understood.

As a part of this unit, the specialized worker not only relieves the physician of a host of time-consuming duties, but also offers special skills and facilities. Only with cooperation between physicians and paramedical workers will comprehensive health service be made generally available.

In most cases, paramedical workers are used more effectively by physicians in group practice than by those in individual practice.

Growth and Development of Paramedical Groups

THE RESPONSIBILITY for developing training programs has been assumed to a large extent by hospitals, colleges, and universities. Some training is also provided in specialized proprietary institutions. However, many individuals are still trained by the apprenticeship method, and in the school of experience.

As paramedical personnel have grown in numbers and assumed diverse responsibilities, a certain pattern of growth has become evident. Presumably the pattern which applies to established groups will apply to many of those fields even now striving for full growth.

When a particular field is established and the duties and responsibilities of its personnel are defined, groups of workers band together in a local professional association or league. Later, several such local organizations coalesce, and a national body is formed. The primary purposes of such associations are educational. Periodic meetings are held and these and other forms of communication encourage the exchange of new ideas.

Then, the national or State organization usually sets standards of eligibility for its members, e. g., the successful completion of an acceptable course of training or comparable experience.

Next, the association becomes concerned with the establishment and maintenance of high standards of training and sets up an accreditation program. Training schools are inspected and their courses periodically appraised. Almost without exception, the associations improve the usefulness of their members by favorably influencing training curricula, through postgraduate educational activities, professional journals, and the like.

Often a registry of members is created, permitting an accurate, quick and convenient check of qualifications for vacant positions. Qualification is usually based upon satisfactory completion of formal training in an approved school and sometimes on membership in the professional society. Unfortunately, the critical shortage of trained personnel has made it difficult to prevent the employment of any person —registered or unregistered, trained or untrained.

In many fields of paramedical service, physician specialists take an interest in the training programs and the activities of the associations. For example, the American Society of Clinical Pathologists is closely allied with the laboratory technicians' association, and radiologists have a continuing concern in the training of X-ray technicians.

Certain paramedical specialties already have attained a level of maturity and a few (e. g., midwifery) have entered a definite decline. Such changes obviously parallel current trends in medical and public health practice. Directors of training programs should attempt to anticipate such development within their specialty and to adapt the content of their program to such trends. For example, one of the major laboratory procedures before the advent of chemotherapy was the determination of pneumococcal types in order to insure the use of appropriate type-specific sera. Today, an insignificant number of such tests is performed. In contrast, routine Rh testing of blood was unheard of 15 years ago, while today it is an indispensable part of the technician's armamentarium. . . .

FURTHER READINGS

The Physician

Altenderfer, Marion E. and Pennell, Maryland Y. *Health Manpower Source Book.* Section 5: *Industry and Occupation Data.* Publication No. 263, Public Health Service. Washington: U. S. Government Printing Office, 1954. 215 pages.

Ashford, Mahlon (ed.). *Trends in Medical Education.* New York: Commonwealth Fund, 1949. 320 pages.

Association of American Medical Colleges. *Preventive Medicine in Medical Schools.* Chicago: The Association, 1953. 123 pages. (Includes references).

Binger, Carl. *The Doctor's Job.* New York: W. W. Norton, 1945. 243 pages. (Includes references).

Deitrick, John E. and Berson, Robert C. *Medical Schools in the United States at Mid-Century*. New York: McGraw-Hill, 1953. 380 pages.
Dickinson, Frank G. and Bradley, Charles E., in cooperation with Cargill, Frank V. *Comparisons of State Physician-Population Ratios for 1938 and 1949*. Bulletin 78, Bureau of Medical Economic Research, American Medical Association. Chicago: The Association, 1950. 15 pages.
Josiah Macy, Jr. Foundation. *Administrative Medicine*. Transactions of the First Conference. New York: The Foundation, 1953. 176 pages.
Stern, Bernhard J. *American Medical Practice in the Perspectives of a Century*. New York: Commonwealth Fund, 1945. 156 pages. (Includes references).
Weinfeld, William. *Income of Physicians, 1929-49*. Reprint from *Survey of Current Business*. United States Department of Commerce. Washington: U. S. Government Printing Office, 1951.

The Dentist

American Dental Association. *The 1953 Survey of Dental Practice*. Chicago: The Association, 1954. 38 pages.
Carr, Malcolm W. *Dentistry: An Agency of Health Service*. New York: Commonwealth Fund, 1946. 219 pages. (Includes references).

The Nurse

American Nurses Association. *Facts About Nursing*. New York: The Association. (Issued periodically).
Bridgman, Margaret. *Collegiate Education for Nursing*. New York: Russell Sage Foundation, 1953. 205 pages. (Includes references).
Brown, Esther Lucile. *Nursing for the Future*. New York: Russell Sage Foundation, 1948. 198 pages.

The Social Worker

Association of American Medical Colleges and American Association of Medical Social Workers, Joint Committee. *Widening Horizons in Medical Education*. New York: Commonwealth Fund, 1948. 228 pages. (Includes references).
Cabot, Richard C. *Social Service and the Art of Healing*. New York: Moffat, Yard and Co., 1909. Reissue, New York: Dodd, Mead and Co., 1928. 192 pages.
Cannon, Mary Antoinette and Bartlett, Harriett M. "Medical Social Work," in *Medical Addenda: Related Essays on Medicine and the Changing Order*. New York: Commonwealth Fund, 1947. (Includes references).
Goldstine, Dora. *Expanding Horizons in Medical Social Work*. Chicago: University of Chicago Press, 1955. 274 pages.

CHAPTER VI

Hospitals

ALTHOUGH HOSPITALS have been known for at least five centuries, the modern hospital does not date back much more than one hundred years. Its appearance followed close on the heels of the discovery of anesthesia and asepsis, and on the development of modern nursing.

As modern diagnosis and therapy has demanded more complicated and expensive equipment, and as increased medical knowledge has advanced specialization, the hospital has become more and more the center of medical research, teaching, and care. Always a haven for the seriously ill, the hospital of today is frequently a center for the diagnosis and treatment, on an inpatient or outpatient basis, of people who are not necessarily severely ill, but who need services beyond the capacity of the private practitioner's office.

While formerly these services were generally restricted to persons of limited means, today they are more and more becoming a resource for the entire community. Today, too, the resources of the hospital are being made available not only to those who are ill, but to the apparently healthy person seeking preventive services.

The development of extra-mural services which extend the resources of the hospital not only to other hospitals and health centers but to patients' homes has centered new responsibilities on the hospital and its staff. The rapid strides made in the past few years in regionalization of medical care and towards the integration of curative and preventive services (See Chapter VII— "Coordination of Facilities and Personnel") have still further strengthened the position of the hospital as a vital factor in medical care.

This chapter deals primarily with the history, present position, and needs

255

of the general hospitals in the United States. It also discusses the relatively new and still changing concept of the health center.

Hospitals for mental disease are dealt with in Chapter X.

A. *History and Development*

39. The Hospital as a Social Institution *

From simple beginnings the hospital has developed into one of the most complex institutions of man. In fact it has become so complicated and costly an organization that the elemental human reason for its existence is likely to be obscured. In its essence a hospital is nothing more than a group of persons working day and night to relieve the distress and suffering of their fellow men. All skills and resources at the command of this group are directed toward insuring survival of the individual. While the hospital has added other functions, this basic purpose of the institution has remained the same. Indeed, it might be said that the germ of the hospital came into being when primitive man found refuge in a cave or crevice where some companion might bind his torn flesh or bring water to still his thirst.

Based as it is on elemental human needs, the hospital has always been closely knit to the daily life of man. Its variations in form have been shaped by the economic conditions that rule simple daily affairs. As men have enjoyed abundance or suffered scarcity, as they have found leisure or labor, their hospitals have been affected correspondingly. Whether man was urban or rural, sessile or migratory, determined the shape taken by the hospital in the particular environment or decided whether it was to exist at all.

The structure of society that arises from the foundation of economic conditions is ever changing. It is made up of intangibles, such as the attitude of man toward his fellow, of class toward class; and is molded by the political ideologies and events of the age. These structural elements give form to the culture of a society. They, as well as basic economic conditions, give shape to its religion, its learning, its arts, and its science. At times the hospital has been closely identified with one or another of these cultural expressions of society or has shown the effect of their combination. But as an institution concerned with human distress and survival, its taproot extends far below the level of what is commonly considered as the cultural expression of a society. It finds anchorage deep in the subsoil along with the primitive needs for food, shelter, and personal defense.

* Reprinted by permission of the publishers from N. W. Faxon (ed.), *The Hospital in Contemporary Life;* Cambridge, Mass.: Harvard University Press, 1949. (The excerpt reprinted, with omissions, is from Chap. I, "The Development of the Hospital," by Edward D. Churchill, M.D.) Dr. Churchill is John Homans Professor of Surgery at Harvard University Medical School and chief of the general surgical service of Massachusetts General Hospital, Boston.

An attempt to trace the development of the hospital by examining those institutions that have been concerned with the care of the sick in the past reveals so many variations of form and function that the thread of continuity soon is lost. To present in chronologic sequence the predecessors of the present-day hospitals and imply that there has been a steady transition from the primitive to the simple and from the simple to the complex would create the illusion that the hospital has an autonomous destiny and a momentum of its own. Actually, it is but an organ of the society that creates it.

A complete history of the hospital would require a broad delineation of the economic conditions and the structure and culture of society itself for each example under consideration. Only by such documentation could the form taken by the hospital at any particular time or place be understood—not by connecting it with an earlier example and projecting it to a succeeding one. The history of the hospital passes over the political boundaries of nations; a complete history would pass beyond those boundaries of societies that separate civilizations. . . .

The Hospital as an Expression of the Christian Virtues

THOSE ATTRIBUTES of man that seek to find expression in the Christian religion have provided the most powerful single stimulus to the development of the hospital. The character of the hospital of today cannot be comprehended without an understanding of its Christian baptism and upbringing. Nor can it be interpreted without an equal understanding of the weaknesses and mistakes of "what has been passing for Christianity during these nineteen centuries." During this period Christianity has cherished, nourished, and guided the hospital as a traditional and sometimes convenient means of obeying the commandment of mercy and compassion. The mistakes as well as the achievements made in the name of Christianity, however, are but part of the total picture. With these must be measured the confusion and the success of society in dealing with poverty and its consequences, the slender support provided by alms and the generosity of philanthropy, and finally, the long period of impotence of medicine as a healing art followed by the developing power of medicine as a science. . . .

The practical expression of charity through the agency of the hospital began after Emperor Constantine recognized Christianity as the most vital and vigorous religion of the times and established a positive relationship between it and the Roman State. At the Council of Nicaea called in A.D. 325, the bishops were instructed to establish a hospital in every cathedral city. The carrying out of this policy proceeded more rapidly in the Byzantine Empire than in the West. The reason may lie in the fact that medicine itself was in Greek hands, although even then Oribasius (325-403) was expounding the teachings of Galen (131-201), and the long rule of authoritarianism that was to close medicine in its grip for centuries, was beginning. Christian teaching also was degenerating and believers were persuaded to give alms as a means to their own personal gain. . . . The aid to the poor brought by these early hospitals was not a simple act of brotherly love but a complicated device directed toward securing grace and salvation for the alms giver.

There appears to have been some systematic attempt to differentiate the medical and social functions of certain of these early Christian institutions, as the *Nosocomia,* for the care of the sick; *Ptochia,* for the helpless poor; *Gerontochia,* for the aged, and so on. This was a differentiation that was lost sight of later when in the eyes of society the ills of poverty became blended with the ailments of disease.

In the Christian West, the establishment of hospitals proceeded at a somewhat slower pace. The first nosocomium in Western Europe was founded by Fabiola about the year 400, according to Saint Jerome, "to gather in the sick from the streets and to nurse the wretched sufferers, wasted with poverty and disease." Others were scattered from Rome to Arles (542) and Paris, where the Hôtel Dieu is said to have been founded about 660 by the Bishop of Paris, Saint Landry. . . .

Events in England that began with the close of the Middle Ages and culminated in the Reformation ultimately had a more profound effect on the pattern that the hospital was to assume in the new world than happenings on the Continent. The monasteries, by the close of the thirteenth century had accumulated vast riches and the Church, through its rigid conservatism, was insensitive to the great changes in the structure of society that were beginning. As the Western World started to move, ecclesiasticism stood still. The monks lost their religious enthusiasm and spirit of service and became enamoured of luxurious living and self-indulgence. The parish priest was on the whole a dull fellow, bent on holding the peasant in fear of hell-fire. His bishops were preoccupied by their duties as secular officers of the state and neglected their dioceses. The friars of the mendicant orders attacked the ortho-dox clergy with charges of corruption, but instead of practicing their doctrine of evangelic poverty, also amassed wealth and treasure. . . .

With the dissolution of the monasteries (1536-1539) by the Reformation Parliament, acting as the instrument of Henry VIII, the hospital system of England, such as it was, crumbled and disappeared. . . .

Deprived of the charity of religious houses, numbers of poor and sick flocked to London, attracted by its reputation for great wealth. These, added to the burden of the city's own indigent, produced misery and confusion of such degree that in 1538 the Mayor and Commonalty of The City of London petitioned that they might have the "order, rule, government, and disposition of the hospitals or spitals, com-monly called St. Mary's Spital (Bethlem) [later called Bedlam], St. Bartholomew's Spital, St. Thomas's Spital, and the New Abbey at Tower Hill, with the rents and revenues appertaining to the same, for the annual relief of the poor, needy, and sick persons." . . . .[1]

Saint Bartholomew's was handed over to civic authorities and reopened in order that "there might be comfort to the prisoners, visitation to the sick, food to the hungry, drink to the thirsty, clothes to the sick, and sepulture to the dead." [2] At first it was intended to use Saint Thomas's as an institution for the relief of the poor, a

---

1. Henry C. Burdett, *Hospitals and Asylums of the World* (London: J. & A. Churchill, 1893), III, p. 60.
2. Burdett, *op. cit.,* p. 61.

precursor of the workhouse. Later Saint Thomas's received the curable sick and Saint Bartholomew's the blind and impotent, the paralyzed, and pregnant women. The orphans of women dying in childbirth were cared for until they could shift for themselves. . . .

The great voluntary hospitals of eighteenth-century England were not connected with pre-existing institutions, except for Saint Bartholomew's and Saint Thomas's, both of which had become royal hospital foundations but took on the form of heavily endowed voluntary hospitals. The dissolution of the monasteries by Henry VIII had left England practically without hospitals for two centuries. This clean break with the ecclesiastic past gave free opportunity for a fresh start. The motivation and pattern of these institutions did not represent a two-century evolution of the hospital but reflected the change in the expression of Christianity itself that had occurred during this period. The two centuries that followed the Reformation in England had offered little opportunity for the expression of Christian virtues in any form. Religion indulged in a period of feuding and confusion in which Anglican priest and Puritan "saint" vied with each other for the right to punish sin and burn witches. The Civil War of Charles and Cromwell, started in 1642, found a country divided on religious as well as political issues. The establishment of the Puritan rule of the Roundhead Commonwealth (1649-1660) was but a brief triumph, and the Restoration of 1660 was in turn followed by the anti-Romanist Revolution of 1688. From this period of strife between High and Low Church finally emerged the "calm broadminded optimism characteristic of the Eighteenth Century Briton." . . .

Guy's Hospital, the first voluntary hospital in London, was opened in 1728. . . .

A very significant feature of the voluntary hospitals was that almost without exception they were designated as being for *curable* poor people. This at once freed them from responsibility toward the mass of derelict humanity that had crowded the old medieval houses of charity. The philanthropy of the eighteenth century was to be socially constructive, not mere alms giving. The will of Thomas Guy, who made a fortune printing Bibles for Oxford and speculating on shares in the famous South Sea Bubble, was somewhat ambiguous in defining the mission of the hospital that was to be built, but the Governors directed the charity toward curable patients. The long illustrious history of "Guy's" places it with "Bart's" as one of the few hospitals affectionately known throughout the world by its abbreviated name. . . .

The Hospital and the Medical Profession

WHILE SICKNESS may be the result of poverty and always is more pitiable when linked with want, it is by no means confined to any one class in the social order. The medical profession is called upon when sickness occurs in the cottage or in the palace. The hospital, however, was dedicated to the sick poor and it confined itself to this restricted function, for reasons that will be explained, up to the end of the nineteenth century. It is true that medicine, especially after the sixteenth century, based certain important activities, namely, its own practical education and a continuing study of disease, on the hospital; but as a profession it remained independent.

It thus escaped the heavy burden that full responsibility for the building and maintenance of hospitals might have loaded on its shoulders. This historic position of the profession in relation to the hospital stands in contrast to that assumed by the monastic orders and yields an important concept that should be visualized clearly both by society and by the profession. It is likely to be lost sight of today as several forces are at work that tend to blend the duties of the profession with the mission of the hospital.

Historically, the hospital belongs to the social order, and takes the form that the needs of society dictate and that the means of society provide. The doctor is a free member of society. He may attach himself to the hospital; it is part of his tradition voluntarily to contribute his skills to the care of the sick poor; and in recent times, he may use the facilities of the modern hospital in order better to treat the illnesses of the well-to-do. The doctor not infrequently plays the role of the gadfly in urging society to fulfill its obligations to the hospital, but never with the self-interest of the mendicant friar who had to abstract his own meager living from the alms he begged.

Organization of the medical profession came into being quite independently of the hospital. . . .

The hospital emerged from the Middle Ages as society's effort to ameliorate suffering, not in a greatly different form from the early Christian nosocomium but under management of the Crown, the state or some voluntary charitable association. The profession, however, during the sixteenth and seventeenth centuries arose as a composite that might trace its ancestry to many elements of medieval society. It contained the town leech and the itinerant cutter for stone; the compassionate monk tenderly caring for his charges and the charlatan friar pretending miraculous cures; Frère Bibliophile of the scriptorium patiently copying and preserving ancient writings and the worldly abbot making frequent journeys to distant lands; the expounder of classic authority in the university and the natural scientist, the product of the Renaissance, seeing and thinking for himself and devising experiments to test his thoughts.

There were three powerful bonds that welded the physician of the eighteenth and nineteenth centuries to the charity hospital: first, the ethical humanitarian response evoked by a vivid firsthand knowledge of the suffering that accompanies disease; second, the urge for increased knowledge and experience that might sharpen his skills; and third, the responsibilities of a teacher to impart the art to those qualified to continue it. These forces bound the doctor to the hospital or led him to stir society into providing one when it was lacking. . . .

We have seen that the origin and spread of the hospital in Western Civilization was identified with Christianity, and that the institution took various forms as a result of changing modes in the expression of the Christian virtues; but no event in history so altered the relation of the hospital to the social order as one single contribution coming from medical science in the last quarter of the nineteenth century. To understand this change it is necessary to set the clock back seventy-five years and learn the sinister implications of the term "hospitalism," a word that is now happily forgotten. In spite of the compassion of religion and the nobility of ethical motives, and not withstanding an increased understanding of disease and a growing effectiveness of remedies, to enter a hospital as a patient at that time meant taking a calculated and by no means insignificant risk. It was no mere happenstance that the hospital was dedicated to the sick poor. The risks of entering a hospital had to be balanced against the hazards of sickness in the hovel of the pauper, or the inability of the stricken traveler to find shelter and care in a strange community, or the necessity and urgency of some malady requiring the operative skill of a surgeon otherwise unavailable. In the absence of these or similar circumstances of dire necessity, no one in his right mind could consider a hospital a desirable or safe place in which to take up temporary residence.

By "hospitalism" was meant the great danger of cross infection that came from exposure to the infections and infectious diseases of other inmates. It was banished by Lister who applied the discoveries of Pasteur to wounds and devised the procedures of antisepsis and asepsis that were to minimize for all time the hazards of cross infection. . . .

The banishment of hospitalism meant that for the first time in history the door of the hospital was opened to all classes of society. The almsgiver and the philanthropist now could seek the hospitality and care of the institution that they had created as a refuge for the pauper and the friendless. The sick of all classes began once more to make pilgrimages, this time to the hospital as a temple of medical science. They sought knowledge and skills rather than faith and miracles.

The hospital was awakened from a complacent and benevolent existence by loud and repeated knockings on its door. More and more patients were there for admission. Room was required for the well-to-do and for the large section of the community possessed of moderate means. Private and semi-private wings and blocks were erected alongside of the old voluntary hospitals. In this country outlying communities built hospitals sometimes with a few beds designated for the free care of the poor, but with the major emphasis placed on the care of the great middle class. With the growth of the West the pattern of the voluntary hospital, which had been established during the eighteenth century on the eastern seaboard, was dropped. What charity was necessary was provided by governmental units—the state, or more frequently the county or municipality. Private corporations and at times individual doctors built hospitals that were to be run at a financial profit. Private clinics appeared, based on the hospitals of philanthropic associations or through affiliated holding companies controlling the managerial functions of hospitals.

This course of events has based the practice of a large portion of the profession squarely on the hospital. The doctor found the hopsital essential for the proper care of major illness among his clientele and thus for the living that this activity provided him. This blending of the interest of the doctor with the function of the hospital led to a sense of responsibility and ownership. The institution was no longer regarded as an agency of society, but became "his" hospital. One well-known institution is called "The Doctors' Hospital." Society, in turn, has been only too ready to relinquish some of its responsibility and relax its efforts. The doctors are supposed to know what they are doing, and comfort is taken in the attitude that it is impossible for a mere layman to judge of such matters.

This situation has created a disturbing undercurrent of thought that only a few observers appear to notice. Is it well for society or, in the long run, for the profession that this trend continue? Can a not disinterested profession be entrusted with an agency of society that is becoming more vital today than ever before in history? However sincere the efforts of the doctor to provide the best of care for his patients, the fact must be faced that these same efforts provide him with the prestige and comfortable living which he claims. It is possible that the profession is unconsciously drifting into a dangerous position not wholly unlike that in which the Church found itself before the Reformation. . . .

It has been noted that the profession bases two other essential activities on the hospital. One of these is the education of the oncoming generation of doctors, and the other the advance that comes from a continuing study and observation of disease. Translated into biologic terms, these represent the vital functions of reproduction and growth of the profession. . . .

The hospital [has been] called upon [in recent decades] to supply the facilities for careful study and analysis of the disorders of its patients. In this it [has been] aided by the university, but it has never been possible to draw a line between what is care of the patient and what may be investigation of the patient's disease conducted so that more effective care can be provided with greater safety. There can be no line drawn between treatment and cautious modification of treatment that may achieve quicker and more certain results. The hospital [has] thus acquired a real stake in the systematic investigation of the ailments of the patients it serves. This has necessitated research laboratories, special wards for the more complicated metabolic studies, library facilities, and an elaborate system of records not only for the good of the individual patient, but to be used in extending the frontiers of medicine. Only a few of the thousands of hospitals in this country can provide the facilities and personnel for education and research. These, in general, are closely affiliated with universities and are known as "teaching hopitals." But it is on these institutions that the future of medicine itself is based.

There is another trend within medicine that promises to change the historic contribution of the hospital to society. If one were to return today to a House of Pity or even to the wards of a hospital of the nineteenth century, he would be shocked at the distress and suffering occasioned by diseases and complications that are not allowed to develop today. Strictly speaking, preventive medicine deals with measures that prevent the inception of disease. Practically, no sharp line can be drawn between preventive and remedial medicine. In a few decades scientific medicine has pushed back the frontiers so that disease can be recognized and dealt with in early and remediable stages. The undertakings of modern medicine and surgery need no longer be directed toward the relief of distress and suffering if they prevent these results of disease by offering adequate treatment at a time when the patient himself scarcely may be aware that some disorder has obtained a foothold. . . .

But even in the strict sense of the term, the hospital today is preventing far more disease than it is treating. Millions of children have been given the opportunity to live and grow into healthy adults that formerly was denied them. Medical students today complete their education without having seen a patient with typhoid fever, tetanus, smallpox, or many other ancient scourges of humanity that have been abolished. If advancement of medical science is encouraged to continue at its present rate, the hospital of the future will become a center of health instead of a center of disease—a House of Prevention rather than a House of Pity.

The Social and Economic Background of the Hospital

IF THE FORMS taken by the hospital in the course of history are left standing only against the backgrounds formed by changing modes of expression of the Christian virtues and the progress of medical science, the impression created is still unrealistic and incomplete. But it is difficult to place the hospital against the background of social and economic history without risking false interpretations and conclusions. The difficulty lies more in the confusion of the background than in the object being portrayed. It is as fallacious to delineate the social and economic background of a period and ignore religion and science, as it is to describe the manner in which Christian virtues were expressed apart from the social life that generated them and the basic tools that were at hand to give them form. This cyclic nature of the background is expressed in the well-known quotation from Machiavelli: Religion "was one of the chief causes of the prosperity of Rome; for this religion gave rise to well regulated conduct, and such conduct brings good fortune, and from good fortune results the happy success of undertakings."

However, my thesis is that the form of the hospital emerges as a resultant of many forces active in the social order of the times. Also, it is generally agreed that these forces are determined by the actions of man that in turn are based on sentiments that are both intricate and interlocking; and it has been pointed out that man's actions become particularly nonlogical when he is afflicted by or confronted with sickness and suffering. So with this warning, an attempt will be made to show how certain forms of the hospital have been determined by the actual daily life of man rather than by what he felt or thought he ought to be doing. . . .

After the Reformation, Tudor England began to recognize the responsibility of society as a whole toward the miseries of poverty. By the end of Elizabeth's reign a system of poor relief was prescribed by national legislation, and compulsory poor rates were levied. Public relief was paid by and administered through the parish. . . . The Act of Settlement passed by the Cavalier Parliament of Charles II gave authority to the parishes to return newcomers to their native parish lest by chance they should some day fall on the rates. The result of all these measures was a quiet and stable people, in contrast to the swarming beggars and paupers that crowded the streets and hospitals in France and Italy.

For on the Continent affairs were different. Italy, from 1530 to 1796, experienced nearly three centuries of political chaos and economic slavery under foreign powers. The charity of the Church was inadequate, but the hospitals struggled with the ravages of poverty as best they could. France suffered under a succession of unstable or arrogant monarchies, preoccupied with wars and political intrigues. Poverty was rampant, and the people reached the boiling point with the Revolution that brought greatly needed reforms to the confused hospital system. . . .

The voluntary hospital was a concept of eighteenth-century England before the impact of the Industrial Revolution. It was not an outgrowth of experience with the great social and economic changes that were brought by the machine age, but a pre-formed pattern that has struggled valiantly during the nineteenth and nearly half the twentieth century to meet needs and cope with problems that were unknown at the time of its origin. With all its shortcomings and inadequacies, it has performed a mighty service by maintaining standards of ethical purpose and humanitarian ideals during a period of changing values. The blending of these attributes with the scientific medicine that developed so swiftly in the last half of the nineteenth century has established the pattern of Anglo-American medicine for the present century. . . .

As a contrast it is of interest to consider what the course of medicine might have been if set by the government of England at this time. During the eighteenth century in England the government "went on adding statute after statute to the 'bloody code' of English law, enlarging perpetually the long list of offences punishable by death; finally they numbered two hundred." [3] This was the period of iron discipline and cruelty in the Royal Navy and the Army. Any form of the hospital cast in the mold of the state of that century might well have blighted the growth of the medicine that was to come, or warped it with the impersonal and arrogant qualities that were recognizable in the medicine of Germany. But the hospital in England was formed by society acting independently of the state and it was this pattern that was transferred to the Colonies that have become the United States. . . .

The voluntary hospital system of England formed during the eighteenth century was expanded to meet the increased needs brought by the Industrial Revolution during the nineteenth century. The seriousness of thought, self-discipline of character, and self-reliance of the Victorians were woven into the fabric of the institutions they sponsored. Enormously increased wealth from expanding commerce and industry provided for what appeared to be an unlimited extension of facilities by founding hospital after hospital. But by 1851 half the population of the island was urban, and vast areas in the cities were covered by industrial slums. Families were crowded into single rooms or thrust underground into cellars. Sanitation measures lagged. The new Poor Law of 1834 was both harsh and inhumane in its efforts to deal with poverty. Yet the voluntary hospital spanned the century in spite of increasing social needs and perplexing problems. The task began to be too much for it only during the final decades when scientific medicine was rapidly increasing the benefits of health that could be bestowed upon all classes of society. . . .

In 1911 David Lloyd George proposed a scheme of National Health Insurance to the British Parliament. In spite of intense and bitter opposition from many quarters, it was written into law after concessions and modifications had been made. This statute increased the availability of medical care among the poorer classes, and in part stepped up the demand for hospital admission. By the early thirties the lists

3. G. M. Trevelyan, *English Social History, A Survey of Six Centuries; Chaucer to Victoria* (Toronto: Longmans, Green and Co., 1946), p. 348.

of patients waiting for admission to the great voluntary hospitals of London reached astounding numbers. It was not unusual for a single hospital to have a list of three hundred to four hundred waiting for admission for the simple operation of repair of hernia. It took years to obtain admission, and with some complaints, a patient might recover spontaneously, move away, or die long before the hospital could find room for him. . . . Emergency cases, however, were rightly accorded priority.

The administration of the old Poor Law, originally in the hands of the parish, had been transferred to Boards of Guardians of the Poor, elected in each borough. . . . The Local Government Act of 1929 transferred the powers of the Boards of Guardians to the county and borough councils. It also removed the hospital facilities of the workhouse from the provisions of the Poor Law, and gave to local authorities the right to take over the Poor Law institutions, and the obligation to work out and build a hospital system supported by taxation. Patients were required to pay whatever they could afford, up to the cost of maintenance. The London County Council (L.C.C.) took the lead, followed by Middlesex, Surrey, and others. Within a few years the old prejudices against the Poor Law Infirmary that were strongest among the destitute and ignorant, began to be overcome. Standards were elevated, and the L.C.C. hospitals had one great advantage in contrast to the voluntary hospitals—they never refused admission to a patient.

. . . It was not long before the great numbers of patients in the public authority hospitals and the experience they afforded the staffs that treated them began to attract attention. A postgraduate school of medicine was attached to the hospital in Hammersmith. Young physicians and surgeons began to wonder whether these public institutions might not become the hospitals of the future. . . .

During World War II all hospitals of England were fused into the Emergency Medical Service. Many of the voluntary hospitals in London were evacuated and some were partly demolished by bombs. The patients of the old hospitals, including the patients of the private blocks, were referred to any hospital under the National Emergency Medical Service. And now, two years after the war, under the National Health Act of the present government, all hospitals and health facilities of England will pass into the control of the Minister of Health. Special provisions have been made to preserve the teaching and research functions that center in the voluntary hospitals and their affiliated medical schools. Nevertheless, the two century cycle of the voluntary hospital movement in England appears to be drawing to a close. . . .

The Hospital and Contemporary Society

THOSE RESPONSIBLE for the future of our social institutions are searching for frames of reference that distinguish essential functions from what may be organizational fetishes. Only by clarity of vision can a course of action be followed that may safeguard those things that are essential and yet be sufficiently elastic to accommodate for the changing needs and moods of society. Mature minds are seeking to define this course between laissez-faire or random action on the one hand, and a yielding to the gospels of force and uniformity on the other. This quest is such a powerful undercurrent today, that it can be recognized as the most typical event of the post-war world. The hospital is by no means immune to this analysis, and it is hoped that even this cursory review of its history may yield some material for constructing a useful frame of reference.

Rhetorical outbursts in defense of some particular organizational pattern are escapist diversions that are useless and may be more harmful than an attitude of indifference. . . .

It is not only possible, but it seems quite likely that society will increase the participation of government in the managerial and financial affairs of the hospital. It has already moved in this direction to an extent that is not fully appreciated, and at all levels—municipal, county, state, and federal. As a general principle, the more useful and vital a service becomes in the social order, the more certain it is to become identified with the functions of government. The increasing power of medicine to determine the survival of the individual as well as to prevent or alleviate suffering has placed the hospital of today in a position that it has never held before. With this has come the increased complexity and costliness of the medical care that is to be provided to all classes of society. It is important that as much as possible be learned about the hospital because the future of this institution will be determined by society, not by the medical profession. It is never easy to learn to understand any institution and to do so with the hospital is peculiarly difficult because it is an institution that from the earliest history has conveyed an emotional experience to the ordinary man rather than an impression that can be analyzed in the light of reason. There is need to provide a rational basis to identify those services that are of proven value and to recognize undertakings that appear to be capable of developing greater values. Only by study of the hospital from a functional point of view can judgment be made regarding whether its management and finance can be entrusted to government, or what safeguards are desirable should it be decided that this course is the one to follow. . . .

Participation by the state in the affairs of the hospital is not a new happening, and history shows that it has come when existing methods of meeting the demands of society for relief of distress and suffering show signs of inadequacy or failure. The hospital of today has been made vulnerable by the tremendous increase in the demand for its services from all classes of society and by the immediate costliness of these services. The profession also is vulnerable because it is caught in a period of mal-distribution of its manpower, as well as an actual shortage created, in part, by the increased demand for doctors and in part, by efforts to raise educational standards to coincide with an increasing complexity of knowledge. Society may be tempted to impatient action under the guise of an effort to correct these imbalances.

It is even now being urged that the control of the hospital and the medical profession in this country be turned over to the government. The demand comes from a surge within the structure of the society that expresses itself as the "quasi-religious demand for social salvation through state action." It is felt everywhere. Control of medical care through state socialism is a solution that sounds plausible to the masses in their striving for the right to health and better living. But this step taken hastily might destroy more than it could bring. It would be one more surrender of the primacy of the individual—one more yielding of the right of individual man to exert his idealist will power and implement it with thoughtful action.

As a matter of fact, short of disastrous events that bring revolutionary changes in their wake, there is little likelihood that government will move in a direct frontal attack against the existing hospital system. It is more likely that if the system remains inadequate, it will be outflanked by a steady extension of tax supported institutions. This was the pattern followed in England. Governmental assistance in care of the sick, research and education, is steadily increasing. To preserve a balance this assistance should be spread widely to all hospitals and not be confined to those institutions that are under full governmental control. If American life proceeds by orderly change as in the past, there is still time for the independent hospital to find a way out of it present difficulties. As an institution it is basically sound without sign of degeneration of function or deviation of purpose. The urge for governmental control actually has paralleled the ascendancy of hospital medicine as a powerful tool of social welfare—not its degeneration.

It is necessary that the hospital be alert to its position in contemporary society and take vigorous leadership in providing health services to all classes of the social order. It must keep abreast of the needs and aspirations of a society that has become aware of its right to the vital service that the hospital can provide. It can only hold its position by moving forward. Society, on the other hand, must learn more about the values that reside in its hospitals; if it does so, it will not place them in jeopardy by ill-considered action or careless indifference.

B. *Present Hospital Facilities*

40. DISTRIBUTION, UTILIZATION, AND NEEDS

A. *STATUS OF OUR HOSPITAL SYSTEM* *

HOSPITALS ARE at the heart of our modern medical system. To the general public, these complex centers dedicated to fighting disease and to preventing needless death symbolize the new role of high quality medical care in the main stream of American life.

In the past several decades, the hospital system has been swept along on a wave of expanding facilities and functions. As a result, hospitals in thousands of

* From: *Building America's Health,* by the President's Commission on the Health Needs of the Nation; Washington: U.S. Government Printing Office, 1953 (Vol. 1, Chap. IV, "Health Facilities," pp. 22-23). Reprinted with omissions, including initial paragraphs. (Note: Four of the five volumes comprising the Report of the President's Commission on the Health Needs of the Nation were published in 1953; Vol. 1, "Findings and Recommendations," was actually issued in 1952).

communities across the length and breadth of this land are the core of the medical activities in those communities. The modern hospital has developed into the basic institution providing technical facilities for the promotion of health, the diagnosis and treatment of disease, and the rehabilitation of the disabled. More and more, it is becoming responsible for a continuing flow of health services to the community, supplying preventive services in health centers at one end of the line and rehabilitative and home care services at the other end.

Moreover, the hospital has become the most important and most expensive factor in medical education. Medical schools could not exist without teaching hospitals. Nor could the education of nurses and paramedical personnel be carried out without them. There has been increasing realization that the center of all medical educational activities is the teaching hospital. The hospitals also take responsibility for the graduate training of interns and residents. All hospitals which have resident staffs or schools of nursing should be regarded as teaching hospitals, whether or not they are connected with medical schools.

Our people's use of hospital beds has soared in the past generation. In 1930 only 37 percent of all births took place in hospitals, whereas by 1949 this figure had risen to 87 percent. The phenomenal growth of prepayment for hospital care has removed much of the pocketbook terror of hospitals for a considerable portion of the population.

Hospitals are sensitive barometers of the rise and fall of different patterns of disease and treatment. Many diseases which once required long hospitalization now require little or none—pneumonia, for example. The modern onslaught against tuberculosis is already reducing the need for beds for this disease in some areas of the country, although many communities are still far short of tuberculosis facilities. On the other hand, our rapidly aging population is increasing the need all over the country for the care of those with long-term illness.

Alterations in the pattern of medical practice and research discoveries will undoubtedly change the manner in which hospitals are used. Projected programs for hospital construction and operation must be constantly responsive to these fast changing patterns, fully cognizant of the need to make hospitals the best community instruments for promoting health and treating disease. . . .

Because recent trends have attempted to bring services and facilities as close as possible to patients, an increased interest has developed in this country regarding health standards and adequacy of hospital care.* This interest has been shared by both professional and lay groups. A recent development characteristic of this trend has been the formation of the Joint Commission on Accreditation. One of the important contributing elements to the trend is the Hospital Survey and Construction

* From: *Building America's Health,* by the President's Commission on the Health Needs of the Nation; Washington: U.S. Government Printing Office, 1953 (Vol. 2, Chap. VI, "Health Facilities and Services," pp. 192-95, 201-2). Reprinted with omissions, including initial paragraphs, some tables and one figure.

(Hill-Burton) program, with its emphasis on hospitals in smaller communities and their relationships to metropolitan centers.

In order to ensure care of high quality in all hospitals, it is important that serious consideration be given to the question of modernizing the larger hospitals and teaching centers, which are the reservoirs of research, training and the producers of the skills necessary to high quality care. This means that careful planning for the future must be done to meet the problems that exist and those that will rise.

These problems cannot be solved by any one group, either government or private; everyone, including the consumer, must take an active part. The effects of hospital services are far-reaching and the responsibility is general. This is evident from the following facts:

1. Hospital service is one of the 10 major service industries in this country;

2. The 6,600 registered hospitals in this country have about one and a half million beds, admit over 18 million patients annually, have almost 3 million births annually, and employ over 1 million persons;

3. Hospitals owned by local, State and Federal Government agencies provide over one-third of the beds in general and special hospitals, well over nine-tenths of the beds for mental disease, and almost nine-tenths of the beds for tuberculosis;

4. Nongovernmental hospitals care for 13 million of the 18 million persons admitted;

5. The cost of treating these more than 18 million patients was nearly $4 billion in 1951; the payroll alone was over $2 billion.

TABLE 35. *Hospitals and hospital beds in the United States, by type, 1951* *

Type	Hospitals	Beds	Percent of Beds
Total	6,637	1,529,988	100.0
General	4,890	640,207	41.8
Special	341	31,421	2.1
Nervous and mental	596	728,187	47.6
Tuberculosis	430	88,379	5.8
Convalescent and rest	120	7,115	0.5
Other	260	34,679	2.3

Source: The Journal of the American Medical Association, vol. 149, No. 2, p. 150, Table D. (Chicago, Ill., May 10, 1952).

Of the Nation's one and a half million hospital beds, beds in general and allied special hospitals account for less than half—44 percent of the total. A greater proportion, 48 percent, over 700,000 beds, are in mental hospitals. Tuberculosis hospitals have only 6 percent of the beds.

These beds represent a very substantial investment. The country's hospitals had assets of $8.2 billion at the end of 1951 and the hospital plant was valued at more

* Cf. the data in this table with those presented in Table 38, in selection immediately following.

than $6.4 billion. On the average, each bed represented a capital investment of over $4,200. General and special short-term nonprofit hospitals had the highest investment per bed ($6,500). Mental hospitals (non-Federal) with 43 percent of all beds had only 21 percent of the plant assets and 18 percent of all assets.

TABLE 36. *Ownership of hospitals and hospital beds in the United States, 1951*

Ownership	Hospitals	Beds	Percent of Beds
Total	6,637	1,529,988	100.0
Federal	388	216,939	14.2
State	554	683,376	44.7
County and city	1,090	197,405	12.9
Non-profit	2,121	225,903	14.8
Church	1,116	154,053	10.1
Proprietary	1,368	52,312	3.4

Source: The Journal of the American Medical Association, vol. 149, No. 2, p. 151, Table G. (Chicago, Ill., May 10, 1952).

Since mental hospitals are primarily State institutions, it follows that almost half of all hospital beds are owned by State governments. Although nonprofit hospitals represent one-third of all hospitals they had only 15 percent of the beds.

On an average day, about eight people out of every 1,000 are in hospitals, more than half of them in mental hospitals. The utilization of hospital beds—from the viewpoint of admissions—looks very different. Out of each 1,000 people, 111 entered general hospitals in the course of the year 1951, two entered mental hospitals, and one entered a tuberculosis hospital. The people who entered general hospitals stayed on the average 10 days, those who entered mental hospitals stayed on an average over 2 years, and those who entered tuberculosis hospitals stayed 8 months. Patients in governmental hospitals had a longer average length of stay than patients in nongovernmental hospitals. Patients admitted to all private general hospitals had an average length of stay of less than 8 days compared with an average stay in government general hospitals of 17 days.

TABLE 37. *Utilization of general hospital beds, 1931-51*

Year	Beds	Census	Admissions	Percent Occu-pancy	Per 1,000 Population			
					Beds	Census	Admis-sions	Average Length of Stay
1931	384,333	247,560	6,321,861	64	3.1	2.0	51.0	14
1940	462,360	325,160	9,219,496	70	3.5	2.5	69.9	13
1950	587,917	433,364	15,830,170	74	3.9	2.9	104.7	10
1951	640,207	470,692	17,065,821	74	4.2	3.1	111.3	10

Source: The Journal of the American Medical Association, vol. 149, No. 2, p. 155 (Chicago, Ill., May 10, 1952).

General Hospitals.—In the past 20 years the number of general hospital beds had increased much faster than population, and use has increased faster still. In those 20 years the number of beds per 1,000 has increased from 3.1 to 4.2 or about 35 percent while admissions have increased from 51 to 111 per 1,000, or more than 100 percent.

Increased utilization has been made possible by a much shorter average length of stay—a drop from 14 days in 1931 to 10 in 1951; and secondarily by an increase in the rate of occupancy.

Mental Hospitals.—Construction in this field has barely kept up with the population increase. Mental hospitals as reported below include institutions for the epileptic and feeble-minded; preliminary data from the National Institute of Mental Health indicate that at the end of 1950 these institutions had a rated capacity of 116,000 beds and resident patients of about 135,000. In 1940 there were about 93,000 beds and 105,000 resident patients and in 1932 a rated capacity of 80,000 and roughly 93,000 patients. The 1940 and 1932 data are for public institutions only but probably represent about 95 percent of the total.

The Public Health Service reports 384 patients in mental hospitals (exclusive of hospitals for epileptics and the feeble-minded) per 100,000 population in 1950, more than twice the rate found in 1903, the earliest year for which reasonably comparable figures were available.

These hospitals are largely understaffed custodial institutions with an increasingly large proportion of old people. A study in New York State showed that persons 60 years and older made up 22 percent of the population of State mental hospitals in 1915, but 33 percent in 1947....

Outpatient Services and Group Practice.—There is a growing recognition of the importance of good outpatient services and the ambulatory diagnostic and therapeutic services available through group practice. Modern medical trends focus more and more upon the promotion of health services for ambulatory patients, with the following advantages:

(*a*) Medical care is provided for the needs of patients who, under former conditions and practices, would have required hospitalization;

(*b*) Patients' needs are met with less economic family and community stress; and

(*c*) More health needs are met with the existing manpower resources.

Thus, ambulatory services are emerging as an integral type of hospital service. This means that hospitals and health authorities must broaden their scope of operations and keep foremost in mind the fact that the primary function of all health services is to keep well people well.

Unfortunately, in some areas the provision of ambulant care has lagged because of the lack of general acceptance of this concept. It has also lagged because of the absence of community funds to aid in the costs of such care, and the critical shortage of professional personnel necessary to set up outpatient departments. Still other factors include, once again, obsolescence of equipment and lack of facilities.

To date a major defect in the majority of prepayment health plans is that they do not provide for services other than to hospital inpatients.

Home Care Programs.—Hospital home care programs have emerged in several areas of the country as a partial solution to many of the difficulties encountered by hospitals in their attempt to provide suitable medical care to patients with long-term illnesses, while at the same time meeting hospital bed needs for patients with acute illnesses.

Home care programs have demonstrated that patients who are medically and socially qualified do very well when cared for in their home. Such programs are excellent vehicles for integrating hospital services with those of the community. They reduce both medical costs and the need for hospital bed expansion. They encourage coordination of services and serve as excellent educational vehicles for both graduate and undergraduate training programs.

Rehabilitation.—Hospitals are beginning to recognize that rehabilitation services are necessary and integral parts of the function of the general hospital. Sound principles of physical medicine and rehabilitation have been applied over the years in many hospitals but they have not yet been applied on a broad enough scale. A limited number of hospitals, especially large institutions and those affiliated with medical centers, provide semi-organized rehabilitation services of varied and limited degrees.

At present there are plans for the establishment of chronic disease units in close association with general hospitals and for regional affiliation of hospitals for such services. However, there is also need for emphasis upon rehabilitative measures for acutely ill patients. Slow but encouraging progress is being made in the education and training of personnel for rehabilitation programs. Joint planning on a national, State, and local basis can accelerate progress in the fields of ambulatory care, home-care programs and rehabilitation by:

1. Enlisting public interest for the promotion of health maintenance plans;

2. Studying and evaluating existing services for ambulatory patients for improvement and expansion;

3. Utilizing presently available personnel, including general practitioners, and finally

4. Coordinating community services, facilities and resources. . . .

B. HOSPITAL CONSTRUCTION AND BED NEEDS *

HOSPITAL BEDS are symbols of hospital services and are not an end in themselves. They do provide a useful measure of the physical facilities at hand for furnishing

* From: "Hospital Beds in the United States in 1953," by John W. Cronin, M.D., Maurice E. Odoroff, and Leslie M. Abbe; *Public Health Reports* 68: 425-32, April 1953 (No. 4). Reprinted with omissions, including some figures and one table. Dr. Cronin is chief of the Bureau of Medical Services, Public Health Service, Washington, D.C.; the other two authors are, respectively, chief and assistant chief of the Program Evaluation and Reports Branch, in the Division of Hospital and Medical Facilities of the Bureau of Medical Services.

hospital services. The capacity to provide adequate health care in a community or a nation can be gauged substantially by the number of beds available, in relation to the number of people living in the area.

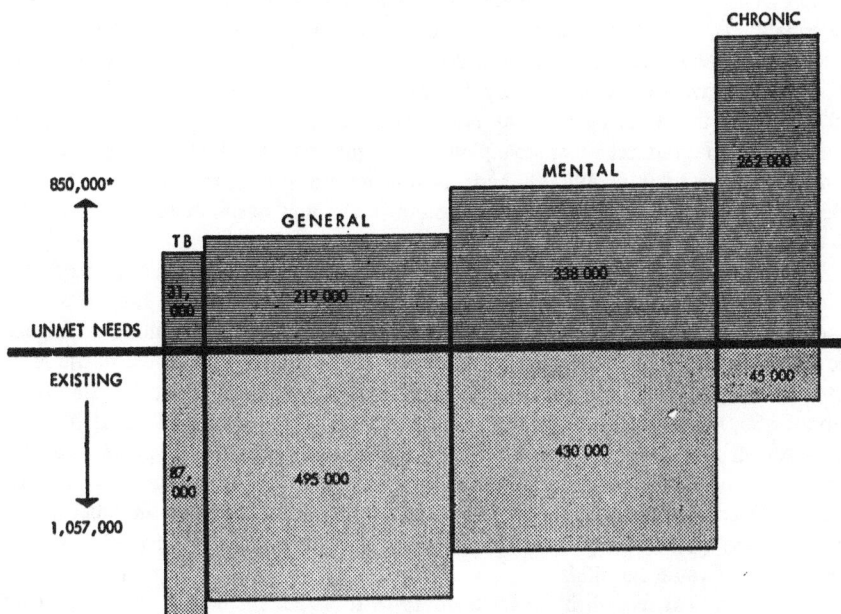

FIGURE 28. Hospital beds in the United States in 1953.
* Exclusive of 117,000 Federal hospital beds. All data in this chart as of January 1, 1953.

Prior to 1946 the building of new hospitals and hospital additions in the United States was sporadic, proceeding slowly in some communities and rapidly in others, according to local pressures and means and without regard to any general pattern or orderly plan. At the same time many communities and sections of the Nation had little or no available hospital care within ready reach. The end of World War II made possible a renewed interest in providing for many domestic needs. Physical facilities for the Nation's health became one aspect of this interest.

A broad program was launched in 1946 by Federal legislation to assist the States to inventory their existing hospitals, to define the total need for hospitals, and to map out a construction program to provide needed hospital and health center services. Financial assistance was included, both for planning and construction. This legislation, the Hospital Survey and Construction Act (Public Law 725, 79th Cong.) has been popularly known as the Hill-Burton Act. Its administration was placed under the Surgeon General of the Public Health Service, as a part of the basic Public Health Service Act. . . .

This report appraises the situation nationally and locally, as reflected by the current State hospital plans under the Hospital Survey and Construction Act. It also comments on the influence of the Hill-Burton program during 5 years of operation and refers to current problems relating to standards of need and standards for the degree of Federal aid now appropriate.

Where We Are Now.—In the Nation as a whole we now have 1,218,000 existing hospital beds, according to State plan inventories as of January 1, 1953. These plans excluded Federal beds. This total is 202,000 more than was recorded in the first Hill-Burton inventory as of January 1, 1948. Of these, however, 161,000 beds are classified by the State agencies as nonacceptable on the basis of fire and health hazards, so that our net acceptable plant for all purposes is 1,057,000 beds. Almost one-half of this total, or 495,000 beds, is in general hospitals; mental hospitals have 431,000 beds; tuberculosis hospitals, 86,000 beds; and hospitals for chronic care, 44,000 beds.

The Hospital Survey and Construction Act establishes standards of need, for planning purposes, in each category of hospital. These standards are limits for construction with Federal assistance and do not preclude State planning to higher levels if warranted. For most States, however, the standards established in the Hill-Burton Act are much beyond the level of existing facilities. By these standards about 850,000 additional beds are needed nationally to provide adequate hospital care for all the people. Of these, 336,000 are needed in mental hospitals, 262,000 in chronic hospitals, 219,000 in general hospitals, and 31,000 in tuberculosis hospitals. Percentagewise, the Nation has 77 percent of its need met in tuberculosis facilities, 69 percent in general hospitals, 56 percent in mental hospitals, and 14 percent in chronic hospitals.

The historical record, by years from 1948 to 1953, for each category appears in table 38. By definition under the present regulations, this inventory excludes beds for civilians in Federal hospitals. These are chiefly in facilities of the Veterans Administration, plus a comparatively small number of beds in the hospitals operated by the Indian Service and the Public Health Service.

During the 5 years for which comprehensive State planning has been carried on, considerable net progress has been made in general hospitals: 107,000 additional acceptable beds are recorded, a gain of 28 percent. Tuberculosis beds have also increased more than 20 percent. Mental and chronic beds, on the other hand, while increasing slowly, are not keeping up with growth in population and obsolescence. In both these categories the remaining need is greater than in 1948. This constitutes one of the major challenges facing the Nation today in meeting the need for adequate hospital services.

National trends and national totals do not accurately reflect the real picture in regard to specific regions of the country. Among the States, wide differences exist as to relative status in providing an adequate hospital plant. Similar differences exist among the major socio-economic regions of the Nation. Generally speaking, the States with large means have the least unmet need, while the least wealthy States have the greatest need. . . . The national average of unmet need is 5.5 beds per 1,000 population. Regionally, the greatest unmet need for general hospitals is still in the southeastern States, although substantial progress has been made here during the past 5 years.

Similar contrasts appear for mental hospitals. The unmet need, nationally, is still 2.2 beds per 1,000 population. In New England it is only 1 bed per 1,000, but throughout the southeastern and southwestern States this need is nearly 3 beds per 1,000. . . .

* TABLE 38. *Civilian hospital beds in the United States and Territories, 1948–53*

Hospital category and year (as of Jan. 1)	Estimated total beds needed A	Existing beds		Acceptable		Estimated additional beds needed
		Total	Non-acceptable B	Number	Percent of total need	
All categories						
1953	1,899,279	1,218,781	161,354	1,057,427	55.7	848,567
1952	1,899,806	1,193,836	176,013	1,017,823	53.6	881,983
1950	1,850,052	1,118,535	166,339	952,196	51.5	897,856
1948	1,776,401	1,016,712	148,752	867,960	48.9	908,441
General hospitals						
1953	714,469	572,493	77,308	495,185	69.3	219,222
1952	708,574	554,084	79,750	474,334	66.9	234,240
1950	682,601	513,814	76,028	437,786	64.1	244,815
1948	652,974	469,398	81,254	388,144	59.4	264,830
Mental hospitals						
1953	766,463	490,598	59,591	431,007	56.2	336,676
1952	755,097	482,733	69,801	412,932	54.7	342,165
1950	725,203	462,859	63,721	399,138	55.0	326,065
1948	690,381	427,201	46,858	380,343	55.1	310,038
Tuberculosis hospitals						
1953	112,075	100,204	13,506	86,698	77.4	30,934
1952	133,899	99,147	11,597	87,550	65.4	46,349
1950	148,936	94,024	12,513	81,511	54.7	67,425
1948	155,987	84,158	13,007	71,151	45.6	84,836
Chronic hospitals						
1953	306,272	55,486	10,949	44,537	14.5	261,735
1952	302,236	57,872	14,865	43,007	14.2	259,229
1950	293,312	47,838	14,077	33,761	11.5	259,551
1948	277,059	35,955	7,633	28,322	10.2	248,737

A As set by Title VI of Public Health Service Act.
B As classified by State agencies, on the basis of fire and health hazards.
Source: State Plans for Hospital Construction.

The Hospital Survey and Construction Act requires that a coordinated system of general hospitals be planned within each State, under which regional hospital centers would provide leadership, specialized care, and consultation for smaller

* Cf. the data in this table with those presented in Table 35, in immediately preceding selection.

community hospitals within the region. Under the Hill-Burton program the United States is composed of 375 such regions, as defined in present State plans. Studies of these regions show that there are actually wide differences as to the level of facilities now available in single hospital regions. . . . State totals may obscure important differences among hospital regions in the present available plant.

For local communities there are also areas of acute need with little or no available hospital plant. A recent check shows 250 hospital areas still without any acceptable hospital facilities. These areas include about 3 percent of the Nation's population and require some 13,000 beds to meet standards for general hospital care. This study also shows that about 5 percent of the population of the Nation live in areas where less than 25 percent of the general hospital facilities needed are available. These facts give some indication of the work yet to be done.

Effect of the Hill-Burton Program.—The act requires a continuous inventory and positive planning of hospital expansion in each State. This has greatly stimulated orderly growth of the Nation's facilities for protecting the health of its people. Its direct encouragement of construction has been substantial, when measured by the dollar volume of hospital construction. During the last 3 years the value of work placed on Hill-Burton projects has averaged about one-third of all non-Federal hospital construction.

A number of additional benefits also have accrued. Perhaps the most significant, in regard to improving the quality of service, have been the very rapid increase in State statutes establishing hospital licensing, improved architectural design, attracting of physicians to rural communities, and creating a greater awareness of the problems of adequate care for chronic illness.

The effect of the hospital survey and construction program is quite significant in regard to the distribution of projects assisted. This is governed by the statutory formula for allocation among the States of the annual appropriation and by the conditions required as to a graduated scale for matching local funds. In each State, the formula for matching is based on population, weighted by its financial ability. As a result, the greatest Federal assistance has been given in the least wealthy States. The record shows that remaining need is still the greatest in these States.

Expressed broadly, the Hill-Burton program in 5 years has assisted in building about 1.0 bed per 1,000 population in the neediest States. These are States where the remaining additional need is still about 8 beds per 1,000 population. A proportionally lesser volume of assistance—about 0.3 beds per 1,000 population—has been accorded States with the least unmet need. In these States the remaining need is now under 3.5 beds per 1,000 population. Comparative study of the relation between remaining need and the degree to which these States are rural in character shows that the greatest need occurs in those States which have the highest proportion of population living in rural areas. In brief, Hill-Burton aid has been distributed to the greatest degree in those States which are least wealthy, most rural, and with greatest proportional unmet need.

Within the several States, distribution of assistance to specific projects has been governed by a priority system based on unmet need, as established in the State plan. In consequence the stimulus of Federal assistance has encouraged many communities where unmet need was the greatest to raise local funds for matching Federal grants, in accordance with the intent of the act. Recent studies have indicated that 38 percent of all general hospital beds added with Hospital Survey and Construction Act assistance have been in places under 10,000 in population; 31 percent in places of from 10,000 to 50,000 population; and 31 percent in metropolitan cities of over 50,000 population. Nearly 600 new projects have been placed in communities which previously had no acceptable hospital. At the other end of the scale, 21 teaching facilities at university medical centers have been assisted in 18 States.

Major emphasis has been placed by State agencies on Hill-Burton assistance to general hospital projects. As of January 1, 1953, general hospital beds added by approved projects amount to 73,168, of a total of 96,428 beds in all types of hospitals.* A gradual change in this emphasis for most States appears important, if a reasonable balance between categories of facilities is to be attained.

The hospital survey and construction program makes funds available not only for hospitals but for public health centers. In the Nation to date 377 such projects have been approved. The largest number of these, 283, will serve the 30,000,000 people in the 11 southeastern States. In this region these projects constitute a substantial increase in facilities available for preventive medicine and extend a means of providing for good health at a very moderate outlay. These projects represent a total expenditure of $28,000,000, or about 2 percent of the estimated total cost of $1,588,000,000 for all projects assisted through January 1, 1953, by Hospital Survey and Construction Act funds.*

Problems Ahead.—After 5 years of active operation of this cooperative Federal-State program, problems are emerging which were not at first anticipated. One group of problems involves the technical aspects of setting more precise standards of need:

1. The standard for tuberculosis beds required, as gradually evolved since 1917, is not on a population basis, but is related to the mortality rate. The mortality

---

* As of May 1, 1956, the total estimated cost of all facilities approved for Federal assistance under the Hospital Survey and Construction Act amounted to $2,284,000,000, of which the Federal contribution represents $740,000,000 and local sponsors' matching funds $1,544,000,000. Approved projects totaled 2,905, of which 2,035—providing 94,566 beds—had been completed and were in operation; 553 projects—providing 24,915 beds—were under construction, and 317 —to provide 11,580 beds—were in the pre-construction stage. The entire group of approved projects adds 131,061 beds to the existing hospital plant, as well as providing 619 public health centers and many adjunct facilities.

Most of the approved projects have been for construction of general hospitals—73 per cent of the projects and 94,928 beds; 3 per cent of the projects have been for construction of mental hospitals; 2 per cent, tuberculosis hospitals; 2 per cent, chronic disease facilities; 19 per cent, public health centers; and 1 per cent, other related health facilities. Twenty per cent of the total funds devoted to the program have gone to teaching institutions, including 37 university medical school hospitals. Of the new general hospitals provided for, 535 are located in areas previously without hospitals; and approximately 55 per cent of the 1,057 new hospitals of all kinds assisted under the program are located in towns of under 5,000 population, while only 11 per cent are in cities of 50,000 or more. ("Hospital and Medical Facilities Survey and Construction Program," by John W. Cronin; *Public Health Reports* 71: 932, September 1956.)

rate for tuberculosis continued to decline rapidly and dropped to a rate of 20 per 100,000 population for 1951. This is in contrast to a rate of 46 in 1940 and 200 at the turn of the century. New cases of active tuberculosis, however, continue to be discovered at a rate which is declining very slightly. It now seems clear that new standards based on incidence of active cases should be substituted for the present basis of planning under the act.

2. One of the important innovations in the Hill-Burton inventory is the distinction made between acceptable and nonacceptable beds. For planning purposes, only acceptable beds are recognized as counting against total need. There is still a considerable variation among State plans as to the degree to which nonacceptable beds have been identified and taken into account for planning. As shown by table 38, nonacceptable beds today amount to about 15 percent of all existing beds in the Nation. In some States only a few such beds have been distinguished. Sometimes this arises from the assumption that facilities licensed must be held acceptable, even though there may be substantial public hazards existing. . . . There is a need for the establishment of practical and comparable minimum standards of acceptability.

3. A third technical problem relates to the role of existing beds for civilians in Federal hospitals. Supporters of the viewpoint that these beds should be included in State hospital plan inventories are increasing. According to last available reports there are existing about 46,000 such general hospital beds for civilians, 55,000 mental hospital beds, and 15,000 tuberculosis hospital beds, which are not now recorded in Hill-Burton plans. These are not distributed uniformly among the States in relation to the population, and cannot all be regarded as reasonably accessible. They still constitute a considerable proportion of the total actual hospital plant. For the present they could probably be added to the record without changing the levels of total need, since many States find these goals greater than the apparent ability of their people to achieve at this time.

A second group of problems relates to broad policy for standards governing the degree of Federal assistance:

1. The Hospital Survey and Construction Act constitutes a fairly advanced form of grant-in-aid principles. It has the practical effect of producing its maximum program in States of minimum income and greatest need. Various proposals have arisen for modifying this distribution of aid among the States and also for requiring State support in addition to local support.

2. Within most States, there are marked differences among hospital areas in need and financial resources. The present Hospital Survey and Construction Act recognizes this situation. An option is provided which varies the percentage of Federal assistance on specific projects, as an alternate to selecting a single percentage for all projects in any one State. Interest in using this option is increasing, as it facilitates actual construction in remaining areas having acute need and restricted means. . . .

C. A PROGRAM FOR IMPROVING SERVICE *

THE NEXT TEN YEARS †

THE NEXT TEN years should see the realization of a third major stage in the development of the nation's hospital services. In the first, the hospitals provided meager care almost exclusively for the sick poor. The second stage witnessed the hospital's evolution into the workshop of medicine to which the sick and injured came largely for curative measures. The third developmental phase, which has already begun, should bring a marked extension of hospital services both into and throughout the country. In the development of this third stage the hospital should become more and more an important health agency, not only in providing the best in therapeutic measures but also in taking active steps toward the prevention of illness. The new hospitals will keep abreast of new developments in medical science and in the changing patterns of the times. Particularly, they will be aware continually of the changing needs for hospital services and will afford the flexibility of operations necessary to adapt the services readily to meet new needs without unnecessary delay. In these and all other activities, the hospitals will cooperate still more closely with members of the medical profession so that the best interests of all will be carried forward in the provision of improved hospital and medical care.

The traditional functions of the general hospital have been care of the patient, research, and medical education. In the new stage at least two more functions should be added. These are preventive medicine and public health education.

Care of the Patient.—Care of the patient is the primary function of the hospital, and it is also an area in which considerable development may be expected in the years ahead. General hospitals should strive continually to provide essential services for all physicians and patients through adoption of the newly developed techniques and the acquisition of more efficient equipment. The general hospital should provide as far as possible for all types of illness. Such service would include facilities for the treatment of acute communicable disease, nervous and mental disease, tuberculosis, and long-term illness. The inclusion of all possible types of cases in the general hospital service has many obvious advantages. Few patients suffer from one condition exclusively. The general hospital staff is in a better position to treat the patient as a whole than is the specialized staff of the special hospital.

Beyond question, one of the greatest needs today is for facilities for the care of the patient with a long-term illness. This need will increase progressively in the years ahead. . . . By 1980 it is expected that the number of persons over forty-five will constitute nearly half of our population. This change will add enormously to medical and hospital care requirements.

Much attention has been directed to the great need for more adequate care of

* From: *America's Health: A Report to the Nation by the National Health Assembly;* New York: Harper, 1949 (Chap. III, "What Is the Nation's Need for Hospital Facilities, Health Centers, and Diagnostic Clinics?" pp. 49-56). Reprinted (with omissions, including initial paragraphs) by permission of the publishers.

† I.e., the decade 1948-58.

the mentally ill. Careful and comprehensive study should be given to this problem. General hospitals should be stimulated to provide facilities and personnel for the diagnosis of mental diseases and for the treatment of those patients who are not in need of long-term institutional care. Mental hygiene clinics should be established in the outpatient departments of general hospitals wherever competent professional service is available. Due attention should be given to the need for expansion of the services of special hospitals for nervous and mental diseases.

The problem of providing an integrated service for the chronically ill is a complex one. Most general hospitals accept chronic patients, although relatively few have specialized departments for their care. Not only are these patients an economic drain on the hospital but they occupy beds badly needed for acute cases.

Many or perhaps most chronic-disease patients require intermittent acute care. This fact points to the advisability of providing chronic facilities either as a part of or under the supervision of the general hospital. Also, in view of the increasing incidence of chronic illness, its study should become of increasing interest and importance to the general hospital staff.

Medical social service will likewise become increasingly important, especially in connection with the care of all chronic illness. Hospitals should establish medical social-work departments or activities to assist patients in meeting social and economic problems relating to their illness, to help them carry out the physician's instructions, and to provide physicians with helpful information regarding the patient's socio-economic environment. The medical social worker should function with the doctor in research, either as part of a medical research project or in the study of social factors in illness. She also shares in the hospital teaching program in supervising the field work of medical social-work students and in teaching the social component in illness to the professional groups—nurses, dietitians, undergraduate medical students, interns, and residents.

Research.—The research activities of hospitals should continue at an even faster tempo. The spectacular discoveries and developments of medical science over the past few years have aroused public interest in research activities to an all-time high. The physician in his day-to-day contact with hospital patients is in an excellent position to add to the sum total of medical knowledge. The present emphasis on research in great specialized institutions in no way lessens the need for clinical research in hospitals.

Medical Education.—The expanding pattern of hospital and medical services throughout the country requires an ever increasing number of physicians, dentists, nurses, technicians, and other professional personnel. Since hospitals are essential to the training of such personnel, the teaching resources of hospitals should continue to be used to the fullest possible extent.

Preventive medicine.—Although preventive medicine in its narrowest sense is usually considered the function of official public health officers, it is in fact a function of every physician and every health organization, including the hospital. With a realization of economic value as an important end result of disease prevention and the promotion of health, hospitals and out-patient departments should concern themselves with the support and maintenance of worthwhile programs in this field. This function may be exercised effectively in many areas such as out-patient services, diagnostic clinics, community services, and cooperation with local health departments.

Public Health Education.—Few hospitals have any planned community-wide programs of health education. This field has been left almost entirely to organized departments of public health and voluntary health organizations. Increased effort should be directed toward achieving a better community understanding of the value of hospital care and other means of illness prevention. A better public understanding of hospital values will result in greater utilization and public support of hospitals. The individual should be made aware that better hospitals mean better care for himself and his family. He must understand that the skill of his own doctor and that of other physicians can be developed only in a good hospital.

Staffing and Licensure.—The boards of management of voluntary hospitals should be composed of members who are broadly representative of the public. Definite liaison arrangements should be made among the members of the managing board, the administrator, and the medical staff for the discussion of professional affairs and the establishment of administrative and professional relationships.

Until relatively recent times formal training in hospital administration has been almost unknown. Training at best has been almost entirely by the apprenticeship method. The complex organization of the modern hospital and the enlarged scope of its function demand that the administrator be a well-trained, competent individual who will insure provision of the essential services as well as efficient administration. The first formal scholastic course in hospital administration was established by the University of Chicago only fourteen years ago. More recently eight other universities have also instituted formal courses in hospital management. One state has already enacted laws requiring the registration of hospital administrators, such registration contingent on their fulfilling certain qualifications. This may well become a trend which will make the value of formal administrative training even more immediately apparent. Formal training in hospital administration prepares the individual not only for institutional management but also for a broader field of medical administration in which opportunities are continually on the increase.

In view of the hospital's responsibility to the community for the provision of a high quality of care, it is essential that it have a formal staff organization. Formal medical-staff organization is essential to assure the best care of the patient in any hospital, as well as to insure supervision and evaluation of the medical care provided.

Over the years through which the hospitals have served the American public, they have remained remarkably free from any governmental controls. No other public service agency has been so favored. This fact is a tribute to the character of the men and women who have built our hospital system. The great majority of the hospitals have not and do not now need any official regulations to insure the best possible service. Nevertheless freedom from control, desirable as it may be in principle, has permitted some abuses in hospital practice. These can be corrected effectively only through the enforcement of minimum standards by means of the mechanism of licensure. Hospital licensure statutes should be such as to develop an effective hospital service adequate to meet the public need and to provide maximum opportunities for the training of medical and nursing personnel. The effective administration of licensure statutes should be directed primarily toward the education of hospitals in the essentials of good practice. The police power of licensure should play a minor role in the main purpose of the procedure.

Out-Patient Services.—Care of the ambulatory patient in the out-patient department should be extended as a means of preventing hospitalization and providing service to the general public as well as to patients before or after their stay in the hospital. Such services provide advice, supervision, assistance, and direction for convalescents and the chronically ill who do not need institutional care. The follow-up services are valuable to both patient and physician in determining the effectiveness of the therapy provided during hospitalization and ambulant care. Out-patient service provides one of the best means for hospital participation in preventive medicine, particularly in the fields of mental illness, venereal disease, tuberculosis, and dental care. The out-patient department, incidentally, is one of the most effective public health educational devices a hospital can use.

Diagnostic Clinics.—Medicine as taught today by the medical schools is best practiced in group organizations such as the diagnostic or group-practice clinic. The trend toward specialization in medicine creates an ever increasing need for consultation if the patient is to receive complete service. Comprehensive diagnostic service can therefore be furnished most effectively in a group-practice or diagnostic clinic where all the specialties are represented. The facilities available in a modern hospital lend themselves to this type of service and greatly increase the hospital's opportunity to serve its community.

Co-operation with Local Health Departments.—Hospitals and health departments have a common responsibility in promoting the health of a community. They should seek every method for co-ordinating their efforts and integrating their functions. This can be done in part through the joint use of certain personnel and of such facilities as laboratories, out-patient departments, and other diagnostic equipment and, wherever it appears logical and feasible, through the use of common physical facilities. Such co-operation lends itself particularly well to maternal and child-health programs, communicable-disease control, tuberculosis, and mental-hygiene case findings. The integrated activity should include the general health education of the community, the visiting nurse service, and social service programs. At the present time about 25 per cent of all organized public health departments carry on some of this work in local hospitals.

Health of Minority Groups.—There are in the United States a number of large minority groups. Their health needs are greater than those of the population as a whole, and in general there is not now available to them the same quality or quantity of medical and hospital care as there is for the balance of the population. The need for an expanded and improved health service for these groups, and particularly for Negroes, is recognized. They should have the same high quality of professional and institutional care as all other segments of the population, and there should be an increased and broadened opportunity for the education and training of professional personnel to serve them.

The Rural Problem.—Because of the social and economic conditions surrounding rural life, special problems are involved in providing good rural hospital care.... Medical care is for all practical purposes almost non-existent in many rural areas today. The question therefore is one not of hospitals alone but of hospitals and medical care.

The problem of extending medical care and the services of the modern hospital into rural areas is one which requires careful planning and coordination of effort on the part of all concerned—the professions and the general public. Public health services, health centers, community clinics, and small hospitals—all properly correlated and integrated with the diagnostic and therapeutic services of larger hospitals and their specialized personnel—appear to offer the best solution of the problem.

CONCLUSIONS AND RECOMMENDATIONS *

FULL RECOGNITION is given to the vast strides made by the American hospital in attaining its present vital and strategic place among the nation's health resources. Yet much remains to be accomplished in achieving the ultimate aim of adequate services for all people without regard to race, creed, color, or economic circumstances. In order that maximum progress toward this goal may be realized in the next ten years, it is recommended that:

1. The program under the Hospital Survey and Construction Act should be continued and extended under a policy of flexibility permitting such adaptation as may be required to meet changing needs. The present authorization of $75,000,000 per year should be increased in view of the urgent needs for the establishment of additional hospital beds and clinics and health centers in many areas of the country.

2. The program under Public Law 725 and the hospital program of the Veterans Administration should be closely integrated in the interest of good planning.

3. Hospitals within service areas should be functionally or organically associated with one another so that the patient may benefit from the resources of all.

4. The full cost of hospital services for those patients for whom governmental agencies have assumed responsibility should be paid from tax funds. This same principle should be observed by nongovernmental agencies purchasing hospital care.

5. Hospitals, health departments and all other health agencies should seek

---

* Adopted by the National Health Assembly Section on Hospital Facilities, Health Centers, and Diagnostic Clinics, at the Assembly's meeting in Washington in May 1948.

every method for co-ordinating their efforts and integrating their functions in the interests of greater efficiency and service to the patient.

6. Diagnostic clinics, out-patient services, and home medical care and allied programs should be developed more extensively in extending health services for all.

7. Hospitals should intensify and extend their basic activities in research and education.

8. Preventive medical and dental service and public health education should be carried out more widely as regular functions of the modern hospital.

9. As far as possible, the general hospital should provide facilities for the care of all types of illness and should give increased attention to the care of the patient with a long-term illness.

10. The pressing need for additional facilities for the care of the mentally ill and those suffering from chronic diseases in general hospitals makes it necessary that special emphasis be given to this problem in the original state hospital plans and any revision of these plans under Public Law 725. A careful study to develop recommended standards is needed in this area for the guidance of state organizations under this Act.

11. In order to develop and adequately meet good standards of patient care, it is recommended that all hospitals, nursing homes, and other facilities for the care of the sick should meet at least minimum standards through the mechanism of licensure.

12. The control of local facilities should be exercised by the people in each locality on a co-operative or community basis, where possible with an elected board of directors representative of both lay and professional groups.

13. Lay and professional organizations and governmental agencies should join in conducting a health education program and in developing plans for adequate facilities and health service which will include well co-ordinated and highly integrated networks of mobile units, clinics, community hospitals, district hospitals, regional hospitals, and great medical centers.

41. Economics of Hospital Service *

In the following pages I want to discuss four sets of problems which, it seems to me, have the most serious implications for hospital management:

1. Hospital costs and income, especially the growth of hospitalization insurance;

2. Utilization of hospitals, new construction, and capital financing;

3. The progress of federal aid and the need to coordinate resources in order to promote efficiency in operation and improved quality of service;

* From: "Economics of Hospital Service," by Herbert E. Klarman; *Harvard Business Review* 29: 71-89, Sept. 1951 (No. 5). Reprinted (with omissions, including initial paragraphs) by permission of the author and publishers. The author is the associate director of the Hospital Council of Greater New York.

4. Most important of all, the relations of the hospital to people—its owners, its employees, and its customers (the patients).

The Hospital System as a Whole

BEFORE DISCUSSING these problems in detail, especially as they pertain to the general hospital, it may be helpful to sketch certain background information for the hospital system as a whole at mid-century.

In 1950 there were more than 18,500,000 hospital patients in the United States. On an average day, there were 1,250,000 patients in hospital beds; in addition, there were more than 150,000 patients visiting hospital clinics.

According to the American Hospital Association, hospitals employed 1,057,000 full-time persons in 1950. This number is supplemented by private-duty nurses, 65,000 in total, most of whom saw service in hospitals; physicians in active private practice, some 150,000, the large majority of whom rendered some medical care in a hospital; and more than 70,000 volunteer workers.

Finally, and certainly not least, it is estimated that more than 30,000 civic-minded citizens were supervising the operations of the 2,000-odd nonsectarian, nonprofit hospitals by serving as members of the boards of directors—in addition to the many others who were serving in an advisory capacity to the administrators of governmental and church-owned nonprofit hospitals.

The financial stake of the public in the hospital system is equally as impressive as the manpower picture. As taxpayers, charitable donors, and consumers of hospital care, the American public in 1950 spent $3,650 million in hospitals and another $800 million on hospital construction. The value of the public's investment in hospitals in 1950 is estimated at approximately $7,800 million, of which $5,650 million is the value of plant. . . .

As shown by statistics for the year 1950, there are marked differences between the long-term and the short-term hospitals which are significant from the standpoint of management:

The long-term hospitals are characterized broadly by (1) long duration of patient stay, (2) slow turnover of beds, and (3) relatively less active medical care. For these several reasons the long-term hospitals are more likely to (4) be the responsibility of government; (5) accommodate a smaller percentage of the total annual patient load; and (6) cost less to operate.

Correspondingly, the short-term hospitals—chiefly the general hospitals—are marked by (1) short duration of stay, (2) rapid turnover of beds, and (3) relatively active programs of medical care. The short-term hospitals are therefore likely to (4) be to a considerable extent the responsibility of nongovernmental agencies, mostly nonprofit organizations; (5) accommodate the bulk of the annual patient load; and (6) be relatively costly to operate.

Some figures will lend precision to this broad comparison. As much as 94% of all long-term hospital beds are owned by units of government, while only 40% of all short-term beds, including the general hospitals operated by the armed forces and by the Veterans Administration, are owned by units of government. The long-term hospitals contain 58% of the approximately 1,450,000 beds in this country, but because of their higher rate of occupancy they furnish 64% of all patient-days of care. However, the long-term hospitals care for less than 10% of all patients.

The long-term hospitals are staffed by fewer than 35 full-time persons per 100 patients; the short-term hospitals are staffed by 178 full-time persons per 100 patients. Similarly, the average cost per patient-day of care is approximately $3.50 in the long-term hospital and $15.65 in the short-term hospital.

Position of the General Hospital

THE TYPICAL hospital on the American scene is the general hospital. By and large, this is the kind of hospital we shall be discussing. It is—and this is no slight to the importance of the other types of hospital and to the problems they pose—the center of hospital service. Currently, the general hospitals accommodate 93% of all hospitalized patients, and the trend is toward an increase in this percentage. On the one hand, the general hospital is absorbing the special short-term hospital. On the other hand, the general hospital is broadening its mission by adding certain facilities and services for long-term patients. The general hospitals are also the primary centers for education of the various categories of medical personnel and for clinical research. . . .

What will the general hospital be like tomorrow? It will be more general, wider in scope and in range of service. Here are some of the developments worth watching:

(1) More general hospitals are offering a wider range of services, replacing services formerly rendered by special hospitals and adding needed services that were not rendered. Thus, several leading hospitals have added units for rehabilitation and mental illnesses in recent years.

(2) The concept that a hospital is a teaching and training center is continually broadening. Today it applies to all phases of medical education—undergraduate, graduate (internes and residents), and postgraduate. The general hospital also plays a predominant role in the education of nurses and technicians.

The idea that the hospital is interested in the continual education of all physicians practicing medicine in the community has many implications. The hospital is now the haven of the specialists. It must also welcome the family physicians, the general practitioners—those who perform the bulk of medical care in the community and need help and guidance from an organized medical staff such as is available only at a hospital. Staff appointments in hospitals serve this purpose by acquainting physicians with advances in medical knowledge and application.

(3) Much remains to be done to expand diagnostic, rehabilitative, and follow-up services for ambulatory patients. General hospitals in large cities, especially in the metropolitan centers of the eastern seaboard, maintain out-patient departments for the "sick poor." In small cities and in the country the sick poor, if ambulatory, are likely to receive medical care in physicians' offices. There is a marked shortage of

diagnostic services to assist practicing physicians in caring for complicated or obscure cases among ambulatory patients.

Even for paying patients there is no substitute for comprehensive evaluation by the family physician in consultation with specialists who have modern hospital equipment at their disposal. The hospital can perform the task of diagnosis at less expense and more effectively than other agencies because the skilled personnel is already available and the expensive equipment provided by the public to serve in-patients need not be duplicated. It is important, however, that the savings in cost attributable to the higher utilization of the hospital's equipment be passed on to the in-patients.

Administration is the key. As the Hospital Council of Greater New York found in a recent survey, the problem of diagnostic services in a hospital is primarily one of program and organization rather than of personnel and facilities. A number of general hospitals in New York City which have not been doing so could provide diagnostic services to assist the practicing physicians in the community if they made appropriate arrangements for space, flow of records, organization of the medical team, and scheduling of the use of equipment.

(4) The scope of the general hospital is also extending beyond its walls. Several leading metropolitan hospitals operate organized home-care programs. They send into the patient's home whatever medical and ancillary services may be needed. A hospital bed is not the sole alternative to out-patient care; the bed at home may be equally acceptable in many cases.

The immediate cause for the adoption of home care by the municipal hospitals in New York City was the postwar pressure on existing capacity. For the municipal hospitals, home care furnished a means of partially overcoming shortages of bed capacity and personnel, on the one hand, and the constantly rising demand for hospitalization, on the other. Yet the solution was adopted only because it had previously been found beneficial elsewhere on medical and social grounds.

The ratio of per-diem cost of home care to per-diem cost of hospital care is reported at less than one to four. This ratio is probably too low, because the relevant index of cost at the hospital is not the average cost per patient-day but something lower. In any case, there is no denying the fact that by staying at home the patient avoids duplicating the cost of his room and of some portion of nursing care. True, these costs are in part thrown on the family of the patient, but in large measure they are absorbed in the overhead cash expenses of maintaining the family unit and in direct noncash expenditures of effort contributed by relatives and friends.

(5) Several movements are afoot to coordinate administrative, educational, and other services among hospitals. Undoubtedly such programs result in some gains in economy, efficiency, and quality of service rendered to patients. To date they have enjoyed support from philanthropic foundations. It remains to be seen whether the hospitals themselves will agree, or be able, to assume financial responsibility for any substantial program unless it promises to yield direct monetary savings and can be reflected in an immediate reduction in the patient's hospital bill. . . .

A great many of the managerial and administrative problems of hospitals are common to other fields—business, government, the military, and so on. But certain special problems are also present, especially in the voluntary (nonprofit) hospitals:

(1) Legally, the directing force in a voluntary hospital is the board of directors (trustees), who represent the business and social leadership of the community. The board selects and appoints the administrator, whose daily activities it continues to supervise closely. In many instances, administration of the hospital is still in the hands of committees of trustees. It is believed, however, that the trend is toward administration by the hospital director, superintendent, or administrator.

(2) Most of today's hospital administrators have risen from the ranks or have transferred from certain related fields, such as medicine, accounting, or hotel operation. The largest number of administrators, especially in the small hospitals, are nurses. As a field for professional training, with its attendant status, hospital administration is in its infancy. The first university course was offered at the University of Chicago in 1934. Gaining headway after the war, the course is now offered in 12 universities.

(3) An unusual and complicating factor in hospital operation is the special status of the doctors. Although it is considered unsound practice to appoint doctors as trustees, they frequently exercise control over an institution indirectly through the high prestige enjoyed by the profession. While the organized medical staff is properly concerned with professional matters, doctors in their individual capacities may influence nonmedical decisions.

Limitation of the role of the hospital, especially with respect to the care of ambulatory patients, is attributable in part to the unwillingness or inability of most boards of trustees to depart from the wishes of their medical staff members. It has been suggested that desirable as such a relationship is with respect to matters that require professional competence and judgment, it may prove injurious in managing a hospital for the welfare of the community as a whole.

It seems evident that the enhanced role of the hospital calls for stronger, more purposeful management and administration. It would be helpful if the locus of policy-making authority were the board of trustees; the instrument for carrying out decisions, the administrator; and the source of counsel on professional matters, the medical board.

Financial Problems

THE CENTRAL ECONOMIC fact for hospital management is the rise in costs during the past decade. This has raised many serious questions about sources of income. Which groups will pay what share of the increase in the bill and how? Hospitalization insurance, which assumed major importance in recent years, has also brought in its wake new problems. Let us look at the relevant factors in some detail.

First, what is the extent of the rise in hospital costs? Nationwide, it is estimated that expenditures by all hospitals, including military, rose from $1,100 million to $3,650 million between 1940 and 1950—an increase of 230%. Only part of the increase can be attributed to the fact that the public was receiving more hospital care (because there were more hospitals and hospital beds, as well as because more people went to them); actually, the number of patient days of care rose only 20% (from 375 million to 450 million). The larger part of the increase in total expenditures—nine tenths of it—is clearly attributable to the rise in the average cost per patient-day of care.

What caused the increase? Although it is difficult to make an exact apportionment, the following factors probably accounted, among them, for most of the increase:

(1) *Shorter length of patient's stay*—During the last decade the average length of a patient's stay in the general hospital declined from 12.9 to 10.0 days, or 22%. Because most patients require a more or less fixed volume of special services, a shorter stay spreads the cost of these services over a smaller number of patient-days. The increase in per-diem cost attributable to this factor is therefore a price paid for medical progress.

The reduction in length of stay in the general hospital is, in part, the result of the introduction and use of costly new drugs, first the sulfas in the late 1930's and then the antibiotics in the later 1940's. Early ambulation after surgery and childbirth has also contributed to the shorter stay in the hospital.

(2) *Shorter working hours*—Another factor underlying the increase in the cost of hospital care is the improvement in the status of hospital employees. They used to be markedly underprivileged. . . .

In the last 20 to 25 years, hours of work for professional nurses have declined substantially. In 1927 the average hospital nurse worked 58 hours a week. By 1941 the average had declined to 48 hours a week. In part, this decline was the result of the decline in working hours that had taken place throughout industry and governmental agencies. . . .

The latest data are for the year 1949, for which the American Nurses Association reports an average work-week of 44 hours. Since then the 40-hour week has become increasingly common. . . .

Just as institutional nurses gained shorter hours owing to competition from industry and public health agencies, their gains, in turn, served to improve working conditions for other hospital employees. . . .

(3) *Higher wages*—During and after the war, salaries of hospital employees rose. It is estimated that between 1940 and 1949 base salaries of staff nurses in hospitals rose from $105 a month to $205, or 95%. This is a lower rate of increase than that experienced by employees in manufacturing, but it exceeds the rate of increase in most clerical and professional employments. The largest part of the 95% increase served to maintain the purchasing power of the income, since the cost of living increased by 70%. . . .

Since the remuneration of other hospital employees tends to be aligned with that of nurses, it follows that the pay status of all hospital employees was relatively improved.

(4) *Fringe benefits*—Certain fringe benefits have also raised hospital costs. Employees gained vacations with pay during the last decade. The requirement of working a split shift grew less widespread. Approximately 12% of the voluntary (nonprofit) hospitals also offered retirement plans to their employees, who were

excluded from coverage by the Federal Social Security system prior to January 1, 1951. . . .

(5) *Personnel shortage*—There is reason to believe that postwar hospital costs would have been higher than they were—and would have risen faster—had it not been for the shortage of personnel. Both during and immediately after the war it was necessary to shut down certain units in general hospitals. Since then a large number of functioning units are said to be operating with staffs that are too small to provide the best possible quality of care to patients. Whereas during the war shortages in paid staff were offset, at least in part, by volunteers who contributed many hours of labor, after the war contributions of volunteer labor ceased almost abruptly and have remained low until recently. Total costs have been kept down by the inability of hospitals to hire qualified workers to replace the departed volunteers and to compensate for the slowly declining work-week. . . .

In the long run, hospital costs are more likely to rise than to fall. Salaries paid to employees are by no means equal to those paid in comparable occupations elsewhere. Continuing reductions in the work-week will also raise costs. Moreover, if more nurses and ancillary workers eventually become available to the civilian economy, they will be hired to raise hospital staffs to a more acceptable ratio of personnel to beds. There also seems to be a prevailing tendency to convert from ancillary to more costly professional workers whenever financial circumstances permit and the more highly trained type of personnel is available. Finally, a reverse movement in a downward direction is not likely to occur because salaries have been constituting an increasing percentage of total hospital costs; it is well known that it is much more difficult to reduce wages and salaries than other prices.

Fortunately, certain partially offsetting developments may be expected. As employment in hospitals comes to resemble employment in other occupations, efficiency of operations is bound to improve. Many hospitals have found that cheap help is by no means the most inexpensive help; substandard wages may well go with substandard working capacities. The fact remains that the continuing rise in the level of hospital costs and the unlikelihood of a reversal are of crucial significance.

The fact that per-diem hospital costs have more than doubled since 1940 has necessitated greater recourse to more fruitful and flexible sources of income. For most governmental hospitals the choice has been fairly clear: they have made larger requests for tax funds. But for the voluntary (nonprofit) hospitals and the governmental general hospitals in smaller cities (which serve as community hospitals, accommodating both paying and indigent patients), higher costs have necessitated greater recourse to income from patients. Endowments yield a lower rate of return (and the same amount of income buys less than one half as many patient-days as in 1940); and increases in charitable contributions from individuals and Community Chests, while substantial, have not matched increases in costs. Hence, income from endowments and charitable contributions constitutes a smaller percentage of total income than in the past. . . .

Usually depending on their financial capacity to pay for hospital and medical care, hospital patients occupy three grades of accommodation: private, semiprivate, and ward. Differences among the three sets of rates charged to patients are seldom related to differences in the cost of providing services. Ability to pay is the usual criterion. . . .

Regardless of its merits, it may be said that the policy of price discrimination in effect renders the aggregate demand for hospital service inelastic. This means that the total volume of hospital care utilized by the public is relatively unresponsive to an ordinary shift in average charges, upward or downward. The reason is that the patient may select an accommodation he can afford and need not forego the service completely just because his ability to pay falls below the average cost of rendering the service.

What is true in the aggregate also tends to be true in particular instances. While there is no reason in theory why the demand for the services of an individual hospital cannot be elastic, in actuality such demand does tend to be relatively inelastic, whether for lack of neighboring—and competing—hospitals or because the patient tends to go to the hospital at which his physician has staff privileges. It is seldom that a patient is in a position to choose his hospital according to its level of charges.

Hospital bills customarily consist of two elements: charges for room and board (inclusive of routine nursing services) and charges for special services. Included among special services are X-ray examinations, laboratory tests, anesthesia, oxygen, blood, and so on. Charges for room and board are incurred by every patient as long as he remains in the hospital. Charges for special services vary greatly, depending on the volume and types of service required by the particular patient. On the average, charges for special services constitute 27% of a bill from a voluntary general hospital in New York City. In actuality, the range is wide, varying from hospital to hospital and from patient to patient. Most patients incur relatively small bills for special services, while a small minority incur large bills. In the latter instances, the total bills also are large.

It has been urged by some students of hospitals that separate charges for special services impose a hardship on patients with complicated or serious illnesses who require such services in large volume. As they point out, the situation is aggravated by two particular factors that operate to raise the prices of special services: (1) The number of special services is large and many of them are rarely used. Consequently, there is less price competition among hospitals with respect to these items than with respect to room and board. (2) Prices of certain special services are usually kept at about the same levels as those charged by specialists in private practice, in order to avoid the allegation of unethical competition with private practitioners.

During the war and postwar periods, under the impact of rising costs, hospitals tended to raise charges for special services at a greater rate than for room and board. . . .

Currently, hospital rates are being raised once again. This time, however, charges for room and board seem to be rising by a higher percentage than those for special services. This may be in part a corrective adjustment. It may also reflect an effort to blunt the allegation that hospitals earn profits on their special services, thereby depriving the physicians in charge of those departments of their just earnings.

As a solution to the special charges problem, among others, some students of hospital care have urged adoption of an inclusive rate—a total charge for a day's care in the hospital. Such an inclusive rate operates to spread the cost of hospital care more equally among patients; proponents call it similar in its effect to hospitalization insurance. However, the differential cost of providing a unit of special service is small, the major element in cost being overhead. It seems only fair to spread the total cost of the special services among all persons who may avail themselves of the services, rather than to penalize those patients who actually need them.

As a policy applied directly to self-paying patients, the inclusive rate is losing ground. Its current importance stems from its use as a method of reimbursement by third parties . . . who arrange by contract to purchase care on behalf of patients. . . .

Hospitalization Insurance

HOSPITALIZATION insurance is an important development from the viewpoint of both hospital management and the public. It developed in this country only recently, being about two decades old. In one sense it is a depression phenomenon, marking a banding together of people in hard times for mutual aid and support. The hospitals sponsored it because they were simultaneously faced with shrinking incomes and fairly rigid costs. The public rallied to it because apppreciation of hospital care was growing widely, while the rise in hospital costs made paying the bill at the time of illness increasingly burdensome. The program was feasible because the incidence of hospitalization for a large group of persons is predictable with reasonable accuracy.

Two kinds of insurance plans developed side by side: the nonprofit Blue Cross plans, a large majority of which provide service benefits, and the commercial plans providing cash benefits. . . .

Although hospitalization insurance covers about 50% of the population, it meets a much lower percentage of the public's expenditures for general hospital care. The reasons are two: (1) some insurance policies provide restricted benefits; and (2) a subscriber may select more desirable accommodations than those provided in his insurance contract (in which case he pays the differential charge himself). . . .

To the extent that insurance pays for substantially less than 100% of the individual hospital bill, it offers only partial or limited protection against the risk of a stay in the hospital. The purposes of voluntary insurance are two: (1) to induce policyholders to save toward the cost of illness and (2) to divert the savings of those who avoid hospitalized illness to those whose own prepayments are inadequate to finance the cost of their illness. If the prepayment and pooling of resources fail to yield adequate protection, the public may not care to engage in them.

The hospitalization insurance plans are faced with the problem of increasing benefits so that the fraction of the bill paid by the patient does not prove burdensome. The aim should be to minimize the subscriber's payments after premiums.

The insurance plans are also faced with the continuing task of expanding enrollment into certain geographic areas and among certain social and economic groups. At the same time they must exert increasing effort to retain their present policyholders. (Actually, too little is known about cancellations and transfers of enrollment.) . . .

. . . In order to avoid repeated increases in premiums, some plans have made use of the co-insurance feature, under which the patient agrees to pay part of the bill. Some people reject the co-insurance feature in principle, while others question its application in practice. As for the latter group, approval is more likely to be given to co-insurance of the bill for room and board than of the bill for special services.

Another way of enhancing the appeal of hospitalization insurance is to increase the benefit value of a given subscriber dollar by reducing the fraction retained for administration, reserves, taxes, or profits. As a plan matures and grows, the fraction retained for nonbenefit purposes tends to decline. However, cognizance must be taken of differences that exist among the several types of insurance plan. Dr. Dean A. Clark reports that in 1949 the Blue Cross plans had an average retention charge of 15% of the subscriber dollar. In the same year the commercial insurance companies estimated their retention charge at 20% for group insurance and 45% for individual insurance. Comprehensive plans report retention charges of 7% to 20%.

In an effort to provide adequate protection, commercial insurance plans can do no more than economize in their own operations and raise rates to subscribers. But the Blue Cross and other plans that provide service benefits are also confronted with their responsibility to the hospitals to make adequate payment for the services received. As the volume of enrollment in these plans increases, their responsibility toward the hospitals increases at a greater than commensurate rate. They become vitally concerned with the effect of their payments on the efficiency of hospital operations, the range of service, and the quality of service.

In practice, this concern on the part of Blue Cross plans does not result in involvement in internal operation, because of the close ties that exist between the management groups of the two sets of institutions. In the absence of such ties and a community of interests, there could readily ensue a tendency to interfere with the operating independence of hospitals. It is obvious that any insurance scheme which goes beyond cash indemnities and offers service benefits is seriously concerned with the costs of hospital care. Asking at first for uniform accounting and reporting, supplemented by a routine audit, such plans are likely to exert direct pressures for lower costs when their members make up most of the patient load. Since they offer insurance on a voluntary basis, they may press for efficiency in operations all the more ardently; their enrollment (hence their continued prosperity) is vitally linked to maintaining low premiums for subscribers.

Hospital operations may be infringed on also in other ways. To retain the membership already enrolled, the insurance plan must provide services of adequate quality. Accordingly, insurers may exert their influence to promote a wider range of service in some hospitals while discouraging it in others. Methods of reimbursing hospitals which recognize differences in the range of services offered are still in the experimental stage.

From the financial standpoint, the existence of the Blue Cross plan may have aggravated the difficulties of the hospitals during the early postwar years. In the past, the stability of the voluntary hospital system used to be threatened by the drops in income that occurred during depressions. But in 1946 and 1947 the trouble arose because income from contractual sources, such as Blue Cross plans, constantly lagged behind rapidly mounting costs. Hospital rates had lost a degree of flexibility as increasing segments of hospital income became subject to negotiation with third parties. . . .

While most Blue Cross plans provide for hospitalization in semiprivate accommodations, several plans have experimented with a cheaper type of contract providing care on the ward (a room with four or more beds). The sale of more than one type of contract assures a degree of flexibility to the purchaser, but it should not obscure the difference between lower premiums to subscribers and lower costs to the hospital. From the standpoint of the hospital, the cost of ward service is close to the cost of service for the other types of accommodation. Where premiums are low to ward subscribers, they must be raised to the other subscribers if the hospital's income from patients is to meet its revenue needs.

Hospitalization insurance may result in unnecessary utilization of the expensive facilities of the hospitals. That is, with the insurance plans concentrating on protection against the cost of hospitalized illness, there exists an incentive for the subscriber to seek care in the hospital as a bed patient rather than to take treatment on an ambulatory basis which is not covered by insurance. This is undesirable. Unlike many other services, such as education or recreation, hospital care is not good in itself. Hospital care is useful only as a means to better health, and there frequently are superior means to that end. This fact deserves recognition from hospital planners.

In addition to their importance for hospital management and planning, the insurance plans have significant implications for the doctors. The existence of such plans has made access to the hospital on the part of the doctor more important than ever. The increasing number of patients who have become self-paying through the help of hospitalization insurance are also expected to become self-paying from the standpoint of the doctor. . . .

Simultaneously with the expansion of Blue Cross enrollment, and at least in part under its impetus, there has been a marked shift in utilization from ward to semiprivate accommodations. This shift is significant for several reasons.

The character of the voluntary hospital is changing. By catering increasingly to semiprivate patients, the hospital is stressing its nonprofit aspect over its charitable aspect. Since it is customary to set semiprivate rates at or near cost, a hospital breaks even or earns a slight profit on this service.

Traditionally, the voluntary hospital's *raison d'être* has been to render free care, in full or in part, on the ward. With few exceptions, the quoted ward rates, which are maximum charges subject to substantial discount, fall below the cost of care. Nor are most ward patients expected to pay the quoted rates. Charges to patients take into account the individual patient's ability to meet the extraordinary expenses of hospitalized illness. Every hospital has its own way of making this determination, with due consideration for the patient's income, assets, estimated duration of illness, and other commitments.

Traditionally, also, the cost of rendering free care on the ward has been met in part by charging private patients above cost. Before the war, when the level of costs to which hospital rates were geared was less than one half the present level, the profit from three days of private-service care bought two days of care on the ward. Today, at the higher level of costs, it is more difficult to earn the same dollar amount of profit on the private service; and even when earned, the same dollar amount buys less than one half the ward care it used to.

... For various groups associated with the hospitals, in management or otherwise, these changes are of major consequence:

(1) One evidence of the new nonprofit emphasis is the demand widely made by the voluntary hospitals that all governmental agencies and jurisdictions pay the costs of care given to public charges. This demand is steadily gaining acceptance, however grudging, on the part of public welfare authorities.

(2) The shift from ward to semiprivate patients is important also to the medical profession. Financially, it implies an increase in its income. A semiprivate patient always receives a bill from his doctor, while a ward patient frequently receives care from the staff doctors whom he does not pay. It follows that in the future increasing financial significance will be attached to a doctor's connection with a hospital.

Professionally, the doctor will have to consider the implications of this shift for medical education and training. It has been suggested that as the number of ward patients declines, it may be necessary for more hospitals to consider private (paying) patients as clinical material. This raises certain problems concerning the organization of medical education in the hospital which require a great deal of thoughtful study and imaginative adjustment.

(3) Apparently the growth of hospitalization insurance has not only shifted utilization between accommodations but has been accompanied by an increase in per-capita utilization of hospital facilities by the community. ...

It may be anticipated that, everything else being equal, per-capita utilization of hospital facilities among the population as a whole will increase as insurance coverage continues to spread. The experience of the Saskatchewan Hospital Services Plan, for instance, seems to support this expectation.

Determining Need for Hospital Beds

ONE OF THE fundamental questions of policy facing any community is whether its hospital facilities are adequate. How can the needs for hospital beds and facilities be determined?

This kind of question has troubled economists for generations. Indeed, the general problem of determining people's needs for real facilities and services has always been a thorny one, no matter what field of activity is concerned. How do we know what the needs are? How do we measure them? What about the cost involved, in terms of alternative uses of resources? In the case of hospitals, what about the possibility of substituting services on an ambulatory status for in-patient care, given the present state of medical knowledge and application? . . .

The validity of [the purely medical] approach to the problem of defining need for hospital care has been questioned on the ground that economic considerations cannot be disregarded. To allocate resources to hospital care is to forego their employment elsewhere. It cannot be contested that for the economy as a whole, as well as for individuals, there are many and diverse uses for income, some of which are just as compelling as hospital care or other kinds of medical care. Medical personnel and medical facilities cannot be given an absolute priority regardless of other circumstances.

Nor should they be, since hospital care is not by itself a desirable object of consumption. The health of a people is more likely to be served by a balanced pattern of expenditures than by the dominance of any single item or set of items. Among the other objects of expenditure that need to be considered are nutrition, clothing, housing, education, and recreation. (Perhaps there is a question whether even the pursuit of good health can be acknowledged as an absolute goal.)

The pure "medical" approach to the estimation of needs for medical facilities being unacceptable, the need for hospital beds is now most commonly estimated on the basis of past utilization experience. This approach rests, at least implicitly, on certain definite assumptions regarding public policy and on criteria governing the allocation of resources to hospital uses. Some of these assumptions and their implications deserve to be spelled out:

(1) All components of medical and health care are "affected with a public interest," thereby subjecting themselves to some degree of public supervision or control. But in contrast to other components of medical care, such as medical or dental services, hospital care has long been considered a social enterprise. Only 6% of the general-hospital beds in this country, or less than 4% of all hospital beds, are operated by owners for private gain—the balance, including those in all hospitals with considerable reputations, being operated either by nonprofit associations or by units of government. . . .

(2) In light of the tradition of public investment, hospital care seems to be viewed as a service to which every citizen is entitled. A fee is paid by those who can afford it in accordance with their financial capacity. Nobody is to be deprived of the service for lack of a fee or a portion of one.

(3) Another assumption is that health—hence hospital care—is a national problem with a high order of priority. It is not just a local problem, because the shortcomings of one community ultimately descend upon the others. . . . The result is that communities in every region of the country are expected to offer a certain minimum amount of hospital care. . . .

(4) What is the level of this minimum? Given the prevailing state of medical knowledge, application, and practice, the minimum can be ascertained at any given time in communities in which there are no obvious financial or physical obstacles to admission to a hospital. On the financial side, in such communities large segments of the population are covered by insurance with adequate benefits; as for those unable or unwilling to buy insurance, they are freely subsidized by the hospitals or by

public welfare agencies. On the physical side, waiting lists for admission to hospitals are not excessive. (As a matter of fact, waiting lists for elective care, if not too long, are desirable in order to minimize normal seasonal fluctuations in the utilization of hospital services.) Utilization of hospital facilities in such communities may be accepted as the guide to planning hospital facilities in all communities, if allowances are made for local differences.

However, this utilization approach fails to recognize the probable effects of preventive medical services and the potentialities of ambulatory services. The prevailing emphasis on insurance against the cost of hospitalized illness may render difficult the realization of both possibilities.

Perhaps the best material for a study of need for general-care beds would be furnished by the experience of a well-defined group of people who voluntarily buy comprehensive medical services on a modest budget. The experience of such a population would yield information on the need for hospitalization after preventive services and ambulatory care have received maximum opportunity. It would also give us a pure figure for hospital care, unaffected by the extended stay in hospitals that poor patients often undergo because of unsuitable homes.

The need for hospital facilities is expressed in terms of beds for lack of a better unit of measure. Actually, the average hospital devotes to beds only 20% of its space, more or less. A hospital contains much equipment for diagnosis and treatment. The need per bed for ancillary equipment varies with the type of in-patient load served by the individual hospital, as well as with the number of patients served on an ambulatory basis.

In recent years the bed-death ratio method for estimating requirements for general-hospital beds has gained wide acceptance. The method consists of two variants, devised independently by the Commission on Hospital Care and by the Hospital Council of Greater New York. It should, of course, be understood that neither variant is to be employed mechanically.

The bed-death ratio method stems from the high correlation that the Commission on Hospital Care found to exist between hospital utilization and deaths in hospitals. Specifically, the variables in question were occupied beds per capita and deaths in hospitals per capita. Since the average number of occupied beds is the total number of patient-days divided by 365, the relationship can be expressed as the number of days of hospital care per hospital death divided by 365. The value of the numerator was found to be 250 days. The value of the fraction, i. e., the bed-death ratio, is, therefore, 0.7 beds occupied per hospital death ($250 \div 365 = 0.685$). To obtain the number of beds required, this ratio is multiplied by the number of deaths that are expected to take place in general hospitals in a progressive community (death rate $\times$ population $\times$ percentage of total deaths that should occur in general hospitals rather than elsewhere).

The formula of the Hospital Council dispenses with the notion of an optimum percentage of deaths taking place in hospitals. Instead, it applies a utilization factor based on experience to the number of resident deaths of a community yielding a total bed requirement at a given time. In order to project bed needs, this bed requirement is related to the size of the population served during the base year. The resulting ratio of bed requirements to population can be applied to the estimated population at a future date to obtain the number of beds needed at that time. A birth factor is employed to determine the number of obstetrical beds and does not affect the total bed requirement.

It may seem odd that deaths and death rates serve as bases for estimating requirements for hospital care. Information on injuries and illnesses would be more suitable but is not currently available by frequency and type on a comprehensive basis. Those who developed the bed-death ratio and related formulas were aware of the desirability of employing characteristics of the living population to estimate bed requirements. Age, income, cultural level, degree of urbanization, marital status, economic level, and other factors were tried and found inconclusive. On the other hand, the data on deaths did yield clear-cut patterns of relationship with data on the utilization of hospitals.

While the best tested formulas currently available should be used, it is essential at the same time to press the search for methods that reflect more directly the hospital utilization pattern of the living population. Several developments can be cited illustrative of the dynamic changes taking place in hospital care:

(1) For certain medical conditions, such as pneumonia, treatment at home is frequently considered superior to treatment in a hospital. This change, affected by the sulfa and antibiotic drugs, has substantially reduced the number of hospital admissions for this condition.

(2) On the other hand, it is an established fact that the number of admissions to general hospitals is steadily increasing relative to the size of population. Between 1940 and 1950 the population of the United States increased 15% while the number of admissions to general hospitals increased more than 70%. There must be more of certain types of cases being admitted to hospitals than in the past.

The best example is the increased number of admissions for maternity care. Between 1940 and 1950 the number of births in hospitals rose from 1.2 million to 2.8 million or by 133%. . . .

(3) For those admitted to a hospital, the average length of stay has declined. The major cause is, as noted, the combined influence of the sulfa and antibiotic drugs and of early ambulation after an operation or childbirth. But there also are several other factors—for example, probable inclusion of a larger percentage of short-stay cases among the increased number of admissions. There is also reason to believe that the shift toward semiprivate accommodations has played some role because the average duration of patient stay in these accommodations has always been shorter.

The average length of stay may, however, rise at a future date, when the influence of the older segment of the population makes itself more strongly felt. . . .

(4) Another factor to consider is the attitude of hospital administration. For a given size of average patient load, the number of beds required is lower than was formerly believed possible. It is true, of course, that utilization of beds in a hospital is never completely flexible, owing to the differences among patients in sex, age, medical condition, and financial status, and that some allowance must also be made for seasonal fluctuations in occupancy. However, it is now considered good manage-

ment to plan for and maintain the utmost flexibility between beds in ward and beds in semiprivate accommodations, converting from one type of accommodation to the other in response to changing demand.

(5) The average rate of occupancy—the ratio of the average number of patients to beds in a given period—has been significantly higher in recent years than before the war. As a result, the idea of what is a normal rate of occupancy has changed. Not only is 80% occupancy no longer universally regarded as an upper limit; the average rate of occupancy is now seen more clearly as a function of the size of the hospital. Given the size of the average daily census, the number of beds required is approximately that census plus 4 times its square root. . . .

(6) With the provision of preventive, diagnostic, and therapeutic services to increasing numbers of ambulatory patients, requirements for hospital beds may decline. Some authorities stress the desirability of keeping people out of hospitals.

(7) Finally, it is noteworthy that the current phase of hospital planning and construction, promoted by the Hospital Survey and Construction Act of 1946 (known as the Hill-Burton Act), intentionally disregards the facilities operated by the Veterans Administration. . . .

. . . Although these facilities may not impinge materially on over-all planning for general-care beds in this country, they are significant in particular localities. In addition, they are clearly important in the field of long-term hospitalization and must be taken into account by planners. . . .

These several reservations seem to point to a policy of caution in new construction. Construction of additional general-care beds is expensive, not only because of the capital outlay, but also because of the high average cost of operation per patient-day when beds are vacant. The overhead cost per unit of service increases, and the direct expenses of operation also increase. A hospital cannot adjust its staff and other items of expenditure to daily variation in the patient load. If the increase in bed capacity is excessive, therefore, an increase in the supply of beds may not reduce the price of hospital care at all. Rather, the price is likely to rise because most hospital units will remain in operation at lower levels of utilization. A particular drain on hospital beds occurs if there is a lack of flexibility in the use of the several types of hospital accommodation.

Fortunately, hospital construction does take time. As new beds come into operation, it is possible to arrive at a more accurate practical evaluation of the true local bed shortage and to adjust construction programs accordingly.

New Construction and Replacement

IF DIFFICULTIES in estimating the community's true need for hospital facilities make a policy of caution wise with regard to new construction, they also put a premium on initiative in planning and coordination. For example, if the number of hospitals is kept at the minimum necessary and the average size increased, lower costs and improved quality of care are made possible. Again, by limiting the construction of new beds so that the total is in conformity with true requirements, the number of vacant beds will be reduced and operations made more economical. Coordination in the use of facilities is equally important. It is advisable to concentrate the services of certain specialists and costly equipment in selected hospitals where they will be available to the residents of other communities or neighborhoods.

To pave the way for coordination of hospital services, there must be foresight in planning the initial construction. In practice, this means promoting organizations with responsibility for planning all hospital facilities in a community or region and with the necessary prestige to lend authority to their plans.

. . . The principal danger is that the various members of the planning organization, who frequently are affiliated with several different hospitals, may support the special pleas of one another in return for favors. Accordingly, it is especially desirable to select members on the basis of individual ability rather than affiliation with an organization.

With the foregoing considerations in mind, let us analyze some of the problems of building and replacing facilities where the need for them exists. . . .

As originally contemplated, the Hill-Burton Act was aimed at assisting hospital construction in areas of greatest need, particularly rural areas and small towns. Despite the fact that almost 80% of the federal monies have gone to communities of 5,000 and over to assist in the construction or expansion of larger hospitals, the facts show that the purpose of the act has been adhered to. An overwhelming percentage of all new general hospitals built under the stimulus of the Hill-Burton Act are small—85% under 100 beds, 61% under 50 beds, and 23% even under 25 beds.

But is this a desirable development? Consider these facts:

(1) Appearances notwithstanding, small hospitals are costly to operate. Published statistics usually show that cost per patient-day increases with the size of a hospital. But this is due to the fact that larger hospitals offer a larger variety of services, which are costly. The relative inefficiency of the small hospital is thus obscured.

(2) The small hospital suffers from lack of flexibility. Its average number of vacant beds is high, and the rate of occupancy is low. In a 25-bed hospital the expected occupancy rate for the year is as low as 45%. In addition, the small hospital incurs a fixed overhead expense, which is spread over a small volume of service. Moreover, in an attempt to reduce costs, less efficient—hence more costly—administrative personnel is hired.

(3) Inability to staff more than the basic services may lead to poor quality of care. The temptation exists to retain the patient rather than refer him elsewhere, to perform services for him beyond the skill of the medical staff. Only close affiliation with larger, more specialized institutions will reduce this temptation.

What about the fact that in the first three years of the program construction did not always take place in the rural area with the highest priorities? It took place, rather, where community interest was greatest, where local leadership succeeded in activating public sentiment in favor of a general hospital. This situation is not necessarily deplorable, since many other areas which had high priorities indicative of serious need for new construction actually enjoyed access to suitable hospital facilities in neighboring communities. Unavoidably, the planning in many states has been done on the basis of political units, such as counties, rather than on the basis of hospital service areas. Some of the communities designated as in need of hospitals would have little use for them and might be duplicating existing hospital plants if they undertook to build.

On the other hand, it cannot be assumed that every priority area which fails to build a hospital has no need for one. More frequently, the reason in such cases is lack of capital for the initial undertaking coupled with a doubt as to the area's ability to finance the cost of operations. Not to be overlooked also is the difficulty of staffing the new hospitals in certain areas; planning for the building of facilities has been independent of any planning for the training and distribution of personnel.

Note that only 55% of the projects for general hospitals involve new hospitals. The other projects are additions to or replacements of existing plants which are regarded as unsuitable for long-term needs. . . .

The problem of financing replacement is more serious in hospitals than in business because, at least until recently, hospitals did not include an allowance for depreciation in their costs and charges. This has been of little consequence for government hospitals, which are able to draw on the revenue-raising and borrowing powers of the sponsoring jurisdiction. But voluntary hospitals have had to resort to public appeals for capital contributions, the results of which are not always certain. . . .

To some extent the problem is eased if the location of hospital beds is made to correspond more closely to the availability of capital funds. . . . With high-speed communications and transportation, it cannot be validly urged that every neighborhood or community must be self-sufficient in hospital facilities of every type. . . .

Just what arrangements can be made to provide for future obsolescence? In particular, what about depreciation charges? Just because depreciation accounting is a standard practice in business, it need not be avoided by nonprofit institutions, such as hospitals. The wear and tear of plant and equipment is as much a cost of operating a hospital as are outlays for salaries, food, and supplies. . . .

Voluntary hospitals have tended to shy away from the idea that they must be businesslike in their operations. That may sound consistent with the ideal of service to the public. A hospital is not devoted to earning income but to serving the health needs of the community. Yet a hospital can remain in operation and render service only so long as it maintains a reasonably dependable and adequate flow of income.

In recent years there has been a tendency among hospitals to introduce an allowance for depreciation into their costs. But the corresponding increase in hospital rates has been questioned on the ground that, unless the depreciation is funded, hospitals would dissipate the money on current expenditures, and inevitably resort to public appeals when the need for capital funds arose. In other words, the belief is that depreciation charging by a hospital is dishonest unless accompanied by depreciation funding. As for the business practice of charging depreciation without necessarily funding it, the answer is that a business is bound to operate efficiently (if it is to continue) and cannot appeal to the public for funds when it fails to do so. Whatever the merits of these contentions, as a practical matter they must be reckoned with.

Funding, which is within the discretion of the board of directors or trustees, thus becomes of great importance with regard to policies for financing the acquisition of new plant and equipment. Of course, even with depreciation, a public appeal may be necessary to make up for past years when charges were not made or for increases in the price level. But charging for depreciation should be of considerable help.

It goes without saying that the position of the general hospital is grounded in the facts of medical knowledge and practice. Yet the hospital is also an economic institution with an important social mission in the community. Certainly its effectiveness in the field of health and medical care depends to a large degree on its financial strength as well as on its ability to understand and cope with the needs of the community served.

In both of these phases the role of management is paramount. . . .

42. STANDARDS OF CARE *

VARIOUS PROFESSIONAL associations have adopted "minimum standards" upon which they evaluate hospitals for registration or approval. These standards furnish those responsible for the provision of hospital care with measuring rods by means which they can appraise their institution's facilities and certain phases of its organization. In a few states similar requirements are prescribed by the laws regulating the establishment and operation of hospitals.

In general, these standards pertain to the physical structure and availability of certain services, the medical staff organization, and the nursing school organization, faculty, and curriculum. They deal primarily with tangible factors which readily permit an evaluation or measurement.

Registration by the American Medical Association

THE AMERICAN MEDICAL Association through its Council on Medical Education and Hospitals has published *Essentials of a Registered Hospital* with which hospitals must comply in order to be included in the *Register*. These essentials relate to governing board, chief executive officer, physical plant and equipment, medical staff and its organization, pathology and laboratory diagnosis, autopsies, radiology, anesthesia, nursing service, dietetics, pharmacy, medical records, and medical ethics.

These essentials enunciate sound principles basic to the conduct of hospital service of proper quality, rather than detailed specifications.

* Reprinted by permission of the publishers and the Commonwealth Fund from The Commission on Hospital Care, *Hospital Care in the United States;* Cambridge, Mass.: Harvard University Press, 1947. (The excerpt reprinted, with omissions including initial paragraph, is from Chap. IX, "Maintenance of Standards of Service," pp. 129-35).

Standards for Intern Training

THE COUNCIL HAS ALSO published *Essentials for an Approved Internship*. These requirements concern only those hospitals, admitting at least 2,500 patients or more per year and having a daily average of at least 85 patients, which desire to undertake and receive approval for the training of interns. Such hospitals must comply with the requirements for registration and must meet additional specifications as to medical staff, clinical records, laboratories, radiology, medical library, organization for the content of teaching programs, and conduct of intern service.

Essentials for Residencies and Fellowships

THE COUNCIL, in cooperation with the various American Boards representing the medical specialties, has also published *Essentials of Approval for Residencies and Fellowships*. Approved residencies and fellowships are now offered in thirty branches of medicine.

Previous admission to the *Register* is prerequisite for the hospital that seeks approval for this type of advanced training. These standards exceed those of either [of the] categories previously discussed. They lay greater emphasis upon the organization and qualifications of the medical staff, particularly in the respective special fields. They also place greater stress on the departments of radiology, pathology, medical library, and medical records, on the number of necropsies, and on the educational programs in the specialty.

Admission of a hospital to the *Register* is usually achieved through correspondence and the submission of detailed data concerning the institution. Approval for internship or resident training is granted only after inspection and interview with the responsible authorities and members of the staff in the respective specialty. While the number of hospitals eligible for approval for internships and for residencies is limited, the quality of professional service implied by these "Essentials" is that to which all hospitals should aspire.

Standards for Technician Training

THE COUNCIL has also published requirements governing schools for the training of medical record librarians and various types of technicans. Hospitals which conduct such training courses are required to comply with the standards before approval of such courses is granted.

Hospital Standardization by the American College of Surgeons

THE AMERICAN COLLEGE of Surgeons has conducted a program of hospital standardization since 1918. Through this program of inspection and approval, the College has contributed greatly to the improvement of the quality of service in American hospitals.

The College publishes a *Manual of Hospital Standardization,* which contains a detailed explanation of the principles upon which these standards are based. Its program pertains to all hospitals with a capacity of 25 or more beds. A continuing inspection is carried on and a list of approved hospitals is issued annually. In recent years the College has extended its minimum standards to include other adjunct services, such as out-patient departments, cancer clinics, physical therapy departments, as well as pharmacies, nursing, dietary, social service departments, and medical libraries.

These programs are all helpful to hospital authorities in developing a high quality of hospital care. It is recommended that: (1) Hospitals of all types, regardless of size, should comply with the essentials of a registered hospital promulgated by the American Medical Association. (2) Hospitals which offer educational programs for interns and residents and those which conduct schools for medical record librarians or for technicians should comply with the requirements for approval prescribed by the American Medical Association. (3) Hospitals of all types, regardless of size, should comply with the standardization program of the American College of Surgeons.*

Nursing Education

THE APPROVAL PROGRAMS of the National League of Nursing Education, the National Organization of Public Health Nursing, and the Association of Collegiate Schools of Nursing evaluate a school of nursing upon the basis of administration, financial support, number and qualifications of faculty, terms of admission and graduation, curriculum, records, library, and classroom and clinical facilities.

These requirements exceed those prescribed by many of the state examining boards for nurses. Material improvement in nursing education would ensue if all hospitals which conduct schools of nursing would conform to these standards. Also, the quality of hospital care generally would be enhanced. It is recommended that: Hospitals which conduct schools of nursing should comply with the approval programs of the three national professional nurses' associations.†

Appraisal of Quality of Care

As WAS PREVIOUSLY indicated, these several programs of standardization provide for the measurement of certain basic tangible factors essential to good hospital care. They are important as guides to hospital authorities, but they do not provide an adequate or comprehensive basis upon which to evaluate the quality of hospital care.

Various efforts have been made to develop an appraisal form or schedule pro-

---

* These three recommendations are numbered 123-125 in original text.
† Recommendation number 126 in original text.

viding a basis upon which the work of an institution might be evaluated and upon which the work in one hospital might be compared with that in another. The American College of Surgeons is engaged upon another such endeavor and is testing a plan of this nature at the present time. Thus far, however, none of these efforts has been successful. . . .

The professional work in an institution can best be appraised by means of a careful review and analysis made by a competent committee of the medical staff. Such an audit involves painstaking study, keen discretion, and judgment. The diversities of conditions, symptoms, and course of illness among patients afflicted with the same type of disease are great and do not readily permit of comparisons. Any worthwhile appraisal, therefore, requires an intensive study of the clinical records of individual patients. For such purpose records must be accurate and complete.

The medical audit is the best method thus far devised for the appraisal of the professional work in a hospital and for the maintenance of a high quality of service. This procedure, however, is predicated upon the medical staff's conception of acceptable standards and upon its willingness to deal frankly and without bias with the findings of the audit. Though it does not lend itself to comparison with the work of other institutions, it has much merit. This method of audit also could be used advantageously in nursing and other hospital services. It is recommended that: The medical staff in every hospital should regularly conduct an audit of the professional work. The findings of such audit should be published to all staff members and should be transmitted to the governing authorities of the hospital in terms which are understandable to the layman.*

Assurance of Good Professional Care

A MEDICAL STAFF organization is of fundamental importance. To the staff should be entrusted the full responsibility for the medical and surgical professional care of patients. There should be a chief in charge of each of the special departments—medicine, surgery, obstetrics, and others. Appointments to the staff should be made by the governing board of the hospital only after consultation with the staff. There should be regular and frequent meetings of the staff, attendance at which should be required for the purpose of discussing all matters which relate to the professional care. At these meetings special emphasis should be placed upon the results of the professional work based upon a detailed report of the causes of death, a demonstration and discussion of surgical specimens, reports of accidental infections, and any other matters related to the quality of the medical care.

In a general hospital the quality of the professional work is approximately proportional to the percentage of autopsies. Both the medical staff and the administrator should encourage to the utmost efforts to obtain a high percentage of postmortem examinations. Any member of the staff who discourages autopsies on his patients should be regarded with suspicion.

* Recommendation number 127 in original text.

Every hospital should have on its staff a competent and fearless pathologist who will not only assist in completing the diagnosis, but will also unhesitatingly call the attention of the staff, in so far as possible, to errors in diagnosis and treatment as revealed by the examination of autopsy and surgical pathological material. The hospitals should have a full-time pathologist; the small ones, through cooperation with other near-by hospitals, can generally arrange for the part-time service of one.

The presence of a staff of interns, and, if possible, residents is one of the best assurances of a high grade of professional service. The intern should be regarded as a graduate student who has come to the hospital from the medical school for further instruction. If the staff provides good instruction, the hospital will attract good interns. Conversely, these young men are quick to detect sloppy, obsolete, and questionable practices. They should, therefore, be encouraged to have a constructively critical attitude. Although expected to render some service as a part of their education and as compensation for the opportunities which the hospital offers them, they should not be exploited as servants.

The maintenance of good and permanent patients' records, including the records of the pathologist, is another important factor in the assurance of good professional service. Moreover, such records are often the basis of important clinical research.

A high degree of proficiency of the medical staff can be assured if the members are alert to changing methods of practice and to the values of continuous study and education. Certification by the respective specialty boards and membership in the American College of Surgeons and the American College of Physicians are measures of skill and achievement. Many hospitals are now requiring that the senior members of their staffs must demonstrate special competence in their respective fields of medical practice. It appears that such regulation is in the interest of assuring a high grade of professional care.

In view of the handicaps under which small hospitals operate, it is urged that they develop affiliations with larger hospitals through which consultation and other professional and administrative service may be made available to the small institution and a better quality of hospital care may be developed.

Personalized Service

BUILDINGS, equipment, organization, administration, competent personnel, and a qualified medical and nursing staff are all essential factors in the provision of good hospital care. The primary purpose of the institution is to restore the patient's health as thoroughly and rapidly as possible. However, professional service may be coldly efficient and unsympathetic. Though the patient's needs may be adequately served as far as diagnosis and therapy are concerned, the attention given to his personal needs and to his human relationships may leave much to be desired. It is incumbent upon the governing authorities, administrator, and personnel in all categories (professional, technical, and general service) to see to it that a kindly, humanitarian spirit pervades the entire atmosphere of the institution. The most proficient professional service with be unsatisfactory to the patient in an environment which is cold and unresponsive to his personal needs and desires. It is recommended that: Hospital authorities and administrators should give keen attention to the development and maintenance of those human relationships that will inspire all engaged in the service of the institution to put forth their best efforts in the interest of the patient and the general public.*

C. *The Physician in the Hospital*

43. WHAT IS A HOSPITAL STAFF? †

THE RELATIONSHIP between the members of the medical staff and the administration of the hospital can best be developed when it is based on the relationship of these groups to the patient in whose interest the hospital has its reason for existence. To the casual student of hospital organization this remark may seem hackneyed and may perhaps indicate too much solicitude, but to those who know or would examine deeply into the functioning of the modern hospital, the fate of the patient is of sufficient concern to call for a policy of eternal vigilance during the organization of hospital relationships and their subsequent adjustment. I shall begin, therefore, by stating that the governing body (variously referred to as the board of trustees, the most descriptive name of all, of directors, of managers, or of guardians), the administrator, and the medical staff, and all others in the hospital whose relationships must be considered in the scheme of organization, have a primary obligation to the patient which must be dominant in all their activities and must serve as the touchstone for the entire plan of hospital organization. The relative position of these groups to each other will be clear if we plan it according to the relation of each of them to the patient.

Members of the governing board, who are the prime movers of the enterprise, are responsible for the creation and maintenance of the hospital. They are among the representatives of the health and medical interests of the community, and their trusteeship makes them responsible to the community for the humane conduct of the institution. . . . Under these circumstances the trustee must be considered primarily as a social worker whose interests are specialized in behalf of the sick. The administrator, too, whether he is a physician or a layman, is a social worker with business functions rather than a business manager with incidental social functions. The proper point of view is important and should be established at the outset.

* Recommendation number 128 in original text.

† From: "Staff Relationships that Focus Service on the Patient," by E. M. Bluestone, M.D.; *The Modern Hospital* 36: 83-86, June 1931. Reprinted (with omissions) by permission of the author and publishers. The author is a consultant for Montefiore Hospital, Bronx, New York.

The medical staff, with its complement of specialists and consultants for diagnosis and therapy, has a specialized task which also carries a cooperative responsibility, for there is social service to be rendered besides purely medical service. In fact medical service, historically viewed, is a specialized form of social service. Under the medical staff and subject to its instructions are such divisions as the house staff and the nursing staff, which need not be considered separately for the purposes of organization. The patient is the individual on whom all service is focused. He is the social entity without whom our three groups would have no reason for existence.

... How shall we plan for the individual patient in his relation to these groups? Shall we, for example, make the rule to fit the needs of the patient, considering him as an individual, or make the patient conform to the rule, considering the interests of the group only? In the hospital we do not often deal with situations that fit into a universal pattern. Hospital relationships with the patient must in fact be adjusted to situations that are for the greatest part unprecedented. To state questions like these is to answer them, if the fundamental purpose of the hospital is borne in mind. Decisions rest fortunately with the governing board, for in this body there are no axes to grind and here singleness of purpose has its greatest opportunity. . . .

While the three groups which we are considering—the governing board, the administrator, and the medical staff—in their relation to the patient should be guided only by the welfare of the sick, in actual practice there are exigencies that are permitted to modify and color this attitude. One example . . . is the relation of the individual to the group in hospital practice. Another is the financial relationship between the patient and the hospital and between the patient and the physician. Where is the happy relationship that will bring the greatest good to the greatest number? A proper spirit in the hospital means a contented patient in so far as this can be effected in those who are physically ill. One of the most satisfying visits that I have ever made to a hospital occurred several years ago when I visited the British Ophthalmic Hospital, Jerusalem, an institution that made no charge for service to patients either in the wards or in the out-patient department. In other words, it did not fine the patient for seeking relief as we do in more civilized parts of the world, where the social machinery for effecting this purpose is somewhat elaborate. Happy is the hospital organization where the financial factor has been reduced to a minimum.

The governing body has for one of its most important functions the selection of an adequate and competent staff. This happens to be one of the moral obligations of the hospital that is also a legal obligation, for the hospital, as a charitable institution, is open to legal suit for malpractice in those cases where proper care has not been exercised in the selection of the staff. As will be pointed out later, the governing body, in the matter of selection, would do well to seek counsel from its medical board as well as from the medical profession at large beyond the walls of the hospital. Whether the hospital should be open to the medical public to assume responsibility for the care of patients or closed except to a selected and highly qualified few is a question for the governing body to decide. But whatever the decision, it must be based on the interests of the patient, which must be supreme, rather than on the personnal interests of those selected to serve him. So it is with the staff after appointment. The legal obligation has now disappeared but the moral obligation persists. The duty of the board does not cease with the process of selection, for the members of the staff should be required by their conduct to prove their right to retain favored positions. This means a positive attitude toward the patient in accordance with the fundamental purposes of the hospital. The medical staff inside a hospital, at least, should maintain the highest type of ethical as well as scientific medical practice and thus light the way. The point of this remark will be obvious in a medical world that lacks an adjusted social program and has become somewhat demoralized by commercial influences and pseudoscientific competition.

Following the appointment of an adequate and competent staff the board is called upon to provide facilities and equipment, another problem in philanthropy. Physicians serving in hospitals are often entitled to much more than they receive for their work. But this presumably is a matter for negotiation, in which again the interests of the patient should prevail.

In the larger question of facilities another problem arises, namely, the current practice of limiting the stay of the patient in the wards or out-patient department according to the duration of his illness. The chronic, the so-called incurable, and the aged are forgotten. In planning for the adequate care of the sick, how many members of the medical staff stop to consider that the right to prescribe involves the obligation to follow up, that the scientific and humane care of the patient (synonymous terms which I am using only to emphasize my meaning) requires that he be kept under observation till the natural history of his illness has run its course? Here is a problem in hospital relationships that is a standing challenge to the student of hospital organization.

In its relation to the governing body the medical staff is responsible for related medical service to the patient (special diagnosis and therapy) as well as for direct medical service. In addition it has a cooperative function that has special meaning in an institution for the sick which draws on a variety of services for its existence. Furthermore, the fundamental functions of the hospital in the realm of (a) preventive medicine, (b) curative medicine, (c) medical education, and (d) medical research are largely in the hands of the medical staff acting with the support of the board. How to strike a proper balance in these four important functions is a problem in hospital organization that can be solved in individual instances by these two groups acting in harmony in accordance with the principles that we have described. The popular and in many respects the best method of conducting such negotiations is through a conference committee composed of the executive officers of the governing board on the one hand, and the executive officers of the medical board on the other.

One can enumerate many instances that require fine adjustment in the relationship between the medical staff and the governing board, but the interest of the patient as a criterion is the best guide in organization. If the governing board has determined its fundamental policy in this respect, the problem of organization is thereafter simplified. One must remember that the social and medical exploitation of the ward (charity) patient in our age is made easy because of his poverty and the weakness of his protest and that this matter requires the constant vigilance of those who plan for his care. He is too often considered public property, whereas adequate medical service is his right and privilege as a self-respecting member of the community.

In its relations with the medical staff the board must also consider its relations to physicians outside the hospital, the general practitioner in his organized and unorganized form. No hospital can successfully isolate itself from the medical world without, any more than it can successfully isolate itself from the social world, for the hospital must have the good will of the community, including the medical community, to ensure its existence. Whatever the internal relationships of the hospital, the practitioner has a definite place in the clinical biography of any patient who is subsequently transferred to the medical staff of the hospital. The more fortunate member of the hospital staff cannot afford to overlook the general practitioner who saw the patient during the earlier stages of his illness. It has been pointed out above, in a general way, that the hospital has an educational obligation. This should include the general practitioner, if we would prevent the establishment of a vicious circle in which the practitioner, disregarded, is deprived of the stimulus to a higher medical education and as a result becomes more and more out of favor with his more fortunate colleagues within the hospital.

Another group that must be seriously considered in the plan of organization, though it is a part of the medical staff as indicated above, is the resident staff, who should be ready at all times to serve the best interests of the patient and toward whom there is an obligation to teach good social and medical habits in the treatment of the sick. From the point of view of relationships, the members of the resident staff should be fully responsible to their seniors for all work that is of medical nature and to the office of the director for matters of an administrative nature. Personal interest on the part of the board in the future of the younger generation of doctors has its rewards. . . .

In its relation to the medical staff the board must deal with individuals and groups in their organized and unorganized form. In the scheme of organization this problem is readily solved by considering the medical board, presumably constituted of the senior members of the attending staff, as the advisory body to the governing board in all matters medical, and the governing board is wise that is willing to accept such advice in its conduct of the medical affairs of the hospital. In doubtful cases recourse may naturally be had to public medical opinion outside the hospital, but this should not be sought without the best of reasons. A typical instance would be one in which the interests of the patient and the personal interests of the staff seem to conflict. The medical staff should be made to feel that it is engaged in a cooperative enterprise and is partner to all hospital activities. I do not doubt that the most fruitful sources of difficulty will be found in the variance that unfortunately exists between the professional and the economic interests of the physician. This must be taken into account in considering relationships under the scheme of medical organization.

The question as to whether the medical staff is to serve on a full-time (paid) or part-time (voluntary) basis is a communal problem which extends beyond the boundaries of the individual hospital but which may be individually adjusted by the governing board, depending on the need and the available funds. In its final analysis the decision depends on the economic environment in which the hospital is cast. Public health is indeed purchasable within reasonable limits. But regardless of the reward that the hospital may be able to give the physician financially, in practical opportunity, in prestige, or in all of these, the relationships remain unchanged and the individual members of the medical staff are looked upon as men of science on whom the hospital must depend for its most important function of all, the humane care of the patient.

Up to this point I have tried to give a few random thoughts on the subject of the relationship between the governing board and the medical staff on the one hand and the patient on the other. An important position in the scheme of hospital organization and in a practical sense the key position in the study of relationships is the office of the director (administrator, superintendent, secretary, or medical director). The director of the hospital, besides being the administrator, is the coordinator of all hospital activities, varied as they are. He is the liaison officer between the governing board on the one hand and the staff and the patients on the other, in all matters that affect the conduct of the hospital. He interprets the staff and the patients to the trustees at the meetings of the board if he attends them, or, if he does not attend them, to the executive officers and the trustees individually. At the meetings of the medical board he has the opportunity of interpreting the board to the medical staff; if he does not attend these meetings, he interprets the board and its wishes to the individual members of the staff.

If these tasks are performed honestly and in the interests of the patient primarily, the administrator reaches the point of maximum usefulness. Since the social point of view must prevail, business management is secondary, though important, and the wise administrator knows how to assemble a group of expert heads of administrative departments to advise him in the same manner that he is advised by physicians in medical matters. The conception of the director's office as a clearing house for all hospital activity provides practical interrelationships, when the administrator is competent to act and is willing to be impartial in his dealings. Centralization of this kind in the modern hospital is essential and should be provided for in the scheme of organization, it for no other reason than to prevent confusion and duplication of effort. If the administrator is himself a physician, so much the better, but the important factor is not so much his clinical knowledge as his social spirit and understanding.

There is reason for disappointment over the failure of our medical schools to place more emphasis on social medicine and on the opportunities for social work and medical organization that hospital administration offers. Training for such work is preferably by the apprenticeship method with proper academic support. The study of medical organization and administration, which are such an important part of medical practice, should not be left to chance factors, and a greater effort should be made by organizations like the American College of Surgeons, with its hospital standardization conference, to train and to hold a competent group of administrators who will round out the proper relationship between the trustees, the staff, and the patient.

44. "CLOSED" VERSUS "OPEN" STAFFS *

HOSPITALS THAT ARE not under the control of medical schools may think that in the matter of medical education theirs is only a subordinate and unimportant part. But in fact, their position is not only important, it is supremely important; for, while the medical school may sell the student his admission ticket to the play, seats are not ordinarily reserved, and it remains for the hospital eventually to usher the medical graduate to his place.

With respect to clinical organization, it is more helpful to classify hospitals as staff and open hospitals than to consider them as hospitals connected or not connected with medical schools, for whether there is such a connection or not, adoption by the hospital of an aristocratic or exclusive form of medical organization implies an obligation to teach and to aid in the advancement of medical science. To the many learners in the noncollege staff hospital, one more group is added in the college hospital, namely, the undergraduate student group; this addition, however, does not fundamentally change the character of the staff hospital or vitally affect its organization. The open hospital, on the other hand, has a distinctly different purpose and significance, and it may well be argued that in this country there is need for both open hospitals and staff hospitals.

While the open hospital can perform a very useful service, the promotion of medical science is essentially a function of the staff hospital. And the most efficient form of staff organization is that in which several clinical departments operate for an unbroken period of years under the leadership of able men, conscientiously chosen by an impartial board.

The hospital in which men holding equal rank as heads of clinical departments rotate in office every three, four, or six months offers no warm hospitality to the scientific spirit. Every staff hospital should make constant contributions to medical science and should be organized with this end in view. The frequent interruption of clinical leadership and authority is apt to involve a damaging interruption of the progressive study of disease. We have witnessed the actual inauguration of valuable investigations and have seen such investigations continue uninterruptedly under the same leadership for three, five, or even ten years. If the improvement of medical science be one of the acknowledged objectives of a staff hospital, there is much to be said against and very little in favor of an interrupted or rotating service.

* From: *On Hospitals,* by S. S. Goldwater, M.D.; New York: Macmillan (copyright 1947). Reprinted with the permission of The Macmillan Company. (The excerpt reprinted, with omissions, is from Part 2, Chap. V, "Hospital Privileges for Doctors," pp. 123-27). The author was the commissioner of the New York City Department of Hospitals from 1934 to 1940; at the time of his death in 1942, he was president of Associated Hospital Service of New York.

It is true that uninterrupted service, too long continued, has its disadvantages, and that the hospital in which so-called continuous service prevails should do everything possible to guard against the danger of continuing in office the head of a department who has ceased really to guide and inspire his subordinates. While continuous service is desirable, the possibility of interrupting it for adequate reasons should be safeguarded. This can be done by the automatic retirement of heads of service by means of a prescribed age limit; by limiting the official term of the head of any service (a five year limit, which some have suggested, is too short; a term of not less than ten and not more than twenty years is preferable); and by making all staff appointments for two or three years, subject, however, to renewal up to the limits of the maximum term referred to above, or up to the pre-established age limit.

Nevertheless, staff or closed hospitals should from time to time reconsider the basic principles of their organization. Wherever hospitals set up a privileged class of practitioners, a natural resentment is aroused, which will not down. Even where, for the moment, no flaming antagonism appears on the surface, opposition smolders beneath, and thus every closed hospital may eventually be compelled, publicly and conclusively, to justify or to abandon its exclusiveness. For a number of years, the perilous state of the family physician, and especially of the country practitioner, as well as the strong and ever stronger disinclination of medical graduates to lead lives of professional isolation, has been conspicuously reflected in every general discussion of medical education.

It is to the credit of the open hospital that it brings into touch with an organized medical institution many physicians who, under a more restricted or exclusive hospital system, would be deprived of those helpful and stimulating medical contacts, without which they are in danger of deteriorating in medical knowledge and proficiency from the moment they graduate from medical school. Another point in favor of the open hospital is that it enables the paying patient to choose his physician or surgeon with the utmost freedom. Granting that an open hospital is of necessity a relatively loose organization, in which uniformity of procedure is difficult to attain, and from which the most systematic and illuminating study of groups of cases by organized teams of clinicians and laboratory men is ordinarily excluded, the open hospital nevertheless affords far better opportunities for fruitful clinical study than can be found in the lonesome and dreary circumstances of private practice.

Proceeding from the basic idea that a physician of ordinary talents cannot mentally thrive without a hospital connection, or, at least, that he is in grave danger of contracting loose habits of thought and of becoming careless and superficial in his clinical methods, it follows that it is the duty of physicians to seek hospital connections, and that it is equally the duty of those who control hospitals to facilitate such connections. It is unreasonable for a community, depending for its own safety and for the maintenance of its health on a high grade of medical practice, to permit a double standard of practice to exist, due to the fact that one group of physicians enjoys hospital connection and is thus aided by an uninterrupted process of progressive education, while the other is deprived of that opportunity. If anything can be done to liberalize the closed hospital without destroying its efficiency as a teaching and research center, it should be done; if any suggestion can be offered that will tend to improve the character of the service in open hospitals, it should be adopted; but these steps, however important in themselves, are of far less importance than the following, namely, that the need of a hospital connection for every practicing physician should be the controlling factor in all community hospital organization.

Let us consider, first, counties or localities that are entirely without hospitals. At first blush, it may seem idle to talk about providing hospital connections for all the physicians in such districts, since without hospitals there can be no hospital connections; but it is precisely in these localities that the opportunity exists for attaining the desired end with the least difficulty. These counties are without hospitals today, but at any moment a hospital project may be launched in any one of them; indeed, next year, or the year after, some of them are certain to appear on the hospital map in a new color. Let each new hospital that begins with a clean slate be organized for the benefit of the entire medical profession of the locality. New hospitals can do this with comparative ease, for no entrenched privileges block the way. . . .

Let us consider, next, a community in which one hospital has already been established on rigid staff lines, and which proposed to establish another. In the absence of any guiding principle, the second hospital is likely to copy the methods and organization of the first. If, however, the doctrine of universal hospital association is accepted as valid, the second hospital will be organized as an open hospital, and will offer a common meeting ground for the entire local medical fraternity. Its aim will be not to compete with the pre-existing staff hospital on the latter's ground, but to round out the community's medical organization and in its own way contribute to the spread of sound clinical practice. Even in an open hospital it is possible to set up certain minimum standards and to see that clinical practice is supervised by physicians who know what that practice should be.

I have visited communities where a small group of physicians, perhaps the only group existing when the community was young, had managed to get possession of a hospital plant and set up a staff organization. In time, the community grew and other physicians of later vintage came into the community—men just as well qualified as was the original group; but the latter fought against new staff appointments. They were enjoying an advantageous monopoly, both from the standpoint of gaining exclusive professional knowledge and from the pecuniary standpoint.

What bearing, if any, has the principle under discussion on the closed hospital? To me it suggests that without sacrificing those elements of strength which are characteristic of the well-organized staff hospital, the closed hospital should utilize every possible means for widening its professional influence. Staff positions should be created for as many clinical and laboratory assistants as the service can healthfully absorb—and the number of men that can be comfortably tucked under the blanket of a hospital staff organization is truly astonishing. The appointment of temporary volunteers who are capable of carrying on intensive studies beyond the capacity or the available time of the regular staff should be encouraged. The practitioners of the neighborhood should be invited to attend clinical and pathological conferences. Formal postgraduate teaching should be organized—under university auspices, if possible; independently of any medical school, if necessary. In some cases, facilities for the treatment of private patients may, without detriment to the hospital, be placed at the disposal of an associate or 'courtesy' staff. Diagnostic aid should be extended to unattached practitioners. Encouragement and practical assistance should be given to open hospitals that are sincerely striving to improve the quality of their work. The educational efforts of the county medical society should be seconded. A reasonable rotation in office should be ensured by the adoption of rules prescribing age and service limits. The hospital should lend a willing ear at all times to unattached physicians who believe themselves the victims of an unduly narrow hospital policy, and who offer suggestions for extending the privileges of the hospital to a larger group.

These are not fanciful or farfetched suggestions; they are all questions of policy and procedure which come up from time to time in actual hospital administration. I have indicated the manner and the spirit in which I believe such questions should be handled; and I hold that they cannot be treated otherwise by any hospital that is sincerely seeking to stretch its educational service to the widest practicable limits. . . .

45. MEDICAL PRACTICE AND THE HOSPITAL *

IT HAS BEEN claimed that a hospital which employs a roentgenologist, a pathologist, or any other physician on a salaried basis practices medicine in violation of law or of professional ethics. It has been further demanded that hospitals be prohibited by law from providing medical services under any and all circumstances.

In the following discussion, which this claim and demand have prompted, wherever the term "hospital" is used it is intended to apply to hospitals of the nonprofit or community type and not to business corporations conducting hospitals for profit. No attempt will be made here to defend profiteering on medical service. . . .

An attempt will be made to answer the questions: (1) What is a hospital, and what are its proper functions? (2) What is the essence of medical practice? (3) What are the legal and ethical rights of the physicians practicing in institutions? (4) Is the salaried employment of a physician in a hospital necessarily injurious to the public and to the medical profession? (5) Is it desirable or practicable to forbid the employment of salaried physicians in nonprofit hospitals under the exigent and complex conditions of modern medical practice?

A hospital is an institution for the care of the sick and infirm; hospital care is the care of the sick and infirm in a hospital; and hospitalization is the provision of hospital care. Law, custom, and common sense require the hospital to furnish

* From: *On Hospitals,* by S. S. Goldwater, M.D.; New York: Macmillan (copyright 1947). Reprinted with the permission of The Macmillan Company. (The excerpt reprinted, with omissions including tables, is from Part 2, Chap. VI, "Medical Practice and the Hospital," pp. 131-39).

reasonably adequate care. The services included in reasonably adequate hospital care are determined by the state of contemporary medical science, by prevailing standards in the practice of the art of medicine, by nursing standards established by law or local custom, and by legally defined or generally accepted requirements for the safety, protection, and comfort of the sick in hospitals or for the satisfaction of their essential needs.

The adequacy of hospital care may be weighed by the test of negligence. If the omission of an act or the failure to satisfy a need of a hospital patient would constitute negligence, either legally or logically, it is incumbent on the hospital to perform the act or to satisfy the need. There is no dispute about the obligation of a hospital to supply proper shelter, nursing, food, dressings, and ordinary room service; the current discussion revolves about the participation of the hospital in certain auxiliary medical services which are bound up with or closely related to medical practice.

The essence of medical practice is diagnosis and treatment. Hospital care divorced from diagnosis and treatment is inconceivable, but no institution can "diagnose, treat, operate, or prescribe." Making a diagnosis, or ordering or administering treatment, is a personal act. Medicine is practiced *in* a hospital, never *by* a hospital.

When the courts say that a public or charitable hospital may practice medicine because it is expressly organized for that purpose, they can only mean that such hospitals, to the extent authorized by law, may employ or appoint physicians to treat the sick. The hospital employs or appoints the physician; the physician diagnoses, prescribes, or operates.

The prevailing rule is that a hospital physician is responsible for his own professional acts unless specifically exempted by law; the hospital which employs or appoints a physician is only required in law to exercise due care in his selection. The legal exemption of physicians from responsibility for the result of their acts in hospitals is rare. The courts seem to know quite well who "practices medicine"; so does the discriminating patient.

The act of diagnosis or of treatment is a personal act; such acts, constituting the essence of medical practice, are of the same professional nature whether performed gratuitously, for an individual fee directly paid by the patient, or as part of a salaried service. Confusion arises when the business of medicine (the pay of the physician) and the art or profession of medicine (the act of diagnosing, prescribing, or treating) are indiscriminately spoken of as medical practice. In the United States, the conditions of the practice of medicine as an art are invariably fixed by law; but practicing physicians may donate their services if they choose, or may exact such fees or salaries as they see fit.

The term "practice through another" has been used in some states as descriptive of a function of a charitable hospital or public dispensary; but it is the "another," the physician, who actually practices, not the hospital or dispensary. The theory that an institution can take the place of a thinking and acting human being is presumably based on a legal fiction which under certain circumstances regards a corporation as a "person." We must not permit ourselves to be confused concerning the naked facts of medical service by a fiction of this kind.

Some physicians, charitably inclined, perform gratuitous services in hospitals; some are paid for their hospital services directly by patients, some are compensated by hospitals out of funds collected by the hospital from patients, others by hospitals out of moneys derived from voluntary contributions or from taxes. In all cases, the services rendered by physicians to the sick are or should be those required by patients without regard to the special business relationship.

It is impracticable to carry on the work of a modern general hospital with a completely uncompensated staff. Notwithstanding the great volume of medical work that is freely given, it is not equal to all that patients need or all that responsible physicians require. Medical salaries, negligible in most community hospitals a generation ago, now represent a substantial and unavoidable item of expenditure in hospital administration. Full-time physicians (resident and others), and many part-time physicians performing time-consuming, indispensable hospital services, cannot be expected to exist without compensation for such services, and investigation will show that the universal substitution of individual professional fees for hospital salaries is not practicable. The unattached family physician or staff member who sends his patient to a hospital for a "work-up" would soon rebel if a separate medical fee were demanded for each medical service rendered to his patient.

A hospital, required to give adequate care, must arrange for medical service, and it can only do so with the co-operation of medical practitioners. Co-operation between hospitals and physicians authorized to practice medicine assumes many forms. A conceivable form, but one encountered only in hospitals of the most primitive type (usually proprietary), is that in which a privately compensated physician individually performs all the medical service the patient receives, the hospital furnishing only lodging, room service, board, dressings, medicines, and nursing.

The dangers inherent in such primitive hospital service are recognized by the medical profession and by law; medical organizations and local government authorities, undertaking to define minimum standards of a safe and acceptable hospital, demand that hospitals furnish or arrange for competent auxiliary professional services. Typical requirements include resident physicians, qualified laboratory diagnosticians, and certain categories of therapeutic specialists.

Sharply contrasting with the primitive hospital, which is really only a boarding-house for the sick, is the government, university, or research hospital in which all or nearly all medical service is performed by salaried physicians. A mixture of paid and unpaid staffs in varying proportions characterizes most community hospitals.

If the employment of a physician by a hospital for any medical purpose is the practice of medicine by the hospital, the Federal Government, every state in the Union, many hundred cities and counties, state and private universities, ecclesiastical hospitals of many denominations, and nonsectarian community hospitals, are engaged in the practice of medicine.

A hospital which employs a salaried physician may in some cases donate, in other cases charge for identical medical services. If it be held that the hospital practices medicine only when it collects a fee for medical service, not when it employs physicians but donates their services gratuitously, then the argument really is that the collection of a fee is the essence or determinant of the practice of medicine

—a palpable absurdity. As has already been said, a hospital never actually practices medicine; in the nature of the case, a hospital cannot diagnose, prescribe, operate, or treat, quite apart from any legal restriction or ethical consideration.

While in any common-sense view, a hospital does not, notwithstanding the phraseology of state law, "practice medicine through another," since medicine as an art is practiced only by the physician, and not by the hospital which is permitted to employ him, it might be said that a physician "practices medicine through another" when he reports his opinion on a laboratory finding or a clinical condition to another physician, who in turn reports the findings or conclusions to the patient and gives the necessary orders. These proceedings, clinical throughout, are clearly distinguishable from the corporate or administrative acts of a charitable hospital. . . .

A physician whose compensation is received from an employer other than the patient, whether payment is made in the form of a fee for a single service, or as part of a salary for multiple services, does not "practice medicine through another" if he gives his professional opinion directly to or maintains direct and independent professional relations with the patient. The making of a diagnosis or the recommendation or performance of any therapeutic procedure completes, in essence, the act of medical practice. Academic freedom, professional prestige and dignity, and all the legitimate rights and privileges of medical practice can be and are maintained under varied forms of organizational and administrative business arrangements. The legal safeguards which surround medical practice aim at the protection of the public and are not intended to foster a monopoly for practitioners who believe in and adhere to a particular business method.

To the distinction between medical practice and business transactions incidental to it must be added the distinction between the practice of medicine and technical aids to medical practice. . . .

Reports of chemical or bacteriological tests influence the judgment of the practitioner, but do not take its place, nor are they on the same intellectual or professional plane. No serious objection has even been raised against employing highly trained nonmedical assistants to make scientific tests. From the standpoint of medical art, the most abstruse and complicated chemical laboratory test is of the same order of evidence as the taking of the patient's temperature with the aid of a clinical thermometer—a diagnostic aid universally rendered by nurses with complete medical approval.

Physicians employ aids in therapy as well as in diagnosis. Actual treatment is given when a nurse administers a drug prescribed by a physician, or when x-ray therapy is applied by a technician under medical direction and control, but the courts have justly held that the performance of these controlled procedures by workers subordinate to and directed by physicians does not constitute the practice of medicine. Similar services are performed by nonmedical assistants in doctors' private offices, and no serious objection is raised. Can it be seriously maintained that a hospital may employ nonmedical personnel for these services without practicing medicine, but that when identical services are performed in a hospital by paid medical personnel the hospital is engaged in the practice of medicine? Or that a hospital may properly be the vendor of a technical service when the performer of the service is a layman, but may not act in the identical capacity when the performer of the service is a medical graduate?

A hospital might conceivably collect a charge for inclusive hospital care of a patient and might retain an undue part of the proceeds, thus depriving medical staff workers of their just reward. It is alleged, and it is probably true, that such profiteering has occurred. The remedy for the abuse lies in a more equitable business arrangement, not in destroying types of hospital organization that have been developed in response to the demands of the medical profession itself and in deference to felt social needs.

Putting aside questions of law and principle, and limiting attention to the naked demand that every fee charged for diagnosis and treatment be paid directly to the participating physician, one may ask whether it is practicable to conduct an adequate hospital service in the manner proposed. The complexity of modern medical service apparently presents insuperable obstacles to the proposal.

How many physicians actually participate or may participate in the hospital care of a single patient? Examination of a series of clinical histories in a well-conducted hospital reveals that in some cases as many as twelve or fifteen separate medical functions were performed in the process of diagnosis alone; the number of required services is further increased by therapeutic indications.

Services of a medical nature required in hospital practice may be supplied directly and exclusively by physicians; others, of a fact-finding character with clinical bearing, may be furnished by nonmedical personnel, who in turn are supervised by physicians. Some of the required services are grave and time consuming; some are slight and of brief duration; but all reflect the demands of medical practitioners and are presumably indispensable to effective practice. . . .

How many patients would care to enter a hospital and submit to the confusion and agony of indefinitely extended professional relations, not to speak of the exaction of an alarming array of individual fees? . . . The intolerable conditions which would be created under the multiple fee system would give an enormous impetus to the demand that all hospital medical practice be organized by the state. Is that what the advocates of the multiple fee system want?

The necessities of modern medicine call for extensive co-operation in hospital practice—co-operation among physicians on the one hand, and physicians and the hospital on the other. The complexity of modern medical practice is such that a high degree of physical, professional, and business organization is required if hospitals are to furnish adequate medical care. The indefinite multiplication of individual professional fees would make hospitals unworkable, and is not essential to the preservation of the integrity of medical practice.

The brilliant success of hospital service subscription plans on a nonprofit basis indicates the fulfillment of a public need. To be successful, such plans must supply adequate hospital care. They can do so without destroying tested forms of hospital organization, without injustice to medical practitioners, without sacrificing any medical right or privilege. . . .

There is no good reason why an ethical plan, acceptable to the physicians of a particular city, should be modified to conform to the preference of physicians in other localities. Compensation for medical service is a business matter which concerns both doctors and the public. Hospitals are justified in entering into any arrangement for the payment of fees which members of their staffs find acceptable, provided it involves neither exploitation nor coercion and promotes adequate medical care. If hospital administrators believe that the direct payment of a separate medical fee to every physician contributing directly or indirectly to diagnosis or treatment would diminish hospital efficiency, obstruct adequate medical care, and embarrass physicians who are primarily responsible for treatment and on whom patients directly depend, they not only have the right to oppose but are under moral obligation to combat the multiple fee system.

Responsibility for making hospital care adequate is not the responsibility of the trustee or lay branch of hospital administration alone; it is equally the responsibility of hospital medical staffs and of the medical profession.

Hospitals do not, hospitals cannot, practice medicine; hospitals can and must participate in the organization and business-like administration of hospital medical practice in order to meet the demands of their visiting staffs and fulfill their obligation to provide adequate hopital care. It is inconceivable that an intelligent medical profession will refuse to co-operate with hospitals that are eager to serve the public, and that propose to do so in a manner which rigidly excludes profiteering and which is not only acceptable to but is actually responsive to the needs of their staff members.

46. OUT-PATIENT SERVICES *

Clinics Old and New

THE OUT-PATIENT Clinic [1] is as old as the hospital in America. The first clinic was established in 1752 by the Pennsylvania Hospital of Philadelphia, America's oldest hospital. The Philadelphia Dispensary was established in 1786; the New York Dispensary in 1790; and the Boston Dispensary in 1796, eight years prior to the founding of the Massachusetts General Hospital and sixty-eight years prior to the establishment of the Boston City Hospital. The methods of operation of these early clinics, or dispensaries, as they were usually termed, were described as follows:

The way of the sick poor was much harder a century ago than it is today, for the sufferer could not then go directly to one of these dispensaries and see the doctor. First, he had to seek out one of the donors to the dispensary and convince this charitable person

* From: *Better Hospital Care for the Ambulant Patient* (Report of the Special Committee on Hospital Clinic Services), by the Hospital Association of Pennsylvania; Harrisburg, Pa.: The Association, 1946 (Chap. I, "Clinics Old and New," pp. 2-7; Chap. III, "Observed Defects in Out-Patient Clinics," pp. 28-43). Reprinted (with omissions, including initial paragraph) by permission of the publishers.

1. The term Out-Patient Clinic, as used in this Report, refers to an ambulatory clinic operated for the care of free and part-pay patients.

that he was not only poor and sick, but also "worthy." For at that period it was the privilege of the "donors," or those who contributed five dollars or more to the maintenance of the dispensary, to designate persons they considered eligible for treatment. For each five dollars contributed, one or two persons might be cared for. If the donor had not already reached his quota of "worthy poor" when our sick man applied, he might be given a card of recommendation and be admitted to the dispensary. There he had to join a slowly moving line and eventually found himself before a bearded and bespectacled doctor seated at a desk behind a large ledger. After the doctor had inspected the permit from the contributor, he entered the name, address, age, sex, and complaint on one line in his ledger. He inspected the sufferer's tongue, felt his pulse, probably inquired about his appetite, sleep, and bowels, and then wrote a diagnosis in his book, with several numbers indicating medications. These numbers were copied on a slip and handed to the patient, who was told to report back if not cured when the medicine was gone.

The patient next passed to the pharmacy where the numbers were interpreted into prescriptions. If the medication consisted of herbs to be steeped at home, he usually carried it away in his hat, or, if a salve were indicated, was expected to produce a clam shell or other container to receive it.

There was little attention to physical examination and little respect for the patient's privacy. The doctor felt obligated to name the condition, however, so that he could enter a diagnosis in his ledger. This need of a name made it to his advantage not to individualize his cases lest he could not define the condition by a single term. The old case books and the annual reports are full of such "diagnoses" as rheumatism, plethora, ague, and so on, which are only symptoms and not diseases.[2]

It is a far cry from these early "prescription mills" to the modern, first class hospital Out-Patient Clinics, whose medical staffs have at their command the formidable array of diagnostic equipment necessary to a scientific determination of the nature of the patient's malady.

The growth in the number, scientific equipment and scope of the diagnostic facilities available in the modern hospital spelled the death knell of most of the early dispensaries. Thus, for example, of the three independent dispensaries which were established and operated in Philadelphia for many years, only one remains—the Southern Dispensary, of 318 Bainbridge Street.

In New York City the dispensaries (many of which had changed their names to "clinics" to keep pace with the development of medicine) unattached to hospitals, numbered about 240 in 1926. Thirteen years later there were less than twenty....

We who are in the hospital field and the public at large must constantly keep in mind that since 1929 we have lived in a highly abnormal period in which little progress could be made in the improvement of the hospital plants and facilities in America. In these momentous years tremendous advances have occurred in the art and science of medicine, but these changes, in large measure, have not been reflected in the facilities and methods of the voluntary hospitals for the treatment of ambulant cases—particularly as regards the full utilization of the potentialities of modern medicine for such cases.

2. *New Clinics for Old,* Michael M. Davis and Anna M. Richardson. New York: The Committee on Dispensary Development of the United Hospital Fund of New York. 1927. Pp. 1-2.

The subject matter of this Report, in reality, is to determine and measure the extent of these deficiencies and to indicate the direction in which the hospitals should proceed to exploit fully the possibilities inherent in modern medicine to improve the care and treatment afforded to the ambulant patient. . . .

Observed Defects in Out-Patient Clinics

IN THE PROSECUTION of this investigation a careful study was made of certain outstanding clinics in Pennsylvania, New York, Massachusetts and elsewhere in which notable innovations are in operation. There are wide differences in the handling of out-patients in various hospital clinics. The Committee is impressed with the fine quality of clinic service in the majority of hospitals visited. On the other hand, the Committee is critical of conditions in some clinics for the reasons hereinafter stated:

(a) In too many Out-Patient Clinics the general atmosphere, furnishings and equipment do not reflect credit upon the institution, are not conducive of good public relations and should be improved in the postwar programs of such hospitals.

(b) Too often the scheduling of Out-Patient Clinic appointments is either non-existent or is poorly planned and handled, in consequence of which patients who can ill afford time off from their work or household duties are kept waiting, sometimes for hours, before they are examined or treated. This not only is wasteful of the patient's time but is subversive of good public relations for the hospital.

(c) Dr. Osler, while working in the Johns Hopkins Clinic, was impressed with the fact that, after patients were discharged as cured, they frequently returned some months later with the same maladies and in many cases in just as bad condition. In seeking for an explanation he discovered that disease was often the product of environmental conditions in the home; that in curing the disease, the clinic staff had not corrected the home conditions which had again produced it. The effort to correct these fundamental conditions produced the medical social worker. Too many hospital Out-Patient Clinics do not get at these fundamental conditions and thus are required to do the same work over and over again. . . .

(d) In many cases, the system employed in assigning members of the medical staff to service in the Out-Patient Clinic is ill-advised. The abler members are assigned to ward service; clinic assignments too often are given to certain physicians who, for various reasons, do not "measure up" to ward service, or to young members of the staff of limited experience. While the chiefs of the various specialties are nominally in charge of the clinic as well as the ward service, in many cases they do little or no work in the clinics and seldom visit them. The Committee finds that the outstanding authorities are in general agreement that such practices are subversive of the interests of the patient and of the hospital.

(e) The attitude of some clinic doctors toward the out-patients is unfortunate. The physician's demeanor eloquently conveys the fact that he has no sustained interest in the patient; that the examination and treatment are chores to be gotten through with as rapidly as possible. In other words, the human element is completely lost sight of in the physician's approach to the patient's illness. . . .

The Human Element in Hospital Clinics

OF ESSENTIAL importance in the organization of hospital Out-Patient Clinics is the human element, the factor which determines whether the clinic is merely a scientific establishment or a living, human institution perpetuating the primary objective of the inception of dispensaries—charity in its truest sense.

To maintain the human spirit in the clinic, the entire personnel must approach the problem in a sympathetic and intelligent manner; they must make the personality of the individual patient the central idea on which all thought and action are concentrated.

There is a tendency at the present time on the part of hospitals to feel that, when a well-organized medical social service department is established in connection with a clinic, the human element is well taken care of. This may not be the case.

In this discussion, it is assumed that there is a medical social service department equipped, as Dr. Haven Emerson points out, to secure a knowledge of and to supply treatment to social environmental factors and social psychological conditions of significance in the diagnosis and treatment of the sick. This department is an integral part of the clinic and supplements the work of the physician and the program of medical care. Its chief objective is to contribute to the patient's restoration to health or to the best possible social adjustment in the light of his condition.

The organization of a medical social service department in the clinic does not relieve the management of the responsibility of seeing that the personnel of the clinic—physicians, nurses, admitting officers and students—are imbued with the spirit that should animate the social service worker. Too often, the human element is disregarded and responsibilities belonging to the doctor, nurse or admitting officer are turned over to the social service worker.

Everyone employed in the clinic must have a full comprehension of the intrinsic value of the human personality and must acknowledge that this intrinsic value so endows the individual as to give him a place of preeminence in the world—in other words, must understand the dignity and sacredness of the human personality, regardless of age, color, physical ability, mental ability or economic status.

It seems that in some instances the human spirit, which motivated those who organized the clinic, is overlooked in the course of scientific advancement. It may become still more obscured unless we realize that science alone cannot alleviate the ills of our patients. Science is the handmaid of the human element, and when these two are united all abuses which may destroy the ideals of the medical profession and the institution disappear.

The clinic, more than any other department in the hospital, demands an understanding of all types of persons. Patients come to the clinic under the gravest crises of their lives. They are waiting for the doctor to diagnose their illness, and what a momentous time in the life of a person!

The doctor's findings will foretell their life or their death. Unquestionably there is no other department in a hospital so well equipped and with so genuine an opportunity to influence the thinking and feeling of the patient at this critical time. Everyone in the clinic must know how to deal with all types of humanity. The attitude of the materialist—any lack of the appreciation of the dignity of mankind —cannot be tolerated in the clinic. A human attitude is one of the prime essentials.

All patients should be met with a gracious approach, because their problems go far beyond physical disabilities. There is a definite nervous aspect accompanying their illness and they need definite psychological care. Nothing should be done to add to the patient's mental and physical discomfort.

The survey shows also that often patients are required to wait a long time, due to the fact that they are instructed to report early so as not to keep the doctor waiting.

As a result, the patient is tired and increasingly apprehensive before the doctor examines him. Too often the patient must sit on a hard bench in a crowded admitting room in company with some who are very ill, others walking with the help of crutches, some with bandages or dark glasses, babies who are crying. It requires little imagination to realize the depressive effect of a long wait in this atmosphere on the clinic patient.

Some clinics now have arrangements whereby patients are taken care of by appointment, except emergency patients. Other hospitals have done much to modernize the clinic and have especially dignified the waiting rooms so that they no longer resemble bus stations but have a more comfortable, home-like atmosphere. Other hospitals have abandoned the white paint heretofore considered essential for cleanliness and have adopted a color as a means of adding a human touch to their clinics, realizing that color frequently has a psychological effect. Yellow, for instance, suggests sunlight and warmth; blue is a cool color, and green has the characteristics of both blue and yellow and has, therefore, an almost universal appeal. Used with discrimination, color can go a long way toward creating a psychologically helpful atmosphere.

Frequently other improvements can be made by simple means—the rearrangement of equipment, the removal of a door or the installation of a partition may give an otherwise old-fashioned room a modern appearance. All of these changes have an effect on the patient and contribute to the upholding of the human element.

We should never lose sight of the fact that the hospital is a quasi-public institution and that the patient has the right to demand that we serve him. It is our duty to awaken confidence in our clinics and do what we can to break down the tradition of aloofness which, for some reason, we have created.

Our problem is to maintain the public's faith in our clinics by proving that we believe in the intrinsic value of the human personality; that our personnel is responsive to the patient's needs; that the patient's time is valuable as well as that of the doctor; that we appreciate the need for attractive surroundings and adequate facilities and, last of all, that we realize the importance of the human element in all our relationships with our patients. . . .

Recommendations

IN THE LIGHT of [the Committee's] findings, the following recommendations are made:

(1) The five fundamental criteria for the proper organization of an Out-Patient Department, developed by the Associated Out-Patient Clinics in New York and adopted by the American Hospital Association in 1927, are sound. In effect, they are: (a) Out-patient and bed service should be closely associated and the medical staff should be unified as much as possible. (b) The hospital should limit the number of patients which it will accept for care to a volume that can be adequately served by the facilities which are available, or which can be provided, the controlling limitations being the medical and lay staff, the space and the equipment available to do good work. (c) Accurate and complete medical records, including social and scientific data, should be written on all patients and should be filed and cross-indexed in such a manner as to be readily available at any time for reference, restudy and statistical and clerical research. (d) Clinical, laboratory, X-ray and other diagnostic and therapeutic services of the hospital should be available for out-patients wherever such services are required. (e) Adequate nursing service, medical social service, clerical service, etc., should be provided as needed.

(2) Out-Patient Clinics must be modernized; the rows of hard wooden benches should be discarded and more comfortable accommodations provided for the patients; better equipment and facilities should be installed and clinic quarters made more cheerful and attractive.

(3) An intelligent system of scheduling patient appointments should be installed and carefully followed. Our investigation convinces us that patients can be handled just as expeditiously and in as large numbers by arranging individual appointments at stated times and by firmly impressing upon the patient the necessity for being prompt.

(4) But in addition, hospitals must modernize their methods of conducting their clinics. Attention is called to the plan quite recently instituted at the Vanderbilt Clinic (for patients unable to afford a private physician) of the Columbia-Presbyterian Medical Center, New York City. Effective April 1, 1946, a group clinic was established at the Vanderbilt Clinic to handle all patients requiring a general workup, the new clinic being a diagnostic and treatment clinic. It is contemplated that this clinic will eventually replace the present Medical, Surgical Diagnostic, and Neurological Clinics. . . . The introduction of the group clinic does not change the handling of emergency cases, nor does it interfere with the operation of the special study clinics which now exist in most departments and which afford the means for the concentrated study of the large number of patients with particular diseases, thus furthering medical knowledge and the training of medical students, which is one of the primary functions of the Vanderbilt Clinic—the Out-Patient Department of the Columbia-Presbyterian Medical Center.

Under the new system those patients who formerly needed five or six appointments in various specialized clinics, are examined in one day by a team of specialists. The so-called Group Staff consists of nine specialists in Internal Medicine and two surgeons, as well as specialists in Dermatology, Ear-Nose-and-Throat, Gynecology, Neurology, Ophthalmology, Psychiatry and Urology.

Those out-patients who require comprehensive examinations are seen by such of the specialists of the Group Staff just mentioned as are required for a thorough and complete examination. To the maximum extent possible these specialists confer after succeeding examinations of the patient. Successive visits of patients to various clinics—frequently four or five—necessitating the loss of several days' pay for clinic patients who are able to work, are obviated. There is an earlier and more accurate diagnosis of diseases and a great saving of time to the patients and to the hospital.

Dr. Robert R. Cadmus, Director of the Vanderbilt Clinic, informed the Committee that this is the first application of the group practice principle to a large metropolitan dispensary; that while it is too early to reach final conclusions with respect to the experiment, the initial reactions of patients, doctors, medical students and the administrative officials of the clinic are that it has produced marked advantages to all concerned. Among these advantages are the following: the clinic administration benefits by the sharp curtailment in the detailed procedures (delivery of histories; Record Room bookkeeping; retaking of temperatures, pulse rates, and weights, etc.) inherent in sending patients to a number of clinics; the ordering of unnecessary laboratory procedures has been reduced; valuable experience will be gained as a guide to the introduction of a semiprivate group practice, if such a move seems advisable in the future and, finally, through this pioneering improvement in dispensary practice—an improvement of far-reaching importance —the prestige of the Vanderbilt Clinic has been greatly enhanced. The Committee believes that a generally similar plan can be instituted with great profit by many other hospitals in their Out-Patient Clinics.

(5) Every hospital should operate a well-organized, carefully supervised medical social service department in connection with its Out-Patient Clinic, to investigate the environmental conditions contributing to the patient's illness. The Out-Patient medical staff should supervise this work in the home.

(6) Attention is called to the following from the *Manual of Hospital Standardization of the American College of Surgeons:*

It is absolutely imperative that the out-patient departments have one or more medical social workers. Each applicant for treatment requires a complete social case study which should be obtained by persons specially trained for this work. The medical social worker can also do a great deal to prevent what is known as "clinic abuse."

The nursing staff and the non-professional personnel of the out-patient department must have as high qualifications as those in other divisions of the institution. A sufficient staff of skilled assistants should be provided in order that the medical staff may be free from administrative duties and routine tasks.

Medical records in the out-patient department, just as for ward cases, should give an accurate picture of the patient's condition and should contain all the facts bearing on the case. The record system should be so arranged that a patient's record can be removed at any time to accompany him if he is transferred to other departments of the hospital. In this respect the central system of medical records is most practical. This will prevent duplication of laboratory examinations, history taking and treatment, and will serve to co-ordinate all forces of the hospital in the care of the patient. Similarly, when the patient is able to leave the ward, his medical record should be sent to the out-patient department as an aid in follow-up. In this way the scientific services of the hospital are correlated.

In many instances the medical staff appears to have no clear conception as to what the medical social service worker is for, or how to utilize her services effectively. The staff will not refer patients to her if she is isolated in some small office "under the stairs," as some of them say.

The Committee has observed that many clinics put the medical social worker in the clinic itself, where she is in constant touch with all the patients and all the doctors. Where the clinic is so large that the social service worker cannot cover the entire clinic, interesting experiments are being tried in concentrating her floor work in certain places, such as the Medical, Psychiatric, Heart, Pediatric and Diabetic Clinics, where more consideration is given to the individual as a person.

(7) The voluntary hospitals now make substantial use of the Public Health nurses maintained and supported by the Public Assistance Division of the Department of Health of Pennsylvania in providing home care for ambulant patients and bed patients who are on relief—those patients being classified as indigent, as distinguished from those who are medically indigent—following their discharge while they are confined to their homes. These Public Health nurses, where required, make daily visits to the homes of such patients to give them nursing care, such as bed baths, where it cannot be provided by members of the patient's family. Frequently, a more effective liaison between the Public Health nurse, the medical social worker and the officials of the Out-Patient Department of the hospital is desirable. Public Health nurses perform a valuable and necessary function both as regards the after-care of indigent bed patients and home care for ambulant patients in the Out-Patient Clinics, and in providing such care, when required, for indigent patients treated in Group Clinics operated in conjunction with the voluntary hospitals.

(8) Present methods of assigning medical staff members to service in Out-Patient Clinics should be radically changed. The chiefs of service should take an active part in the conduct of the clinic. Dr. J. A. Curran, President and Dean of the Long Island College of Medicine and an outstanding consultant on medical and hospital problems, informed your Committee that he regularly attends the Medical Clinic of his hospital, taking his turn with other members of the staff, for two reasons: first, because of the influence this has upon young doctors in impressing upon them that the Out-Patient Clinic service is, in fact, a *privilege*—not a *chore* —owing to the greater variety of cases available for intimate study in the clinic as compared with the wards; and, second, because of the stimulating effect which such first-hand contact with clinic work has upon its efficient operation.

Dr. Curran and others with whom the Committee discussed this matter advocated that assignments to duty of the members of medical staffs not now adhering to such a plan be revised, so that each member of the staff, from the chief to the intern, would have a regular tour of duty in the clinic and would be required scrupulously to adhere to his schedule.

(9) The same high type of service afforded to private patients in the hospital should prevail in its clinic. It is the responsibility of the board of trustees to see that these principles are carried out and that no clinic patient is treated in a cavalier fashion.

The hospitals and their staffs should ask themselves the question: What will the out-patients do if the Murray-Wagner-Dingell Bill (S. 1606; HR 4730, entitled "The National Health Act of 1945") should pass in substantially its present form, thus providing them with the means of paying for their medical care? Will they continue to turn to the hospital for such care, or will they turn to some outside doctor or group of doctors, because of the kind of treatment they have heretofore received in the hospital's clinic? Will they not avoid a hospital which has permitted its medical staff to patronize and humiliate them?

The Committee believes it is high time that the hospitals set their clinic house in order. The foregoing suggestions are founded upon what is now being done in certain clinics—particularly in the Group Clinics—where no distinction is made between the free patient and the pay patient. In some of the most celebrated Group Clinics in the United States, people of affluence and those in humble circumstances sit side by side in the waiting room and are treated without distinction by the same doctors and in exactly the same manner. . . .

If the plan which is recommended were made universally effective in Out-Patient Departments, the quality of medical care of patients would be substantially improved. The hospital authorities should see to it that the case-load per doctor is not too great; that patients are seen by appointment only; that appointments are skillfully scheduled so that they can be adhered to; that new patients are given as much as forty-five minutes for the first examination and return patients at least fifteen minutes; that the Out-Patient Clinic is properly equipped; that first-class diagnosticians and specialists examine the patients, determine the clinical procedure to be followed, diagnose the case, and prescribe the treatment. The interns, fellows, and young doctors should assist the experienced men, observing their methods and learning from them by observation and individual instruction; they should not be assigned to clinic patients to do as they, in their limited knowledge and experience, deem best.

FURTHER READINGS

Hospitals: Facilities and Services

American Hospital Association. *Cumulative Index of Hospital Literature.* Chicago: The Association. (Issued semiannually).

Bachmeyer, Arthur C. and Hartman, Gerhard (eds.). *The Hospital in Modern Society.* New York: Commonwealth Fund, 1943. 768 pages. (Includes references).

Bachmeyer, Arthur C. and Hartman, Gerhard (eds.). *Hospital Trends and Developments, 1940-1946.* New York: Commonwealth Fund, 1948. 819 pages. (Includes references).

Bridgman, R. F. *The Rural Hospital: Its Structure and Organization*. Monograph Series No. 21. Geneva: World Health Organization, 1955. 162 pages. (Includes references).

Commission on Financing of Hospital Care. *Financing Hospital Care in the United States*. (3 vols.). Vol. 1: *Factors Affecting the Costs of Hospital Care*. New York: McGraw-Hill, 1954. 300 pages. (Includes references).

Dickinson, Frank G. and Raymond, James. *Some Categories of Patients Treated by Physicians in Hospitals*. Bulletins 102 and 102A, Bureau of Medical Economic Research, American Medical Association. Chicago: The Association, 1956. 27 pages. (Includes references).

Joint Commission on Accreditation of Hospitals. *Standards for Hospital Accreditation*. Chicago: The Commission, 1956. 12 pages.

McGibony, John R. *Principles of Hospital Administration*. New York: G. P. Putnam's Sons, 1952. 540 pages. (Includes references).

Reed, Louis S. and Hollingsworth, Helen. *How Many Hospital Beds Are Needed?* Publication No. 309, Public Health Service. Washington: U. S. Government Printing Office, 1953. 73 pages.

The Physician in the Hospital

American Academy of General Practice. *Manual on General Practice Departments in Hospitals*. Kansas City, Mo.: The Academy, 1951. 10 pages.

American Hospital Association. *The Board's Control of Hospital Medical Care*. Chicago: The Association, 1950. 47 pages.

American Medical Association. *Relation of Physicians and Hospitals*. Chicago: The Association, 1953. 15 pages.

CHAPTER VII

Coördination in Health and Medical Service

D IFFICULT ORGANIZATIONAL problems are created by the increasing complexity of the apparatus, knowledge and skills of modern medicine. The efficient and economic use of all of these resources to provide a high quality of medical care demands that they somehow be brought together and yet remain available wherever they are needed. In Chapter V, we were introduced to the concept of the medical care team, one of the essential devices for the coordination of the personnel resources of medical care. This chapter presents several of the processes through which coordination of personnel, facilities and services may be achieved.

The time is not long past when it was possible for one physician to carry in his head and two hands a major share of the knowledge and skills available; when this one physician was health advisor to his patients and to the community and ministered to the ails and aches of all the family; when no one thought much about the need for hospital services way out in the country— since you could be sick and die more comfortably at home. But this time is past. We are in a period of specialism, required by the tremendous extent of our knowledge. (Specialization has artificially separated the parts of the body; the body from the mind; and prevention from cure.) The hospital, and its many tools for the diagnosis, treatment and prevention of disease, is needed for good practice in the country as in the city.

To recreate the whole patient and bring to him the composite resources of the physician, the process of group practice has been devised. Some of its many forms and its problems are described in this chapter. Also included is a discussion of how the large, up-to-date hospital, physically based in the city, can make its resources available through the more rural hospitals of its area to physicians and their patients who live outside of the city. Both group practice and hospitals offer possibilities for achieving the reintegration of the preventive and curative aspects of medicine.

A. *Medical Group Practice*

47. PATTERNS AND PROBLEMS *

THERE HAS BEEN a radical revolution in medical science, which is now being followed by a gradual evolution in medical practice. Group medical service is being developed to coördinate the specialized knowledge and skill of individual practitioners, and to utilize effectively the public's investment in diagnostic and treatment facilities, including hospitals. . . .

Group Medical Practice is a program for prevention, diagnosis, and treatment, the essential characteristic of which is a *common interest by a number of physicians in the care of individual patients.* The doctors share their knowledge and skill in determining and providing the necessary services. Observable features of group practice include: specialized professional qualifications of the practitioners; contiguity of professional offices with availability for regular and frequent consultations concerning individual patients; joint use of supplementary services; some joint ownership of equipment, apparatus, or buildings; coöperative, rather than competitive division of total income among the group.

Origins of Group Medical Practice

Group practice is a process, rather than a form of organization. The central theme —a common interest in the patient—is always present. But the variations are numerous. Some group practice may be *intermittent,* rather than continuous, as in the exchange of opinion during ward-rounds in a hospital. Some group practice may be *part-time,* rather than full-time, as in the sessions attended in a hospital outpatient department, or office appointments at a clinic serving prepayment contract patients. Some group practice is for *diagnosis* only, with treatment procedures becoming the responsibility of individual doctors. Some group practice is limited to *special groups,* such as contract patients, rather than the general public. Some group practice is limited to *referred cases* with no acceptance of patients who do not have a personal physician. Some group practice is limited to economic classes, such as persons of *moderate means* or those unable to pay current established fees.

* From: "Patterns and Problems of Group Medical Practice," by C. Rufus Rorem; *American Journal of Public Health* 40: 1521-28, Dec. 1950 (No. 12). Reprinted (with omissions and original italics) by permission of the author and publishers. The author is the executive director of the Hospital Council of Philadelphia.

The evolution of group practice was inevitable. The *development of specialization* in medical knowledge and skill has forced a degree of coördination in medical practice. This trend is similar to that which occurred in private business when artisans began to specialize in detailed processes of building construction, the manufacture of clothes, or the preparation of food. As medical knowledge deepens in specific areas, it must be shared through conference and observation; otherwise, its values are not effectively utilized in prevention, diagnosis, and treatment. Medical service has become characterized by an *increasing reliance upon capital investment* for adequate diagnosis and treatment. Illustrations are x-ray apparatus, laboratory equipment, operating rooms, and complete hospitals for bed cases. Even if one doctor could finance the purchase of such plant and equipment, he could not personally perform each professional or technical service. He would need to rely upon subordinate or coördinate practitioners for most of the work, who, in turn, would be required to coördinate their services by conferences, records, and reports.

Specialization in knowledge and skill and the use of capital investment in medical practice are *causes,* not *results,* of group practice. The scientific and economic aspects of present-day health service make it necessary that the various phases of diagnosis and treatment be coördinated. *The general hospital is the natural site for the greatest development of group practice in America.* The medical specialists are already spending a great deal of time at hospitals in the care of patients who need bed care during a portion of their diagnosis and treatment. The hospitals contain the greatest portion of specialized equipment for diagnosis and treatment, together with a full-time staff trained to use the facilities under medical supervision. . . .

Patterns of Group Practice

THE PATTERNS OF group practice in the United States may be classified by several standards, such as degree of full-time paticipation, degree of hospital affiliation, scope of health services offered, groups eligible for service, or other bases. The following listing emphasizes the administrative characteristics of various forms of group practice. It does not include the hospital outpatient departments conducted for the "worthy poor."

Private group clinics.—This form of group medicine includes a number of individual practitioners representing several specialties, who work together in adjacent offices, most of them on a full-time basis. They usually rely upon local hospitals for the bed care of their patients and for provision of the more unusual types of scientific apparatus and equipment; but they may own and operate radiological and pathological laboratories and may perform minor operations at the central offices. They are in economic competition with other doctors, but not with each other.

The headquarters may be in office buildings or separate structures which are owned or rented. The doctors are usually organized in partnerships, but corporations may be established for the ownership of property and the employment of the doctors. Ordinarily, the clinics are open to the general public for all types of service, but a certain number of cases are referred by other doctors. They may have special contracts with insured patients, but most groups rely upon such revenue only to a limited degree.

Private clinics tend to be located in the smaller cities, and the medical personnel ranges from 3 to 300 individuals. The largest number have been organized west of the Mississippi River, in part through the influence of the Mayo Clinic at Rochester, Minn. The number of such groups is variously estimated at from 300 to 500, depending on the standards used for the listing.

This form of group practice represents the pattern most easily applied to present-day medicine by a group of physicians desiring to coördinate their efforts in the prevention, diagnosis, and treatment of disease and in the study and development of a positive health program. Some of the private clinics established to serve individual patients have relied greatly upon prepayment contracts with groups of employees and their dependents or with employers for the care of industrial compensation cases. An example of this type of clinic is the Ross-Loos Medical Group in Los Angeles, organized in 1929. It now includes 115 physicians and serves about 110,000 people on an insurance contract basis, as well as the general public. Hospital care is obtained in local institutions.

Full-time hospital staffs.—The outstanding example of this type of group practice is the Ford Hospital, established in 1915 at Detroit, Mich. Other significant examples are the Cleveland Clinic and Hospital, the Geisinger Hospital at Danville, Pa., the Guthrie Clinic and Robert Packer Hospital in Sayre, Pa., the Hitchcock Memorial Hospital, Hanover, N. H., the Underwood Hospital, Woodbury, N. J., and the Trinity Hospital, Little Rock, Ark.

These groups merge the outpatient and inpatient professional services at the hospital; the physicians are engaged on a full-time basis for annual salaries; the institution is open to the general public for both general and specialized care and for referred and walk-in patients. An exception is the Pratt Diagnostic Clinic and New England Medical Center Hospital, Boston, which are limited almost exclusively to cases referred by other physicians.

This form of full-time closed staff has seldom developed (if ever) from a community general hospital with an attending and courtesy staff. Usually, the institutions have established closed staffs at the time of their organization. In some cases, a private clinic has obtained control of an existing hospital or has constructed bed facilities for its own use. Combined institutions with full-time closed staffs have seldom been the recipients of city-wide philanthropy. But a number control endowment funds provided by an original donor or accrued from the net earnings of the private medical practice.

These organizations may accept insurance patients on the same basis as other practitioners and hospitals, but typically they do not rely upon group prepayment for their financial support.

In this group may be included the full-time medical faculty of the University of Chicago Clinics which accept diagnostic and treatment cases from all income levels in the general public, and which utilize all patients as teaching material when they are suitable for the purpose.

Medical groups organized for insured or other special groups.—Within the past three decades a number of clinics have been established to serve special groups of the general public. These include the full-time staffs of industrial plants, such as the Endicott-Johnson Company and the many private clinics in the Pacific Coast States which have contracts with employed firms to serve their employees and dependents.

More significant for the future are the groups established in connection with consumers who have provided capital facilities on a coöperative basis with small contributions from each member eligible to medical service benefits. Examples are the Elk City Hospital in Oklahoma, the Labor Health Institute in St. Louis, and the Group Health Co-operatives in Seattle and the District of Columbia. The clinics typically accept patients from the general public, and some of the practitioners are engaged on a part-time basis for service at the clinic. But the final objective in most instances is the development of a full-time staff devoted to a program of constructive health service on a prepayment basis.

The "giant" in this category of group practice is the Health Insurance Plan of Greater New York, which has aided in the establishment of 30 medical groups, with a total of 900 physicians, to serve the now 250,000 * participants in a comprehensive prepayment program for prevention, diagnosis, treatment, and health education. This organization began services to patients in 1947, and was aided in its establishment by grants from several foundations. H. I. P. is one of the few organizations which began with a three-dimensional program, namely: full-time group practice by doctors; group prepayment for entire families; comprehensive service in the home, office, and hospital. Most other organizations established either group practice or group prepayment independently of each other, and usually limited the service to specialty work or the coverage to catastrophic illnesses.

Part-time medical groups.—These groups are usually limited by the character of service provided or the method in which cases are accepted. Examples are the Mt. Sinai Diagnostic Clinic in New York for referred patients of moderate means; the Vanderbilt Clinic in New York for diagnosis and treatment of patients of limited incomes; the Benjamin Franklin Clinic of the Pennsylvania Hospital in Philadelphia for flat rate diagnostic service to referred patients of any income level; the Private Out-Patient Service of the Johns Hopkins Hospital, Baltimore; the Boston Dispensary which provides home care, as well as office service.

The part-time clinics have not grown rapidly in number, although some have increased their volume of service greatly, as the public has become aware of the available benefits. As a general rule, "reference" clinics have relied upon cases referred by doctors outside the immediate private practice trading area. This form

---

* The Health Insurance Plan of Greater New York employed in its medical groups, in 1956, approximately 1,000 physicians to serve a subscriber population numbering close to 500,000. For a description of the structure and functioning of the Plan, see Selection No. 84, Chapter XII.

of organization tends to become a general service available to walk-in patients, or to remain a limited activity for the convenience of the member physicians rather than the general profession and population. Diagnosis and treatment are inseparable in the patient's mind, and attempts to maintain a division are not approved or accepted by the general public.

Private ambulatory service.—The most prevalent, but least spectacular, group practice is the intermittent or regular use by individual doctors of hospital personnel and facilities in diagnostic service for private patients. This may take the form of reference of a patient to the hospital for x-ray films, examination, or treatment, for laboratory examination, or for conference with various medical specialists. The doctor may utilize hospital consulting rooms on a regular or intermittent basis for conferences with his patients and the various members of the hospital staff.

This trend represents "group practice *a la carte.*" The solo doctor may carry it *as far as* he wishes, and *when* he wishes. But the practice is growing rapidly. In total volume this work probably exceeds that of organized group practice by full-time and part-time clinics throughout the country.

Some physicians have viewed this trend with alarm, as placing the hospital in the practice of medicine, and making the solo doctor dependent on hospital personnel and facilities for the conduct of his practice. But service to private ambulatory patients may be more accurately regarded as a protector of individual practice, the absence of which would require direct hospital control over much diagnostic and treatment service. The alternative would be for the solo doctor to continue hand-bag medicine without regular contacts with specialized knowledge, skill, and facilities. Moreover, the regular contacts by general practitioners with hospitals may lead to appropriate staff appointments for such physicians and their integration with formal group practice which may develop at such institutions.

Physicians should be guided by enlightened self-interest in their decisions to participate in group medical practice. The "fate worse than debt" for the physician is the loss of self-determination in the practice of his profession. Statistics indicate that, on the average, physicians fare better financially under group practice than individual practice. But specific individuals (often the ones with the administrative genius to organize a group) might earn more income "on their own," and also be free from the trials of holding a medical group together. *Leadership is the missing link in the growth of group practice, for those best able to organize a group often have the least financial incentive to do so.*

Problems of Group Practice

THE FOLLOWING LIST of problems facing the establishment and continuance of group medical practice does not cover all opportunities and difficulties which must be faced, but they are submitted as representatives of some of those which will be faced at one time or another:

1. *Motivation.*—A clinic may be established for any of a variety of reasons, such as: the improvement of quality of medical care; the lowering of costs to patients; the increasing of income to physicians; the stabilization of working conditions for doctors; the training of subsidiary personnel; a demonstration of the advantages of coördinated practice; the freeing of physicians from direct concern about economic problems; etc. In the writer's opinion, *the sustaining motivation for physicians must be their personal self-interest, not social reform or demonstrations in medical economics, or even the avoidance of socialized medicine.*

Self-interest cannot be measured exclusively in terms of current income or future estate. More important is the *opportunity for personal and professional self-realization.* Group practice must expand rather than contract the doctor's opportunity to work as an individual and a professional man. The economic security of group practice must be accompanied by personal freedom to care for patients in accord with their needs, and to practice medicine at the highest attainable level of quality.

Much discussion of group practice has assumed that it is a form of revolution in the field of health service. From a logical point of view, a medical group is no more revolutionary than a baseball team. Each member has his position to play, and effectiveness depends upon team work rather than star performance. In the long run, group practice must reward individual doctors more adequately than does individual practice.

2. *Provision of working capital.*—Group practice involves less "per capita" investment by medical practitioners than does a group of individual private offices. The borrowing power of a partnership is enhanced by the demonstration of willingness to coöperate in professional activity. Vendors of scientific apparatus and equipment are typically more willing to extend credit to a group of physicians than to individual doctors. A group of physicians who have determined to carry on group practice seldom face difficulties in obtaining necessary working capital. Moreover, they can begin with partial facilities and arrange for temporary use of special apparatus on a rental or fee basis from other organizations.

3. *Selection of site.*—There is no one best location for a private clinic, geographically or as to type of building structure. Downtown offices, separate suburban buildings, portions of a hospital plant—all have advantages and limitations. Other things being equal, a medical group should not be "too far" away from the patients to be served or the related facilities (such as hospitals) which are utilized from time to time. But the public will soon discover the source of good service.

4. *Scope of service.*—Medical groups should be prepared to deal with all types of illness and any member of the population. If the group does not include the specialized knowledge and skill for certain treatment, arrangements should be established for other physicians and institutions to furnish necessary care. As a general rule, a clinic should direct patients to proper medical service, rather than merely refuse to accept certain categories of illnesses or of the population.

The number and specialties within the medical group are influenced by a variety of factors such as size of the community, available supplementary facilities, and the prospective amount of "referred" work as contrasted with care of minor ailments.

An important factor is the degree to which a medical group utilizes subordinate personnel for routine diagnostic or treatment procedures, as well as personal contacts with patients.

5. *Fees to be charged.*—A medical group should not be a "cut rate" organization, but should be able to offer a patient (or group of patients) more for his money than an equal number of competing practitioners. It is the total cost, rather than the detailed charges, which interests the prospective or actual patient. Composite fees established in advance give a sense of security and gratitude to the patient. He often will pay in full because of the certainty as to the amount. Medical groups are particularly equipped to establish composite fees for a variety of different services, since the total income accrues to all practitioners.

6. *Distribution of income.*—Most defunct clinics have prospered financially, as far as total income is concerned, up to the point of dissolution. Without exception, their greatest difficulty was the determination of each physician's share in the net earnings of the group. A medical group cannot distribute net earnings to physicians solely on the basis of each one's volume of service.

Variables to be recognized in establishing a doctor's share in the net income of group practice include the following:

a. Degree of administrative responsibility
b. Amount of capital investment
c. Length of service with the group
d. Demonstrable popularity with old patients
e. Demonstrable "pulling power" with new patients
f. Contribution to quality of service through research or teaching ability
g. Interest in health conservation and health education
h. Relative scarcity of his special knowledge or skill
i. Ability to perform an unusual volume of high quality service.

7. *Relations with individual practitioners.*—A medical group is both a supplement and a competitior of the practice of individual doctors. Even referral groups are a potential threat to the economic security of non-member physicians. Competition based on quality, rather than price, will ultimately win the respect of many individual doctors. The maintenance of cordial professional and personal relations with non-group physicians requires considerable effort and attention.

8. *Relations with hospitals.*—These problems are continuous for medical groups and often very difficult. Under ordinary circumstances, use of a voluntary hospital is preferred to the purchase and management of a proprietary institution. In the long run, it is more rewarding to make peace with the local medical profession concerning use of an existing hospital than to run the risk of excessive facilities by establishment of a new institution.

9. *Use of subsidiary personnel.*—The medical supervision possible in a clinic permits nurses and other technically trained employees to perform many procedures which otherwise consume the time of a physician. This applies particularly to the use of nurses in response to house calls and the performance of follow-up procedures prescribed by a physician.

It is desirable that a nurse should not "practice medicine." But it is also important that a doctor should be freed from the necessity of performing nursing procedures.

Group practice should permit specialists to use their knowledge and skill to the greatest degree. General practitioners and non-medical personnel should be colleagues rather than competitors.

10. *Varied administrative problems.*—Group medical practice faces many administrative problems in its development and growth. Some of them are:

a. Care of patients during personal absences
b. Need for intensive service to cases requiring special study
c. Old age and retirement allowances
d. Full-time use of young physicians
e. "Tapering-off" of services by older physicians
f. Attention to health education
g. Skillful and humane handling of malingerers
h. Attention to psychological factors in treatment and recovery
i. Responsibility for home calls and night service
j. Recognition of unusual knowledge or skill
k. Scheduling the use of apparatus and equipment
l. Informal consultations in diagnosis or treatment
m. Authoritative contacts with regulatory bodies
n. Interpretation of services to the general public
o. Sub-contracting with prepayment organizations, particularly for home and office calls which involve a substantial degree of "moral hazard"
p. Periodic appraisal of quality of service
q. Study of medical records
r. Statistical analysis of services performed and results achieved.

Conclusions

1. The development of group medical practice will be dependent upon the degree to which doctors consider such activities as favorable to their immediate and long-run self-interest. Opportunity for unfettered professional service is a greater factor than size of total income.

2. Doctors with a genius for business organization are also usually successful private practitioners. The main administrative need in group practice is an attitude of common concern for the patient's recovery and health maintenance. This is more important than brilliance in the field of management, or unusual scientific knowledge and skill. In group practice the whole is greater than the sum of its parts.

3. Courage and determination are more important than plant and equipment or working capital. The public stands ready to provide working capital for responsible medical groups by one of several processes:

a. Contributions by patients who expect to be served, such as members of a coöperative or insurance organization

b. Private loans from commercial banks or vendors of medical equipment

c. Offers of the use of public facilities in hospitals or health agencies

4. An important area for the development of medical group practice is the gradual transformation of hospital out-patient departments from limited service for the "worthy poor" to general service to the entire public.

5. "Restrictive" group practice will probably not become a significant phase of medical service in the United States. This prediction applies particularly to diagnostic or referral clinics, as well as medical groups limited to service to industrial firms or single insurance corporations.

6. The public does not distinguish between functions of diagnosis and treatment and wishes to receive complete medical care from the same medical organization.

7. Group medical practice is a way of life and an attitude toward health service, not merely an administrative device to increase quality, reduce costs, or to stabilize medical income.

8. Group medical practice is a process of "evolution" which is developing gradually. It is following upon a series of "revolutions" in medical science. Specialized knowledge and skill in the field of medicine require the use of group practice in their application to prevention, diagnosis, and treatment. But a "cultural lag" still remains between what is *known,* and what is *being done* about it.

48. ADVANTAGES *

IT SEEMS to me that group medical practice *per se* tends toward improving the quality of medical care because of the incentives it brings about in two separate, though intimately related, areas, namely the professional and the economic. In professional matters, the qualitative advantages of the group method arise from factors such as the following. The individual physician has easily available to him, in a medical group, the varied skills of his medical colleagues and associated personnel. He usually has access to technical facilities, such as laboratory, x-ray, and physical therapy equipment, vastly superior to what he as an individual could afford or could efficiently utilize. These associations stimulate and educate the physician as a member of a team. His specialized colleagues may be called in at a moment's notice; his daily work, in the nature of things, is constantly under the scrutiny of other physicians of the group, senior and junior. In such circumstances, any man wants to do his best—and he expects their best from his associates. Other professional advantages work toward the same end. A group may arrange systematically for free time for its individual members, whether for recreation or study. The young

* From: "Improving the Quality of Medical Care: Group Medical Practice," by Dean A. Clark, M.D.; *American Journal of Public Health* 39: 321-28, March 1949 (No. 3). Reprinted (with omissions, including initial paragraphs) by permission of the author and publishers. The author is the general director of Massachusetts General Hospital in Boston.

physician in a group may immediately exercise, under suitable supervision, the full range of his professional capacities instead of being obliged to wait, as is all too common in individual practice, for patients to accumulate while his hard-earned skills grow rusty. It is thus clear that the professional influences in a medical group provide an inducement to the improvement of the quality of service rendered by its physicians, individually and collectively.

In the economic area, the influences are no less conducive to our purpose. First, the group method, by its very character, makes for economies which aid rather than hinder professional quality. The ability of a group to obtain at relatively low cost to each individual physician, better technical equipment and personnel than its physicians could afford separately has already been mentioned. Additional economies are achieved by the fact that this equipment and personnel can be used to greater advantage by the group than by an individual physician. Many a general physician, for example, has in his office costly x-ray and physical therapy equipment which he can use but a few hours each day, but in a group such equipment can be kept busy to the limit of its capacity.

Second, physicians in group practice are apt to earn, whether because of the economies achieved or for other reasons, much higher net incomes, on the average, than those in individual practice. A recent study by "Medical Economics," for instance, showed that in 1947 whereas physicians in solo practice received an average gross income of approximately $18,000 and a net of $11,000 physicians in partnership or group practice averaged $27,000 gross and $16,500 net. While amounts of earning are obviously not necessarily commensurate with quality of care, the possibility of a better living would seem bound, in the long run, to aid in attracting the better trained physician to group practice. The advantages of steady income and, in many groups, of a planned retirement system are other influences of the same character. The joy to a physician of being relieved of the tedious burden of business management, of hiring personnel, purchasing, setting and collecting fees, offered by a medical group through its business manager, is a third advantage in the economic area which not only attracts the best type of physician but leaves him free to devote his full time and energy to his professional work.

But above all, from the standpoint of quality of care, the financial arrangements of group practice induce coöperative rather than competitive effort on the part of the physicians of a group. A healthy competitive element exists over the years, of course, in any group, because each physician wants to demonstrate his value to the group as a whole and thus his right to a larger share of the proceeds—even this is a stimulant for high quality in a physician's service. But for the daily work of rendering medical services, the economic as well as the professional incentives in group practice lead toward coöperation and, therefore, improved quality. For in a group, the good work done by any individual physician reflects credit on the whole group. Discredit for the whole group obviously results likewise from any physician's poor work. Therefore, all physicians of a group, if only from purely economic motives, are constantly stimulated to do good quality work themselves and, equally important, to urge their associates to attain the same ideal.

In most existing medical groups, the physician's share of the group's net income is based upon his competence and his general value to the group as a whole. These shares are usually not determined primarily by the number of patients seen or the number of services rendered by a given physician, although such matters may be taken into account. As a result, individual physicians in a group lose no income when they refer a patient to another physician, and have no financial incentive to "hold on" to a case personally. Rather, the financial interest of each physician is best served if the most thorough and satisfactory job possible is done for the patient by the group as a whole, so that the group as such may attract and keep a good clientele. Thus, the economic incentives of group practice encourage physicians to make use of the varied skills of their colleagues and of the group's laboratory and x-ray services for diagnosis and treatment as fully as may be medically desirable for the patient's benefit. Such teamwork medicine is of course the essence of group practice, and is obviously necessary to produce a high quality of care amid the complexities of modern medicine which cannot conceivably be grasped by any one physician alone. So we see that economic incentives for high quality, as powerful as the professional ones mentioned earlier, spring from the nature of the group method itself.

The value of group medical practice in improving the quality of medical care is not limited, however, to the positive advantages to be found within a medical group. It arises also in a negative sense, from the fact that group practice, and as far as can now be ascertained only group practice, will serve to correct many of the evils apparently inherent in the individual, competitive practice of medicine on a fee-for-service basis. These evils are in large part of recent origin and do not spring primarily from any malign intent on the part of the physician as a person but rather from the sane scientific advances which have made teamwork in medicine necessary and desirable. Some of these evils have been referred to by implication in describing the advantages of group practice. The waste by duplication in individual offices of often inadequate but nevertheless costly technical equipment and associated personnel, rarely used to their fullest effectiveness, is one example. Another is the waste of the time and skill of the young physician in individual practice who must frequently spend much time in idleness before his talents can be fully utilized. The expensive equipment and highly skilled associated personnel and the long and costly training of the young physician, all of which are in part wasted in solo practice, are, of course, necessitated by the tremendous advances in medical science. All are too precious to waste. Group practice, especially in association with better training of personnel, regional planning, and sound administration can go far toward eliminating this waste.

But of all the evils of individual practice which the group method can eliminate, the most serious is the chaotic state of the relationships of the general practitioner and the various types of specialists with each other and the effects of these relationships upon the care of patients. Clearly, from the patient's point of view, he should be referred to the various types of specialists and provided with laboratory and x-ray examinations as frequently as necessary for the management of his case according to the best standards of scientific medicine, but no more so. Obviously, the exact optimum for such referrals is often impossible to determine in any given case but, over the long run, something very close to it can be achieved in a well organized medical group or on the wards of a teaching hospital. There is no doubt that the optimum can be and sometimes is achieved in solo practice, especially for relatively well educated and well-to-do patients. But the barriers to a proper use of teamwork in individual practice make attainment of this goal exceedingly difficult at best.

On the one hand, the physician in isolated practice may refer his patients to others too infrequently. He may fail to use others' services, for one thing, simply because his years in solo practice have so limited the horizons of his knowledge that he does not even realize that his patient might gain from special tests or consultants' opinions. He may hesitate, too, to refer a patient for consultation or other special service because of the cost to the patient. This may also be true in group practice, of course, but to a lesser extent because, in the first place, the group can control the fees for *all* the services the patient needs and can temper the wind when necessary, while the individual practitioner usually cannot greatly influence the fees set by the individual consultants to whom he refers patients. Second, it is the practice in many medical groups—and a good practice for improving quality—to make no charge for consultations; specialists' fees are charged only when the patient has been transferred to the specialist for continuing study or treatment.

But probably the strongest motive against utilizing referral services to full effectiveness in individual practice is the competitive element. In its crudest form, this means that a physician may not refer his patient to another physician for fear that he may "lose" his patient (and his fee) permanently to the second doctor. More subtly, it means that a physician may fear that by calling for frequent consultations he will undermine the patient's confidence in his own ability. He may believe that his reputation for self-reliance, broad medical knowledge and skill will suffer among his colleagues if he calls on others too much. Most of all, perhaps, he may fear that the consultant will find errors in his work and "show him up" to both the patient and the profession.

For all these reasons and for at least one more, namely, the sheer physical inconvenience to the patient of going about from one office to another, making numerous appointments with varying periods of delay before seeing the different doctors, there is an inevitable tendency in individual practice not to employ the full medical team to the extent it should be used for realizing the full potential of modern medical service of high quality. The physician in solo practice, therefore, is often obliged to try to perform a range of service up to and sometimes beyond the limits of his technical capacity. This, of course, adversely affects the quality of service obtained by the patient and, in the long run, tends to produce in the physician a habit of superficial performance, trusting to luck and nature that his lack of thoroughness and of specialized knowledge will not cause errors resulting in serious disablement or death. On the other hand, somewhat paradoxically, the physician in individual practice may under some circumstances refer his patients too *frequently* to other physicians. Here the practice of fee-splitting rears its ugly head. Fee-splitting, like the other evils mentioned, does not occur because of any desire of physicians to perpetuate a harmful practice, but arises almost inevitably out of the character of the individual practice system. I dare say it will continue, in spite of all the laws and professional pronouncements that can be devised, as long as this system is the prevalent method of practice. Here again, the basic reason is the advances in medical science which make specialization a necessity. One can hardly expect the general physician who has correctly diagnosed a case of appendicitis on a $10 house call not to feel that he deserves a lot of the credit for saving the patient's life and not to gaze at the surgeon's $200 or $300 fee with some envy. Moreover, one can understand that the specialist (particularly the young one, just starting in practice) in a fiercely competitive situation may yearn to reward tangibly the general physicians who most assist him in building up his practice by referring cases to him.

But it is not the act of splitting a fee that makes this practice an evil and an impediment to a high quality of medical care. It is, rather, the fact that the split is unknown to the patient and unregulated in amount and volume. Thus, the patient does not know, when he buys a pair of eyeglasses from an optician, for example, that part of what he pays may go back to the doctor who referred him to that optician. The same is true, of course, for x-rays, surgical procedures, and so on. The result of hidden fee-splitting is that if a sizeable split is in the offing the physician may be tempted to refer patients more frequently than is medically necessary and to send his cases to the doctor or laboratory or optician who gives the biggest kickback rather than the one professionally most competent to handle the case. The magnitude of the practice of fee-splitting may perhaps be gauged by the fact that more than 4,000 eye specialists—about one-half of those in the United States—were involved when the U. S. Department of Justice sought to stamp out rebates in the optical industry.

The utter futility, under our individual practice system, of expecting the medical profession to cope with this evil is illustrated by what occurred in New York City in the fee-splitting scandals under workmen's compensation a few years ago. Almost 2,800 physicians were charged with participation in the fee-splitting racket. One hundred and seventeen were definitely exonerated. More than 1,000 were definitely found to have been implicated. A few lost their licenses to practice medicine. But a diligent, personal search of the published records of all medical societies in New York fails to disclose a *single* instance in which any of the remaining 900 "definitely implicated" physicians were suspended or expelled by a medical society. This is a commentary not only upon the durability of fee-splitting in the individual practice system, but also upon the ability of medical societies to set and maintain professional standards in general. It is in interesting contrast with the promptness and vigor displayed by medical societies in disciplining members who participate in group practice associated with prepayment plans for comprehensive medical care.

Group practice is sometimes considered to be a type of fee-splitting. This is *true* in the sense that a patient's payment is divided according to the group's internal administrative provisions, and does not go exclusively to the doctor or doctors who treated that particular patient. But group practice most emphatically is *not* fee-splitting in the sense that this open division of income among the physicians of a group is *never* a kickback paid for favors received. The patient knows all along that he is paying the group for his service, not an individual physician, and he fully expects the group to divide its income equitably among its members. So division of income by the group method completely eliminates the evils of the hidden kickback system and yet, at the same time, provides a distribution of income among general physicians and specialists more equitable than is possible in solo practice unless fees are split. . . .

49. DISADVANTAGES *

CRITICS OF GROUP practice deny some of these advantages categorically but generally take the stand that the advantages are theoretical and that, although they may be true for a few groups, the great majority of groups not only fall far short of the theoretical ideal but also replace alleged advantages with actual faults. The most important criticism is that most patients can be adequately treated by an individual practitioner with the equipment that any physician would have in his office and that it is inefficient, time consuming and unduly expensive to give every patient the questionable benefit of being treated by two or more physicians in offices fitted out with all the latest diagnostic and therapeutic equipment. This sort of treatment should be reserved for the approximately 15 per cent of patients who really need more than the general practitioner can give them. In addition, the physician in a group is deprived to some extent of independence of judgment and action, and his professional growth is stunted by constant supervision. A physician may get some stimulation from his intimate associations within a group, but he thereby cuts himself off from association with the larger number of physicians in his community, so that he actually suffers a net loss in this respect. The prospect of higher income in group practice is illusory and materializes only for the physician with poor training or personality who could not succeed in individual practice: the well trained physician can make more in individual practice. (This claim, incidentally, is concurred in by many of the advocates of group practice, who contend that group practice is the best way to practice honest, satisfying medicine, but is not the way to make the most money.) The group's claim for ease of consultation and availability of laboratory service is conceded to be of value in medically undeveloped regions but is said to be of decreasing importance as a region develops specialists, hospitals and laboratories, which enable the practitioner who is not allied with a group to pick the best consultant or laboratory to care for the particular illness of the particular patient, whereas the group physician is limited in his referrals or laboratory work to the available specialists or equipment within the group. Mechanization of medicine, with undue dependence on a dragnet type of laboratory workup, and referral of patients without adequate medical reason are alleged. Allied to these are the allegations that in some groups every patient is "sent through the mill" of referrals and laboratory work, that "made work" is thrown to the less busy members, or that consultations are ordered

* From: "Medical Group Practice in the United States," by G. Halsey Hunt, M.D.; *New England Journal of Medicine* 237: 71-77, July 17, 1947 (No. 3). Reprinted (with omissions, including initial paragraphs) by permission of the author and publishers. The author is chief of the Center for Aging Research, in the National Heart Institute, Public Health Service, Washington, D.C.

with an eye on the fee rather than for any medical indication. The obvious advantages of concentration of equipment and the handling of finances by a business manager are often more than counterbalanced by the economic necessity of making the large investment in building and equipment pay its way and by the interjection of business persons untrained in medical ethics into the relations between patient and physician, with the results that unethical promotion and publicity policies often develop. The patient-doctor relation is further disrupted by the fact that a patient does not have "his doctor" who knows and understands him, but has a whole set of physicians, each of whom concerns himself with only a fraction of the patient's person. (Advocates of group practice are somewhat divided regarding the desirability of having a "personal physician" for each patient, but they all agree that such a relation can be maintained in group practice as easily as in individual practice.) The patient's choice of physician, which is ordinarily present in his original choice, is lost as soon as referral becomes necessary, since he is limited to the specialists within the group. Furthermore, many groups that set themselves up as giving complete specialist coverage actually have inadequately trained physicians posing as specialists. This is claimed to apply especially to groups having prepayment plans.

These controversial and contradictory sets of statements may be roughly divided into those having to do with medical care per se and those having to do with medical ethics. It will be noted that the former are by implication largely concerned with the practices of service groups. Reference groups receive tacit approval if their specialists are of reasonably adequate caliber and if they avoid unethical practices. The statements that seem to attack group practice as such apply principally to the practices of service groups and with double force to the service groups that have prepayment plans. On the other hand, some of the advantages claimed for group practice also apply to the larger groups with diversified well trained specialists rather than to the small service groups.

It may be said, then, that whereas the fundamental question in group practice concerns its ability to provide medical care, as compared with that afforded by individual practice, realistic consideration of this problem requires that it be broken into two parts—the provision of general medical care and the provision of specialist care. It is essential to determine the extent to which groups carry out each of these functions and to evaluate their success in each case. To what extent does a specific group act as (and replace) a general practitioner, and to what extent is it a specialist? What are the trends in a given group or set of groups—toward increasing reference work or toward a greater volume of general-medical-care work?

Analysis of the controversy from this point of view, and in the light of the preceding paragraphs, shows that the real differences of opinion about group practice center around three basic considerations: whether the great majority (80 to 90 per cent) of sick people suffer from illnesses that can be adequately treated by a well trained general practitioner without consultation; if so, whether it is not wasteful to set up a group organization, with specialists and laboratory equipment, to take care of these ordinary and easily treated illnesses; and whether the 10 to 20 per cent of patients who need specialist care will not receive better care if their physician is free to refer them to the best specialist (or reference group) available for their particular illness, than if he has to refer them to the specialist within his own group, even though better specialists are available outside the group.

Answers to these questions and to such related and subsidiary questions as the role and functions of the individual general practitioner in service groups involve some degree of interpretation and therefore will never be supplied by any simple accumulation of facts; until the questions can be discussed in terms of facts rather than theories and impressions, however, little progress toward their elucidation can be made....

50. GROUP PRACTICE AND FREE CHOICE *

EVER SINCE THERE has been organized care of the sick, the medical profession has been fighting for the right of the patient, no matter what his social position, to choose his own doctor; the right of the individual physician to participate in programs for the sick; and the right of the professional association to be consulted in selecting the physicians to be admitted to service. The medical profession has been, and is, maintaining that the preservation of the principle of free choice is basic. Freedom of choice, it is asserted, benefits the patient because confidence in the ability, integrity, and discretion of the physician plays a most important part in the care of the sick; serves the interests of the profession because it offers all competent members opportunity to work; and is to the advantage of the public at large because it safeguards the quality of care. However, even the staunchest supporters of the free choice principle admit limitations upon its application to be indispensable to the successful operation of any program of medical care no matter how it is financed. It is widely acknowledged that the family doctor should be chosen from among those practicing within the geographical area in which the patient resides, that specialists ordinarily should be consulted only on referral from a general practitioner, and that a change from one doctor to another during the same illness or within a certain period of time should be contingent upon presentation of valid reasons.

All these principles can be maintained—and strengthened—by proper organization of group practice.

Obviously if all local physicians work together in a center, the patient is as free to select his family doctor as under the system of individual practice. All he has to do is to state his preference at the center, if he has not already established a relationship before.

If in the same community some physicians belong to groups and others are engaged in individual practice, then, indeed, difficulties may arise. Presuming that free

* From: *Public Medical Care: Principles and Problems*, by Franz Goldmann, M.D.; New York: Columbia University Press, 1945 (Chap. VI, "Planning for Medical Care," pp. 177-78). Reprinted (with omissions, including initial paragraphs) by permission of the author and publishers. The author is associate professor of medical care at the School of Public Health, Harvard University, Boston, Mass.

choice is as fundamental as the vast literature and legislative action in its favor indicate, then there cannot be any "ifs" and "buts." A patient who wants to choose a group of physicians as such rather than a doctor in individual practice must be free to do so. Physicians who wish to offer their services as a group must have as much right to participate in a community program as their colleagues conducting their practice in the traditional form. A community must be permitted to select the method of organization best suited to its conditions. Objective interpretation of the principle of free choice precludes its use as an argument against group practice. But it cannot be denied that the operation of group clinics in communities where there are also a number of physicians in individual practice may pose a problem. At its core is the question of competition rather than that of free choice, and this fact must be recognized. The natural way out of this dilemma is to offer the opportunity to practice in groups to all qualified physicians in a community.

To finance the building and equipment of medical centers and to organize the payment for professional services a variety of methods may be employed. There is no innate relationship between group practice and methods of finance. As W. J. Mayo said: "Properly considered, group medicine is not a financial arrangement, except for minor details, but a scientific cooperation for the welfare of the sick." However, group practice will only gain in value if the savings it affords are passed on to the "consumer". . . .

51. A MEDICAL GROUP IN OPERATION *

THE SUMMIT [N. J.] group stemmed from the large private practices of its founders, Drs. Maynard G. Bensley and William H. Lawrence, who felt they could do justice neither to their patients nor to themselves without associates. Today, a staff of eighteen physicians, including five general practitioners, offers a comprehensive service embracing office, home, and hospital care. Specialties represented on the staff include general and orthopedic surgery, internal medicine, cardiology, obstetrics, gynecology, pediatrics, ophthalmology, ENT, urology, allergy-dermatology, anesthesia, X-ray, and physiotherapy.

About 50 per cent of the group's patients live in Summit, a residential community of some 20,000 people, and its surrounding area. The rest are drawn by the group's reputation from other parts of New Jersey and in a measure from outside the state.

Patients referred to the Summit group by family physicians are returned to the referring doctors after diagnosis has been established. If surgery or specialized care

* From: "The Summit Medical Group," by Arthur E. Soderberg; *Medical Economics* 23: 78-85, June 1946 (No. 6). Reprinted (with omissions, including initial paragraph) from *Medical Economics* by special permission. Copyright 1946, Medical Economics, Inc., Rutherford, N.J.

is indicated, the family doctor is so advised. In sum, the code of ethics is rigidly observed; only those patients who come of their own accord are accepted for full care.

Referrals average around 15 per cent of the total patient load. Approximately ten out of every 100 patients come to the group for a general diagnostic work-up requiring the services of several specialists.

In its two-story, eighty-room medical building, the Summit group handles about 300 ambulatory patients a day. Another 75 or so are seen daily in homes and in the three nearby hospitals with which the staff physicians are associated.

The group conducts itself as a limited partnership: Ten physicians, each with a capital investment, are group shareholders and, as such, are guaranteed an annual return of 8 per cent on their investment. In addition, these men divide the net income of the group with seven non-shareholders on a pre-established percentage basis. (The remaining member of the staff, a physician on a part-time basis, also shares in the profits.)

Each department—surgery, obstetrics, general practice, etc.—is charged 25 per cent of its own gross income for group overhead, plus an additional 5 per cent which goes into a reserve fund for future expansion. The net is then divided between the department's senior (or seniors) and its associates, if any, on the pre-established percentage basis.

The group has no established fee schedule; each doctor sets his own fees, basing them on his patient's ability to pay. Investigation of a patient's financial status, when needed, is made by the business office. Fees charged by members of the group are comparable to those of the more successful solo practitioners nearby.

Patients are billed in the name of the group, and bills are itemized only on request. About 25 per cent of the accounts are handled on a cash basis. Bad debts average only 2.5 per cent. All collections are taken care of by the business office.

Approximately 4 per cent of the patients are indigents referred to the group by private welfare organizations which foot the bills—at substantially reduced rates.

Office hours are maintained from 8 A.M. to 6 P.M. and from 7 to 9 P.M. daily, except Sundays, and the majority of patients are seen by appointment. Emergency care, however, is available twenty-four hours a day, with the G.P. staff handling all night and Sunday calls.

Staff members work about eight hours a day, five days a week, and are on call the sixth day. Certain specialists see patients during the evening hours once or twice a week.

Each partner's equity in the group is protected by a life insurance policy. If he dies or retires he or his estate receives a cash settlement, representing his full investment, in return for a release to the group of the deceased's equity in the partnership. The terms of the partnership make it impossible for a lay person to become a shareholder through the death of a principal. If a physician-partner retires without disposing of his equity to another doctor, he continues to receive his annual 8 per cent return.

In the event of the death of a partner, his accounts receivable are carried in his name for a period of six months, and the proceeds therefrom are paid to his estate in the regular departmental division of net income. At the end of that period, the receivables are purchased by the group at a stipulated rate of thirty cents on the dollar.

At present, the group has no retirement or annuity program for its staff members. It is, however, contemplating a waiver of the 30 per cent expense and sinking-fund charge after the completion of twenty years' service. It is also considering some form of protection for physicians who suffer permanent disability.

Administrative control is in the hands of an executive committee which determines professional and business policies; there is no administrative officer and no medical director. An executive committee, a finance committee, and an expansion committee take care of other administrative matters. To settle any major issues which arise, the executive committee may call an open meeting at which all physicians, whether partners or not, have a voice in determining policy. Any staff physician is eligible for election to any of the committees. The executive committee meets weekly, and two group meetings a month are devoted to business matters.

Ownership of land, building, and equipment is lodged in a holding company controlled by the partnership. Thus the laws which forbid the practice of medicine by a corporation are in no way violated by the group.

To become a member of the group's specialty staff a physician must be a specialty-board diplomate or demonstrate to the satisfaction of the entire staff that he possesses education, ability, and experience equivalent to that of a diplomate. He must also be a member of organized medicine. During his first two years with the group, he is on probation; after that, he becomes a permanent staff man and may not be ousted except by unanimous consent of all members of the group.

All physicians are required to attend weekly group meetings of the staff. Formal post-graduate study is not required, but the average Summit physician spends one month each year taking such courses and another month on vacation. As yet, the group has no teaching program of its own, but soon hopes to inaugurate one for the benefit of its members.

The auxiliary staff includes twelve registered nurses, three laboratory technicans, and three X-ray technicians. The business office is headed by an office manager who works under the close supervision of the finance committee; he has three clerical assistants. Four secretaries take care of the doctors' correspondence and records; one of these secretaries doubles as case historian. There are three receptionists; and four switchboard operators are required to handle the day and night calls.

The Summit group accepts pre-payment patients who are subscribers to the state medical society's voluntary plan. Also under consideration is a plan to provide service to patients on a postpayment budgetary basis. . . .

The [group's medical] building houses an extensively equipped laboratory and X-ray department, as well as all necessary equipment for EENT work, physiotherapy, electrocardiography, and basal metabolism.

The original structure was erected on land owned by Dr. Lawrence. For some five years,* the founders operated the group as a two-man partnership, employing

* That is, from the founding of the group in 1928, to 1933.

physicians on a salary-plus-bonus basis. In time, it was felt that the individual practitioner's stake in the group could be enhanced and his income increased through his own efforts if he had a vested interest in the enterprise. With this in mind, the present shareholding plan was adopted in 1933.

At first, the group encountered considerable hostility from the local county medical society and from practitioners in the area. But the feeling waned as the group demonstrated both its ability to practice good medicine and its strict adherence to the code of ethics. Some seventy-five physicians practice independently in the same area; consequently, earlier charges of "monopoly" are heard only rarely today.

According to staff physicians, the Summit form of organization disproves completely the widely held feeling that group practice is a refuge for doctors who can't quite make the grade by themselves. "The man coming into our group," explains one specialist, "knows that we are really operating as individuals, but on a collective basis. Moreover, he knows that in our group he must possess the same requisites in the way of education, ability, and experience that he would need for success in solo practice.

"In addition, he must have the sort of personality that will enable him to function well as a member of a smooth-running team. If he can fill the bill in these respects, he will benefit in many ways: His medical knowledge will be advanced by close association with men in various fields; he will earn more money than he probably would as a solo practitioner; he will have adequate time for post-graduate study; he will have no bookkeeping and collection worries; he will have access to the best type of diagnostic and therapeutic equipment; and he will be less vulnerable to malpractice suits. In my opinion, he will also find that the doctor-patient relationship is definitely enhanced in group practice—for group specialists, particularly the obstetrician and the surgeon, invariably enjoy the same sort of respect the patient and his family have always accorded to the general practitioner." ...

B. *Regionalization*

52. THE REGIONAL CONCEPT *

MANY CURRENT problems in the field of medical care, medical education and public health, account for the increasing trend toward regional coordination of health services. In turn, many of the needs in widely different fields of professional activity

* From: "Regionalization of Medical Services," by E. Richard Weinerman, M.D.; *Annual of the Western Branch* (American Public Health Association), 1949, pp. 38-48. Reprinted (with omissions, including initial paragraphs) by permission of the author and publishers. The author practices internal medicine in El Cerrito, Calif.

can be approached through such careful planning. Current problems which may be met, at least in part, through the regional concept include:

1. The need to correct the present haphazard, unrelated conglomeration of hospital facilities.

2. The need to improve the inadequate and low quality resources available to medical practice in many outlying and underprivileged areas of the United States.

3. The need to modify the maldistribution of doctors, hospitals, and the like, which now reflect the economic status rather than health needs of a community.

4. The problem of the isolation and professional and technical limitations of many small hospitals.

5. The need for improvements in patterns of undergraduate professional education, and the need for development of a continuous system of postgraduate education.

6. The hope that new institutions being constructed under the Hill-Burton Act may some day function in real coordination with existing facilities.

7. The need to delineate health service areas according to natural trade lines and normal population movement, rather than only in conformance with existing boundaries or political jurisdiction.

8. The need for greater integration of public health and clinical medical services.

It seems clear, then, that current public health, medical care, hospital service and professional education problems can all find common ground in this regional approach.

Social and political scientists have long recognized the advantages of utilizing natural geographical and trade areas rather than the unwieldy boundaries of political units. In a recent issue of the *American Journal of Public Health,* Professor J. E. Ivey stated that "Regionalism as a science is concerned with the measurement of existing environmental capacity and with the social engineering of potential environmental capacity."

The medical service region, then, within which health facilities are to be coordinated can be carefully planned in accordance with a number of important factors. These include: (a) population density and movement, (b) natural and geographical characteristics, (c) income, occupation, and other socio-economic data, (d) cultural traditions and characteristics of the area, (e) regular marketing patterns and lines of trade movement, (f) transportation and communication facilities, (g) supply and distribution of medical personnel and hospital facilities, (h) lines of patient-flow and physician-referrals, (i) supply and adequacy of medical and related teaching facilities, and (j) boundaries of existing political units and their administrative jurisdiction.

Throughout the nation such health service regions can be delineated by the proper analysis of such factors. Each health service region can develop within itself the elements of a self-sufficient and comprehensive health system. The outlines of such a concept have long since been worked out by economists and sociologists, and have been given specific medical coloration in studies conducted by the American Medical Association, the United States Public Health Service, a Senate War-time

Committee on Health and Education, the National Commission on Hospital Care, State agencies responsible for the operation of the Hill-Burton Act, and many interested foundations and universities. In our own State of California the recently submitted report on the Survey of Hospital Facilities concluded with a strong recommendation for coordinated district planning.

Here in the County of Los Angeles, a brilliant coordinated hospital plan has recently been worked out by James Hamilton and his associates and remains on file crying for some kind of implementing local action.

Elements of the Regional System

WITHIN CAREFULLY delineated health service regions, medical facilities of all kinds can be coordinated. The elements of the network include the metropolitan *medical teaching centers* as the base or the nucleus. Specialty hospitals, chronic care institutions and rehabilitation facilities can be appropriately coordinated with the medical center. Peripheral to the base institution are the larger and smaller *community hospitals* of the region, sometimes referred to as *district hospitals*. *Community health centers* or small *rural hospitals* constitute the outpost facilities of the system. At every level of the network, public health units should and are being correlated. All such facilities more completely approach the concept of real community medical centers as individual and group practice offices of private physicians and dentists are included within the local facility.

The Medical Center.—Wherever possible the central regional institution is based in a teaching medical center, preferably in a university. Here are combined the medical, dental, nursing, public health and hospital administration facilities necessary for an all-inclusive regional center. The center includes all resources necessary to the region for service, consultation, training and research.

The District or Community Hospital.—The hospitals of the moderate size communities in the region, ranging from fifty to two hundred beds in the community hospital, or two to four hundred beds in the district hospital, form the next echelon of the network. Here all *basic* medical and surgical services would be provided, including necessary laboratory and x-ray facilities, with training opportunities for interns, residents, nurses, and certain technicians. The community hospitals would include (or affiliate with) certain specialized institutions such as tuberculosis sanatoria or mental hospitals. These community hospitals would service the smaller units peripherally and, in turn, obtain certain aids from the larger base at the medical teaching center.

The Community Health Center.—The key unit of the entire network is the community health and medical center—to serve residential urban communities as well as suburban and rural areas. This is the place where the basic relationships between the population and the health service teams occur. Ideally, the community health center should include clinic and laboratory facilities; a small number of hospital beds sufficient only to care for emergencies and, perhaps, for obstetrical cases that are uncomplicated; facilities for the local public health department and voluntary agencies in the community; plus the private offices, wherever possible, of individual or group practitioners. In this way the facility becomes, in fact, a health center for the entire community.

Functions of the Coordinated Hospital System

FOR ALL THE scientific delineation of regional cases, and for all the fancy network of hospital and health center buildings, the entire purpose and importance of the concept depends upon what happens functionally within the system. Here we must recognize the potentialities for a continuous two-way flow of personnel, materials, and, to a minor degree, patients among the various specialized levels of the network.

In the first place, the standards and practices of *hospital operation and administration* can be inordinately enhanced. Administrative consultation, joint conferences, and continuous training programs can be, and are being, organized. Uniform cost accounting and other procedural methods can be worked out for all the hospitals in the area. Improved and coordinated record systems, joint purchasing operations, standardized training courses for auxiliary and technical personnel, all are possible of achievement. New construction in the area or expansion of existing facilities can be planned on an over-all basis as is not possible in individual operations.

The second important function involves the *extension of diagnostic and other medical services*. In a coordinated system, the specialized personnel and the complex equipment of district and regional hospitals can be utilized by the smaller community institutions that are unable, within themselves, to provide adequate laboratory, x-ray, pathology, EKG, anesthesia, and other services that their patients need. Not only may laboratory specimens, x-ray plates, and the like be sent forward for interpretation and reporting, but specialized personnel from the higher centers can regularly visit the outlying institutions for consultation and service.

The third important feature is that of *continuous professional and technical education*. Within such a system teaching and consulting personnel from the bigger centers can regularly visit the outlying institutions and conduct ward rounds, teaching clinics, conferences, and the like. A systematic consultation and referral system is possible. At the same time, local personnel can visit the bigger centers for long and short refresher and specialized training courses. This is true not only of physicians, but of nurses, laboratory technicians, and other specialized personnel. Only in such an organized regional program is it possible to send itinerant substitute technicians or locum tenens physicians to take the place of the local personnel studying at the center who might not otherwise be able to get away. A tremendous advantage in such a system is the ability of the medical, dental, nursing, and other professional schools to utilize the entire system in their teaching program, thus to orient their students to the full complex of health needs and health services. Similarly, interns and residents can rotate through the system, broaden the entire base of their training, perhaps become stimulated to settle in some of the suburban and rural areas of the region, and—at the same time—bring to the practitioners of the local community hospitals the fresh point of view and the new concepts from the teaching centers.

The final feature of the system is the possibility of *referring particularly difficult or specially characterized patients* to such higher echelons of service as may be deemed necessary by the attending physician. While this concept does make the full facilities of the largest medical teaching center available to all the patients anywhere in the region, it is *not* particularly a desired aim of this sort of program to move everybody out of the local communities into the big metropolitan area. On the contrary, by making available so many specialized services to the local physician and hospital, far more patients can be handled adequately and completely in their own community.

The two-way flow, therefore, of administrative activity, of medical extension services of professional and technical personnel, of laboratory and other diagnostic specimens and of patients is the feature that breathes the life into the entire system.

Financial Arrangements

REGIONAL SYSTEMS now operating are able to call upon the resources of a centralized fund and can utilize this money for the financing of those educational, consultative, and service features which characterize the regional plan. In addition, participating hospitals can and do pay part or all the cost of the services which are being made available to them. In the last analysis it is, of course, the patient, whether through prepayment devices or regular charges, who supports the great bulk of the actual services provided.

It is this matter of financing which today causes the primary problems which regional systems have not yet been able to solve. In the first place, most operating programs today are financed as demonstration activities by various of the philanthropic foundations. This, of course, cannot be considered a permanent basis for financing such a movement. On the other hand, no matter how efficient and desirable this new pattern of service may be in an area, those patients now unable to obtain needed medical and hospital services do not reap the benefits of the higher standards achieved. Furthermore, physicians taking care of privately paying patients are reluctant to ship them off to distant places and competing specialists. The individual patient, moreover, is not always able to undertake the cost of all the regional services, the travel, and the other features involved.

The need would seem clear, then, to integrate this entire concept of regional planning into the two great patterns of financing which are developing in this country. One is to make this sort of development the basis for the federal-state program of hospital construction, as embodied in the Hill-Burton Act. The second is to integrate this concept into whatever over-all system of medical care financing we finally adopt in this country, so that those financial barriers to proper patient movement and physician referral within the region will no longer operate. It is in this connection that we can see that the regional organization of hospitals within natural health service regions not only elevates the general quality of medical care available to the individual patient, but makes it possible for him to receive a greater scope, range, and quantity of needed medical services—especially in nonmetropolitan places.

Public Health Aspects

CURRENTLY THERE is an unfortunate separation between many public health and medical service activities. Most of us would agree that the line between prevention and cure in health services is rapidly disappearing. Medical care programs, on the one hand, are placing insufficient emphasis on prevention and public health programs, on the other, are missing many opportunities in the community control of disease due to their isolation from existing treatment and diagnostic facilities. By coordinating both the facilities and the functions of preventive and curative medicine in this regional hospital concept, this long delayed "rapprochement" can be achieved. This trend is in direct line with a recently issued joint statement on coordination of hospitals and health departments released by the APHA and the American Hospital Association.*

Current Regional Plans and Planning

WHILE THIS regional concept is not new, neither is it untried. A sketch of a few of the successfully operating current regional systems may be of interest. . . .

The Bingham Associates' Fund in New England.—With the financial support of the Bingham Associates' Fund and the Rockefeller Foundation, a regional program has been operating in New England ever since 1931. The base medical center here is the Pratt Diagnostic Hospital affiliated with Tufts Medical College and it maintains typical regional affiliations with two or three district hospitals in nearby smaller cities. Through them over twenty small community facilities in Maine and western Massachusetts are affiliated. Patients are referred centrally for diagnostic and therapeutic aid, local doctors and auxiliary personnel move to the district and Boston institutions for consultation and instruction, while a peripheral flow of technical aides and teaching personnel proceed concurrently. Emphasis is placed upon the continuous education of the community physician through detailed case reports, follow-up literature, visiting ward rounds, conferences, and refresher courses. Laboratory and diagnostic assistance is available to the outlying unit. Plans are developing for the rotation of medical and surgical residents through the community hospitals. Full-time pathologists and other medical specialists are made available to the cooperative community hospitals.

The Rochester Plan.—A similar regionalization project has been financed by the Commonwealth Fund, centered around the University of Rochester Medical School and the six larger hospitals in the City of Rochester, New York. Whereas the Bing-

* See, for text of this joint statement, Selection No. 54C (in Section C of present chapter).

ham program is merely a loose and informal affiliation of hospitals, the Rochester system has been formally organized into the definite Council of Rochester Regional Hospitals. It is interesting to note in this connection that the medical director of the council is also the health officer of the City of Rochester. Some twenty-six community hospitals are affiliated in this program, which involves a good deal of coordination of administrative procedure, the promulgation of a voluntarily accepted manual of medical staff procedures, a program of visiting professional consultants and teachers from the central hospitals, a series of special courses in the Rochester centers, rotation through local hospitals of interns and residents from the city hospitals, extension of x-ray, pathology, anesthesia, and other services, establishment of a regional blood bank, and the granting of funds for capital construction and improvement purposes out of the central regional treasury.

Other Plans.—Many other programs, including a greater or lesser number of the features potentially possible in such a system, have been operating throughout the country. A small plan, but one similar to the Rochester system and also financed by Commonwealth has been developed around the Medical College of Virginia in Richmond. The New York University Medical School has recently announced teaching and service affiliations with seven suburban and rural hospitals in its vicinity. The Kellogg Foundation is supporting this program. At the University of Michigan teaching affiliation with some nineteen outlying hospitals throughout the state has been going on, at least in part, ever since 1927. Other medical schools developing such programs in affiliation with community hospitals include the Colorado University Medical School, the medical schools at Minnesota, Tulane, Bowman Gray, Iowa, and some others. Here in our own state, some preliminary conferences have been held with the Deans of both medical schools in Los Angeles and with the Professor of Medicine at the University of California Medical School in San Francisco. Their interest in this trend has been manifest. Particularly comprehensive planning which has not yet been translated into operation is under way at the University of North Carolina, at the Long Island College Medical School and more recently at the Massachusetts General Hospital. . . .

C. *Integrating Prevention and Cure*

53. PREVENTION AND THE PRACTICING PHYSICIAN *

WHEN WE SPEAK of "preventive medicine" we are very apt to think primarily of the brilliant sweep of modern public health science across the country, reducing or even

* From: "Group Practice in Preventive Medicine," by Dean A. Clark, M.D.; *American Journal of Public Health* 37: 264-68, March 1947 (No. 3). Reprinted (with omissions) by permission of the author and publishers. The author is the general director of Massachusetts General Hospital in Boston.

eliminating water-borne and milk-borne infections, venereal diseases, malaria, yellow fever, or typhus. Or perhaps we have in mind the prevention of the ravages of diphtheria through mass immunization. But usually we put as distinctly secondary the innumerable preventive measures for the individual that must so largely be carried out by the practising physician. Yet today it is these individual preventive measures which constitute the main hope for the prevention of disease and disability.

As a matter of fact, if we are to understand the potential scope of prevention by modern techniques, we must agree that "Any procedure which serves to ward off disease or maintain health is to be considered preventive medicine." This definition, phrased by William Davis [1] is broad indeed but none too broad to make clear the real issues we are facing. Davis continues: "Such preventive procedures defy classification into rigid groups, for they range from the impersonal measures of environmental sanitation to curative medicine for the individual. Is the hospitalization and treatment of a woman with typhoid fever to be called curative medicine for her or preventive medicine for the community? Should the early treatment of syphilis be classified under contagious diseases or under the prevention of mental disease? If a man has a job where he eats irregularly, is tense, and has indigestion, and he sees his doctor and as a result gains insight into his anxiety, is placed at a different job in his industry, goes on a better diet and gets well, is this a triumph for gastroenterology? or industrial hygiene? or nutrition? or psychosomatic medicine? And is it curative of anxiety or preventive of a stomach ulcer?"

The point is, obviously, that preventive and curative medicine are no longer separable (if indeed they ever were); both must be included in anything we would wish to recognize as complete medical care. The health officer and the practitioner are both involved in preventive medicine today—in fact, the larger share now belongs to the practitioner, although many in both the public health and the medical professions fail to recognize it as yet.

Take, for example, the prevention of communicable disease, traditionally the realm of the health department. In the case of measles, it is the practitioner who must first take steps to administer gamma globulin if the new-born infant is to be spared this serious disease, caught from his older brother or sister. Even where the technique of prevention is largely through mass measures, the attending physician must be relied upon to recognize the disease, properly isolate and treat his patient, and report the case, say, of diphtheria, malaria, dysentery, or indeed venereal disease, tuberculosis, and smallpox.

But, in the fullest sense, prevention is not confined to stopping the *communication* of such diseases; it is equally concerned with the prevention of their complications or sequelae. It is the practitioner who is responsible for the prompt and efficient treatment of pneumonia or scarlet fever or meningitis if his patient is not to have life-long crippling effects from them.

The physician's rôle in prevention can be even more easily seen in diseases which are not communicable. Only the expert diagnosis and intelligent treatment of the physician can prevent the otherwise almost certain destructiveness of cancer,

1. Davis, William A., M.D., Assistant Professor of Preventive Medicine, New York University College of Medicine. Unpublished paper.

diabetes, hyperthyroidism, glaucoma, the allergies, and emotional disorders. More general recognition has already been given to the preventive functions of practitioners in pregnancy and in infancy.

The techniques used by the physician in his preventive activities run the whole gamut of medical science, from a careful history and physical examination to the most complex laboratory, x-ray, or instrumental procedures, from thyroid surgery to health education. Indeed, every type of skill and every technical device known to medicine has its preventive as well as its diagnostic or curative rôle to play.

The preventive medicine of today, then, is inextricably bound up with the quality and distribution of medical care. It is safe to say that at least three-fourths of the preventive work made possible by present-day medical science must be carried by the practising physician. It follows, obviously enough, that any health officer or other public health worker who desires materially to increase the effectiveness of preventive medicine today must devote a major portion of his effort to improvement of the organization of medical, dental, and nursing services, and to their adequate application for the benefit of the individuals of the community. . . .

54. New Approaches to Integration

A. THE ROLE OF THE HOSPITAL *

THE TERM "preventive medicine" is a dialectitian's delight. A review of the definitions that have been given to it would fill a book, and to discuss the connotations of the term would occupy tedious days of exegesis. Some would limit it to individual activities, and assign its practice to the family doctor, separating preventive medicine from the mass activities of public health. Others, emphasizing the limitation imposed by the adjective and the negativistic connotation, would abolish the term and substitute some new word meaning the promotion and fostering of health, or the construction and reconstruction of health. For the purposes of this paper and in accordance with a habit of thought, I would define preventive medicine, in the words of General Simmons, as "the sum total of all those services required to prevent disease and keep well people well." This broad conception is expressed also by Smith and Evans in their definition of preventive medicine as "all medicine that seeks to alter the course of disease or to better the patient's physiological status." Preventive medicine in this sense has been called "an alliance with nature to prevent disruptive forces." Furthermore, there is no real dividing line between curative medicine and preventive medicine. It is natural, therefore, that the hospital should be a

* From: "The Hospital as a Center of Preventive Medicine," by Stanhope Bayne-Jones, M.D.; *Annals of Internal Medicine* 31: 7-16, July 1949 (No. 1). Reprinted (with omissions, including initial paragraphs) by permission of the author and publishers. The author is the director of research, Army Medical Research and Development Program, Office of the Surgeon General, Department of the Army, Washington, D.C.

center of preventive medicine for the extension of medical service and the raising of the health level of the individual.

None of these ideas is new. They have been newly expressed, however, in recent important publications.* . . .

If I may add anything new to the discussion, I believe it will be in the presentation of a list of the chief preventive medicine activities which are now carried on either extensively or partially from the hospital as a center, or which might be developed from the potentialities of the hospital as a center of health service. Statements about hospitals as centers of health service have been rather general and I have not found an assembled listing of these activities and possibilities. In offering it, I do not wish to imply that it means exclusive centering of these activities in hospitals, but present it as an indication of the specific part that hospitals have to play in the total concern that individuals, practitioners of medicine, lay, governmental, and professional organizations—from the simplest to the most complex system—share in fostering health. It seems to me that the best examples of preventive medicine centered in hospitals are those provided by the teams in pediatrics and in obstetrics and gynecology. Almost all elements are included in their programs.

While divisions of the material are convenient, they are not really natural, because all these activities are integral parts of the whole. Divisional arrangements, in fact, may do harm by strengthening the existing departmental barriers which present some obstacles to communication and concerted effort. With these reservations, and a frank admission of incompleteness, the following listing, with some comments on requirements, is suggested:

1. *Attitude.*—There appears to be a wide acceptance among bodies that have studied modern hospitals that the hospital is a social institution with special capacities and obligations to function as a center of medical care and health services, and that in this conception preventive medicine has an "over-all significance." While this is a point of view of some administrators, some medical professional groups, and many trustees or responsible officials, it is not universally accepted and is opposed by portions of the medical profession and by some organized medical associations. It is suggested that more than respectful attention be devoted to it. If that were done, artificial divisions between curative and preventive medicine would disappear, certain services would be strengthened, new services would be developed, relationships would be extended and co-ordinated, and a unified effort would be made in the common purpose of having the hospital participate to the fullest possible extent in contributing to comprehensive medical care.

2. *Facilities, Equipment, and Construction.*—One of the difficulties in the way of developing hospitals as centers of health services is that they have been built and equipped primarily to take care of sick people in beds within the hospital or in clinics for the ambulatory in their outpatient departments. Not only additions, but construction in accordance with enlarged conceptions will be needed. This construction will involve particularly outpatient departments, doctors' offices, laboratories,

* The author cites here, among other publications, the 1947 reports of the Commission on Hospital Care and the Committee on Medicine and the Changing Order of the New York Academy of Medicine.

accommodations for special services, space for occupational therapy and rehabilitation, more space for all functions of nursing, central offices for a large group of related agencies, interior traffic and external transportation, space and equipment for records and statistical work, accommodations for specialties, more space and equipment for education and research. At present many of these activities and services are crowded, usually without systematic arrangement, into the buildings constructed in accordance with the limited ideas of an era now past. Taking a lesson from this rigid past, it would be well to devise construction and arrangements sufficiently flexible to be adaptable to changes in ideas and activities as they develop in the future.

3. *Education.*—All hospitals are inevitably concerned with education through the very nature of their daily services, which bring together all sorts of workers, patients, doctors, medical students, and nurses. . . . There remains, however, to be developed in the hospital greater educational emphasis on preventive medicine, the significance of group practice, education of patients in the carrying out of instructions for their own good, adult education, health education, and educational influence upon curricula of medical schools and resident training through the exhibition of the changing experiences of hospitals, such, for example, as is occurring through increase of types of diseases characteristic of an aging population. An appreciation of the social science aspects of medicine will bring into the clinics as parts of the medical team psychologists, sociologists, cultural anthropologists, and possibly also economic, legal, and religious advisers. Public education in general and along lines of preventive medicine could extend from the hospital in many directions.

4. *Research.*—The opportunities for investigations in the whole field of medicine and human biology centered in the hospital are too obvious to require elaboration. There are, however, unrealized possibilities for research in preventive medicine in almost every department of a hospital.

5. *Relationships.*—There is no person, group, or agency in the community as a whole that may not be related in some manner to the hospital. If these relationships are not cultivated by the hospital, they will be imposed. No relationships are more natural or close than those concerned with public health, preventive medicine, and general welfare. At present they are increasing with federal, state, and municipal health agencies, with regional relationships between hospitals, and with hospital, medical, and health insurance plans, whether voluntary or supported by money derived from taxes or imposed contributions. The hospitals have a central position in the current discussions of all systems of medical care. The more these systems provide for comprehensive medical care the more will preventive medicine become important in the hospital's relationships with these plans.

Professional relationships are in the very center of all the internal and external activities of the hospital. Although they present difficult problems, it is to be hoped and expected that each party concerned in these professional relationships will be moved by inclination and demonstrated needs to provide enlarged services of preventive medicine.

Although some details have been included in the list of general functions and considerations, a large number of special activities need to be designated separately. Among these are the following:

1. Diagnostic clinics, with services available to all persons of all economic levels.

2. Consultation services available to all.

3. Extension of connections with physicians of a community, particularly general practitioners and family doctors.

4. Periodic health examinations for the well, in general diagnostic clinics, or in clinics equipped and oriented for the detection of cancer or other diseases. Early detection of chronic diseases is a new essential for preventive medicine.

5. Child welfare and child development clinics, including nursery schools. For preventive medicine, the full development of modern pediatrics is of incalculable importance.

6. Prenatal clinics and postnatal clinics, maternal welfare, and facilities for advance and application of knowledge of human reproduction, emphasizing preventive medicine. Departments of obstetrics and gynecology have led the advance, but the activities and points of view should be shared by other departments.

7. Preventive dentistry and oral hygiene, with inclusion of modern stomatology, capable of recognizing in oral lesions the superficial and deep evidences of a wide range of diseases.

8. Health services for the institution's personnel and associated staffs and groups.

9. Concern with industrial medicine. This may be developed by examinations of persons sent to the hospitals, or by examinations at plants through arrangements with the hospital, by personnel trained not only in general medicine but also in the recognition of industrial hazards.

10. Follow-up clinics, and continuity of care.

11. Treatment and prevention of communicable diseases, by maintenance of service for treatment and education; by immunizations; and by linking the community's programs for control and prevention of tuberculosis and venereal diseases (and other diseases) with the activities of the hospital.

12. Nutritional advice and supervision.

13. Social service departments, enlarged and more integrated into the medical team.

14. Co-ordination of hospital activities with services of visiting nurses and public health nurses.

15. Development of group practice centered either in the hospital or in relation to medical groups of the community.

16. Development of programs for convalescent care and home care, centered in the hospital, motivated by a sense of continuity of service.

17. Development of record keeping, mortality and morbidity statistics and reports, particularly morbidity reports, to utilize to the full extent the hospital's capacities to serve as a center of epidemiology and control of disease.

It is admitted that this list includes nearly all of the functions of a hospital, and perhaps some not yet undertaken. However true that may be, it was not presented in this manner to stake out an overambitious program for preventive medicine, but to draw attention to the fact that there is an element of preventive medicine in almost every activity of the hospital, and that if hospitals are to fulfill their destinies as centers of health services they will need to strengthen many existing arrangements and develop new ones. . . .

B. THE ROLE OF THE HEALTH CENTER *

THIS ARTICLE features types of physical accommodations that may be utilized under different circumstances for coordination of community health efforts; a discussion of administrative schemes required for implementing various functional concepts is reserved for another occasion.

From the standpoint of structure there are at least four patterns along which health centers may be developed.

(a) Those designed exclusively for use by public health agencies.

(b) Those that provide space for public health functions to be performed in the hospital.

(c) Those that furnish accommodations for the health department and the practicing physicians.

(d) Those that bring together in one building, or in a group of related buildings, the health department, the hospital, and offices for practicing physicians. . . .

Among the major shortcomings of many existing health center facilities are inadequate parking space, insufficient room for expansion, and rigidity of structure. Choice of a sufficiently large site will solve the first two problems. Flexibility, which is the capacity of the plan to adapt itself to certain functional changes, must be designed into the building at the start. Changes in community health programs often necessitate alteration of health center space requirements. The use of light demountable partitions will readily permit simple revisions in the arrangement of space to accommodate for such changes. In small health centers flexibility also may be obtained by planning rooms to serve dual purposes, thus varied activities can be carried on in them at different hours.

When several distinct health organizations are housed together, the benefits of such a combination must be obtained without interfering with primary functions. This is achieved most readily in a one-story building by providing complete segregation in separate wings with direct entrances for health center clientele, private physicians' patients, and for staff members. Clinic rooms and physicians' offices are most convenient for patients when located on the ground floor; however, if patient areas are located on upper floors, elevators should be provided.

The traditional type of health center, and that best understood by the general public is [one that] houses the health department [primarily]. In such a building

* From: "The Health Center: Adaptation of Physical Plants to Service Concepts," by Joseph W. Mountin, M.D., and August F. Hoenack; *Public Health Reports* 61: 1369-79, Sept. 20, 1946 (No. 38). Reprinted with omissions, including initial paragraphs and illustrations. Dr. Mountin was, at the time of his death in 1952, chief of the Bureau of State Services, Public Health Service, Washington, D.C.; the co-author is a supervisory architect for the Division of Hospital and Medical Facilities of the Public Health Service.

provision is made for discharge of functions common in orthodox public health programs. Work which is essentially administrative in character requires little more than ordinary office space. An activity closely allied with administration is that of popular health instruction. For its performance the health department needs suitable space to display pamphlets, posters, exhibit materials, and films, and for conducting demonstrations. On occasions people need to be assembled in a group, and to accommodate them a small auditorium is essential. Almost without exception health departments operate preventive clinics such as: immunization, maternity and child hygiene, also clinics for the diagnosis and treatment of venereal diseases and tuberculosis. Each of these clinics has its own set of requirements, although considerable interchange of facilities is possible and in the interest of economy. To complement these clinics and otherwise aid in the program of the health department, the laboratory is maintained. Where the health department has responsibilities in addition to those [that have already been referred to] suitable alteration in building design or space arrangement would be indicated. Likewise the capacity or number of rooms may be increased or decreased depending on size of the population served. As stated previously, clinic and demonstration rooms may be used for a number of related purposes.

In rural sections and in large metropolitan areas it is not always practicable for the health department to conduct all of its operations from the headquarters building. Decentralization can be accomplished by development of neighborhood health centers. These may resemble the headquarters building except for size; likewise some accommodations may be omitted if corresponding services are not provided. . . .

A thought often expressed is that health centers in areas remote from general hospitals might be designed to include a few beds—perhaps eight or ten. Implicit in this idea is their use for ordinary emergencies and obstetrical cases. Irrespective of how inappropriate the facilities actually provided may be, there is likely to develop a strong urge to use them for purposes that should be carried out only in a good general hospital. Proposals for the inclusion of a few beds in outpost health centers therefore should not be adopted without due reflection on the responsibilities entailed. In a word, such responsibilities are little short of those attached to full hospitalization of patients. Quite another matter is the combination of a health center with a general hospital of size sufficient for efficient operation and suitable staff organization.

In varying degrees joint housing of the hospital and the health department is both practicable and desirable. Where a community maintains only a single small public hospital and a correspondingly small health department, unity of structure, function, and management should be sought. . . .

As a usual thing several hospitals, each operating under separate auspices, will be found in a single health jurisdiction. If the headquarters of the health department were to be accommodated by any one of the hospitals, an additional structure, very likely, would be required. For reasons of policy, the health officer might not desire intimate association with a particular hospital to the exclusion of others, especially if he does not have administrative responsibility for its operation. A preferable arrangement for the health department is one whereby all hospitals make specified service contributions to the general health programs. Suitable physical accommodations further this scheme, since the essential purpose to be accomplished is making technological resources of hospitals available to the community at large. Units of any hospital particularly involved in such a relationship are radiology, physiotherapy, and laboratory. These units need to be placed so that they are readily accessible to ambulatory patients without causing disturbance to bed patients or otherwise interfering with necessary hospital routines. A point often overlooked is that patients coming to a hospital for service on a visit basis present requirements that differ in many respects from patients who are admitted for bed care. They should not be subjected to the usual admission routines. Their passage through the several diagnostic and treatment units also should be scheduled and expedited. Comfortable waiting space and dressing rooms represent essentials that are often skimped even in new designs. If it is desirable for an existing hospital, designed originally to serve only bed patients, to meet the added requirements of general community service, it may be necessary to concentrate units for use alike by bed and ambulatory patients in a new section constructed especially for the purpose.

Particularly in remote areas, where the establishment of a hospital is not contemplated at all or within the near future, improvement of both medical practice and public health organization should be promoted by pooling of local personnel and physical equipment. Accomplishment of this end often can be advanced by bringing personnel into that close association which is made possible by joint housing. . . . The degree to which functions may be separated or, on the other hand, integrated, depends on the desires of occupants and needs of those who apply for service. In any case, combined use of laboratory, radiological, and other types of equipment together with technical personnel involved in their operation, is contemplated.

The fourth basic service plan mentioned earlier contemplates bringing together in physical as well as operating relationship the health department, the hospital, and the practicing physicians. Where the entire population of an area is tributary to a single community hospital, and all local physicians are represented on the staff, this arrangement should be present no great difficulty from an administrative standpoint. Structurally the plan may be executed in a single building, especially if an entire new development is contemplated. . . . If the service scheme must take into account a pre-existing hospital, then erecting additional buildings on the same or adjoining sites may be the only feasible arrangement. Even so, the hospital might require essential alterations so as to make selected units readily available for ambulatory patients.

Throughout this discussion emphasis has been placed on structural design with a view to facilitating operating relationships among occupants participating in the services afforded. This consideration, while of primary importance, should not be allowed to overshadow others of equal weight—especially general location and site characteristics. Unless it is necessary to relate new construction to existing buildings, health centers should always be placed so as to assure maximum accessibility to the population served. The site itself should be chosen with a view to beauty as well as utility. Not alone is ample space essential to those ends, but in no other way is it possible to provide for orderly expansion of accommodations. . . .

. . . The community should not be unduly critical if the type plan selected originally does not fulfill every expectation. Health organization is now passing through an evolutionary stage, and no person can be certain of its ultimate form. In the final analysis a health center, like any other physical structure, will be no more than an instrument for accomplishing a purpose. First of all, the purpose must be conceived as clearly as possible, and second, those who are responsible for its execution must exercise that degree of patience and persistence which always is required in the conduct of delicate human relationships.

C. HEALTH DEPARTMENT-HOSPITAL COORDINATION *

THE AMERICAN HOSPITAL Association and the American Public Health Association have prepared this statement to define the areas in which fuller cooperation and integration of hospitals and health departments may be achieved. The statement is confined to an exploration of these areas and does not concern itself with other aspects of either hospital management or community health organization. It is hoped that hospitals and health departments will find it a useful guide to their attainment of closer working relations in the interests of greater efficiency and improved health service.

Among the foremost institutions which today serve the health of the community is the general hospital. . . .

Because of its important position the general hospital's responsibilities in the total community health picture have been constantly expanding. In addition to the provision of facilities for medical care of high quality, its functions now include training of medical and allied personnel, medical research, and participation in local public health activities.

Profound changes and advances in the activities of health departments have paralleled this expansion in hospital functions. The achievement and maintenance of ever higher levels of community sanitation is making it possible for health departments to turn increased attention to developing programs to improve individual health through immunization, education, and health supervision; at the same time they have found it essential to provide therapeutic services if communicable diseases such as tuberculosis and syphilis are to be effectively prevented. Health departments have begun to recognize the important public health implications of such major health problems as cancer, heart disease, and other long-term illnesses and to combat them by providing certain facilities to aid in early diagnosis and treatment. In order to secure maximum effectiveness for these campaigns they have begun to

* From: "Coordination of Hospitals and Health Departments" (Joint Statement of Recommendations), by the American Hospital Association and the American Public Health Association; *American Journal of Public Health* 38: 700-8, May 1948 (No. 5); published concurrently as a separate pamphlet, under the same title, by the American Hospital Association (Chicago, 1948; 9 pp.). Reprinted (with omissions) by permission of the publishers. (Note: This document has been adopted as an official statement of the two associations).

develop increasingly closer relationships with hospitals and practicing physicians.

Preventive and curative medicine have reached the stage where they are no longer separable, and it is necessary at the present time to bring them together physically and functionally. The close physicial and organizational association of health departments and hospitals will provide a valuable step toward this essential goal.

Hospitals and health departments have a common interest in providing the best possible technical facilities and administrative tools for the further development of both the preventive and therapeutic aspects of medical practice. The expression of this relationship in terms of greater coördination of the activities of hospitals and health departments has already occurred in some communities, but a great deal still remains to be accomplished in this direction.

Housing of Hospitals and Health Departments.—Since a considerable increase in the construction of hospitals and public health facilities may be expected in the next few years, it is appropriate that certain advantages of joint housing be pointed out at this time. It is strongly recommended that, wherever circumstances justify and permit, there should be joint housing of hospitals and health departments, and, if possible, the offices of physicians and dentists.

Although coördination of the activities of hospitals and health departments can be accomplished even if they are not closely integrated physically, it is most feasible when there is joint housing of the hospital and health department. The common use of laboratory and clinic facilities, which is difficult to achieve when the two institutions are physically separated, occurs readily when they are housed together. The planning of integrated programs is facilitated by joint housing and their administration is made smoother and more efficient.

The health needs of rural areas which are isolated, thinly settled, and unable to support a general hospital may be met by the construction of outpost health facilities. These facilities would house the offices of physicians and dentists, diagnostic facilities, the office of the local public health nurse, public health clinics, and in some areas a nursing unit for maternity care and minor illnesses.

The physicians whose offices are located in the outpost facility should be members of the medical staff of the nearest general hospital. Arrangements should be made for transportation of patients from the outpost area to the hospital and for consultation visits by the hospital staff to the outpost facility. Otherwise the outpost personnel may deteriorate professionally owing to their medical isolation or the outpost facility may attempt to undertake functions belonging properly in the general hospital.

The establishment of hospitals and public health facilities in many rural areas will require entirely new construction. It is recommended that in these areas hospital and health department facilities be constructed as an integral whole. It is particularly recommended that physicians' offices be included in the new structures so that the time and effort usually expended by private practitioners in shuttling back and forth between office and hospital would be minimized. This arrangement would facilitate laboratory and x-ray examinations of the physicians' patients, prevent unnecessary duplication of expensive technical equipment and make it easier for physicians to consult with their colleagues.[1]

Many advantages to the public, the health department, and the hospital may be derived from joint housing of hospitals and health departments. A single health and medical center means greater convenience and continuity of service for the public. The pooling of resources resulting from joint housing enables the community to obtain more adequate facilities and better trained personnel than it could otherwise afford.

Through joint housing the hospital achieves greater prestige as the community center for all health and medical activities; it is able to hire a more competent staff by virtue of its increased financial strength and can therefore offer more comprehensive and effective service. Joint housing facilitates follow-up by public health nurses of patients after they leave the hospital, while the medical staff benefits from closer association with public health programs. Furthermore it may stimulate increased public interest in the hospital since more people will visit the institution for health promotion and preventive services rather than as a last resort.

The health officer likewise benefits professionally from more intimate association with physicians engaged in clinical medicine. His health programs receive added impetus from the increased knowledge and interest in public health gained by practising physicians, interns, and nurses. Case finding for public health programs in the hospital wards and outpatient department is facilitated. The health department attains new stature, dignity, and public understanding.

Where the general hospital already exists and health department facilities are needed, it is recommended that the latter be constructed as an addition to the hospital or adjacent to it, and that an understanding be reached between the two agencies concerning joint use of certain facilities in order to avoid unnecessary duplication. This plan, however, may not be practicable in some instances because of the isolated location of the hospital.

While it is administratively easier to combine the rural hospital with health department facilities when both are public institutions, there is little reason why joint housing of voluntary hospitals and public health facilities cannot be achieved.[2]

In small cities with one existing general hospital it is recommended that health department facilities be constructed as part of or adjacent to the hospital wherever feasible. It may be more difficult to arrange for joint housing in cities with more than one hospital. Nevertheless, the difficulties are not insurmountable.

In larger cities public health facilities should, in so far as it is logical and possible, be built as part of or adjacent to general hospitals. Of course this will not be feasible in neighborhoods which do not have hospitals. Where joint housing can be achieved it will have an important effect in improving the coordination and effectiveness of hospital and health department activities.

1. The joint housing of hospitals and health departments has already been effected in a number of areas such as Sonoma, Monterey, and Kern Counties, Calif., and Washington, Charles, and Wicomico Counties, Md. . . .
2. In several counties of Maryland, for example, the health department pays rent for that portion of the hospital which it occupies, and the arrangement has proved highly satisfactory.

The cities in which medical schools are located present a special situation. In such cases the principal public health facility should be built on the grounds of the teaching hospital.[3]

Personnel and Administration.—There are many ways in which health department and hospital personnel can work together effectively. In urban areas, for example, coöperative arrangements between hospital social workers and public health nurses can prevent duplication of services and increase efficiency. In rural hospitals and health departments, although medical social workers are not generally employed by the separate institutions, it should be possible to employ a medical social worker to serve both agencies where there is combined housing of the health department and hospital.

In urban as well as rural areas the public health nurse can provide continuity of care for discharged hospital patients by carrying out the treatments recommended by the physician and giving home nursing care and supervision. This is true not only for patients with communicable diseases but for all hospital patients, whether ambulatory or not, who require further home supervision or care. Physicians, hospitals, and health departments should together agree on and carry out simple and effective referral systems.

In many areas the shortage of public health nurses limits the possibilities of this type of service. Nevertheless in some rural communities the public health nurse is able to perform a substantial amount of bedside nursing care. In the cities there has been a significant trend toward the amalgamation of voluntary visiting nurse services with those furnished under the health department program, thereby improving service and increasing the potentialities of physician-hospital-health department coöperation in this field.

There are several ways in which the medical staff of the hospital can contribute to the activities of the health department. Arrangements may be made for members of the visiting staff to conduct specific health department clinics on a part-time salary basis. Members of the visiting and resident staffs can instruct public health nurses in current medical advances and assist in the health department's educational program by lecturing to community groups. Such service by physicians contributes to the building of a close partnership of physician, hospital, and health department to meet the overall health needs of the locality.

Consideration should be given to broadening the concept of intern or resident training to include a definite period of time spent in a public health department approved for this purpose. This would improve the physician's understanding of the preventive approach to medicine and acquaint him with services available to the public through the health department and other community agencies.

The achievement of closer administrative relationships between hospitals and

3. This is the plan followed in Louisville, Ky., where the medical school, teaching hospital, and public health department form a single, integrated medical center. In New York City, five of the municipal public health centers are adjacent to medical schools. The health officers hold positions in the medical schools, and medical students serve clinical clerkships in the public health centers....

health departments does not come about automatically but requires careful and continued planning as well as administrative finesse. Where the health department and the hospital are jointly housed but under separate administration, joint conferences should be instituted and definite fields of administrative coöperation outlined to further closer and more harmonious relationships.

In those areas which have a small community hospital and health department the appointment of a single administrator for both organizations may be considered. There is need for further experimentation in this field.[4]

Closer coördination of the training of health officers and hospital administrators is needed to familiarize health officers with hospital problems in view of their increasing responsibilities for hospital planning, construction, inspection, and licensure, and to develop hospital administrators and health officers who have sufficient understanding of each other's activities to coördinate them effectively. This would also make available personnel competent to direct combined hospital-health department units. Several schools of public health have already recognized the importance of such coördination by requiring one basic course of training for both groups and permitting specialization subsequently in either public health or hospital administration.

Prevention of Communicable Disease.—The control of tuberculosis, venereal disease and other communicable diseases affords numerous opportunities for joint action by hospitals and health departments. Tuberculosis and venereal disease clinics belong properly at the general hospital, not at the city hall or some other non-medical institution. Likewise rapid treatment centers for syphilis should, in so far as possible, be housed in general hospitals rather than organized separately.

With present knowledge of the control of cross-infection there is very little reason for establishing special hospitals for the care of acute communicable disease. With the possible exception of large urban centers such special hospitals are economically wasteful and seldom provide services which meet the total medical needs of the patient. A more rational approach is to use general hospital beds for the care of patients with communicable disease and to obtain the assistance of the health department in developing effective isolation techniques. Such coöperative action will be facilitated if the hospital appoints the health officer to its medical staff as consultant in communicable diseases.

Routine chest x-rays as well as serological tests for syphilis ought to be undertaken by all hospitals. The interest of the health department in these health protection activities should take the form of substantial financial and technical aid. With such assistance every hospital can become a strategic center in the community attack on tuberculosis and venereal disease.

Close working relationships between general hospitals and tuberculosis sanatoria are necessary to afford sanatoria patients the advantages of modern surgical therapy

4. In Branch County, Mich., for example, the health officer is also director of the voluntary general hospital. This arrangement has made it possible to offer sufficient compensation to attract a competent physician. It has also proved highly advantageous in achieving greater coördination of hospital and health department activities and a better quality of administration.

as well as consultation services. For similar reasons a portion of the newly established hospital beds for tuberculosis should be located in or closely connected with general hospitals.

Laboratory service is essential to communicable disease control as well as to the proper functioning of hospitals. Health departments and hospitals have a vital interest therefore in the planning and development of adequate laboratory service.[5]

In some states hospital as well as health department laboratories are approved by the state department of health which, in addition, holds an annual educational meeting of laboratory directors and supplies them with current bibliographies on technical subjects. Marked improvement in laboratory standards has resulted from such procedures and they have been well received by hospital laboratory personnel.

Programs for Non-communicable Disease.—With the progressive conquest of many communicable diseases attention has shifted to other major causes of disability and death. Heart disease, cancer, and mental illness are rapidly becoming recognized as having significant public health implications. The epidemiological study of such diseases—their prevalence and relation to socio-economic, environmental, and constitutional factors—can shed much light upon their origin, prevention, mitigation, and treatment. The social effects of non-communicable diseases, their chronic nature in many instances, their increasing importance as the population ages and the huge expense involved in their care put them beyond the scope of the individual physician or hospital alone and mark them clearly as among the most important public health problems of the day. Accordingly, there have been renewed attempts to construct adequate systems of morbidity reporting and greater emphasis has been placed on health education as a preventive device in the management of non-communicable disease.

Hospitals provide an effective environment in which to educate the public in health matters. In addition hospitals are repositories of much valuable information on the incidence of disease which should be studied and utilized in the development of control programs. They occupy an important position in relation to plans for controlling heart disease and cancer and are natural locations for cardiac and tumor diagnostic clinics. The recent development of cancer detection clinics, in which apparently well persons receive thorough diagnostic examinations, promises to encourage greater concentration of this type of preventive activity by the staffs of general hospitals.

It has long been recognized that psychiatry suffers through its isolation from general medicine. Similarly the average physician, having received little or no training in psychiatry, is handicapped in his ability to recognize, treat or prevent mental disease. The importance of mental illness is indicated by a recent estimate that approximately 1 patient out of every 28 new admissions to general hospitals, and

---

5. In some of the rural counties of Maryland, the use of a joint laboratory has been found to be advantageous, since the additional financial resources allow the utilization of better trained personnel. In small cities with more than one hospital as, e. g., Jamestown, N.Y., it has been found effective to have a single director administer the health department laboratory as well as the several hospital laboratories. . . .

1 out of every 16 new admissions to outpatient departments presents problems requiring the services of the psychiatrist.

Owing to the passage of the National Mental Health Act a large-scale development of research facilities and clinics for mental hygiene may be expected. In many areas the local and state health departments will be responsible for administering the mental health program and integrating it with other health activities. It will be to the best interests of psychiatry and medicine in general if hospitals welcome the establishment of mental hygiene clinics and incorporate their functions as part of a general hospital service. Large general hospitals should establish psychiatric services for observation and treatment of mentally ill patients and, wherever feasible, the medical staffs of general and mental hospitals should develop liaison in order to provide consultation services to patients of mental institutions and to furnish the patients of general hospitals with skilled psychiatric assistance. In this way a more fully generalized and comprehensive service to the community would be achieved.

Maternal and Child Health.—Maternal and child health clinics should be easily accessible to the persons served and many must be conducted in communities or neighborhoods which do not have hospitals. Nevertheless, there are numerous instances where the general hospital is easily accessible but is not utilized for such services. This situation, which has arisen from the separate development of hospital and health department facilities, prevents both hospital and health department from operating at their maximum effectiveness in the protection of maternal and child health. Health department prenatal clinics for the adjacent neighborhood should be conducted in the general hospital in order to insure continuity of care, easy transfer of records, and adequate postpartum follow-up. Similar considerations apply to well child and pediatric diagnostic and treatment clinics. The maternal and child health clinics conducted by health departments in areas not easily accessible to hospitals should be affiliated with the central hospital clinics for referral of complicated cases.

Still other opportunities exist for closer relationships between hospitals and health departments. The latter can supply educational literature to hospitals for distribution by physicians to their maternity patients. The state department of health in particular can furnish consultation services by medical, nursing, nutrition, and other staff members. Hospitals can enlist the aid of the health department to prevent outbreaks of infant diarrhea and to develop comprehensive programs and facilities for the specialized care of premature infants, and should coöperate with the health department and practising physicians in their review of maternal and infant deaths. The health department can assist hospital laboratories to make determinations of the Rh factor by furnishing consultation services, providing typing sera, or actually performing the tests.

All too often the public health nurse receives notice of the birth of a child several weeks after its occurrence and the mother is thereby deprived of her advice and assistance during the period when they are most important. This problem has been solved in some areas through coöperative arrangements by which the health department is informed of the birth before the mother and child leave the hospital. In many communities arrangements have been made with physicians and hospitals for the public health nurse to see the mother while she is still in the hospital as well as make a preparatory visit to the home, thereby establishing the best possible conditions for adequate home follow-up.

The proportion of home deliveries is still too high in many areas. Hospitals should give serious attention to the provision of sufficient maternity beds to meet the needs of the entire community, particularly for the care of complicated cases.

Medical Care and Hospital Services.—A number of specialized medical care programs, including those for communicable disease, tuberculosis, venereal disease, and crippled children, are recognized responsibilities of health departments, and it is desirable that they be entrusted with new programs of community medical care which may be assumed by various levels of government. It would seem wise therefore for hospital and health authorities to undertake intensive research on several mutual problems. One of these, for example, is the creation of a satisfactory cost accounting system which will be equitable to both the hospital and the health department.

The experience of the last few years, particularly with the Emergency Maternity and Infant Care Program, has established the important principle that the hospital receive full cost for the care of patients for which government assumes full responsibility. This precedent should be followed in all public medical care programs provided that an agreed standard of care is established and there is proper cost accounting.

In approximately three-quarters of the states the state health departments have been given the responsibility for hospital surveys and planning incident to the Federal Hospital Survey and Construction Act of 1946, and it is expected that they will be given similar administrative responsibilities with respect to the construction phase of the program. This will inevitably encourage much closer relationships between hospitals and health departments than have ever existed in the past.

Hospital licensure laws have already been enacted in most states and with few exceptions the state department of health has been designated as the responsible agency. Much of the activity of the agencies administering such laws is of an educational character, designed to assist hospitals in improving standards of service to the public.

A significant expansion in the number of full-time local health departments as well as in the scope of their activities may be expected in the next few years. Similarly the nation's hospital system will be extended to many areas which now lack adequate facilities and greater emphasis will be placed on the community responsibilities of the general hospital. It is important at this time that hospital and health department administrators plan to achieve maximum coordination through joint housing, coöperative use of personnel, and the development of active programs to safeguard and promote the health of their communities.

FURTHER READINGS

Group Practice

American Medical Association, Bureau of Medical Economic Research. *An Annotated Bibliography of Group Practice, 1927-1950.* Bureau Bulletin 85. Chicago: The Association, 1951. 72 pages.

Clark, Dean A. and Katharine G. *Organization and Administration of Group Medical Practice.* New York: Twentieth Century Fund and Good Will Fund, 1941. 109 pages.

Dickinson, Frank G. and Bradley, Charles E. *Discontinuance of Medical Groups, 1940-1949.* Bulletin 90, Bureau of Medical Economic Research, American Medical Association. Chicago: The Association, 1952. 11 pages.

Hunt, G. Halsey and Goldstein, Marcus S. *Medical Group Practice in the United States.* Publication No. 77, Public Health Service. Washington: U. S. Government Printing Office, 1951. 70 pages.

Medical Administration Service, Inc. *Benefits of Group Practice.* New York: The Service, 1949. 40 pages.

Portfolio of Articles on Medical Groups and Partnerships. Oradell, N. J.: Medical Economics, 1956.

Weinerman, E. Richard and Goldstein, George S. *Medical Group Practice in California.* Berkeley, Calif.: School of Public Health, University of California, 1952. 28 pages (processed).

Other Devices for Achieving Coordination

Ciocco, Antonio and Altman, Isidore. *Medical Service Areas and Distances Traveled for Physician Care in Western Pennsylvania.* Publication No. 248, Public Health Service. Washington: U. S. Government Printing Office, 1954. 32 pages. (Includes references).

Rosenfeld, Leonard S. and Makover, Henry B. *The Rochester Regional Hospital Council.* Cambridge: Harvard University Press, 1956. 204 pages. (Includes references).

Solon, Jerry and Baney, Anna Mae. *General Hospitals and Nursing Homes.* Publication No. 492, Public Health Service. Washington: U. S. Government Printing Office, 1956. 54 pages.

Trussell, Ray E. *Hunterdon Medical Center.* Cambridge: Harvard University Press, 1956. 236 pages.

CHAPTER VIII

Care of Long-Term Illness

THE PATTERN of ill health today reflects the state of social and scientific development of our civilization. In the United States, the major threats to health and to the completion of a "normal" life span are no longer the epidemic plagues and acute infections that until recently took such a heavy toll in death and disability. Now it is the so-called "chronic" or "long-term" ailments that head the morbidity and mortality lists.

As a result of successful control of many major hazards of childbirth and of the earlier years of life, people have been surviving in greater numbers to the later years. Many more of our people are therefore subject to cancer, arthritis, heart diseases, nephritis, diabetes and other long-term illnesses. Further, the very advances in knowledge and in our standard of living which have so improved man's chances for survival and longer life, have contributed new hazards to health. Industrial and traffic accidents, radiation dangers, water and air pollution, obesity and the tensions of urban living emerge as causes of chronic disease and disability.

The long-term diseases constitute, as a group, the most significant health problem of our time. Provision of proper medical care for these disorders calls for the use of the most advanced skills of modern medicine in a balanced and comprehensive manner. The special characteristics of long-term disease give special relevance to three aspects of the organization of health services:

1. First is *prevention* which, in the context of long-term illness, must be interpreted broadly. The concept encompasses not only health promotion and the early detection of disease, but prompt and effective treatment as well. Disability and premature death can be prevented by medical care even though it may not yet be possible to prevent the disease itself.

374

2. The provision of medical care to long-term patients requires a complex array of facilities, personnel and services. In most communities these resources may be sought only from diverse and often unrelated agencies. A logical and consistent relationship among them is much needed. Such *coordination* will help to achieve continuity in appreciating and meeting the needs of long-term patients.

3. Care of the long-term patient is hardly complete when active signs and symptoms are controlled. Medical, social and vocational *rehabilitation* give promise of effective relief of much individual suffering and social waste which have been so often the sequelae of chronic illness.

In this chapter are presented selections on the magnitude and characteristics of the problem of long-term illness; on methods for coordinating services to meet the problem; on the preventive, therapeutic, and rehabilitative aspects of medical care for the long-term patient; and on some of the specialized facilities—nursing homes and home medical care—that play a key role in providing continuity of service for such patients.

55. THE CHALLENGE OF CHRONIC ILLNESS *

THE PATIENT with chronic illness is one of the major challenges to modern society. Sooner or later some form of long term illness affects one or more members in most families of the nation. A conservative estimate suggests that more than one-sixth of the population—some 25,000,000 persons—are afflicted with some chronic disease. Approximately 2,000,000 of our population are chronic invalids at the present time, and the number is steadily increasing. It will increase still more as the control of other disorders which were so devastating heretofore are now being more effectively managed. The mortality rates from acute infections, nutritional deficiencies, glandular abnormalities, are falling. Many patients afflicted with cancer are being cured due to earlier diagnosis and complete eradication.

A report from New York State estimates that seven out of every ten deaths are due to some chronic illness. And while in 1900 chronic disease was the cause of twenty-six percent of all deaths in New York, in 1940 almost seventy percent of the fatalities resulted from prolonged illness. No age is immune. Some forty percent of the patients suffering from chronic illness are under forty-five years of age, and in patients between twenty-five and sixty-four years of age, sixty percent

* From: "The Chronic Invalid," by Edward L. Bortz, M.D.; *Journal of the American Medical Association* 138: 745-47, Nov. 6, 1948 (No. 10). Reprinted (with omissions) by permission of the author and publishers. The author is the chief of Medical Service "B" at the Lankenau Hospital, Philadelphia.

of the reported cases of long term illness are found. Chronic illness is also found among children, adolescents, and those in the young adult years.

The extent of this problem is expanding. Inadequate individuals, such as persons with mongolism and other unfortunates, formerly were frequently removed by a severe infection or some nutritional discrepancy. Now the control of these maladies is carrying over larger numbers of individuals who are charges on society. The strain on family budgets and household organization is mounting. It therefore becomes necessary for planning on a much broader scale to meet the challenge of chronic invalidism.

The need for comprehensive planning to meet the challenge of chronic disease must be emphasized. While the economic and social aspects are of vital importance, the highlights in the problem of the chronic invalid are prevention, management, and research. Since each year approximately 1,000,000 deaths are due to chronic illness, and a billion days are lost from productive activity, it is high time that concerted action on a broad plane be directed to counteract this huge loss to our social existence.

As more persons are living longer, there is more opportunity for chronic illness to develop. To this extent aging of the population may be regarded as a contributory factor. However, it should be kept in mind that aging and chronic invalidism are not synonymous by any means. The misconception that old age is constantly visited by chronic invalidism must be dispelled. Many individuals now have a vigorous and enjoyable senectitude free of prolonged illness.

Long term illness is one of the principal causes of economic hardship. The presence of a chronically ill patient in the family frequently alters the psychological atmosphere within the home. When an attitude of defeatism is adopted by the patient and those around him, the outlook is likely to be hopeless.

The Major Chronic Illnesses

THE MAJOR chronic illnesses are as follows: cardiovascular disorders, including arteriosclerosis, apoplectic stroke, rheumatic heart disease, and syphilitic heart disease; the arthritic and rheumatic disturbances; mental diseases; advanced cancer; tuberculosis; diabetes; gastrointestinal disturbances of organic or functional origin; disorders of the genito-urinary tract; the allergic states; and chronic alcoholism. Some 4,000,000 invalids are suffering from chronic heart disease. Vital statistics indicate that approximately 600,000 lives are lost each year as a result of a breakdown of the cardiovascular system in the form of cerebral hemorrhage, coronary occlusion, or chronic heart failure. It has been estimated that approximately ten percent of all chronic disease cases fall into the group of cardiovascular disorders.

Arthritis and rheumatic disorders stand second on the list of the most common disabling afflictions; the exact number of invalids suffering from arthritis is not known. Available statistics are not satisfactory. This is because of the variation in terms and lack of exactness in diagnosis. There is a great need today for state-wide surveys which will give a clear picture of the magnitude of the problem of chronic disease. With arthritic and rheumatic disorders, for instance, it is important to know the number of patients suffering from degenerative joint lesions, those suffering from acute infectious arthritis, and the number in which a metabolic abnormality, such as gout, is the underlying factor. To know the extent of the problem is the first essential in a program of combating the ravages.

According to a recent summary there are 641,331 beds for general hospital cases with an average census of 496,527. There are 674,930 beds for nervous and mental cases with an average census of 635,769. With the use of shock therapy for certain types of mental illness the number of admissions to hospitals is increasing, while, at the same time, the length of stay is being reduced.

This year approximately 180,000 lives will be lost because of cancer. It may be conservatively estimated that seventy-five per cent of these patients are bedridden or otherwise incapacitated to such an extent as to be classified as chronic invalids.

With the superb work of various organizations interested in the control of tuberculosis, the death rate is decreasing in those areas where modern health measures have been instituted for its control. According to statistics from the National Office of Vital Statistics, in 1945 there were 52,916 deaths—a ratio of 40.1; in 1944 there were 54,731 deaths—a ratio of 41.3; while in 1943 there were 57,005 deaths—a ratio of 42.6. It is unfortunate that there is no uniform method for reporting cases of tuberculosis. While there are not any accurate data on the total number of persons suffering from tuberculosis, various authorities have estimated that at the present time there are approximately 1,500,000 patients. It should also be stated that tuberculosis is still the captain of the men of death in areas where modern control measures are not utilized.

While diabetes is listed as a chronic disease, and there are probably two million persons with diabetes in the country at the present time, few of these are invalids. Modern control measures have greatly improved the status of the diabetic patient.

The high pressure of social existence at the present time is reflecting itself in the large number of individuals suffering from some form of gastrointestinal disorder— the most frequent being peptic ulcer or colitis. Grouped with disorders of the gastrointestinal tract may be those conditions of chronic involvement of the biliary tract. Here, too, persons ofttimes are not sick and not well, but become chronic sufferers because of low-grade efficiency.

With increasing years approximately fifty per cent of the male population becomes afflicted with prostatic hypertrophy. As the cardiovascular system becomes sclerotic prostatic lesions may be more pronounced.

It is estimated that one and one-half to two per cent of the population are chronic sufferers from some allergic condition, although they may not be incapacitated for long periods of time.

Chronic alcoholism must be regarded as a menace to the public health. Its devastations carry far beyond the destructive effects on the individual patient. A condition which has destroyed so many brilliant careers, disrupted so many homes and caused as much unhappiness as chronic alcoholism, must be regarded as an important problem in the realm of chronic illness. The periodicity of bouts merely emphasizes the chronicity of the condition. While no accurate statistics are available, it has been estimated that there are 75,000 alcoholic addicts in the United States. Although the alcoholic frequently is a social problem with a legal aspect, basically the condition is medical and needs concentrated study, the same as other chronic medical disorders. The National Committee for Education on Alcoholism and the organization known as Alcoholics Anonymous have rendered outstanding public service in emphasizing the need for rehabilitation of the problem drinker.

Social Factors

LONG TERM ILLNESS produces an added burden on the patient's family. It adds one more problem case to the social agencies which exist for the purpose of neutralizing adverse social influences. If the invalid is the wage earner, the family's economic predicament becomes immediately acute, and economic dependency on society may result.

According to the National Health Survey, chronic illness occurs most frequently in families with relatively limited financial resources. The rate of chronic illness found in families on relief in 1937 was about double that for families with incomes of $2,000 to $3,000 per year. The New York State Health Preparedness Commission in 1944 found in their investigation that some thirty-seven per cent of persons receiving old age assistance were afflicted with some form of chronic illness, just double the average for their age group. As pointed out by Howard Rusk, long term illness depletes earning power at a time when the patients are called upon to pay more for their care than those who are suffering from an acute illness. An important additional burden is the common tendency on the part of the invalid to become a permanent dependent. Psychological factors, such as boredom, lack of initiative to improve one's status, and the acceptance on the part of relatives that the condition cannot be bettered, are some of the chief obstacles which must be removed if the chronic invalid is to be rehabilitated. Too many patients accept their illness with resignation, and appear to be willing to become charges on society. A rehabilitation program has much to offer these persons.

Although chronic illness may occur in any age group, it is likely to be more devastating for older persons in society. Rusk has emphasized the fear of chronic disease and disability as the most haunting specter of increasing age. In 1936 the National Health Survey indicated that fifty-eight per cent of all persons sixty-five years and over suffer from some form of chronic illness or physical disability. It should be emphasized that there are many persons with some physical infirmity who are useful and productive members of society. It has frequently been pointed out that some form of chronic illness may teach persons the advisability of living a restricted existence, thereby enabling them to live out their normal life span. A psychological atmosphere of defeatism and fear of the future is a major detrimental influence in perpetuating chronic illness. Greater attention to the patient's attitude and the creation of a buoyant and hopeful atmosphere are the first step in a sound rehabilitation program. . . .

56. THE ANSWER: COMPREHENSIVE PLANNING *

THERE IS A GREAT need for comprehensive planning to insure that the widespread interest in chronic disease [1] is channeled into sound and effective activity. Such planning requires the mutual cooperation of the agencies and professions most vitally concerned with the problem. For this reason, representatives of the American Hospital Association, the American Medical Association, the American Public Health Association, and the American Public Welfare Association have considered the experience already accumulated and have prepared this statement as a guide in the development of community programs. . . .

Prevention

THE BASIC approach to chronic disease must be preventive. Otherwise the problems created by chronic diseases will grow larger with time, and the hope of any substantial decline in their incidence and severity will be postponed for many years.

There is a need to intensify health department programs to control chronic communicable diseases such as tuberculosis, syphilis, hookworm, and malaria. Accident prevention programs—in industry, on the farm, and in the home—should be greatly expanded to reduce the incidence of physical handicaps.

The promotion of optimal health throughout life is an important factor in the prevention of chronic illness. Child and school health programs need to be strengthened. Wide expansion of nutrition, mental health, and housing programs can have important effects in decreasing the incidence of chronic illness.

* From: "Planning for the Chronically Ill" (Joint Statement of Recommendations), by the American Hospital Association, American Medical Association, American Public Health Association, and American Public Welfare Association; *American Journal of Public Health* 37: 1256-65, Oct. 1947 (No. 10); *Hospitals* 21: 108-12, Nov. 1947 (No. 11); *Journal of the American Medical Association* 135: 343-47, Oct. 11, 1947 (No. 6); and *Public Welfare* 5: 218-24, Oct. 1947 (No. 10). Reprinted (with omissions, including initial paragraph) by permission of the publishers. (Note: This document has been adopted as an official statement of the four associations.)

1. The term "chronic disease" is susceptible to various definitions. An administrative definition of chronic disease has been suggested as follows: "A disease that may be expected to require an extended period of medical supervision and/or hospital, institutional, nursing, or supervisory care." (Rogers, E. S.: "Chronic Disease: A Problem That Must Be Faced," *Am. J. Pub. Health* 36:345, April 1946.) In the National Health Survey, chronic disease was defined for statistical purposes as "a disabling or non-disabling chronic pathological condition known to the informant, the symptoms of which had been recognized for at least three months." (Perrott, G. St. J.: "The Problem of Chronic Disease," *Psychosomatic Med.* 7:22, January 1945.) Another definition is that used for survey purposes by the Public Welfare Council of Connecticut, "A disease or condition of the body or personality which has been present at least six months and which interferes with one's occupation and normal physical and social life." (*Need for a State Infirmary for the Care and Treatment of Aged, Infirm, and Chronically Ill Persons,* Public Welfare Council, Hartford, 1944, p. 4.)

The success of programs to conserve the health of infants and children suggests the possibility of achieving effective health programs directed to adolescents as well as adults. The health programs of our high schools and colleges, including medical examinations and correction of defects, physical fitness and recreational programs, and health education require intensive development.

The periodic medical examination of apparently well persons needs to be explored on a new basis, including selective laboratory and clinical examinations chosen for particular age, sex, geographical, and occupational groups. These include serology, chest x-ray, urinalysis, electrocardiography, ophthalmoscopic and other examinations.

Industry and labor can play an important constructive role in this connection by encouraging health examinations of employees, including laboratory procedures, on a much larger scale than at present.

The recent development of special phases of the health examination, particularly in the fields of tuberculosis control and cancer detection, is especially noteworthy. The great interest shown by the medical profession and the public in chest x-ray surveys and in the establishment of diagnostic centers to examine apparently well persons for early signs of cancer represents a distinct advance in preventive medicine. It may well initiate a basic shift in emphasis in the medical care of adults comparable to that which has occurred in obstetrics and pediatrics, in which preventive supervision and examination of presumably well persons is a major requirement of good medical practice. There is a need to explore the practical possibilities of preventive examinations to discover all possible disease, making full use of the diagnostic aids developed by modern medical technology.

Research

FURTHER ADVANCES in the prevention as well as the treatment of many chronic diseases are dependent on research. Although a good deal of research is now being carried on in chronic diseases, only a fraction of the total need is being met.

War experience in medical research has made it clear that we must broaden our vision and think in terms of research planned and organized on a much larger scale than any now contemplated. This requires the training and support of a much larger corps of medical scientists, and the development of teams of research workers to carry forward coördinated programs. The greatest emphasis must be placed on those diseases which are the most important causes of death and disability, such as heart disease, high blood pressure, arteriosclerosis, arthritis, kidney disease, cancer, diabetes, and asthma.

Research institutes in chronic diseases, associated with clinical facilities, may well become the basic units of such a program. In New York City, the research services of the Goldwater Memorial Hospital have carried on important research in kidney disease, arteriosclerosis, malaria, and cirrhosis of the liver. In Illinois, the State Commission on the Care of Chronically Ill Persons is considering the advisability of developing a state supported university research institute for the study of chronic illness which would, in addition to suitable research facilities, provide beds for 200 patients and an outpatient service for 15,000 patients a year. The National Institute of Health is formulating plans for intensive laboratory and clinical research in heart disease, geriatrics, cancer, and mental disease.

There is a great need for administrative research, for more precise information on methods of providing the necessary services for the chronically ill. Basic research on some of the administrative problems is already being undertaken, but the field is a relatively new one and requires intensive study and development.

Research is also necessary in the social and psychological aspects of chronic illness. The influence of these factors in the development of specific chronic diseases needs to be more fully determined, while the effect of chronic illness on the individual's social relationships needs further study.

Medical Care

IN THE PAST, the approach to chronic illness has been primarily concerned with institutional care for advanced stages of disease. There is need for a new orientation which places major emphasis on the early stages of chronic illness with a view to preventing or at least delaying the progress of the disease process.

Diagnosis and treatment of illness at its inception is essential to the control of chronic disease. Competent medical supervision, if brought into play early enough, can have an important preventive effect. The most dramatic expression of this fact is found in cancer control, where diagnosis of early symptoms and prompt treatment may be a life-saving measure, Early diagnosis and proper management of diabetes prevents the serious complications of infection, gangrene, and coma. Similarly, early diagnosis and treatment may prevent complications or prolong the lives of persons with heart disease, hypertension, rheumatic fever, peptic ulcer, and other chronic diseases.

The barriers to early competent diagnosis and treatment must be removed. This requires the construction of hospital and laboratory facilities to cover all our communities, with coordination of facilities to insure a maximum of diagnostic and therapeutic effectiveness for the individual patient. Health and medical agencies need to plan to fill the great needs for personnel as rapidly as possible. Means must be found to remove the basic economic barriers to early diagnosis and therapy.

Health departments, which have carried on excellent educational activities in communicable disease, should turn in increasing numbers to the larger field of chronic illness and teach the public the facts about heart disease, cancer, diabetes, and other chronic diseases, with special emphasis on early signs and symptoms and the importance of early and continued medical supervision.

The concept of medical care must be broadened to include the social factors which play a vital role in the progress of chronic illness. Physicians have learned, for example, that it is not enough to cure a patient with minimal tuberculosis and send him back into the community. On the contrary, he must be observed carefully over a long period of time for signs of reactivation of the disease process. Even more important, the physician must draw on community resources in order to change the patient's environment to prevent breakdown. If the patient's previous occupation called for strenuous physical exertion, he should be retrained for office work or some other light occupation so that he can live with his tuberculosis or other chronic disease. Occupational retraining and job placement are essential therapeutic and preventive measures.

Several general considerations should be borne in mind in planning to provide adequate medical care for the chronically ill.

First, the care of the chronically ill is inseparable from general medical care. While it presents certain special aspects, it cannot be medically isolated without running serious dangers of deterioration of quality of care and medical stagnation.

Second, major emphasis must be given to coördination and integration of services. The person who is chronically ill will receive the type of care which he specifically needs only if provision has been made for the highest possible degree of coördination. Since the medical condition of the chronically ill person is not static but changes with time it is essential to develop smoothly operating mechanisms for referral from one type of care to another.

Third, facilities for the care of the chronically ill should be planned for the community as a whole and not for the indigent alone. Chronic disease strikes all sections of the population, and the lack of facilities is as great for those who are able to pay as for those who are not. The facilities for chronic disease should be community institutions serving all sections of the population. They will in this way achieve a greater degree of financial stability because of the additional income from those able to pay, and will be able to furnish a higher quality of care.

Fourth, the services and facilities necessary for the medical care of the chronically ill require considerable and continuing financial expenditures in order to maintain the quantity and quality of care offered. Good medical care for chronic illness cannot be purchased on an "economy" basis.

Fifth, and most important, the goal of medical care is to maintain and restore the chronically ill as independent and self-supporting members of the community. Major emphasis should be placed on home and office care, with hospital care, convalescent care, and rehabilitation serving where possible to return the chronically ill to productive community life, and with nursing home facilities providing for those whose medical condition is such that they cannot remain in their home environment.

Home Care

THE MAJORITY of persons who are chronically ill can best be cared for in home, office, and clinic.

It is unwise as well as impractical to consider a separate home, office, or clinic service for the chronically ill; their needs are best met by inclusion in the general community medical care program.

Ready access to diagnostic and specialist service is essential to adequate care for chronic diseases, since many of them are difficult to diagnose and treat.

One of the most pressing needs is for an expansion of public health nursing service to provide bedside and other nursing services for the chronically ill. Most rural communities and small cities do not have sufficient public health nurses to provide adequate bedside nursing care. Some of the larger cities have well organized bedside nursing programs, but even here the number of nurses is generally below the estimated minimum of one nurse per 2,000 persons to carry out all public health nursing activities including bedside care. In addition to increasing the number of public health nurses, there is need to train them to provide valuable assistance to physicians in the time-consuming task of educating the individual patient in the proper understanding and management of his chronic illness.

Much wider use should be made of practical nurses and nurses' aides, working under the supervision of the public health nurse, for duties which do not require the training and experience of a graduate nurse.

Housekeeper service should be widely encouraged; there has already accumulated ample experience to show the value of the visiting housekeeper in the home care of chronic illness. Housekeeper service performs the important social function of enabling the chronically ill patient to remain at home, and has an economic value in helping to reduce the need for expensive institutional facilities.

Other measures which enable chronically ill persons to be cared for at home include improved housing, supervised boarding homes, medical-social service, recreational and occupational therapy, and vocational rehabilitation. Social security measures to maintain income such as disability insurance, old-age insurance, and public assistance are likewise of vital importance.

Hospital Care

THE LARGE number of chronically ill persons in general hospitals who require long-term care represents a serious problem to hospital administrators.[2] The general hospital as at present constituted is often unsuited to the care of long-term patients, since it is geared primarily to the therapeutic and general requirements of the acutely ill. It may lack adequate departments for physiotherapy, occupational therapy, and rehabilitation, as well as sun porches, recreational facilities, educational facilities for children, and an understanding of the social and psychological needs of the chronically ill.

The average long-term patient requires less costly care than that provided in the

2. The percentage ranges from 7 to 10 per cent, depending on the area surveyed. In New York City, in 1928, a fifth of the ward beds in both private and municipal general hospitals were occupied by chronic patients. (Jarrett, M. C.: *Chronic Illness in New York City*, Columbia Univ. Press, 1933, vol. 1, p. 119.) In New Jersey, in 1940, 38 general hospitals reported that 7 per cent of the total number of patients were chronically ill. (Frankel, Emil: "New Jersey Studies Problems of Care for the Chronically Ill," *Hospital Management* 50:19, August 1940.) The findings to date in the Illinois State Health Department's survey of hospital facilities indicate that about 15 per cent of the beds in the general hospitals of the state are occupied by chronically ill patients (unpublished data).

acute general hospital.[3] To continue to care for the long-term patient in the acute general hospital is wasteful; it provides care which is more expensive than he actually needs, and which is often unsuited to his requirements.

The construction of hospital facilities for the chronically ill has been encouraged by the passage of the Hospital Survey and Construction Act, which provides federal aid for such facilities up to a maximum of two beds per 1,000 population.

There is already evident a tendency in some localities to build chronic disease hospitals in areas remote from the medical center and the general hospital and with no relation to them. This trend unfortunately follows the pattern already laid down in the construction of our tuberculosis and mental hospitals, a pattern which has resulted in many instances in the medical isolation and stagnation of these special institutions.

Hospital facilities for long-term illness should be built in the very closest relation to teaching centers and general hospitals.

The specialized chronic disease hospital is suitable in large cities, where it can be located on the grounds of or very closely related to a medical school or teaching general hospital. Special consideration should be given to planning the facilities for children who are chronically ill. While an official or voluntary organization may be responsible for the construction and maintenance costs, the medical school should provide the attending and resident staff and utilize the facilities for research and medical education in chronic disease.

It is important that the specialized chronic disease hospital serve as the consultation center for chronic disease in its medical service region. It should maintain formal professional affiliation with general hospitals in the region that care for chronic patients, in order to provide consultation and teaching visits from the center to the general hospitals as well as the referral of patients to the center for special study.

Most patients with chronic illness who require hospitalization are best cared for in a unit of the general hospital especially designed to meet their needs. This arrangement encourages patients to seek and use care since it is near their homes, families, and friends; makes available to them the existing facilities of general hospitals; provides opportunity to internes, nurses, and staff for experience and teaching in chronic disease; avoids expensive duplication of existing general hospital facilities; and affords the most ready means of transfer to and from the acute and chronic disease sections of the hospital when needed. Further, it allows for greater flexibility in hospital planning by making it possible for future, unforeseen shifts in the relative proportions of patients with acute and chronic diseases to be met by changing the designated use of either chronic or acute beds in the same hospitals.

Many advantages of this plan would be lost if the chronically ill were simply

3. The cost at Montefiore Hospital, a high standard voluntary chronic disease hospital in New York City, is more than two-thirds the cost in acute general hospitals. (Communication from Dr. E. M. Bluestone, Director.) In 1945, the cost at Goldwater Memorial Hospital in New York City, was one-half the average cost in the acute general municipal hospitals. (Communication from Dr. E. M. Bernecker, Commissioner of Hospitals of New York City).

intermingled with all other patients in general hospitals. The provision of a special wing or floor devoted to long-term patients insures that the special needs and problems of chronic disease are not lost sight of in competition with the more urgent and dramatic needs of the acutely ill. It makes possible the planning of the special unit in conformity with its special purpose, both as to architecture and staff. It makes it easier to provide occupational and recreational therapy, special physical therapy, rehabilitation and other services essential to the care of long-term patients. It facilitates a more economical use of nursing personnel, the utilization of a larger proportion of attendants, and less intensive medical staff attendance than is needed in the section of the hospital devoted to patients with acute illnesses.

Under no circumstances should chronic disease hospitals or units be limited to the indigent. The lack of facilities is felt by all sections of the population. High standards will be maintained most effectively if the facilities are geared to meet the requirements of the entire community. Also, the admission of patients who are able to pay will reduce the need for tax funds. It must be recognized, however, that prolonged illness exhausts the financial resources of many patients, necessitating payment from tax funds for their care.

Care in Nursing Homes

CHRONICALLY ILL persons who need active and continuous medical care should be treated in a hospital. On the other hand, there are many chronically ill persons who are more or less disabled by their illness, whose requirements for care can be met by practical nurses and attendants with medical and nursing supervision, and who cannot or should not remain at home. Care for such persons should be provided in nursing homes.

The following example may make the difference clear. A person who has suffered a cerebral hemorrhage with paralysis of one side of his body requires hospital care. This care will extend over a period of weeks and months during which time he will receive intensive physical therapy to restore the maximum possible use of his muscular system. When no further improvement can be obtained by medical treatment, and he is left with a good deal of disability which makes it impossible for him to be cared for at home, he is eligible for care in a nursing home.

Nursing homes, both private and public, should be brought under state licensure laws in which provision is made for minimum standards and regular inspection. The minimum standards should require continuing medical supervision, including complete medical examinations of patients prior to admission to the nursing home and follow-up examinations at definite intervals, as well as physician visits on a regular basis and on call. The standards should call for a sufficient number of practical nurses and attendants to meet the full needs of the patients. They should provide for at least one full-time graduate nurse in charge of nursing care. The standards should require facilities for recreation and occupational therapy, for a maximum of privacy and individual attention, and for cheerful and homelike surroundings. Construction should meet adequate standards of safety and sanitation.[4]

Private Nursing Homes.—Experience has demonstrated that improvement in the quality of private nursing homes cannot be obtained merely by passage of a licensure law. The power to inspect and license nursing homes carries with it the responsibility for carrying on an intensive educational campaign, working with the individual nursing homes to improve the care given. The device of placing each new nursing home on a six month probationary period, during which time there is a great deal of educational assistance from the licensing agency, has been demonstrated to be an effective method of raising standards.

It is suggested that wherever possible, the quality of medical and nursing supervision can be greatly improved through arrangement with the medical board of a nearby hospital to provide the necessary medical services.

One of the most serious drawbacks to adequate care by private nursing homes is the low payments made by welfare agencies for clients requiring nursing home care. A sharp upward revision of payments by welfare agencies, to bring them up to the actual cost of care, is an indispensable prerequisite to raising standards. At the federal and state levels, liberalization or elimination of the ceiling on payments for public assistance clients is indicated.

Public Nursing Homes.—The realization that a large proportion of the population of county homes or almshouses consists of chronically ill adults has led to a widespread movement to convert them into public nursing homes.

It is clear that such conversion does not make the almshouse a chronic disease hospital, but rather a nursing home for the chronically ill.

County homes should be converted into public nursing homes only if their physical facilities are adequate, if they are within reasonable distance of general hospitals with which close medical relationships are maintained, and if the responsible authorities are prepared to meet the minimum standards described previously: namely, adequate medical and graduate nursing supervision; sufficient personnel to meet the full needs of the patients, including medical-social service if possible; provision for privacy, a cheerful and homelike atmosphere, recreational and occupational therapy; and construction which meets safety and sanitation requirements. Many county homes cannot meet these conditions and should therefore not be considered for conversion.

It is suggested that conversion be planned on a state-wide basis, with the most careful evaluation of the suitability of individual almshouses for conversion. Financial and technical assistance by the State to localities planning conversion will make it possible to achieve higher standards of care. Public nursing homes should be included in the provisions of nursing home licensure laws.

A factor which will help obtain increased community interest, better administra-

4. A detailed description of minimum standards of nursing home care is given in *Institutional Care of the Chronically Ill*, a report issued by a joint committee of the American Hospital Association and the American Public Welfare Association in January 1940.

tion, and higher quality care in public nursing homes is the admission of patients able to pay part or all of the cost of care. There is a considerable demand for public nursing home care on the part of patients able to pay. By opening its facilities to such patients the public nursing home will not only improve its financial position but will perhaps begin to free itself from the almshouse tradition and serve as a public facility for the entire community.

The Social Security Act should be amended to allow federal matching to states for assistance to patients who wish to enter public medical institutions, including nursing homes, that meet adequate standards. Payment for nursing care in public as well as private homes should be commensurate with the actual cost.

New Institutions.—The shortage of institutions for nursing home care of the chronically ill cannot be met by present facilities or by the conversion of county homes. There is a definite need for new construction.

It is recommended that voluntary and governmental general hospitals which have chronic disease pavilions give serious consideration to establishing nursing home facilities for the chronically ill. These facilities should be built on the grounds of the general hospital or within a reasonable distance. There should be close administrative, medical, and nursing relationships between the hospital and the nursing home.

The specialized chronic disease hospitals located in teaching centers should likewise maintain nursing homes which can be utilized for research and training and will set standards of quality of nursing home care.

The construction of new institutions should be closely integrated with state plans for reconversion of public homes and utilization of private nursing homes in order to prevent an overabundance of facilities in some areas and lack of facilities in others.

Convalescence and Rehabilitation

UNDOUBTEDLY the most neglected aspect of chronic illness is that of convalescence and rehabilitation.

Only recently has there been recognition of the fact that convalescent care is an important feature of the care of the chronically ill. Chronic diseases often run a course of many years, with periods of relative well-being alternating with periods of illness. Following a flare-up of illness adequate convalescent care may lead to complete or partial rehabilitation, and may help delay the progress of the underlying chronic disease. Such convalescent care undoubtedly conserves hospital beds and performs important therapeutic and preventive functions. Examples of chronically ill persons requiring convalescent care would include those recovering from a period of heart failure, an attack of acute rheumatic fever, or a flare-up of arthritis. Then there are persons who have a chronic illness such as diabetes or heart disease, and develop pneumonia or some other acute illness, and need convalescent care after recovery from the acute illness.

There has been a large growth of convalescent homes for children with rheumatic heart disease and other crippling conditions. It is essential that such convalescent homes be located near enough to general hospitals to permit close professional relationships and adequate medical supervision.

Convalescent homes for adults have never been developed to any appreciable extent in the United States. Most convalescent care for adults is now provided in nursing homes which also care for non-convalescent patients. On the whole, there has been insufficient appreciation of the value of convalescent care and rehabilitation in the care of the chronically ill.

Recent experience with planned convalescence and rehabilitation in the armed forces has demonstrated their great potential usefulness. By providing physical reconditioning, educational training, recreational activities, and vocational guidance, it was found possible to shorten the period of hospitalization, reduce the incidence of recurrences, and return a larger proportion of men to active duty.

Planned convalescence and rehabilitation are particularly important in chronic disease. The chronically ill have to be made conscious of their limitations early in the course of the disease, and many of them must be retrained for new occupations so that they may stay within the limits of activity prescribed by their illness and yet maintain their economic independence.

Probably the first steps along these lines will be taken by university hospitals, some of which have already made plans for rehabilitation centers as an integral part of their medical program.

In 1943, Congress broadened the scope of the national rehabilitation program. As a result, state rehabilitation agencies were able to rehabilitate successfully nearly 42,000 persons in 1945. These were generally persons with long standing chronic impairments and illnesses—orthopedic disabilities, speech, hearing, and sight defects, poliomyelitis, tuberculosis, mental disease, heart disease, asthma, hernia, and other conditions. That the need is still far from being met is indicated by the fact that the estimated backlog of persons in need of and entitled to such service is between 1½ and 2 millions.

Of the 42,000 disabled persons who were successfully rehabilitated in 1945, nearly 79 per cent were unemployed at the time of applying for rehabilitation service, and 18 per cent had never been employed. The average yearly income before rehabilitation, including those who received assistance from public or private sources, was $288. The average annual wage after rehabilitation was $1,764. The total income of the group was increased by rehabilitation from 12 million dollars a year to 74 million, a sixfold increase.

In the past, many of the disabled have had to be supported by public or private assistance at a cost up to $500 a person each year. Vocational rehabilitation costs an average of only $300 a person, and this cost is not repeated. On the contrary, rehabilitation changes the individual into a self-sustaining productive member of the community. It is clear that rehabilitation is economically and socially sound.

The results achieved with long standing chronic impairments and diseases point up to the potentialities of rehabilitation instituted early in the course of chronic illness.

Coördination of Services

THE PROBLEM of chronic disease presents many aspects—prevention, research, medical care in home, hospital and nursing home, and convalescence and rehabilitation.

Undue emphasis on any one aspect would be unwise, uneconomical, and ineffectual. For example, to concentrate on the provision of medical care without paying serious attention to prevention and research would postpone for many years any basic attack on the problem. On the other hand, it is impossible to focus sole attention on research because of the very urgent need for medical care. Likewise, to provide hospital beds for chronic disease without making nursing home facilities available would result in many beds being occupied by patients who do not need hospital care. Too great an emphasis on nursing homes would deprive many patients of the specialized hospital care which is necessary for their improvement. Failure to plan adequately for home care or for convalescent care and rehabilitation would defeat the purpose of the program—to maintain and restore the individual as a self-supporting productive member of his community.

There is a great need for coöperation and coördination of the numerous agencies concerned with chronic disease: health, welfare, and education departments, hospitals, medical societies, medical schools, social agencies, rehabilitation services, nursing homes, etc. In some communities this coördination has been achieved through the establishment of central planning and coördinating bodies which study the various aspects of the problem, make the facts known to authorities and the public, stimulate needed services, assist in securing necessary facilities, and act as information centers for patients, physicians, and health and social agencies.

The total problem of chronic disease is not a series of separate problems which can be solved one by one, but rather a complex of interrelated problems which require simultaneous solution. It is recommended, therefore, that coördinated and comprehensive planning be undertaken at all levels in order to achieve effective action to meet the challenge of chronic illness.

57. THE PREVENTIVE APPROACH *

THE TERM "detection" has been used in medical literature in a number of ways. It has been taken to mean early clinical diagnosis, diagnosis of disease in apparently well persons, and the application of screening tests for early diagnosis. It is useful to

* From: "Detection of Chronic Disease," by Morton L. Levin, M.D.; *Journal of the American Medical Association* 146:1397-1401, Aug. 11, 1951 (No. 15). Reprinted (with omissions, including some tables) by permission of the author and publishers. The author is assistant commissioner for medical services, New York State Department of Health, Albany.

confine the term to *the identification of disease which is not causing symptoms or manifest illness.* Detection is thus a variety of diagnosis.[1] It is to be distinguished from the usual form, clinical diagnosis, since this is the determination of the nature of disease that is already producing symptoms or illness. The two forms of diagnosis may be contrasted by saying that clinical diagnosis is identification of disease for which the patient seeks help; detection is diagnosis of disease of which the person is not aware and thus for which he is not seeking help.

Detection, however, in a very real sense has its oldest and most extensive application in clinical medicine, when the physician, examining a patient, looks for disease other than that which is responsible for the presenting illness. The extent to which this is done distinguishes the thorough from the superficial practice of medicine. I can recall a striking example of the failure to practice clinical detection: A woman was examined within a few months by a distinguished surgeon because of a thyroid enlargement and by an eminent cardiologist because of symptoms of heart failure; both examinations failed to detect a malignant tumor in the right breast, which was diagnosed by a general practitioner a few weeks later. Possibly, had the tumor been in the left breast, the cardiologist might have detected it during the course of his examination. Had this diagnosis been made as part of a screening program or in a detection clinic, it would have been an example of nonclinical detection.

There are thus two chief varieties of detection, clinical and nonclinical, and both are forms of definitive diagnosis. "Screening," which is sometimes mistakenly used as synonymous with detection, is the application of presumptive tests to determine whether there is a need for the application of more definitive diagnostic procedures. It may be used in clinical diagnosis, in clinical detection, or in nonclinical detection. Screening is not a form of diagnosis but one of the steps toward diagnosis. Diagnosis is of course a medical judgment or decision and can be reached only by one qualified to render such judgment—a physician.

To complete this attempt at a definition, it is necessary to point out that although detection is early diagnosis it is not the same as early clinical diagnosis. Early clinical diagnosis refers to the identification of the nature or cause of illness early in its clinical course, i. e., as soon as it produces symptoms or illness. Detection, on the other hand, is the diagnosis of disease before the clinical course has begun.

We have now, in attempting to clarify the subject of detection, distinguished three different types of diagnosis, or identification of disease, early clinical diagnosis, clinical detection, and nonclinical detection—and a fourth procedure, screening, which may be used in connection with any of the three. The distinction between the three diagnostic processes is justified since they refer to three different situations. For example, with reference to tuberculosis, early clinical diagnosis can be practiced only on persons who have symptoms of tuberculosis, clinical detection on persons

---

1. The Committee on Early Detection and Screening in Medical Practice at the National Conference on Chronic Disease (Commission on Chronic Illness), Chicago, Mar. 12-14 [1951], defined detection as "the identification of ordinarily unrecognized disease or defect by application of screening tests, examinations and diagnostic procedures."

who have symptoms suggestive of some other disease, and nonclinical detection on persons who have no symptoms. In any of these three, one may proceed directly to procedures leading to definitive diagnosis, such as taking a 14 by 17 inch chest roentgenogram or a sputum examination and culture, or the screening procedure for tuberculosis, which is the taking of a small photofluorographic chest x-ray, may precede these.

In the control of disease, particularly chronic disease, all these types of diagnosis must be considered. The first, early clinical diagnosis, does not belong in theory to the subject of detection; in practice it has been found that some people attend centers for nonclinical detection because of the presence of symptoms. This in part accounts for the higher than expected number of cases of disease often found among the presumably "well" persons examined at detection centers. Although persons with symptoms of disease do not, strictly speaking, belong in a detection center, they do go there, and to that extent a detection center serves to advance early clinical diagnosis. This may indeed be its most important function. For many important chronic diseases no reliable detection procedures are known, and early clinical diagnosis is the chief control method. The "yield" of new cases found is highest in this procedure, and it is probably still the most important single control measure in chronic disease. The medical literature continues to groan with complaints from various specialists on how late in the course of disease patients reach them. The validity of these complaints, expressed in terms of the general population, is supported by a recent state-wide study in Michigan. In this study of a sample of the population (exclusive of Wayne County, Michigan), 41 per cent had one or more of 26 symptoms indicative of chronic disease, and of these one in three, or 14 per cent of the population, had received no medical care whatever during the six months preceding the survey. If this study is at all representative of the whole country, it would indicate that additional efforts to achieve early clinical diagnosis of chronic disease are needed with respect to approximately 21 million persons in the United States.

Detectable Chronic Disease

SOME FURTHER indication of the importance of the chronic diseases today is given by the fact that almost four out of five deaths occurring in the United States in 1948, or 1,127,228 deaths (table 39), were attributed to a chronic disease. Of these about one-fourth, or one out of every five deaths, were caused by a disease which could be considered detectable (table 39). . . . Both the feasibility and the ultimate value, to the patient and the community, of detecting each of these chronic diseases vary. Certainly, with respect to pulmonary tuberculosis, syphilis, and certain forms of cancer and heart disease, the importance and value of detection is well established. With respect to many other of the diseases listed, what would be gained, in prolongation of life and prevention of progression of the disease process, by bringing these diseases under medical care before they cause symptoms is not so much questioned as not precisely known. The necessary data to determine this can best be gathered by detection and long-term observation of a sufficiently large and representative sample of such cases. Thus, in many instances, determination of the value of detection depends on giving it an organized, systematic trial.

TABLE 39. *Mortality from chronic disease, United States, 1948* [A]

Cause of Death	Number	Per Cent
All causes	1,444,337	100.0
Chronic diseases	1,127,228	78.0
Detectable chronic diseases *	320,646	22.1

[A] Deaths and crude death rates for each cause: United States, 1946-1948, Vital Statistics Special Reports, Federal Security Agency, United States Public Health Service, National Office of Vital Statistics, Vol. 35, No. 11, May 15, 1950.

The number of deaths from detectable chronic disease is not necessarily a good index of the number of cases at a detectable stage which exist at any given time. Many important chronic defects and diseases do not appear in mortality statistics. Also, annual mortality is not usually an accurate index of annual incidence. Even if it were, one must remember that the number of new cases of a detectable chronic disease which can be discovered during the first examination of a population is a product of the incidence of the disease and the length of the detectable period. If this detectable period exceeds one year, the number of cases found during the first examination is correspondingly increased. For example, from data on the annual incidence of carcinoma of the uterine cervix (a detectable form of cancer) the number of new cases expected in a representative group of women over 40 years of age would be 62 per 100,000, or approximately 16,000 cases if the entire female population of this country were examined.[2] However, there is evidence that carcinoma of the uterine cervix may remain in the nonclinical but detectable stage for as long as five years. This would increase the number of cases expected *at first examination* to 310 per 100,000, or 81,000 cases in the entire female population over 40 years of age. At a subsequent examination of the same group, however, the new cases found should approximate the annual incidence, assuming that examinations were made at yearly intervals. We have little data regarding the duration of the detectable period for most chronic diseases. Information on this point would be a valuable by-product of further experience in detection of disease in large samples of the population.

Estimates of the prevalence of detectable chronic diseases or defects also will necessarily vary with the number of conditions included, the age and sex distribution of the population considered, and the basic figures on incidence of the various diseases and defects employed. In table 40 are presented two such estimates and one figure based on actual experience in a multiple-detection project involving 235,191 persons in Atlanta. The estimates vary from 27 to 260 per 1,000 persons. The

* The author lists, in a table omitted here, the following as the "detectable" diseases causing the more than 300,000 deaths indicated: chronic nephritis; epilepsy; syphilis; idiopathic hypertension; respiratory tuberculosis; cancer of various sites; heart disease (congenital malformations and chronic valvular); diabetes mellitus; hypertrophy of prostate; and non-malignant uterine tumors.

2. Based on annual incidence rates furnished by the New York State Department of Health, ⌐eau of Cancer Control, 1945-1947.

estimate of Chapman is for persons 15 years and over. If visual defects, hearing loss, and obesity are included, Chapman estimates that 976 diseases or defects (not persons) would be found per 1,000 persons examined. Without these conditions Chapman's estimate is 260 per 1,000 persons, and this is somewhat higher than the observed number of 208 per 1,000 found in the Atlanta detection project reported by Bowdoin....

TABLE 40. *Some estimates of detectable chronic disease*

Author	Estimated Number per 1,000 Examined	Conditions Excluded
Chapman, A. L.	260	Visual and hearing defects and obesity
Bowdoin, C. D.	208	210 per 1,000 in need of dental care
Smillie, W. G.	27-47	Serious pathological

If dental defects in need of treatment are included, the Atlanta figure becomes 418 per 1,000 persons examined. Smillie estimates that, in an "adult" population, previously undetected cases of active tuberculosis, active syphilis, heart disease, cancer, diabetes, and "other serious diseases," would total 27 to 47 per 1,000. These estimates are probably closer to what might be expected in an unselected white population at first examination, but not on subsequent examination. However, the practical facts are that, until the entire adult population is examined, most detection programs will be, in effect, first examinations, and most groups examined will not be unselected samples of the population. Whether we consider the minimum estimate of 27 or the maximum of 418 cases of significant chronic disease and defect found by detection examinations, there can be little doubt that to find these cases and bring them under medical care would be a substantial contribution to the better control of chronic disease. Two questions are frequently raised with respect to this objective: 1. Can it best be accomplished by clinical detection or nonclinical detection? 2. Should detection programs be concentrated on single diseases, as in the past, or should tests for several diseases or conditions be applied at a single examination?

Multiple or Single Detection

SOME DETECTION procedures, though aimed at a single disease, are inherently or potentially multiple by reason of the kind of examination required to detect that disease. For example, in cancer detection a fairly complete examination is needed because cancer may affect any part of the body. Consequently, cancer detection centers discover many non-neoplastic as well as neoplastic conditions and are, in effect, "multiple" detection centers. In chest roentgenographic surveys, although examination of the roentgenogram is often limited to determination of the possible presence of significant tuberculosis, the same roentgenogram can be used to look for evidence of lung tumors and abnormal heart shadows. The inclusion of tests for several detectable diseases, such as tuberculosis, syphilis, heart disease, diabetes, and cancer, in a single examination session is a logical expansion of the single-disease-screening technique. The first organized attempt to conduct multiple screening and detection was carried out in 1949 at San Jose, Calif., as a joint project of the County Medical Society, the State Department of Health, and the City Department of Health. It has since then been extensively applied on a mass scale in the cities of Richmond, Va., and Atlanta and in the state of Alabama.

A number of objections or questions have been raised with respect to multiple screening or multiple detection. One such objection is that many borderline deviations from some arbitrary norm may be uncovered whose clinical significance is doubtful or uncertain. The same objection might, of course, be raised to single-disease screening or, for that matter, to many diagnostic tests or procedures employed in clinical medicine. So long as final interpretation of the test rests with the physician, we may rely upon him to exercise the same skill and judgment in this situation as he would exercise in the clinical setting. Another objection which has been raised is that wide-scale multiple testing would prevent the otherwise more successful application of single-disease-screening tests. This may be true in some communities. It has not been found true in others (such as Atlanta) where mass multiple screening has been tried and widely accepted.

Whether or not detection, or its screening phase, should be single or multiple would seem to depend on the primary purpose of the procedure. One may conceive of situations in which it would be necessary, or at least desirable, to concentrate on a single disease. For example, tuberculosis may be the major health problem in a community, and all available health resources may be needed to attack it alone. Or, one may wish, for publicity or fund-raising purposes, to focus public attention on a single disease. If the purpose of detection is health maintenance and the prevention of chronic illness, then it would seem reasonable to include in the detection examination, as a minimum, all procedures and tests known to provide reasonably accurate evidence of the presence of diseases for which effective control measures are known. Others might be added for investigative purposes.

One gains the impression that a good deal of the objections to mass multiple screening rest on two factors: (a) its widespread application to the apparently well population and (b) the possibility that it may be applied chiefly by governmental health agencies, e. g., health departments, and thus would represent an extension of the scope of governmental health programs. The first objection is hardly valid if it can be shown that the apparently well population would benefit from the application of multiple screening and detection. The validity of the second objection depends on the relationship between the voluntary health agencies, including the medical profession, and the official health agencies in a given community and may be considered a matter for local option. From the standpoint of medical ethics, it would be difficult to defend, as a general principle, the viewpoint that would oppose any new health measure, regardless of its public health value, simply because it would be carried on by a governmental health agency. However, there is no reason why multiple screening could not be carried out by hospitals, voluntary health agencies, health departments, the organized medical profession, or all of these agencies together. Certainly in clinical detection, when the objective is to obtain all pertinent information regarding the health status of the patient, the physician should prefer to apply all the detection tests which are practicable and useful.

Clinical Detection

THE OPPORTUNITY for the practice of clinical detection of chronic disease, in people who seek medical care for illness, is indicated by the number of persons who visit a physician or are admitted to a hospital during a given period. . . . It would probably be conservative to say that within a 12-month period an opportunity to carry out clinical detection of chronic disease exists for approximately 50 million persons, or one-third of the population.

At the recent National Conference on Preventive Aspects of Chronic Disease, held in Chicago, March 12 to 14, 1951, the Committee on Early Detection and Screening in Private Practice concluded that "the best way to detect chronic disease in its early stages is for every doctor to practice detection in his own office." The committee recommended that office examinations for detection of chronic disease include a history; physical examination; tests for visual acuity, hearing loss, and increased intraocular pressure; laboratory examination of a blood sample for the hemoglobin and glucose content; serologic examination for syphilis; x-ray of the chest, and urinalysis. It was recommended also that detection procedures be applied to all members of a family in which there was discovered a case of rheumatic fever, diabetes mellitus, hypertension, arteriosclerosis, blindness, deafness, epilepsy, tuberculosis, or syphilis.

Recognizing that this type of examination is an ideal difficult to achieve under present conditions, the committee went on to say:

. . . the tremendous demands on the doctor's time and the great expense of doing many of these procedures on an individual basis require the development of techniques which will lighten the burden on the doctor and be economically feasible. Such techniques are utilized in mass screening. . . . Since the doctor must follow through suspicious cases to definitive diagnosis and treatment, it is important that mass screening programs for communities be cooperative ventures with the physician assuming a major responsibility.

Thus, in effect, the committee's conclusion may be interpreted as a recommendation that clinical and nonclinical detection be combined, with the detection center serving as a laboratory facility to which the physician can refer his patients for screening tests as well as a means of examining persons who otherwise would not seek medical attention and referring them, when indicated, to the physician for definitive diagnosis and care.

The extent to which clinical detection is now being practiced is unknown. Two notable examples of its present practice are the routine chest x-ray examination some hospitals give to all patients on admission and the periodic health examinations some group health plans provide for their clients. The private practitioner of medicine, however, has not been stimulated to utilize either single or multiple nonclinical-detection projects as facilities to which he can refer patients in the first instance. This may be due, to a great extent, to the preoccupation of the voluntary and official agencies sponsoring detection projects with the apparently well population.

We must now consider whether greater gains in the control of chronic disease might not be achieved by shifting some of the emphasis from nonclinical to clinical detection. This would involve cooperative planning on the part of the voluntary and official health agencies to pool their resources to establish detection centers to which physicians could refer patients for rapid screening for those chronic diseases for which reliable screening procedures already exist. Such centers could be used, also, for nonclinical detection at periodic intervals. They could serve as research centers for the evaluation of new screening tests.

Concentration of our efforts on clinical as well as nonclinical detection would avoid the greatest psychological hazard which the latter presents, the difficulty of converting the frame of mind of an apparently healthy person to that of a patient's. Since a large proportion of the population voluntarily seeks a physician's advice each year, it would seem logical to use every effort to encourage the physician to utilize facilities for the detection of chronic disease as a minimum and basic service which he can offer each patient. With proper safeguards as to referral of patients and confidential record-keeping and reporting, such a service should be entirely acceptable to most physicians.

Since such a service should be as inclusive as possible, it should offer a project in which all voluntary and official agencies concerned with the detectable chronic diseases could reasonably join forces. This would undoubtedly increase the effectiveness of individual programs. It would also constitute an important step toward further cooperative efforts in the solution of the many other problems common to the chronic diseases.

58. MULTIPHASIC SCREENING: PROS AND CONS

A. SCREENING PROGRAMS IN ACTION *

DEFINITIONS

IT BECAME apparent early in the present study that a clarification of terms was needed as well as the development of a definition which would most nearly embrace the fundamental concept of multiple screening and minimize misunderstanding. As Levin observed, "... much of the difference of opinion regarding multiple screening and detection has been based on differing concepts of what was meant by the term and the program rather than differences in fundamental philosophy."

* From: *A Study of Multiple Screening: Descriptive Date on 33 Screening Surveys,* by the Council on Medical Service of the American Medical Association; Chicago: The Association, 1955 ("Introduction" and "Survey Summary" sections, pp. 7-14). Reprinted (with omissions) by permission of the publishers.

At the National Conference on Chronic Disease [1] it was agreed that *"Screening is the presumptive identification of unrecognized disease or defect by the application of tests, examinations, or other procedures which can be applied rapidly."* It stated further that "screening tests are procedures which sort out those who probably have abnormalities from those who probably do not," and that "mass screening programs consist of the application of screening tests rapidly and economically to large population groups, to identify those who probably have abnormal conditions, and refer them for diagnosis and, if indicated, for further medical care." Levin has emphasized that "screening is not synonymous with detection," nor is it "... a form of diagnosis ...," but is rather "... one of the steps towards diagnosis." ...

Multiple screening, then, is just what the name implies—"mass screening tests ... applied simultaneously for the discovery of more than one disease." * A fairly complete definition therefore might be: *Multiple screening is the use of two or more simple laboratory tests, examinations, or procedures, applied rapidly and on a mass basis, to determine presumptive evidence of unrecognized or incipient disease or defect.*

BASIC PRINCIPLES

SOME BASIC principles involved in multiple screening are: (1) the screening tests should be simple to administer, (2) they should be easy to interpret, (3) they should be relatively inexpensive, (4) they should require little time to perform, and (5) each test or procedure should meet the five criteria suggested by the National Conference on Chronic Illness, Section on Evaluation of Scientific Data.† These criteria are:

(a) *Reliability.*—"The test must be reliable in that information must be available concerning the reproducibility of results as limited by the technical procedure."

(b) *Validity.*—"The validity of a test is measured by the frequency with which the result of the test is confirmed by an acceptable diagnostic procedure."

(c) *Yield.*—"The yield of a screening program can be measured by the number of previously unknown verified cases of disease among the total population surveyed, the number of persons with previously unknown verified diseases benefited by referral to medical care, and the number of previously known cases not under medical care benefited by return to it ..., and the number of cases of communicable diseases who are prevented from spreading their disease to the family or to the community."

(d) *Cost.*—"The size of the yield of the screening program must be balanced against the cost ... measured in monetary terms and in the relative amounts of time of professional and non-professional personnel."

(e) *Acceptance.*—"Reliability, validity, yield, and cost are essential criteria for evaluation of screening tests and programs. The measurement of acceptance of the

1. Preventive Aspects of Chronic Disease, Conference Proceedings, National Conference on Chronic Disease, March 12-14, 1951, Chicago, p. 63.
    * Ibid., p. 68.
    † Ibid., pp. 64-68.

program by the physicians, individual laymen, and the community is a useful additional criterion of the effectiveness of a screening program."

"The goal of multiple screening is to find those conditions which require early attention from the physician and to obtain the correction of the condition in the physician's office. It is this latter part, the *referral of the patient to the physician's office for early care,* that is the *prime objective of multiple screening."* [2]

STATEMENTS FAVORING MULTIPLE SCREENING

As IN MOST experimental programs, the literature contains statements for as well as against multiple screening. Most of the favorable comments are from physicians concerned with public health programs and having a part in screening surveys, although it must also be borne in mind that at least 24 of the surveys described here were carried on with the approval of the medical society concerned. The following quotations were selected as representative of the favorable comments contained in the literature reviewed for this report:

One of the conclusions reached by Levin and Brightman in a presentation at the 146th Annual Meeting of the Medical Society of the State of New York was that "Multiphasic screening, utilizing presumptive tests to determine whether there is a need for the application of more definitive diagnostic procedures, with proper safeguards, is an excellent preliminary procedure to any form of examination and, by reducing the cost and time factors, may make it possible to extend periodic examinations to significantly larger groups of the population."

The following is a statement from the Conference Proceedings, National Conference on Chronic Diseases [p. 81]: "Screening programs are one of the practical ways of bringing the benefits of early detection to as many people as possible. Designed as an auxiliary to the practicing physician, they can help sort out persons who are apparently well but who in reality may need medical care."

Referring to the Richmond multi-test clinic, one article points out that, "Roughly two-thirds of the clinic visitors later had a physical or clinical examination. This could contribute to better detection of health hazards, and could also serve to make people more health conscious, more aware of the value of regular checks for early detection of disease." [3]

A report on the San Jose screening project states: ". . . the functions of private medicine and public health supplement each other and are not in any sense competitive. It can be demonstrated that cooperative effort will tremendously enhance the effectiveness of each field of medicine toward achieving a vastly improved total community health without interference with the normal processes of private enterprise." [4]

Writing in the Journal of the American Medical Association for March 22, 1952,

2. Getting, V. A., and Lombard, H. L.: The Cost and Evaluation of Multiple Screening Procedures, N.Y. State J. M. 52:2605 (Nov. 1) 1952. [Italics not in the original.]
3. The Multiple Screening Idea—Report on the Richmond Clinic, prepared by the Health Information Foundation, 420 Lexington Ave., N. Y. 17, N. Y.
4. Canelo, C. K.; Bissell, D. M.; Abrams, H., and Breslow, Lester: Multiphasic Screening Survey in San Jose, Calif. Med. 71:409 (Dec.) 1949.

about the Georgia experience, Petrie, Bowdoin, and McLaughlin state that, "No method of health education, other than the multiphasic screening survey, has been demonstrated that will effectively educate as high a percentage of the previously apathetic and medically unsupervised public."

In another presentation before the 146th Annual Meeting of the Medical Society of the State of New York, Getting and Lombard conclude among other things that "The modern concept of multiple screening enables the individual to benefit in a single visit from the most recent developments in preventive medicine and health supervision. Multiple screening enables the physician to do more for his patient by giving to him data which are generally not available to him. Multiple screening causes apparently well persons who were not aware that they might have a progressive disease to consult their physician." . . .

An editorial in the American Journal of Public Health of March 1952 explains that, "While we could probably all agree that the best way to detect disease in its earliest stages is for the doctor to practice detection in his own office, the fact remains that this is an ideal difficult to achieve under present conditions . . . the multiple screening facility can serve a dual function . . . as a laboratory facility to which the doctor can refer patients for screening . . . as an agency to screen persons who have not sought medical attention, and to refer them, when indicated, to a physician for diagnosis and care. Such screening facilities need not be limited to health departments." . . .

Getting and Ryder in discussing "Mass Screening or the Multiphasic Clinic" in the July 1951 Journal of the Michigan State Medical Society state that "Although a mass screening may miss certain physical disabilities when it is applied without a history and without a physicial examination, it has proved to be effective in bringing to the attention of physicians suspected cases of some of the major killers."

Through their experience in California, Breslow says that "Increasing attention is being focused by health agencies, private physicians, and the public alike on early detection as a basic long range approach to the chronic disease problem. The experience of this project indicates that multiphasic screening programs help meet this need. They should be encouraged as effective health education and case finding tools." [5]

Speaking of the Pennsylvania Mobile Health Survey Program the medical director states that "The one prime objective of this health survey plan is to assist in the provision of adequate medical care for the Union members, *through their family physicians*. It is not the purpose of the plan nor the desire of its sponsors to replace or embarrass the private practitioner. The feeling is strong and the conviction firm, that for him and his services there is no adequate substitute." [6]

In an article on "Screening—In the Doctor's Office" in the November 1950 Connecticut State Medical Journal, White is of the opinion that "widespread screening is here to stay," and poses the question concerning the feasibility of it being

5. Breslow, Lester, M.D. See Conclusions section of Los Angeles (Northeast Health District) Multiple Screening Survey of this compilation.
6. Bloom, James, M.D., Medical Director, Health and Welfare Dept. ILGWU, Central and Western Pennsylvania.

incorporated into medical practice. This would be desired rather than having it " 'taken over by outside agencies'." He says that if the laboratory tests, which are now available to the practicing physician only sporadically, ". . . were centralized in such a way that a patient could get them all performed at one convenient spot, the physician could more easily and confidently devote a portion of his time to the seeking out of disease processes in the early or pre-symptomatic stages." White [7] emphasizes in a later paper that there are no short cuts in the relationship between the physician and the patient in the time-honored diagnosis and treatment phase, but he sees possible curtailment of time in the " 'screening' phase for unexpected diagnoses . . . provided office arrangements permit rapid examination and provided 'package' laboratory tests can be made readily available."

OBJECTIONS TO MULTIPLE SCREENING

MANY HAVE QUESTIONED the value of, and expense involved in, multiple screening, others have voiced specific objection to its use. A number of editorials and articles object to such screening or call attention to its inadequacies. The following are comments from the various medical bulletins and journals:

An editorial in the North Carolina Medical Journal of July 1950 calls multiple screening "one glorified medical production line." The author urges the public to seek good medical care regularly and "not be deluded into believing that examination by machine can exclude or detect all incipient disease."

The Columbus Academy of Medicine Bulletin's editorial of June 1950 expresses the belief that "its collectivism could put the physician backstage in the diagnosis of disease." The writer doubts "if multiple screening as presently proposed, or the finding of disease by gadgetry, will work."

In his article in the Journal of the American Medical Association of April 21, 1951, Smillie states that "the great difficulty in multiphasic screening is that the interpretation of diagnostic tests is of little value without a knowledge of the history of the patient, an understanding of his personality and a familiarity with his whole family background." He observes also that, "Some 960 of the 1000 persons who pass through the multiple screening tests emerge with negative results. This group is treated most unfairly. They have a false sense of security. They do not know that negative tests have little value. . . . The tests are not intended, of course, to give the individual a rapid, clean-cut and concise series of comprehensive diagnoses. But that is exactly what the average man thinks they do; otherwise he would not go through with the procedure."

Commenting on the Massachusetts pilot multiphasic screening clinic preliminary to a description of a similar group health survey at the Pratt Diagnostic Clinic, McCombs and Finn cite in an article in the New England Journal of Medicine of January 29, 1953, certain dangers inherent in the multiphasic method. "The most important of these was the sense of false security given to patients who believed that they were free of disease after being examined in the clinic and being told

7. White, Benjamin V.: Practical Diagnosis in Preventive Geriatrics, Geriatrics 7:87 (March-April) 1952.

little when they left. . . . The second major objection was that there was a distinct break between the initial screening examination and the suggestion that follow-up studies by the family physician were necessary."

Levin and Brightman in their discussion of "The Place of Multiphasic Screening in the Chronic Disease Program" review briefly some results of the Richmond, Virginia, program and state that "Although this experience indicates that the objections of false security and unnecessary alarm need not obtain in a majority of cases, nevertheless, their possibility remains, particularly when detection is directed in the first instance to persons who do not consider themselves in need of medical care." . . .

Northwest Medicine's editorial of March 1953 points out that "Promotion of multiphasic screening has come from those who treat humanity as a mass. No discernible enthusiasm has emanated from those who are familiar with the needs of individuals." In conclusion this editorial points out that ". . . there is nothing in the average multiphasic setup not used by every good practitioner. Only he does not apply such tests in a manner of saturation bombing." . . .

In the January 1955 Journal of the Michigan State Medical Society the Council's attitude toward multiple (multiphasic) screening is expressed in a letter by the Secretary: ". . . The Council of MSMS (Michigan State Medical Society) is very doubtful of the program because it has a number of undesirable features similar to those inherent in any plan which places a government agency between the physician and his patient, or takes the practice of medicine out of the doctor's private office. This doubt is based upon the belief that the multiphasic screening program could very possibly affect the future health of the people adversely by: (1) Establishing the questionable concept that the discovery and diagnosis of all disease is a public health responsibility, placing the family physician in the role of a therapist who merely treats patients upon recommendation of a public agency. (2) Discouraging the regular thorough physical examination in the doctor's office by promoting a false idea that a hasty screening program at infrequent intervals is a proper substitute." . . .

"Multiphasic Surveys: Streamlined Diagnosis for the Public" is an editorial in the September 1954 California Medicine with the following comments and objections: "Periodic examinations (referring to multiple screening), when accompanied by positive action on the part of the patient, may be very helpful. However, when not accompanied by intelligent action, it may have the following disadvantages: 1. If the report is negative, the person acquires a false sense of security; while disease may not be evident at the time of survey, it can develop a few weeks or months later, but the person is inclined to pay little heed to symptoms and delays going to his physician because 'he was well at the survey.' 2. It may and does cause undue apprehension in persons with 'false positive' diagnosis. . . . 3. It can result in considerable expense to those who are reported as having findings suggestive of disease, but in whom disease is not confirmed on regular examination. 4. Most multiphasic screening techniques leave no opportunity for appraisal of the 'negative' group by a physician; yet in this group will be persons who need medical attention.

"Diseases of high communicability are recognized public health problems, but diseases of non-communicable nature are the province of regular practice and are undoubtedly most effectively cared for by personal physicians.

"It would seem from the experience to date that multiphasic screening, while superficially appealing, is, in fact, a poor way of improving the public health . . . is an extremely expensive way if all the costs are listed . . . gives the semblance of scientific accuracy on a mass basis, but yields little in concrete improvement for most persons concerned.

"Despite these critical appraisals by experts, some welfare groups and labor organizations in California continue to promote multiphasic campaigns among employee groups. Health and welfare funds are being used to defray part of the costs involved. It is therefore desirable that members of the medical profession be fully informed as to the apparent value of these types of medical screening procedures. If it can be shown that they have had some lasting educational benefit, then the surveys now being completed will not have been altogether in vain."

SURVEY SUMMARY

THIRTY-THREE SURVEYS are included in this report. While these are not all of the multiple screening surveys conducted in the United States, they are all that could supply the information required in the study. . . . The following is a summary of various survey characteristics: . . .

Number Screened.—About 2½ million people were tested in these surveys. The number of persons included in individual surveys ranged from 572 in a small industry in Vernon, California, to 1,376,237 in the state-wide Georgia project. . . .

Time per person.—Calculation of the time used in screening each person is, of course, difficult. However, since this is an important factor, it has been included wherever estimates were available. Time-per-person ranged from 3 minutes to 2 hours varying with the number and types of tests used. In 10 surveys the time required was 15 minutes or less per person; in 6 it was from 15 to 30 minutes; and in 7 it took from 30 to 60 minutes; 1 took 2 hours; and in 9 surveys no figures were available.

Cost per person.—Cost is another important factor, but here the variations are even greater than in time. Wherever available, estimates of cost have been included even though it is recognized that the basis of calculation may have differed so greatly as to prevent comparison. The range in the 18 surveys reporting costs was from $1.03 to $39 per person. Of these 5 were less than $2.00; 3 were from $2.00 to $5.00; 3 from $5.00 to $10.00; 6 from $10.00 to $15.00; and 1 was over $15.00.

Survey Objectives.—Four general objectives characterized the surveys studied: (1) To test the feasibility of administering several tests at one time and place; (2) to test certain aspects of multiple screening procedures; (3) case finding; and (4) health education. Four surveys were primarily as health education endeavors; and 20 had as their objective a combination of the 4 with one-half of these emphasizing the health education factor.

Survey Staffing.—Nine of the surveys studied had one or more physicians in the examining or testing line; the others had medical supervision with physicians available when needed (depending on number and kind of screening tests). Results of many of the tests were interpreted by technicians, but in all cases interpretation of chest films, EKG's, significant points in history and other tests requiring expert clinical judgment were made by physicians.

Tests Used.—The experimental nature of multiple screening has led to a wide variety of testing procedures. Among the 33 surveys the range in tests was from 2 to 15. Ten surveys used less than 6 tests; twelve surveys used from 6 to 11 tests; and eleven surveys used from 11 to 16 tests. The basic tests generally included in the surveys were those for tuberculosis, diabetes, syphilis, cardiovascular disease, anemia, and nutritional status.

Results.—The results of the 33 surveys must be reviewed in reference to techniques used, follow-up methods, testing procedures, type of population surveyed, and other characteristics. These vary in each individual survey, making totals or comparisons a difficult task. . . .

However, a number of relationships can be shown, such as the direct correlation that exists between the number of tests used and the percentage of positive findings. Of the 33 surveys included in the study:

Six surveys using 5 or less tests reported positive findings on 2%, 3%, 7%, 12%, 14%, and 15% of persons screened;

Eleven surveys using from 6 through 10 tests reported positive findings on 14%, 18%, 21%, 26%, 35%, 43%, 51%, 54% (2), 55%, and 56% of the persons screened; and

Six surveys using more than 10 tests reported positive findings on 48%, 60%, 62%, 63% (2), and 67% of persons screened.

Probably the greatest obstacle in any evaluation of multiple screening is the lack of data on diagnosis resulting from follow-up on persons with positive indications of disease. In only 15 of the 33 surveys were such follow-up data available, and even in these instances there was no way of knowing how many of the positive screenees actually went to their own physicians for further examination. Figures on the percentage of positive screenees found to have positive diagnoses cannot be compared until the percentages of persons seeking follow-up are known.

These examples point up very clearly the fact that these screening surveys must be accepted as experiments. To be successful they require the cooperation of both the screenee and his physician in medical follow-up. The question arises, cannot the objective of early diagnosis be best accomplished in the doctor's office without the mass screening step? Some say yes and insist it will be less expensive for all concerned. Others say no, because too few persons who are "apparently well" will ever go to their physician for a check-up.

B. SOME PROBLEM AREAS *

PROGRESS IN reducing the disability resulting from many chronic diseases is dependent in large measure on *early* diagnosis and treatment. In the practice of medicine it is commonplace to be faced with patients who for one reason or another have gone untreated for a prolonged period and whose disease has passed the point at which a satisfactory response to therapy can be anticipated. Nursing homes and chronic disease hospitals are filled largely with patients in whom the disease process has done its damage and for whom no definitive treatment can be expected to result in substantial curative as opposed to symptomatic improvement. Yet many patients would not have reached such advanced states of illness if the chronic disease from which they suffer had been diagnosed early and brought under adequate treatment.

The problem then is: How to narrow the time gap between the onset of a disease and its diagnosis? To what extent is it possible and practical to diagnose asymptomatic or "nonmanifest" disease? In the normal course of office medical practice, some nonmanifest disease is detected. An increasing (yet small) group of physicians in general practice encourage their patients to come in for a periodic health examination. The physician who in obstetrical cases routinely obtains a chest x-ray and serologic test for syphilis is rewarded from time to time by detecting unsuspected disease. As a group, the pediatricians have probably gone furthest in developing the techniques and pattern of practice directed toward early detection of minor deviations from normal (supervision of the "well" infant and child) that may be of importance to the subsequent health of the patient.

Early detection of asymptomatic disease through office practice appears to be substantially limited by three factors:

1. If a physician's examination of a presumably well person is to be useful, it must be thorough, fairly detailed, and supplemented by selected x-ray and laboratory tests. Such examinations are expensive.

2. The great bulk of the population goes to a physician only for the diagnosis and treatment of manifest illness. Except for persons in the upper income brackets who are perhaps more sophisticated in health matters, the American people do not seem impressed with the value of periodic health examinations.

3. A large number of physicians have neither the time for nor the interest in examining well adults. They are overtaxed by meeting the demands of acutely and chronically ill patients and all too often deal as briefly as possible with the person seeking a health examination whom they may regard as "probably neurotic."

Several other approaches to early diagnosis of silent disease have been developed, each of which has strong and weak features. The general public is now familiar with

* From: "Introductory Statement on Screening for Asymptomatic Disease" (part of "Symposium: Screening for Asymptomatic Disease"), by Lester Breslow, M.D., and Dean W. Roberts, M.D.; *Journal of Chronic Diseases* 2:363-66, Oct. 1955 (No. 4). Reprinted (with omissions) by permission of the authors and publishers. The authors are, respectively, chief of the Bureau of Chronic Diseases, California Department of Public Health, Berkeley; and executive director of the National Society for Crippled Children and Adults, Chicago.

the mass chest x-ray surveys using mobile photofluorographic units. Cancer detection clinics, annual diabetes detection drives, school health examinations, routine insurance and employment examinations, are all well-known examples of different administrative approaches to detection of nonmanifest disease. The last decade has seen development of multiphasic screening in which a battery of screening tests is applied to large population groups and the results are sent to the patient's physician. Such programs have been operated, practically always on an episodic demonstration basis, by health departments, hospitals, unions, and medical societies. It is important that the strengths and weaknesses of each of the available approaches to early detection of disease be evaluated objectively. This will necessarily involve a consideration of the reliability and cost of the methods employed, the ease with which procedures can be widely applied to large numbers of persons, and the acceptability of procedures to the patient, the physician, and the community. . . .

. . . The primary purpose of mass screening is to bring persons with disease to physicians at an earlier stage than otherwise would be the case.

. . . The validity of a test is measured by the frequency with which the result of the test is confirmed by an acceptable diagnostic procedure. Four possibilities exist when the results of the screening test are compared with those of the diagnostic tests:

a. "True positives"—those who are selected by the screen and are also found to be positive by the diagnostic procedure.

b. "False positives"—those selected by the screen who are found to be negative by the diagnostic procedure.

c. "True negatives"—those who are not selected by the screen and are found to be negative by the diagnostic procedure.

d. "False negatives"—those not selected by the screen but found to be positive by the diagnostic procedure. . . .

. . . It has become clear that screening programs, while they have accomplished a great deal of good, have not fully met their early promise, probably because of:

1. The general absence of a continuing (as opposed to an episodic or a demonstration) facility for multiphasic screening.

2. The general absence of practicing physicians' interest and participation.

3. Lack of agreement as to which procedures should be incorporated into a screening program for general and special population groups. This disagreement is at least in part based on the following:

4. Lack of accurate knowledge of the yield of disease to be expected from particular screening procedures.

5. Cost. . . .

59. Progress in Treatment Methods *

[There have been substantial] accomplishments already made in the control of chronic disease. These advances have largely occurred in the past 40 years. A few of these highlights may be brought forth by a consideration of some short case histories of patients with chronic diseases which were usually fatal in 1921. They are from the records of the Presbyterian Hospital in New York and tell their own story.

Mary C., a 38-year-old housemaid, was admitted in November 1925 complaining of weakness, weight loss, and soreness of the tongue over a four-month period. On the basis of the physical examination and laboratory data a diagnosis of *primary or pernicious anemia* was established. In spite of all attempts at therapy, she died in December 1925, 7 weeks after hospitalization.

Countless Mary C's since 1926 have been spared this outcome by Minot and Murphy's introduction of liver therapy. And, as you know, this regimen has been followed by the use of folic acid and vitamin B_{12}.

Alfreda T., a 44-year-old housewife, came to the clinic early in 1922 because of known diabetes mellitus of 3 years' duration. She had been treated with a restricted, high fat, low carbohydrate diet during this three-year period and had lost 75 pounds. The laboratory data confirmed the diagnosis of *diabetes mellitus*. Within two days, in spite of all therapeutic attempts, she developed progressively severe diabetic coma, and died.

Since the introduction of insulin, countless Alfreda T's have been spared this outcome by diligent case finding and conscientious care.

Leon A., a 22-year-old student, was admitted to the hospital in November 1935 because of fever and night sweats of 3 weeks' duration. A cardiac murmur had been known to be present since birth and for 5 years he had noted increasing shortness of breath on exertion. A diagnosis of *patent ductus arteriosus* with superimposed streptococcus viridans endocarditis was made. Effective treatment was not available for either the infection or the underlying cardiac lesion and the patient died 4 months later.

Now, antibiotic prophylaxis prevents the superimposed endocarditis in these cases and appropriate treatment usually controls the infection when it occurs.

The introduction by Gross in 1937 of a surgical procedure to ligate the patent ductus arteriosus has resulted in a great benefit to the majority of individuals with this form of heart disease and prevents the otherwise expected heart failure.

* From: "Prospects for the Prevention of Chronic Disease," by David Seegal, M.D., and Arthur R. Wertheim, M.D.; in *Proceedings of the National Conference on Preventive Aspects of Chronic Disease*, Baltimore: Commission on Chronic Illness, 1952. Reprinted from pages 19–22 (with omissions, including initial paragraphs, figures, and some tables) by permission of the publishers. The authors are, respectively, professor of clinical medicine at the College of Medicine, State University of New York, New York; and assistant professor of medicine at the College of Physicians and Surgeons, Columbia University, New York.

Blalock and Taussig, after a series of brilliant experiments in dogs, have demonstrated that a suitable shunt operation will benefit a considerable number of patients with another form of congenital heart disease known as the tetralogy of Fallot.

Rose K., aged 35, who came to the hospital in October 1921 because of backache for a 2-year period, swollen hands and feet for 3 months, and a skin eruption on the face and arms for 1 month. She was considered to have *pellagra*. In spite of attempts at dietary therapy, she became progressively weaker and deteriorated mentally. She died 3 months after admission.

Today most Rose K's do not share the fate of their predecessor because of the introduction of nicotinic acid and its derivatives in 1937. Through public health education since Goldberger's time and economic measures a proper dietary regimen has led to the primary prevention of pellagra.

Let us turn from these special case histories and survey the larger scene. In association with Drs. Colcher and Duane, a wide variety of chronic diseases were catalogued to determine the effectiveness of our present methods of prevention and control. Table 41 lists 17 long-term diseases which may be *largely controlled* if proper preventive, diagnostic and therapeutic measures are employed.

TABLE 41.   *Partially controlled chronic illnesses*

Congenital heart disease	Disseminated lupus erythematosus
Addison's disease	Bacterial endocarditis
Cretinism	Lung abscess
Diabetes insipidus	Bronchiectasis
Acromegaly	Trypanosomiasis
Coeliac disease	Hay fever
Hemophilia	Asthma
Erythremia	Myasthenia gravis
Tuberculosis	Myotonia congenita
Actinomycosis	Familial periodic paralysis
Osteomyelitis	General paresis
Rheumatic fever	Epilepsy
Rheumatoid arthritis	Certain neuroses and psychoses
Gout	

It is impossible to estimate how much human suffering has been alleviated and economic wealth increased by the development of measures which are preventing and largely controlling this group of chronic diseases.

Table 42 contains a list of 27 chronic illnesses which are *partially controlled.*

TABLE 42.   *Largely controlled chronic illnesses*

Diabetes mellitus	Beri-beri
Pernicious anemia	Scurvy
Syphilis	Rickets
Hyperthyroidism	Hookworm infestation
Myxedema	Malaria
Hyperparathyroidism	Amebiasis
Sprue	Thrombocytopenic purpura
"Alcoholic" neuritis	Familial hemolytic jaundice
Pellagra	

It is heartening to view the considerable progress made in the care of this group of illnesses. Although the methods of control are generally not curative, the outlook for the patient with diseases such as diabetes insipidus, Addison's disease, pulmonary tuberculosis, rheumatoid arthritis, and asthma is considerably improved by virtue of the accepted preventive measures and treatment. . . .

60. HOME CARE *

WHEN A HOSPITAL limits its precious facilities to those who have been admitted within its portals, it inevitably invites ineligible patients to hospital beds, who can do as well at home. Such a policy often prevents the hospital from achieving its maximum of usefulness, though this still seems to be acceptable to those who bear the burden of the cost.

But the hospital that serves the public best does not limit its superior scientific facilities to the patient within its walls. It reaches out into the community with its wares because it has a monopoly which is vital to public health progress. Nor does its staff remain forever out of reach of the medical practitioner; it extends a helping hand to him when he needs it.

There is an area of expanding medical opportunity—the patient's home where most pathological conditions originate—which the hospital must take under its wing.

By including the patient's home in its organization the hospital can befriend doctor and patient alike, so that expert medical care will be available to everyone, rich or poor.

Only by a combination of hospital and home care under the same over-all medical management can the hospital employ its unique facilities in the field of scientific medicine to best advantage. And this it can do at less cost to the community in the long run.

Three major reasons for the hospitalization of a patient dominate hospital policy in varying degrees and each one of them should be reappraised at this time in the light of the newer concepts of medical practice. These reasons are, briefly:

First, *scientific necessity*. The problem presented by the applicant for admission may be too difficult for the home, because of the steady need for a highly trained staff of specialists having instruments of precision at their immediate disposal and working with highly concentrated facilities. The hospital staff commands a greater degree of expertness, and has the patient under closer observation and control than is possible to achieve in the home. Major surgery is a typical example. In any case, scientific necessity compels priority in the assignment to the patient of a hospital bed which is expensive both to construct and to maintain.

Where favorable home conditions prevail, or can be made to prevail through the

---

* From: "Home Care: An Extra-Mural Hospital Function," by E. M. Bluestone, M.D.; *Survey Midmonthly* 84:99-101, 133, April 1948 (No. 4). Reprinted (with omissions, including illustrations) by permission of the author and publishers. The author is a consultant for Montefiore Hospital, Bronx, N.Y.

efforts of good social service, this should indeed be the sole criterion for the admission of a patient to a hospital.

Second, *concentration of service to patients.* This reason has some merit, but it is related to the comfort and available time of the staff doctor rather than to the comfort of the patient in cases where a hospital bed might not, under other circumstances, be required. If this reason is established as valid, it will continue to dominate the hospital picture progressively as doctors' offices come closer and closer to the hospital. In an era of mounting hospital costs neither the patient nor the community will be able to finance the item of expense which this policy of concentration will entail. It should, therefore, be reconsidered in view of the possibilities of a less expensive extramural hospital program, in which medical care radiates from the hospital to the home.

Third, *the poverty of the patient.* The social aspects of medical care exert a strong influence on the matter of hospitalization, and patients are often referred for admission to hospitals because the family cannot afford the proper care at home. But poverty can be neutralized as a pathogenic factor in a way which is less expensive, and sometimes more effective, than by the easy expedient of the hospital bed. One might conclude, from the indiscriminate transfer of the poor patient, that the chances for his recovery are better in a well-organized hospital. However, this is not always the case; often we find the reverse to be true.

The hospital, suffering from all of the defects of its virtues, has disadvantages, as well as advantages for its patients. Structurally and functionally it is conducted on the ward principle. The management of the sick en masse, which results from the application of this principle, cannot compete with their management on an individual basis, since the hospital ward is so forbidding to the sensitive patient. And if, as some ward apologists hold, "misery likes company," then we are dealing in our hospital wards with a perverted form of the gregarious instinct.

There would be little cause for complaint about hospital policy in the assignment of beds if reasons like these were weighed carefully and applied in a spirit of justice to the sick. But, to complicate matters, there are not enough hospital beds, if we are to believe what we are told by hospital authorities. In spite of the gains of scientific medicine in recent years, which would seem to reduce the necessity for more hospital beds, we have been misguided into making these beds as popular as they are expensive. In view of prevailing conditions we must now plan to be more thrifty with those that we have.... The question that we must ask ourselves is: "How close must the patient's bed be to centralized scientific facilities and what are the requirements in each specific situation?" The extramural possibilities of the patient's home must be measured carefully and employed to supplement the opportunity provided by the hospital bed.

... Ward care compels the sacrifice of individual comfort and privacy to the interests of neighboring patients in the group. Such sacrifices vary all the way from family separation and minor details like the individual response to ventilation, to the extreme form when patients die in public on open wards.

Moreover, ward care heightens the consciousness of neglect which the patient cannot help feeling when the best doctors, whose ministrations he was led to expect when he left home, pass him by for his more "interesting" type of neighbor and perhaps the one who needed a hospital bed more than he. "There ought to be a rule in every hospital," said the late Dr. Emanuel Libman, "compelling every doctor on ward rounds to sit down for at least one minute by the bedside of every patient."

There is little that one can do about such human situations under the limitations of ward care, but it is interesting to note that the home care patient, far from feeling neglected, knows himself to be the object of the special attention which he craves. The point is that ward care is not always superior to home care, as some might think. The struggle for life, which mobilizes the balance of the patient's energies, should not be handicapped by any adverse arrangements which the hospital planner might impose. He must also remember that sickness is always a humiliating, and sometimes a degrading, experience for anyone to endure and that it is not endured easiest when the patient is surrounded by strangers who might be as sick as he.

Hospital construction is a comparatively expensive type of construction and should be undertaken only after the needs of the community for intramural hospital care have been carefully estimated. At this writing the cost is about $20,000 per bed. . . .

We may find that we already have enough hospital beds for every person who needs one, if those that are available are used intensively, provided, however, that we take advantage of the extramural facilities furnished by the patient himself when he is subsidized medically in his own home under full hospital supervision. A bed in the patient's home, which meets the requirements of a good home-care program can immediately become a hospital bed. It is, therefore, a valuable hospital asset under certain conditions of organization and cooperation.

Hospital maintenance, after construction has taken its toll of the hospital treasury, is high, as anyone can testify who has had to balance a hospital budget. The cost at present is $12 per patient per day in our hospital.* When you think of philanthropy in voluntary hospitals you cannot help thinking of deficits at the same time, without disrespect to those who give so generously. Medical progress seems to have outstripped the ability of the philanthropist to contribute, but there is a way of relieving him of some of the burden, as we now find. . . .

The hospital should never be the court of first resort except under the most compelling clinical conditions. The patient in his home environment is placed where nature intended him to be. You never saw nostalgia associated with the memories of a hospital bed.

The fact that hospital wards are safer today for patients than they were in the earlier chapters of the infectious diseases is a relative and not an absolute achievement. . . .

Our wards are not yet safe enough for comfort, nor can they be made fully safe until more of the warmth of the home is transferred to the impersonal ward

* Dr. Bluestone was the Director of Montefiore Hospital (Bronx, New York) at the time this article was written.

of the hospital. The individual private room for every patient, regardless of his ability to pay, would help, but it would certainly be prohibitive in cost and therefore practically unattainable. Philanthropy cannot associate itself with luxuries for the poor—and it still considers the private room a luxury. We have not yet found the way to individualize the care of patients in hospital wards, but we are already in a position to do it in a home-care program.

The ingredients of a good extramural hospital program present themselves as the logical outcome of applied social medicine. The typical program, and the one with which we have successfully experimented at Montefiore Hospital in New York City since the beginning of 1947, is an extramural program on an extension basis. Ward patients who can do as well in their own homes as they can in the hospital, as determined by specially trained and highly selective doctors and social workers, are returned there with a promise of complete hospital care, either in their own homes entirely or by a return to the hospital as necessary.

For the present, the program is limited to . . . patients who cannot afford the services of a private physician. . . . As this program develops, however, it will add the patient who can afford the services of a private physician but not of the more expensive facilities which his condition demands. This will result in a form of cooperation between hospital and practitioner in which the practitioner will have at his disposal, more directly than ever before, all of the diagnostic and therapeutic instrumentalities in the patient's home which are now available only to the patient within the hospital and its out-patient department.

We believe that this kind of service by the hospital to the practitioner will bring both together and go a long way to resolve the age-old controversy on the relative merits of the "open" and "closed" hospital. Such a cooperative effort, where the patient's resources are limited, has long been the goal of progressive leaders in both fields of activity and, when it is established, we shall witness another triumph for the cause of scientific medicine. We believe that the home is the missing link which those who are trying to forge the chain have been seeking through the years.

For the carefully selected cases in the extramural program, where the social and medical factors are favorable, Montefiore Hospital provides every kind of service that has thus far been available only to the intramural patient. The physicians assigned to the home-care program are full time, salaried, members of the attending staff of the hospital. All of the specialties are available to them and to the patient at home. These doctors serve in-patient, out-patient and home-care patient on an integrated and continuing basis as part of the day's work and they partake of the educational and research program of the hospital, like any other qualified member of the attending staff.

Home-care patients are entitled to "free consultations," as they call them, through participation in the teaching program, arranged as part of the service either in the home (for members of the house staff—the future practitioners—and others) or in the class-rooms of the hospital (for students of the College of Physicians & Surgeons of Columbia University, with which the hospital has an undergraduate and postgraduate affiliation). Research is likewise facilitated, because the patient is under continuous observation over longer periods of time, while occupying what is, for all practical purposes, a hospital bed. As far as the record is concerned, the clinical biography of the patient is continuous and therefore more valuable for scientific purposes.

Nursing is done by the Visiting Nurse Service of New York through a contractual arrangement. Social service is complete and shares a fruitful partnership with the physicians in the program. Housekeeping service is furnished, as it may be required, on a part time basis. . . . The services of the occupational therapy and rehabilitation departments of the hospital, to mention only a few additional services, are also available to the home-care patient. Medication is provided, if the patient cannot afford it, as well as transportation to and from the hospital. It goes without saying that the patient has a priority on a hospital bed if he should require it at any time.

An analysis of cost to the hospital indicates that home care is about one fourth of the cost of maintaining the same patient in a hospital bed. A saving like this should be too tempting for any hospital expansionist to overlook, apart from the other advantages of the program, such as the individualization of treatment in the home environment. The family pays the rent and food costs, among other things, and relieves the hospital of that much of the financial burden. As for the bed which the patient occupies in his home, it costs nothing for the hospital to build and one fourth of the prevailing hospital costs to maintain. Besides, it is immediately available in many cases and has the added merit of flexibility which is not to be found within the rigid walls of the hospital. . . .

The response on the part of hospital, home, and community has been uniformly enthusiastic and encouraging. We now have here a medical care demonstration project of a high order. It is the answer to many a prayer on the part of patient, practitioner, and social worker. When you see a patient whom the doctors consider hopeless enjoying the illusion of hope, so that he can gather up enough courage to do things within the family environment which would have been impossible in the hospital, you know that you are on the right track. The logic of the program justifies itself many times over again through its supplementary achievement in the realm of psychosomatic medicine. In the best sense of the word, here is something revolutionary in the field of medical care.

61. NURSING HOMES *

NURSING HOMES have had an unprecedented growth in the past ten years. Today no one knows just how many there are, although many states have made compre-

* From: "Nursing Homes: Their Part in the Community's Attack On Chronic Illness," by Morton L. Levin, M.D.; *Chronic Illness Newsletter* 2:2-3, Feb. 1951 (No. 2). Reprinted (with omissions) by permission of the publishers. The author is assistant commissioner for medical services, New York State Department of Health, Albany.

hensive surveys. Their growth has been in response to an urgent need. This need has always existed, but the demand for nursing home care was greatly increased by the Old Age Assistance Program, which in 1935 made it possible to grant Federal and State assistance to the aged in their own homes or in private institutions such as nursing homes, but not in hospitals or public homes. Other important factors have been the increase in the number of older persons, the shortage of hospital beds, the general housing shortage since World War II, and the lack of other facilities for the chronically ill and for the homeless aged.

Nursing homes now provide a variety of types of care, of varying quality. These include: substitute home or boarding home type of care; convalescent care for patients who stay only a limited period while recovering from an acute illness; attendant and nursing care for chronically ill persons, varying from minimal help to an ambulant infirm aged person to continuous nursing care for a bed-ridden patient.

Nursing homes have developed in response to two types of need for persons who have no homes or whose homes cannot properly care for them. These are: older persons and the chronically ill.

The relative extent to which nursing homes now care for older persons and for the chronic sick is not known. A recent study in New York State showed that 79% of the patients were over 65 years of age; that 75% were either bed-ridden or required considerable care and 25% were able to care for themselves.

The problems of caring for the *aged* and for the *chronically ill* are often confused, for two reasons; chronic illness is most prevalent in older persons and the combination of chronic illness, indigency and lack of a home is found most often among older persons. It is important to remember, however, that the problems of chronic illness are found in all age groups; that the majority of persons with some chronic illness are not old; i. e. are under 65 years of age, and that old age is not a disease or an illness. It would be a disservice to our older population to assume that the care of the aged is the same as the care of the chronically ill. Indeed, it is one of the great needs of older persons to be helped to maintain an active, useful existence as independent members of the community. Their needs are well summarized in your convention * theme: "A home in which to live; something to do; someone to care."

I would like to emphasize especially that last phrase: "Someone to care." The persons—nurses, attendants, physicians—all those who come in daily contact with patients, should, above all, be people who like people—people who do not dislike sick people—and people who like older people.

This liking is not something entirely within our control—some of us don't have it for reasons not our fault. To some extent it can be cultivated, by trying to put ourselves in the place of the older, and ill person. It is often difficult to understand older persons and by older persons we usually mean anyone five or more years older than ourselves, but it can be done as many of you have demonstrated by the way in which you have handled these problems.

* The first annual convention of the American Association of Nursing Homes, in Omaha, Nebr. (September 1950), at which Dr. Levin delivered this address.

The chronically ill who require care need many facilities and services. These have been well described recently in a study of the needs of terminal cancer patients made by Miss Edna Nicholson and her associates of the Chicago Central Service for the Chronically Ill.

The chronically ill person who has reached the stage where he needs care from others, usually needs: medical attention; nursing care; drugs, dressing and sick-room supplies; housing that is safe, sanitary and comfortable; housekeeping and maintenance services to provide cleanliness, warmth and comfort; preservation of ties with family and close friends; recreational activities and other wholesome use of leisure time consistent with the patient's capacities and interests; special services as needed, including particularly, (a) social workers to help with emotional, economic and social problems and (b) the visits of clergymen and opportunities for religious worship; study and training to help the patient overcome residual disability and to become as self-sufficient as possible.

The chronically ill person needs these services whether he is at home, in a nursing home, a hospital or some other institution. Obviously to provide all these services, in good quality, is not easy and requires organization, personnel and money. How to provide these services on a limited budget is one of the big problems which nursing home operators are continually facing. It is not your problem alone, it is the community's problem and you should be able to look to the community for its help.

Unfortunately, in many communities the services are there but are not used, either because those responsible for the care of the chronically ill patient do not realize that he needs them, that the services are available, or do not know how to get them.

Nursing home operators are busy people and they need help in maintaining contact with and knowledge concerning other community agencies which could provide some of the services which their patients require. Several ways in which this can be done have been suggested: the establishment of a special agency—a central information service for the chronically ill in each community—contacts with social agencies and the churches created by the nursing homes themselves; and the development of a direct connection between nursing homes and hospitals, with hospitals providing guidance, consultation and special services as needed. Each of these methods should be seriously considered by your association.

The dollars and cents aspect of the chronically ill lies underneath a great many of the inadequacies for their care which now exist. In many localities welfare departments need to increase the rates which they will allow for the care of the indigent chronically ill and in some areas they have done so. But what of the many chronic sick who are on the border-line of indigency, who are either too proud to accept public relief or who have some resources of their own which are nevertheless insufficient to provide the full care they need? Part of the cost of their care may, at one time or another, be paid for by a hospital, by a visiting nurse agency, or by welfare. And yet recent studies show that in many cases funds to provide good care are *not* available. The American people each year contribute generously to drives for funds for the control of the major chronic diseases, such as cancer, heart disease, tuberculosis, poliomyelitis and other crippling conditions. To a great extent these funds are expended independently. There would seem to be a definite need in each community, to determine whether by cooperative action between these different agencies, use of more of their funds cannot be made available to provide more adequate care for the chronic sick and whether the funds already available cannot be used more efficiently.

I am sure you are aware that many professional persons concerned with medical care are not too willing to accept the idea that the care of the chronically ill should be considered as profit-making enterprise. They point out that only 3 per cent of all hospital beds in this country are under proprietary auspices. It seems paradoxical that that portion of our sick population least able to pay for care—the chronically ill—should be left largely unprovided for by community supported institutions and programs. Nevertheless, private nursing homes have developed in response to a need which was not otherwise being met. It is reasonable to suppose that there will always be a place for private nursing homes which offer good services at reasonable costs. But the funds to pay for reasonable costs must be made available. Our departments of welfare are justly concerned with standards and quality of services provided by nursing homes to their clients. They must be equally concerned with providing sufficient funds to ensure at least minimum standards of good care for the indigent chronic sick. Nursing homes, on the other hand, must be ever on the watch to maintain high standards. The operation of a nursing home is a professional enterprise, comparable to the operation of a hospital. The maintenance of that point of view is essential to the continued existence of nursing homes.

In each locality there is a need for education so that the public—and its official representatives will appreciate the need for nursing home care and their place in the care of the chronic sick. Then perhaps efforts will be concentrated on help and improvement rather than the present all-too-frequent approach of rigid and narrow interpretation of building code or licensing law. Nursing homes have been deplored—you have been told that you should improve, but it is hoped that state and national plans not only will define the role of the nursing home as it fits into the pattern of institutional care, but will find methods of providing practical guides to achieve your goals more readily.

Licensing can be a positive force—and a help to all—if it is based on practical, desirable and realistic standards. There should be licensing or accrediting laws in all of the states and these laws should be administered with the objective of giving services to operators, the patients and the public.

Finally, nursing homes should adopt the point of view that the function of the nursing home, and of all institutions and agencies providing services to the chronically ill—is not only to give care—but to see that patients are physically or vocationally rehabilitated if possible. . . .

The care of the chronically ill, the aged and the infirm is an important community health service. The welfare of the patient is the primary consideration and goal. Nursing home operators and attendants are gathering invaluable first-hand experience in the every day problems of caring for these patients—experience which others concerned with community health need to know about and will gladly use.

You as nursing home operators therefore should take an active part in advancing community awareness of these problems, stimulating community planning to meet them; making certain that your patients receive the full benefit of already existing community services.

The proper care of the chronically ill can never be advanced solely from the standpoint of operating a business—it is a profession, like hospital administration —and should always be looked at and practiced from the professional and humanitarian viewpoint. . . .

62. THE GOAL: REHABILITATION *

TO THE PHYSICIAN the term "rehabilitation" has long connoted "the restoration of the handicapped to the fullest physical, mental, social, vocational and economic usefulness of which they are capable." In general usage, however, the term itself, during the past few years, has lost much of its significance, for it has been used to describe everything from correctional programs in modern penal institutions to the social and economic rebuilding of war devastated countries. With the developing emphasis placed on the processes of restoring handicapped workers, a new term has arisen which describes such processes more aptly and with more virility. That term is "the third phase of medical care."

The modern concept of this third phase of medicine, which takes the patient from the bed to the job, springs both directly and indirectly from the war. The rehabilitation programs of the military services and the Veterans Administration demonstrated that planned, integrated programs of convalescent care stressing activity as an adjunct to definitive treatment could reduce the period of hospitalization, offset the deconditioning phenomena of bed rest and prevent the harmful psychologic sequelae which often result from extended hospitalization. The technics of physical rehabilitation and retraining for the severely handicapped developed by the military services also have profound implications for the even larger number of our civilian population who are disabled. . . .

* From: "Rehabilitation," by Howard A. Rusk, M.D.; *Journal of the American Medical Association* 140:286-92, May 21, 1949 (No. 3). Reprinted (with omissions) by permission of the author and publishers. The author is chairman of the Department of Rehabilitation and Physical Medicine, New York University College of Medicine, New York. (Note: This article was originally published with the authorization of the American Medical Association's Council on Physical Medicine).

Advances in Rehabilitation

IMMEDIATELY following World War I, as today, there was a developing interest in increasing rehabilitation opportunities for the disabled. Unfortunately, this interest died in many quarters in the years between the wars. From it, however, did come some pioneer institutions and some needed legislation, such as the Federal Vocational Rehabilitation Act of 1920. The failure of the movement to gain sufficient stature to become an accepted part of medicine can be attributed to the fact that it was restricted largely to guidance, trade training and the purely vocational aspects of rehabilitation. Few provisions were made for physical restoration or reducing the physical disabilities of the trainees. When the physical condition became static, a program of vocational rehabilitation was planned, "training around" the disability rather than attempting to reduce or eliminate it through medical procedures. In many instances a comparatively large expenditure of time and money was necessary for vocational rehabilitation when, by the expenditure of a few weeks and a modest sum, the physical limitations could have been substantially reduced with an automatic increase in employment potentials. Such restrictions made it impossible for the state vocational rehabilitation programs operating under the Federal Office of Vocational Rehabilitation to give adequate service to their clients. Such failure is shown by the fact that, until the basic philosophy of this program was changed by the Barden-LaFollette Act of 1943, in twenty-three years only 210,000 persons were rehabilitated, although over 1,000,000 persons were in need of such aid at any given time during that period.

Although the underlying philosophy of the third phase of medical care is based on logic and common sense, basic and clinical research in medical rehabilitation has been minimal until the past few years. Studies done in the military services, the inquiries of Keys, Barr and others into the deconditioning phenomena of bed rest, the numerous reports of Powers, Whipple, Dock, Menninger, Ghormley and others on bed rest as it affects their particular specialties are indicative of an increasing mass of scientific data on which such concepts are based. This evidence has been reinforced by the studies of successful experience with the impaired worker in industry, the economic values of rehabilitation as shown by the Office of Vocational Rehabilitation and the success of the Veterans Administration Medical Rehabilitation Program. . . .

The Extent of the Disability

THE LACK of a systematic approach requiring the reporting of cases of physical disability to a central agency, together with varying subjective interpretations of "what constitutes a handicap," makes it difficult to stake out the boundaries of the field of rehabilitation and services to the handicapped in any quantitative fashion.

Although a census of such conditions has been proposed on several occasions (legislation calling for an exhaustive census of the physically handicapped was introduced in Congress by Senator Johnson of Colorado on March 15, 1948) there has never been a complete survey of the extent of disability in the United States. The most comprehensive source of information at present is the National Health Survey, conducted by the United States Public Health Service in 1935-1936. In this survey, 800,000 families in eighty-three cities and twenty-three rural areas of nineteen states were studied. The reliability of this study has been demonstrated in other extensive surveys on the extent of chronic disease and crippling conditions, and although results are not strictly comparable, because of different methods of enumeration, they bear out the fact that the National Health Survey is probably the best source available for such statistics, although later studies indicate that its results are conservative.

Although the focus of attention has been the disabled veteran, the extent of disability among our civilian population is far greater. There were 20,500 amputations during World War II, but over 120,000 major amputations during this same period among our civilian population. Approximately 1,500 men were blinded while in military service during the last war, but 60,000 civilians lost their sight during this period. Some 265,000 men were permanently disabled as a result of combat injuries during the war, but 1,250,000 civilians were permanently disabled by disease and accidents in the corresponding four years.

There were some 23,000,000 persons in the United States handicapped to some extent by disease, accidents, maladjustment or war. One third of all draftees were rejected as unfit, and more than 1,000,000 had to be discharged shortly after induction. In 1946, 10,400,000 persons suffered disabling accidents, and, of these 370,000 were disabled permanently. It is estimated that there are over 7,000,000 persons in the United States disabled by diseases of the heart and arteries, 6,850,000 from rheumatism and arthritis and 2,600,000 from orthopedic conditions.

These are the numbers, but they cannot tell the story of pain, anxiety, suffering and all the vital secondary problems that disease and disability leave in their wake. Aside from pain and wearing personal and family anguish, the economic costs of disease and disability are staggering. . . .

. . . The physician in the past has thought too much about the physiologic and clinical aspects of the patient's disability. The vocational counselor too frequently has thought only in terms of physical skills which could be utilized vocationally. Between the two, however, there is a wide area through which most physically handicapped persons must go when their definitive medical care is completed but before they are ready to undergo vocational training. In this area lies the physical retraining in skills necessary for the carrying on of the activities inherent in daily living and common to all types of work.

Except in a few isolated instances, the physically handicapped person must be retrained to walk and travel, to care for his daily needs, to use normal methods of transportation, to use ordinary toilet facilities, to apply and remove his own prosthetic devices, and to communicate either orally or in writing. These are such simple things that they are frequently overlooked, but the personal, vocational and social success of the handicapped person is dependent on them.

The Practice of Rehabilitation

THE PRACTICE of rehabilitation for any doctor begins with the belief in the basic philosophy that the doctor's responsibility does not end when the acute illness is ended or surgery is completed; it ends only when the patient is retrained to live and work with what is left. This basic concept of the doctor's responsibility can be achieved only if rehabilitation is considered an integral part of medical service. Any program of rehabilitation is only as sound as the basic medical service of which it is a part. The diagnosis and prognosis must be accurate, for it is on them that the feasibility of retraining is determined.

In addition to the general diagnostic studies, the medical evaluation of the orthopedically handicapped must include muscle tests, determination of joint range of motion and tests for the inherent needs in daily living. In the rehabilitation service at Bellevue Hospital, a check list of ninety-six items is used to determine these factors. They include: (1) bed activities, such as moving from place to place in bed, and the ability to sit erect; (2) toilet activities; (3) eating and drinking; (4) the ability to dress and undress, such as tying shoe laces, manipulating buttons, zippers and other fasteners, and applying and removing braces; (5) hand activities—for example, winding a watch, striking a match and using various door knobs and latches; (6) wheel chair activities, getting from the bed to the wheel chair, the wheel chair to bed, and in and out of the bathtub, and (7) elevation activities, which include the needed abilities for walking, climbing and traveling.

At first glance, such a test list sounds formidable and time consuming, but, in reality, the information may be easily obtained by a therapist, nurse, a well trained volunteer or a member of the patient's family. From special check sheets used for charting the activity accomplishments, information is readily available both on the status of the patient at the time of admittance and his progress while undergoing rehabilitation.

The use of such a check list is particularly helpful if personnel are not available to do definitive muscle testing and accurate range of motion determination, for the daily activities test can be completed in the hospital, the physician's office or the patient's home. The subsequent training program is designed to teach the patient the various skills and activities which he cannot perform.

In Bellevue Hospital and the Institute of Rehabilitation and Physical Medicine, after the basic medical work-up, and the range of motion, muscle and needs of daily living tests, the physician, in conference with other staff members, prescribes a five-hour a day program for the patient. These prescribed activities include training in the ambulation and elevation rooms and the remedial gymnasium, occupational therapy, physical therapy, speech therapy or any other activity which may be helpful in meeting the specific needs of the patient.

In a comprehensive rehabilitation program, vocational guidance specialists should also be available to do guidance and testing, in order that the patient may be started on a prevocational exploratory and work testing program as soon as it is medically feasible. However, good basic rehabilitation can be carried out with the personnel available in the ordinary general hospital, if such a program is properly organized, supervised and prescribed by the physician. . . .

In rehabilitation, the primary consideration in working out a program for the severely disabled is to teach him to live, and, if possible, to work, with what he has left. Those capacities can be determined only through performance testing. It is impossible, through the analysis of the clinical manifestations of a disease such as multiple sclerosis, to determine what the sum total of the remaining physical capacities of the patient can be trained to do in the way of work or self care activities. In addition to general diagnostic studies, the medical evaluation of the patient with multiple sclerosis must include muscle tests, joint range of motion and tests for the inherent needs of daily living. These are of primary importance, for it is on their results that the patient's rehabilitation program is planned.

Too frequently, in rehabilitation, many of the basic skills necessary for effective daily living are overlooked. The patient is given numerous medical, psychologic and vocational services in preparation for employment, but retraining in the basic physical skills of ambulation, elevation and self care activities is neglected, with the result that the patient, being unable to walk, travel or care for his personal needs, is also unable effectively to utilize the other medical, psychologic, social and vocational services which he has received for richer and fuller living.

Retraining in the basic physical skills of daily living is primary; it is simply a matter of "first things first," for daily activity skills are the basis for all subsequent rehabilitation processes. . . .

The physician must also recognize that emotional trauma may be present in any patient who has suffered a severe physical disability. The sudden shock and realization of the possible economic and social consequences of permanent disability frequently produce fear and anxiety which become as handicapping to the worker as the original physical disability. Even at the Department of Rehabilitation and Physical Medicine at Bellevue Hospital, and at the Institute of Rehabilitation and Physical Medicine, where many of the patients have physical disabilities of long standing, it has been found that approximately one third of all patients have concomitant emotional problems of such severity that psychiatric attention is needed. Consequently, the full time services of a psychiatric team consisting of a psychiatrist, a clinical psychologist and a psychiatric social worker have been added to the staff.

When patients present themselves who are in need of psychiatric attention, it is the responsibility of the physician to recognize that need and see that proper referrals are made for such attention. In many instances where emotional problems are of a less severe nature, the general practitioner can resolve such problems. One of his greatest responsibilities with those patients who have severe physical disabilities is motivation—encouraging and convincing the patient that he can be rehabilitated. This motivation, to be most effective, must begin at the earliest possible moment following the accident or illness. The physician who knows something of rehabilitation can start at the time of the accident or crippling illness to allay the fears of his patient by giving him understanding, courage and hope predicated on an accurate knowledge of what can be done. He can interpret to the patient the findings of the specialist in words that are understandable and meaningful. He can explain to the patient the nature and extent of his disability, not in medical terms of the disability alone, but in terms of its effect on the vocational, social, economic, family and personal life of the patient. The physician must practice the art of medicine as well as the science.

Regardless of the type of disability, the responsibility of the physician to his patient cannot end when the acute injury has been cared for. It ends only when the physician has taken the responsibility for seeing that proper referral has been made to those agencies and institutions which are equipped to rehabilitate and re-train the patient with a residual physical disability. The physician who fails to see that those patients under his care receive the full benefits of modern methods of medical rehabilitation and retraining is in the same category as the physician who still persists in using dietary restriction alone in the management of diabetes, when insulin is available, for medical care is not complete until the patient has been trained to live and work with what he has left.

FURTHER READINGS

Boas, Ernst P. *The Unseen Plague—Chronic Disease.* New York: J. J. Augustin, 1940. 121 pages.

Commission on Chronic Illness. *Chronic Illness in the United States.* (4 vols.). Vol. 2: *Care of the Long-Term Patient.* Cambridge: Harvard University Press, 1956. 606 pages (Includes references).

Graham, Earl C. and Mullen, Marjorie M. *Rehabilitation Literature 1950-1955.* New York: McGraw-Hill, 1956. 621 pages.

Hospital Council of Greater New York. *Organized Home Medical Care in New York City.* Cambridge: Harvard University Press, 1956. 538 pages. (Includes references).

Josiah Macy, Jr. Foundation. *Problems of Aging.* Transactions of the Fourteenth Conference, Nathan W. Shock, ed. New York: The Foundation, 1952. 138 pages. (Includes references).

Kessler, Henry H. and others. *The Principles and Practices of Rehabilitation.* Philadelphia: Lea and Febiger, 1950. 448 pages. (Includes references).

National League for Nursing. *Public Health Nursing Care of the Sick at Home.* New York: The League, 1953. 57 pages. (Includes references).

National Social Welfare Assembly, National Committee on the Aging. *Standards of Care for Older People in Institutions.* Section III. New York: The Committee, 1954. 112 pages.

Nicholson, Edna E. *Planning New Institutional Facilities for Long-Term Care.* New York: G. P. Putnam's Sons, 1956. 358 pages.

Rusk, Howard A. and Taylor, Eugene J. *New Hope for the Handicapped.* New York: Harper and Bros., 1949. 231 pages.

Turner, Violet B. *Chronic Illness: Digests of Selected References, 1950-52.* Publication No. 305, Public Health Service. Washington: U. S. Government Printing Office, 1953. 262 pages.

United States Department of Health, Education, and Welfare, Public Health Service. *Illness and Health Services in an Aging Population.* Publication No. 170, Public Health Service. Washington: U. S. Government Printing Office, 1952. 68 pages. (Includes references).

United States Department of Health, Education, and Welfare, Public Health Service. *A Study of Selected Home Care Programs.* Public Health Monograph No. 35. Washington: U. S. Government Printing Office, 1955. 127 pages.

CHAPTER IX

Rural Medical Care

THE PROVISION OF MEDICAL service to people is a social challenge—one least met in the rural areas of the world. Even in our own well endowed nation, the rural areas offer evidence of the difficulties to be faced in providing modern medical services to rural people.

As we have become an urban, industrial society, moving our people, our workers and our wealth to the cities, so have our medical care resources moved and developed—and rural medicine has lagged. The young physicians have come from and have remained in the cities. Hospitals and medical schools have been urban institutions. The specialized skills which they have developed also have remained in the cities. Even public health services have failed to reach much of the rural population.

Recognition of these problems has been relatively recent. Chapters II, III, V and VI include information on the needs and resources for medical care among rural people. This chapter presents some of the special efforts developed to improve the provision of medical care to people living in small communities (less than 2,500 persons) or in the open country.

63. RURAL MEDICINE IN CRISIS *

IN RECENT YEARS there has been a growing recognition in the United States of rural health and rural medical care as fields constituting a special medical-social problem.

* From: "Historic Development of the Current Crisis of Rural Medicine in the United States," by Milton I. Roemer, M.D.; in *Victor Robinson Memorial Volume: Essays on the History of Medicine* (S. R. Kagan, ed.), New York: Froben Press, 1948. Reprinted from pp. 333-42 (with omissions) by permission of the author and publishers. The author is the director of research, Sloan Institute of Hospital Administration, Cornell University, Ithaca, N.Y.

With the rapid industrialization and urbanization of our nation over the last hundred and fifty years, it was natural that medical developments should have been mainly urban and that, indeed, a specialty of industrial medicine, concerned particularly with diseases arising from industrial employment, should have arisen. Urbanization created certain hazards to health, but at the same time it brought about economic and technological resources for combatting them. It was a long time before the other side of the coin was brought into view and the neglected field of rural medical services was seen to demand special control measures of its own.

At one time, of course, all American medicine was what would now be called rural. The Colonial physician, like the country doctor today, worked largely without benefit of facilities, equipment, or auxiliary personnel; he compounded his own drugs and gave nursing care to the sick. With the greater part of the population agricultural, medicine was obviously rooted in the soil, but even in the centers of population there were few advantages that were not available in the most isolated outposts. . . .

Since the little black bag that held the total armamentarium of early nineteenth century medicine could be carried in the country as well as in the city, there was little technological inducement for [medical] graduates to favor urban settlement. More important, the cities had not yet come to represent concentrations of wealth where the doctor's income could be expected to reach higher levels. Add to these factors the rural background of the majority of the medical students, and it will be evident why the distribution of physicians between town and country was probably not noticeably uneven through most of the nineteenth century.

It was not until the period of Pasteur and Koch, when modern scientific medicine began to flower, that a consciousness of the disadvantages of rural medicine began to appear. Somewhat striking evidence of this is found in the appearance in the last quarter of the nineteenth century of at least three journals designed specifically for the country doctor. The earliest of these, entitled The Country Practitioner or New Jersey Journal of Medical and Surgical Practice, was first issued in June, 1879. In 1890, another, entitled The Country Doctor—A Weekly Journal of Medicine and Surgery was published at Arcot, Tennessee and a few years later The Country Doctor, A Monthly Journal of Medicine and Surgery appeared at Sparta, Tennessee. All three were edited by rural physicians. While serving to bring the rapidly expanding knowledge of the period to the attention of the country physician, there was something of a spirit of self-assertiveness about the issuance of these journals, an insistence that—in the midst of bacteriological and chemical discoveries emanating from city laboratories—rural medical experience still had much to contribute. Thus, in opening his journal in 1879, Dr. E. P. Townsend writes that the first reason for the publication:

. . . is to try and add to medical knowledge, by bringing into general use the latent information possessed by every practitioner who is, and has been doing good service in his own immediate circle, fighting out his own difficulties, when out of reach of specialists and scientists, leaning upon his knowledge of general principles, basing his practice upon his good common sense, making his syringes in emergencies from hog's bladders, and filing nozzles for them out of thigh bones of chickens, making surgical splints out of old shingles with his jack knife; working, reading, striving and fighting his way alone through emergencies that would cause some of the great medical luminaries to stagger in their traces.[1]

The dominant notion of the century was that life in the country was highly beneficial to health and the farmer was prey to less illness than the city-dweller. In relation to the disease burden of city life at the time, this was doubtless true and the rural family, therefore, presumably had less need for medical services. . . .

The literature of the nineteenth century does not appear to contain any reference to a relative shortage of physicians or other medical personnel in rural areas. Indeed, there are even references to over-crowding of rural doctors. With the abundant output of doctors by fly-by-night, proprietary medical schools, the resultant field of excessive "competition" among practitioners seemed to be characteristic of rural and urban communities alike. . . .

Toward the end of the century and the beginning of the twentieth century, however, there developed several interrelated processes which up to then had been only embryonic, and which were to have an increasing influence on the relation of rural medicine to urban. First, wealth became appreciably concentrated in the cities and rural areas were increasingly characterized by poverty and subsistence living. The doctor, therefore, was able to make a better income in urban than in rural practice. Secondly, medical science became developed to a point where hospitals, technical equipment, and specialized auxiliary personnel were considered more and more essential to good work. These were resources that could be supported only in urban centers. Thirdly, the cost of medical education gradually rose, so that increasingly only youths from relatively well-to-do city families could undertake a medical career. Such a background hardly predisposed the young doctor to settle in a country village. Fourthly, stringent measures began to be undertaken to reduce the total output and improve the quality of medical graduates, culminating in the monumental report of Abraham Flexner in 1910. The number of poorly trained doctors, who might be satisfied with a simple, isolated medical career, therefore, steadily declined.

The combined effect of these forces was obviously to set into motion an accelerating concentration of physicians and related personnel and facilities in the cities. As early as 1906 it was discovered that only 41 percent of the nation's physicians were located in rural communities which had at the time 50 percent of the nation's population. By 1914, 47 percent of new medical graduates were choosing to settle in cities of over 100,000 population, while at the time less than 26 percent of the national population was in such cities. Comparable rural-urban discrepancies became evident in other respects. Specialists came to be commonplace in the larger cities. Hospitals multiplied in the cities and gradually became places for the care of the affluent, as well as the indigent. Rural hospitals, unlike urban, developed chiefly as private institutions for the care of those who could pay; their growth was

1. Editorial, "To Medical Practitioners," *The Country Practitioner* . . . Beverly, New Jersey (vol. 1, p. 1, June 1879).

accordingly much slower. All municipalities came to be served with some type of public health service, but it was not until 1911 that the first county health department serving a rural district was organized.

Not only did deficiencies in rural medical resources become evident, but the notion that the rural setting represented the healthiest possible environment was becoming modified. . . .

Definite evidence of rural health status being inferior to urban in the United States did not accumulate, however, until quite recent years. In the First World War, for example, rejection rates because of physical or mental defects were higher among urban youth, but in the Second World War, they appear to have been higher among rural youth. The infant and maternal mortality and deaths from most preventable diseases are today higher in rural areas than in large cities. Although both urban and rural health have improved over the last fifty years, the rate of improvement of rural health has been appreciably slower, and we seem to be arriving at a time when the curves of health status are crossing, and the rural record is, on the whole, poorer. While the environmental hazards of city life had their ill effects for many decades, the corrective measures, in the line of public health services and medical care, appear to have more than overcome the liabilities.

Consciousness of special deficiencies in rural medicine was not confined to the professional world, nor did it wait on the testimony of comparative vital statistics. As early as 1911, the Farmers Educational and Cooperative Union engaged in discussion of the difficulties of obtaining medical care in rural areas—especially when agricultural income was low. At its annual convention this organization recommended Federal and State legislation to protect the health of children through "bureaus of child and animal protection." Since that time other farm organizations, as well as the Farmers Union, have shown increasing concern for equitable health services for the farm population.

As with most measures of social control, it was many years after deficiencies became evident before positive steps were taken to meet the situation. The medical disadvantages of rural isolation had to be faced by lumber, mining, and railroad establishments in the nineteenth century; to make physicians available, these enterprises organized group prepayment plans which would assure them a secure income. Improvements in rural sanitation and public health services were begun by such programs as the attack on the hookworm disease in the rural South, launched by the Rockefeller Sanitary Commission in 1909. It was not until the 1920's that official governmental action was taken to remedy the shortage of physicians in rural communities. In that period a number of States passed laws authorizing towns to appropriate funds for the attraction of physicians to rural districts. . . .

In 1935, the Social Security Act provided Federal funds for extending public health services, chiefly in rural districts, and in 1936 the prepayment medical care program of the Farm Security Administration got under way. Governmentally subsidized construction of hospitals in the 1930's, developed chiefly for work relief purposes, benefited urban centers predominantly; it was not until the 1940's that

Federal legislation specifically to improve health facilities in rural districts was introduced in Congress and, as of this writing, such legislation is still pending.[2]

While the process has been slow, we have finally arrived at a time when the special problem of rural medicine is becoming generally recognized. The forces of urbanization have left the rural districts not only with fewer physicians proportionately, but also with physicians of older age levels and less adequate training. The rural medical profession has almost the earmarks of a dying civilization; its members are disappearing and they are not being replenished by new blood. While public health services are being extended, and hospitals are increasing, the relative supply of rural doctors is decreasing. The problem, in any event, is recognized, and remedial measures, on the nation-wide basis essential for effectiveness, are being proposed. The problem is, of course, not peculiar to the United States, but has existed in other countries for many years.

The problem of rural medicine is, of course, a segment of the larger problem of inadequate medical care, related to insufficient or unplanned purchasing power for health services. Yet it is ironic that rural medical patterns, which more than any other reflect the dilemmas of laissez-faire individualistic medicine, are sometimes used to justify opposition to progressive changes. The country doctor, in his most typical form, is a figure who reflects the past and the portrait painted of him is used often in sentimental defense of the ways of the past. While his resourcefulness and devotion to his work win the admiration of all socially-minded persons, he does not present a pattern which can guide us effectively toward the future.

Today rural medical care represents a special issue which must be faced. The solution is probably to be found in developing patterns of rendering medical care that are even more at variance with conventional patterns than those proposed for the urban population. . . .

64. ATTRACTING DOCTORS TO RURAL AREAS *

IT IS GENERALLY conceded that there is no distressing problem of medical care and no difficulty in getting and keeping medical personnel in the more populous rural areas, so our attention and efforts can therefore be concentrated on the larger more sparsely settled areas, where neighbors are far apart, and towns which are large enough to support a doctor are widely separated. It is in such communities that it will be difficult to convince the younger doctor to locate and establish a practice. Some better system of professional, educational, religious, social and economic

2. On August 13, 1946, the National Hospital Survey and Construction Act became federal law.

* From: "Methods of Bringing and Holding Doctors in Rural Areas," by Fred A. Humphrey, M.D.; *Journal of the American Medical Association* 133:778-79, Mar. 15, 1947 (No. 11). Reprinted (with omissions, including initial paragraph) by permission of the author and publishers. The author is a general practitioner in Fort Collins, Colo.

relationship will have to be established in order to hold doctors in such rural communities, once they have located there.

. . . No rules of procedure can be made which will not have to be revised to fit some unusual condition, since there are so many diverse types of rural areas in the United States. A specific program drawn to the measurement of conditions found in the corn belt of the middle West would of necessity need some revision to meet the entirely different type of person and occupation present in the cotton belt of the South or the mining areas of either the Eastern or the Rocky Mountain States. However, a start must be made and a general plan outlined which is flexible enough to allow the changes needed to meet the different conditions found in the various sections of the United States.

In drawing up such a plan, the first things to consider are the changes which should be made by the individual farmers and business men in the small towns which will increase their chance of having a doctor locate in their community. The suggestions made are not unreasonable or difficult of accomplishment. More time, money and energy should be spent on such things as good roads, especially from farm to market, improved sanitary conditions, safer water supply and storage and similar local projects, than in trying to get a hospital located in their community under the provisions of the Hill-Burton Act. Such a hospital should rightfully be located only after a scientific and practical interpretation of a thorough survey of hospital and health needs. The many "ghost towns" scattered in the mining areas of the Mountain states do not present a pleasant picture, but an even more depressing sight would be "ghost hospitals" appearing over the United States in the next few years because of poor judgment now in choosing their locations. If a town and its surrounding trade territory is large enough to support a doctor adequately and wishes to have one, then every effort should be put forth by its citizens to obtain that desire. The initiative is squarely in the lap of the local people, and to secure the goal they may have to offer even further inducement such as the physical facilities which are so essential to a doctor if he is to care properly for the sick. In some cases it may be necessary to take still another step and subsidize the doctor on a monthly basis in order to make his income commensurate with his education and ability. Such subsidies should be financed locally, if at all possible, before application for state or federal aid is made. By all means, after a doctor has located in a rural community its citizens should show their loyalty to him by using him in case of illness and not go to the larger, but more distant, towns for their medical care.

Universal participation in prepayment insurance by farm people will be of definite assistance in bringing and keeping doctors in rural areas and should be incorporated in any plan devised for that purpose.

The medical schools of the United States should be asked to cooperate and join in the attempt to solve the rural health problem. There is no other instrument in organized medicine which can or should lend itself to such a service as easily and efficiently, but a definite program must be submitted to them which will enhance rather than jeopardize the prime purpose to which they owe their existence.

Other medical schools should follow the example of the Colorado university which has established a residency in general practice following the usual rotating internship of one year. . . . After this training it is expected that the doctor will be capable of caring for better than 90 per cent of the patients coming to him should he locate in one of the small towns. Possibly other schools have instituted the same program. If not, they should be advised to do so.

Another change in policy which would relieve materially the present shortage of doctors in rural areas is the requirement of from three to five years in general practice before resident training is begun. Such a plan would be of great benefit to the individual by broadening his clinical knowledge and by giving him a better understanding of the difficulties encountered in general practice and a finer appreciation of the economic features involved. A doctor after such an experience would be more mature and better qualified to choose the specialty for which he has the greatest aptitude and in which he has developed the most interest. Later, should he wish to become certified, some credit should be given for the time spent in general practice. It would also be beneficial, at least in the immediate future, by opening many residencies which could be and would be filled by qualified men who have served in the armed forces and who are now attempting to obtain residencies in order to become certified by special boards. . . .

The final suggestion to the medical schools originates from the statement "You can take the boy out of the country but you cannot take the country out of the boy." In the present condition of many applicants to medical schools to one admission, a certain definite proportion of them should come from the rural areas. A boy who has been born and reared in or near a small town is much more likely to return to it than a boy who has experienced nothing but city life.

As methods of "Bringing and Holding Doctors in Rural Areas," suggestions have been offered both to the rural communities and to the medical profession. The recommendations to be carried out by the rural communities are:

That they build and maintain good roads from farm to market.

That they educate themselves on public health matters and put into practice known disease preventing measures.

That they improve their living conditions.

That they have in their area persons trained in first aid and home nursing.

That in some instances they furnish for the doctor the needed facilities, such as equipment and office headquarters; in some localities even a subsidy may be necessary.

That they apply to the proper agency of their state for assistance under the provisions of the Hill-Burton Act if financial aid is required to carry on their program.

That they participate in prepayment insurance.

That they patronize their local doctor and whenever possible conserve his time by going to his office.

The recommendations to the medical profession are:

That they require three to five years' general practice before resident training is begun.

That certification boards give credit for such time spent in general practice.

That hospitals establish residencies in general practice.

That students from rural areas be encouraged to study medicine.

That hospital staffs be open to men in general practice.

That the system of medical care to soldiers be adapted to rural medical care.

That the rural practitioner be kept informed on advances in medical science by contact with other medical men at county medical society meetings and short refresher courses held in the rural districts.

65. The Kansas Plan *

The United States is faced with a serious shortage of properly trained medical personnel. Doctors, nurses and medical technicians of all types are in very short supply. . . .

The situation in rural areas is particularly acute and all authorities recognize the shortage of adequate medical care in rural communities to be our most pressing national health problem. The rural shortage is due to several factors, including overspecialization by physicians, desire to be near centers where postgraduate training is available, and, most important, local lack of adequate facilities with which to practice modern medical techniques.

The situation in Kansas mirrors the national picture but in some respects is more severe due to the essential rural nature of the state. . . .

In summary, [this situation] is represented by the facts that in the past 42 years, with an increase of 25 per cent in the population, the state has had a decrease of 30 per cent in the physician population, mainly at the expense of the rural communities. The mean age of the physician in the country is much greater than that in the city, which makes the future even darker for the rural citizen. Finally, over 70 Kansas communities plus the eleemosynary institutions are clamoring for well trained physicians, nurses and technicians, and the small hospitals building program when completed will create an even greater demand for such people. Is there any reason why the rural Kansan and his family should be denied the type of medical care his urban neighbor can and does get? Within the limits of practicality, what can be done in Kansas to correct this inequity and thereby make more complete the life of the rural citizens who make up the majority of our people? . . .

PROPOSED PLAN

Point I.—The foundation on which any program for medical care must be built is an adequate supply of raw material. The first point in this program is, then, increased production—doctors, nurses and medical technicians of all types—to make

* From: "Medical Care in Rural Kansas: The Problem and Its Proposed Solution," by Franklin D. Murphy, M.D.; *Journal of the Kansas Medical Society* 49:472-78, Nov. 1948 (No. 11). Reprinted (with omissions) by permission of the author and publishers. The author is the chancellor of the University of Kansas, in Lawrence.

up for an underproduction over the past 30 years as well as to take care of the normal attrition of practicing physicians in Kansas, which is apparently increasing. . . .

In order to maintain its accredited rating and still handle a class of 80 students a year, the medical school has gone on a quarter system, whereby the plant of the medical center is in use the year around. In other words, the medical school is straining its present physical facilities and faculty to the utmost in order to graduate 80 students per year. If the problem of rural health care in Kansas is to be attacked, the medical school must graduate at least 100 students per year, to say nothing of more nurses and medical technicians. There is absolutely no means by which the school can increase its student load and maintain its accredited rating without increasing its physical facilities and augmenting its faculty.

It should be stated at this point that the school fully recognizes its obligations to train men for general practice in Kansas, and drastic changes have been made in the curriculum this year with an eye to emphasizing general or family practice as opposed to specialization. However, the intensity of this general practice-type training is again limited by the lack of adequate facilities in such divisions of the medical center as the Outpatient Department. The members of the faculty of the School of Medicine are increasingly striving to re-dignify the general practitioner, who, after all, makes up the backbone of rural practice.

Point II.—Once having produced enough physicians, it becomes necessary to see that an adequate percentage of the young doctors go to the places where they are most needed, i. e., the rural areas. Detailed questioning of medical students and recent graduates of the School of Medicine clearly indicates that the major deterrent to settling in a smaller community is the local lack of equipment and office space with which to practice modern medicine. . . . It is, therefore, suggested that each community, to attract and maintain a doctor, raise the funds necessary to provide adequate office facilities, including office, examining rooms, reception room, small diagnostic x-ray laboratory and small clinical laboratory. This would be a community project and would have the added advantage of giving every citizen in the community a stake in the health of the community. A young doctor, then, fresh from modern medical training, would settle in this community, paying a fair rental for office space and equipment out of current income, and be able to start to work with the type of tools he has been taught to use. At the end of two or three years, if the community is satisfied with the doctor and he with the community, he would begin to amortize the equipment, probably at no interest, for, after all, the community would not be interested in making money but rather in providing itself with good health service. At the end of a few years, the young doctor would be sole owner of the equipment but would continue to rent office space from the community. If it seemed desirable, the doctor could also buy the office space. There is no reason why this arrangement would not work for more than one physician. For the average small community, $15,000 would probably suffice to provide a modern facility. . . . With such a program, then the community provides the magnet which will draw a young doctor to the area where he is most needed. This, of course, is a mutually benefiting plan because the doctor is able to begin practice immediately with the modern diagnostic tools which he has been taught to use in medical school and with no serious immediate financial hardship. The community, on the other hand, benefits not only in the acquisition of a physician, but also assures itself of up-to-date methods in the diagnosis and treatment of disease. . . .

Point III.—One of the most frequent objections given by medical students and young medical graduates against practicing in remote rural areas is the fact that they feel they will become medically isolated if they settle too far from the cities and medical centers. That is to say, they are reluctant to remove themselves from the opportunities of seeing and learning about the new advances in medical diagnosis and treatment. They desire to maintain professional excellence and feel that it is less possible in a remote rural community.

The answer to this objection is an intensive program of postgraduate medical education. The Medical School of the University of Kansas in conjunction with the Kansas Medical Society and the State Board of Health has already initiated plans to build an adequate postgraduate program in medical education, and early experience demonstrates an enthusiastic response from practitioners of medicine in Kansas for this type of training.

The program consists basically of three different but complementing types of training:

(a) The short refresher course which consists of a two or three-day program given at the University of Kansas Medical Center. Each program relates to one field of medicine, i. e., surgery, internal medicine, etc. Guest instructors are chosen from the leading men in their respective fields throughout the United States. The remaining instructors are made up by members of the faculty of the medical school and leading practitioners of medicine in Kansas. . . .

(b) In the past few years, circuit courses have been carried out in one or two fields of medicine each year. It is contemplated that this year, there will be set up six circuit courses covering at least 12 separate topics in medicine and surgery. Cities in Kansas will be chosen for their strategic geographic location, and teams of instructors, made up of members of the faculty of the medical school and qualified practitioners of medicine in Kansas, will travel from one city to the next giving the newest and most practical information in diagnosis and treatment of specific medical problems. In the beginning, at least six Kansas cities will be covered by this circuit. Here, then, in the form of an extension program, the medical school is bringing education to the doctor rather than making it necessary for the doctor to come to the medical center.

(c) The third and possibly the most important part of the postgraduate program cannot yet be initiated because of limited facilities. This consists of setting up a formal type of training program in the medical center and medical school which would allow the man in general practice to return to the medical center for several weeks at a time and as often as every three to five years. The general practitioner takes care of from 80 to 90 per cent of the nation's illnesses. Yet there is no type of postgraduate facility in which he can actually work, participating in bedside instruction, attending clinics, lectures, conferences, etc. Formal graduate medical education has been from time immemorial the almost exclusive property of the specialist. If this third point in the postgraduate program can be achieved, it will make it possible for the man in general practice, i. e., the rural practitioner, to have the same opportunities for maintaining his professional excellence as the specialist. In order to provide this in-residence experience for the Kansas doctor, at least 100 to 150 hospital beds are needed, to say nothing of the laboratory space which he would utilize.

Once the facilities are available to set up this complete postgraduate medical education program, the student entering the medical school of the University of Kansas will be told upon his admission and told repeatedly throughout his four years of medical work that he is entering upon a 40-year educational program, only the first four years of which end with his graduation from medical school. He will leave the medical school feeling not only the desire but the obligation to participate in postgraduate medical education and will, furthermore, see that he has the opportunity to do just that in his medical school until the day he dies or retires from practice. He will further see that this training experience will be worthwhile and satisfactory because the proper facilities and staff are available to provide it. Thus the young doctor on entering a remote rural practice begins his professional life with the full understanding that the state medical school is keenly interested in his maintaining professional competence and the further understanding that instead of being medically isolated, he actually is in continual contact with the newest advances in medical diagnosis and treatment. The people of Kansas, on the other hand, through this mechanism are assured of the best medical care, both present and future, no matter whether they live in the city or in the country. . . .

66. RURAL MEDICAL CARE PROGRAMS *

CUTTING ACROSS the lines of every aspect of America's problem of medical care are the needs of the nearly 60,000,000 people living in rural areas.[1] Most, if not all, of the problems of organization of medical services are found in their severest form in rural sections, and a large measure of the organized efforts expended in the last two or three decades has been directed specifically to meet rural needs. . . .

* From: "Rural Programs of Medical Care," by Milton I. Roemer, M.D.; *Annals of the American Academy of Political and Social Science*, Vol. 273 (entitled *Medical Care for Americans*), Jan. 1951, pp. 160-68. Reprinted (with omissions) by permission of the author and publishers. The author is the director of research, Sloan Institute of Hospital Administration. Cornell University, Ithaca, N.Y.

1. "Rural" is used here, according to the definition of the U. S. Bureau of the Census, to mean places of under 2,500 population.

Rural Health Needs

COMPARISONS of the health of rural and urban people are difficult because of artifacts affecting reporting and because of sheer lack of data. Space does not permit a discussion of rural health status by diagnostic categories, but for all causes of death combined, the American rural population appears to enjoy an advantage over the urban. Over the past fifty years, however, this advantage has been dwindling, and we seem to be approaching a time when rural and urban age-adjusted death rates will be equal. As for frequency and duration of illnesses, the data are inconclusive but suggest higher rates for the rural population. With respect to physical and mental defects as a whole, the burden seems to be appreciably higher in the rural population, compared with the urban. For those causes of death and disability which are most readily preventable or curable by modern science, the record of the rural population is distinctly poorer than the urban.

Regardless of the health status of rural people, it is generally recognized that they have access to and receive less medical care of virtually every type than do city dwellers. The rural areas are supplied with proportionately smaller numbers of physicians, dentists, nurses, technicians, and every other class of medical personnel except untrained midwives and possibly chiropractors. They are served by fewer general and special hospital beds. While beds for tuberculosis and mental disorders tend to be predominantly on a state-wide basis, the rural states as a whole are far more meagerly supplied than the urban. Laboratories and even drug stores are proportionately fewer in rural sections. Public clinics attached to both hospitals and health departments are relatively less adequate.

To cope with the general inadequacies of medical care for families of low or moderate income, a variety of organized activities have developed throughout the Nation, but the effectiveness of these efforts has, by and large, been far less in the rural sections than in the cities. This applies to programs financed by tax funds or by voluntary charity or by the insurance device. Thus, programs of medical care for the needy, under public assistance agencies, are more meagerly supported in rural counties than in the larger cities. Community chests and other charitable sources of funds for medical care to the "medically needy" tend to be weaker in rural sections. Hospital outpatient departments and wards for inpatients, which give large volumes of "free" or low-cost care to low-income persons in the big cities, are quite unavailable in most rural districts. Voluntary insurance programs, providing either indemnification for medical care expenditures or direct service, reach a very much lower percentage of rural than of urban people. Many governmental programs which provide economic support to help meet the medical needs of industrial workers—such as workmen's compensation, disability insurance, and old age and survivors insurance—do not cover farmers or farm laborers.

Nevertheless, despite these deficiencies in rural medical care as compared with urban, a great many organized efforts have been undertaken designed specifically to meet rural needs. Any scheme for describing these rural programs will yield some overlapping in categories, but a convenient approach is the following: (1)

programs to attract medical and allied personnel; (2) programs to develop hospitals and other facilities; (3) programs to ease the financial support for medical services; and (4) programs to improve the general quality of rural medical care.

Personnel

THE MOST IMMEDIATE and dramatic deficiency in rural health services has long been the increasingly severe shortage of personnel. The problem has been world-wide. In the United States, while there have been gradual improvements in the supply of rural hospitals, the coverage of rural health departments, and even the economic support for general medical services, the relative supply of physicians and other health personnel has actually declined. As a result, there has probably been wider attention to this than to any other facet of the rural medical problem.

Since about 1920 a number of corrective steps have been taken. Direct subsidy to attract physicians has been attempted by small towns in New Hampshire, Vermont, Massachusetts, and Maine since 1923. Frequently the towns guarantee a minimum annual income, providing from local revenues the difference between this sum and what the doctor earns privately. Sometimes the doctor has been offered a rent-free house. In the 1930's the Commonwealth Fund gave fellowships to medical students on the condition that they would practice in a rural community for a few years. Although the results were discouraging—most of the men leaving for an urban area at the end of the period of obligation—the same scheme was launched by state governments in the 1940's. Virginia passed a law for this purpose in 1942, and North Carolina, Georgia, Alabama, Mississippi, Florida, Indiana, and Kentucky have followed suit. It is too early to judge the effects of these efforts, but the number of physicians trained through these programs is small considering the size of the problem.

Still other approaches have been made through the medical schools. The impetus to the establishment or expansion of medical schools in several rural states has in large measure been the need for rural physicians. Alabama, North Carolina, and North Dakota have put large state funds into medical education under this incentive. Some medical schools, like those attached to the University of Tennessee and the University of Kansas, make serious efforts to persuade their students to enter rural practice. No school in the United States has gone as far as Mexico, with its required period of "social service" of six to twelve months in a rural village for all medical graduates; but in Mississippi, Louisiana, Kentucky, and New York State medical students are offered summer positions in rural health departments during their schooling. An increasing number of internships and residencies involve periods of work in small rural hospitals under some supervision by a central institution.

At the national level there has been much planning for the training of more physicians, dentists, and nurses. Bills recently considered by Congress for Federal subsidy of professional schools have been designed, among other things, to increase the over-all national supply of health personnel in order to correct rural shortages.

During and immediately after World War II, a number of Federal programs were undertaken which directly or indirectly were designed to improve or at least stabilize the supply of rural doctors. In 1943 Congress enacted a law to pay transportation expenses and a temporary stipend to physicians and dentists who would relocate in a community needing help. The National Procurement and Assignment Service was the vehicle established to balance the medical needs of the civilian population with those of the armed forces. Although in most rural regions military medical quotas were rapidly exceeded, this program helped to focus national attention on the critical nature of rural medical shortages. The specialized training programs of the Army and the Navy and the Cadet Nurse Corps helped to train an increased number of medical personnel, and enabled many rural youth who otherwise could not have afforded it to undertake medical training. In the immediate postwar years surplus military property was supposed to be offered to rural doctors and hospitals as a means of strengthening rural medicine, but little was accomplished.

The autonomy of the states with respect to professional licensure has been an impediment to the free movement of physicians and dentists to areas of greatest need. Reciprocity of licensure between states is only about 50 per cent effective, and wide discretion is sometimes exercised by medical examining boards to reduce the exchange below this. The National Board of Medical Examiners has made headway in correcting this problem, but it still affects only a small percentage of new graduates. Further assistance to a free movement of physicians has been provided by an Information Service maintained by the American Medical Association's Committee on Rural Health Service. It works through the state and county medical societies and attempts to bring together doctors seeking a place of settlement and communities needing physicians. Many rural communities, moreover, advertise their attractions in medical journals. Whatever other measures are used to correct the maldistribution of physicians, a free flow of information is obviously essential.

Organized efforts to attack other aspects of the rural health problem, like the construction of hospitals and the development of prepayment plans, also have an important influence on the supply of medical personnel.

Facilities

RURAL HOSPITALS, like those in cities, have been built over the years primarily through local community effort. The lower income of rural sections, however, has meant scantier funds and hence fewer hospital beds proportionate to population than in the cities. With more meager resources in both local government tax funds and local philanthropy, the rural deficiencies have been greatest in general hospitals under the control of nonprofit voluntary and governmental agencies. A proportionately higher number of rural hospital beds have been established in proprietary institutions, organized for profit and suffering numerous inadequacies in the quality of service.

Systematic efforts to improve the supply of rural hospital beds have naturally depended in large measure on outside assistance. Philanthropic foundations have provided important demonstrations by giving financial assistance to selected rural communities toward the cost of modern buildings. The work of the Commonwealth Fund, which subsidized fourteen rural hospitals, has been outstanding; the Kellogg Foundation has been a benefactor in Michigan, and the Duke Endowment in the Carolinas.

Outside of financing institutions for tuberculosis and mental disorders, state governments have done little to support hospitals in rural sections. A notable exception is Louisiana, whose state-wide system of "Charity Hospitals" serves low-income and indigent people in all parts of that rural state. Some states, like New York, Connecticut, and Washington, use state funds to pay for hospitalization of public assistance recipients in local hospitals, but the impact of this aid on rural institutions has been slight.

The Federal Government has helped to finance hospital construction since about 1935.... In 1946 a Federal hospital construction program was launched specifically to meet health needs.... [This program] has helped to establish hospitals, on a basis of rational state-wide planning, in hundreds of undersupplied rural counties.

Of special interest in rural areas is the use of the co-operative principle as a means of financing small institutions.... The first co-operative hospital was built in Elk City, Oklahoma in 1929 by the National Farmers Union, in association with a prepayment plan for financing hospital and medical services. Others have been established in Kansas, Minnesota, Washington, Oregon, and especially in Texas. In the last-named state, some twenty institutions have been organized in rural communities on this basis since the end of World War II. The home missions of several church denominations have also set up hospitals in needy and isolated rural districts of the Southeast and Southwest.

In the last five years another approach to rural hospital needs has been emphasized: regionalization of services. Instead of simply adding more independent units of twenty-five or fifty or a hundred beds to the countryside, it has been recognized that rural people could get the best service if they could have access to services not only in local hospitals, but also in the finest urban medical centers in the state. The plan conceives of a flow of patients from peripheral to more highly developed central institutions and a flow of technical and consultant services from the urban center to the rural outposts. While there has been much more discussion than action in this sphere, accomplishments so far will be reviewed below, under "Quality of Service."

Financial Support of Services

MOST GOVERNMENTAL programs for financing medical services have, reasonably enough, applied to all areas in a state or in the Nation, and not solely to the rural sections. However, many of these programs have had only slight impact on rural people. Public medical services for persons receiving public assistance ... are, of course, available to rural people, but—since their support comes primarily from state and local rather than Federal funds—they tend to be less well developed in rural areas than in cities. Cash allowances to recipients of the three special assistance programs, designed to enable them to pay for medical and related services, are usually very low. Vocational rehabilitation medical services are generally available, but the concentration of this program is inevitably on industrial workers in the cities. Workmen's compensation nearly everywhere excludes farm laborers and agricultural processing workers from coverage, and never encompasses self-employed rural people.

Certain national programs for financing medical care, on the other hand, may mean more for rural people than for urban, simply because of the local rural deficiencies. Thus, the Veterans Administration program of medical care probably serves a higher proportion of rural than of urban veterans, since private services are less accessible to the average rural veteran, both because of lack of personnel and facilities and because of insufficient purchasing power. The same probably applied to the wartime Emergency Maternity and Infant Care program, which provided obstetrical and pediatric care to the dependents of servicemen. It is difficult to document either of these statements, since statistical data in these programs are not kept on an urban-rural basis; but they are borne out by casual observations. The marine hospital system, operated by the United States Public Health Service for merchant seamen, renders medical care to men who may live part of the year in rural communities.

Other national programs have served population groups that are wholly or predominantly rural. The Indian Service of the Department of Interior has long rendered tax-supported medical care to the 375,000 Indians in the Nation, nearly all of whom are country dwellers.* For the years 1937-47, a special nation-wide system of medical care was available to certain groups of migratory farm laborers, administered by a series of agencies in the Federal Department of Agriculture. During the construction phase of the dams of the Tennessee Valley Authority, medical services were organized for the entire families of the workers on this great rural project.

One of the most significant governmental efforts to ease the burden of medical expenses in rural areas was the medical care program of the Farm Security Administration operating between 1936 and 1947. This activity, one phase of a general welfare program for farm families, was based principally on the device of voluntary insurance. The Federal Government made loans to help depressed farm families to become rehabilitated, and, among other things, these funds were used for paying membership fees in locally organized and controlled prepayment plans for physicians' care, hospitalization, drugs, and dental care. At the height of the program, in 1942, there were about 620,000 farm people in some 1,100 counties enrolled in these insurance plans. The pressures of the wartime period and postwar legislative

* Provision of health and hospital services for Indians became the responsibility of the Public Health Service on July 1, 1955, under the authority of Public Law 568, signed by the President on Aug. 5, 1954. This legislation did not affect education and welfare programs for Indians, which remained the responsibility of the Indian Service of the Interior Department.

changes brought this program to an end, but it has undoubtedly had widespread impact on the attitude of rural people toward group prepayment as a system for financing medical care.

In a few selected rural counties a special "experimental rural health program" was conducted by the Department of Agriculture from 1942 to 1945, based on the same principle but supplemented with outright grants (instead of loans) to make possible a comprehensive scope of service for a higher proportion of local farm families. The lessons of this experiment are useful in helping to evaluate the strength and the weaknesses of voluntary medical care insurance, fortified by government subsidy for families of low income.

Prepayment plans for medical care under nongovernmental auspices have developed indigenously in rural areas and have also reached rural people from urban centers. Some of the oldest prepayment plans in the Nation had their origins in rural sections—in lumbering, mining, and railroad establishments, where groups of workers were isolated from ordinary community health facilities. Most of these plans still operate, and, while the quality of service rendered under them has frequently been criticized, they furnish rural nonfarm people with services that might otherwise be lacking. Other classes of industry in small towns sometimes have prepayment arrangements with private group-practice organizations.

Among farm people, a scattering of voluntary "co-operative" prepayment plans has developed since the organization of the Community Hospital Association at Elk City, Oklahoma in 1929. Similar plans, usually associated with the ownership of a hospital, have been organized elsewhere in Oklahoma, and in Texas, Nebraska, Minnesota, Washington, and Oregon. These plans under local control are characterized by a fairly comprehensive scope of medical care and by administrative control by the consumer.

In contrast, the prepayment plans organized on a state-wide basis tend to offer limited service and to be under the administrative control of professional or related groups. The most important by far are the Blue Cross plans for hospitalization and the Blue Shield plans for surgical and sometimes nonsurgical services. These insurance plans ... have enjoyed tremendous national growth, but their impact on the rural population has not been great. While a variety of interesting devices have been used to promote rural enrollment—farm bureaus, granges, co-operative associations, rural banks, and so forth—only a small fraction of the Nation's rural population, undoubtedly less than 10 per cent, has been reached. Commercial insurance companies also sell millions of policies for partial indemnification against hospital, surgical, or medical expenses, but they are largely concentrated among industrial workers. While prepayment coverage of all types has had a steady growth in rural areas, the cumulative percentage of the rural population protected is slight, and even among those covered, only a fraction of aggregate medical care expenses is cushioned by insurance.

Quality of Service

IT HAS LONG been realized that the handicaps of rural medical resources in personnel and facilities must yield an inferior quality of service for rural people. To improve the quality of rural medicine, various steps have been taken by physicians, medical schools, private agencies, and governmental authorities.

Most important has probably been the organization by private physicians of group-practice clinics, most of which are located in the generally rural regions of the United States. Since the Mayo Clinic was organized in the small town of Rochester, Minnesota in 1887, the pattern of group-practice clinics has grown slowly but steadily in small towns of the Midwest, the South, and the West—less along the Eastern Seaboard. These clinics offer a device for making specialist services available to rural people, as well as various technical laboratory and X-ray services rarely accessible to the nonhospitalized rural patient. Group practice may be associated with prepayment, but in rural regions it more often is not; nevertheless, economies are possible which are often passed on to the patient in fees lower than the same services would cost from independent practitioners. . . .

Another measure to improve the quality of rural service has been the organization of various courses of postgraduate medical education. Medical schools, medical societies, health departments, and private foundations have sponsored courses to acquaint the rural practitioner with recent developments in the various clinical specialties. Physicians may come into the urban medical centers, or traveling lecturers and consultants may go out to the small towns of a state. One of the difficulties impairing the effectiveness of these courses has been the lack of any organized system of locum tenens physicians, which would enable the busy rural doctor to get away for a solid period of training.

While periodic re-examination of physicians for new licensure has been suggested as a device to encourage rural and urban practitioners to keep abreast of new developments, nowhere has this been tried. Routine inspection and approval of hospitals, however, by the American Medical Association and the American College of Surgeons have served in some measure to maintain the quality of service in rural hospitals. Since 1946, moreover, nearly all the states have enacted hospital inspection and licensure laws which provide a legal foundation for this type of practice.

A culmination of various efforts to heighten the scientific quality of rural medicine is found in the concept of "regionalization of services," promoted in recent years. Recognizing the hospital as the key facility for delivery of complex medical services, the concept envisages a system of interrelationships between rural and urban institutions which would enable any rural person to have access to the highest level of service provided in the greatest urban medical center. Itinerant consultation services, referral of patients, exchange of interns and residents, formal postgraduate courses, pathological or laboratory or X-ray services by traveling specialists, circulation of medical literature, regional blood banks, and other services are all involved. . . . While each element in a regional plan has been tried separately in one place or other for many decades, the combination was launched only recently. . . .

Public Health Programs

IT MUST be realized that the line between prevention and treatment has long faded away. Many "public health" programs in country and city alike constitute advances also in the provision of medical care. Programs of dental care for children in rural schools, for example, provide diagnostic and treatment services, under the auspices of official health or education agencies, which would otherwise have to be purchased privately. Clinics for expectant women and for infants and preschool children offer an organized system of diagnostic services for many families of moderate income. Public services in venereal disease, tuberculosis, and cancer detection, and the general examination of school children, help to meet the personal health needs of increasing numbers of rural people.

Under the "categorical" disease-by-disease approach, much organization of both the payment for and the provision of services has been possible, and has been attended by less controversy than under a comprehensive approach to general illness. Yet the proportion of the total population reached by these specialized programs is usually small, and in rural areas they are usually less well developed than in the cities.

A Social Movement

EFFORTS TO improve rural medical care have taken the form of a special social movement. It is an aspect of a broader movement to better the general living conditions of rural people. Agricultural agencies like the Farmers Home Administration, the Extension Service, and the Farm Credit Administration have directed attention to the problem. All the major farm organizations—the farm bureaus, the granges, the farmers' unions, and the major farmers' co-operatives—have developed plans to extend medical care for their members. In many states, various citizen committees have worked to develop plans for better rural health service, based on both voluntary and governmental efforts. The American Medical Association has promoted the organization of rural health committees in nearly all the states.

When a social movement reaches an advanced stage, it usually becomes crystallized in legislative proposals. In addition to Federal legislation on facilities and personnel, several other bills have been introduced in Congress devoted largely to rural medical care. One bill provided for various forms of assistance to rural communities for public health services, postgraduate medical education, prepayment medical care plans, health centers, and so forth. Another bill would subsidize the organization of medical care co-operatives. In several major bills on nation-wide medical care insurance, compulsory or voluntary, special provisions are made for supplemental assistance to rural areas. The issue of rural medical care remains a live one, socially and therefore politically. It is altogether likely that in the years ahead increasing steps will be taken, both by government and by voluntary groups, to close the gap between the capacities of American medical science and the level of services actually received by rural people.

67. RURAL HEALTH: SUGGESTED PROGRAMS

A. THE NATIONAL HEALTH ASSEMBLY *

TEN-YEAR HEALTH goals for rural America include the development and expansion of the following programs:

Medical and Other Health Personnel.—The center of a modern rural medical service is the general practitioner. The family physician of the future, however, must practice truly preventive medicine through the evaluation and treatment of mental and emotional stresses as well as common illnesses. He can accomplish this purpose only by working as part of an integrated team which makes available the necessary medical specialists, public health personnel, and community agencies. Among the measures needed to provide the desired type of medical and other health personnel are the following:

1. Medical schools should give special consideration to the type of training needed for general practitioners in rural areas. Medical students should be afforded opportunities to work in situations where they can experience physician-family relationships. The system of rotating interns and residents through small rural hospitals should be extended. . . .

2. Medical education must be expanded to train an adequate number of doctors, dentists, nurses, and other health personnel to meet rural needs, both white and Negro.

3. Scholarships or loan funds should be available to enable all qualified rural youths to attend medical and other professional schools. This movement is already developing in many rural states. . . .

4. Scholarships to rural physicians for refresher courses and graduate study should be provided, so that the quality of rural medical practice may be improved.

5. Rural people must have a responsible part in developing plans for medical education. A first step in this direction is that the farm organizations arrange a meeting with representatives of the American Medical Association and other professional groups most concerned. At this meeting, a joint review should be made of all the factors involved in medical education to meet rural needs.

6. Special measures must be taken to attract and hold a sufficient number of both white and Negro doctors, nurses, dentists, and other health workers in all rural areas.

* From: *America's Health: A Report to the Nation by the National Health Assembly;* New York: Harper, 1949 (Chap. VI, "A National Program for Rural Health," pp. 158-63). Reprinted (with omissions, including initial paragraphs) by permission of the publishers.

7. Adequate nursing service, both professional and auxiliary, is essential to the effective functioning of a total health and medical program. This involves improving the quality of nursing schools, licensure for practical nurses, and an integrated system of preventive and bedside nursing services.

Paying for Medical Services.—The over-all goal is to have every rural family enrolled in a comprehensive health insurance plan within the next ten years.

Among immediate steps to achieve this goal are the following:

1. Every effort should be made to extend voluntary prepayment plans to all rural people through the most suitable methods for achieving full coverage.

2. Groups desiring to organize voluntary prepayment plans through cooperative health associations should have full opportunity to do so. To make this possible, the medical profession and medical co-operatives will have to reach an understanding on two points:

   (a) The enactment of enabling legislation (such as that recently put upon the statute books of Wisconsin) establishing the right of co-operative health associations to contract with doctors for professional services; and

   (b) The desire of the medical profession to ensure that the terms of contracts with doctors in these plans be such as to provide the highest quality of medical care.

3. Aid to communities in the form of an increase in the proportion of the cost of hospital construction might do much to bring the current net cost of medical care within the reach of nearly all rural families.

4. Residents of local political subdivisions should have the right voluntarily to tax themselves in order to obtain comprehensive medical services.

5. A Federal tax-supported program to provide health services and medical care for migratory agricultural workers should be enacted.

Hospital Facilities.—Health facilities should be extended to serve all rural people without discrimination with respect to color or economic status.

The aims and progress to date of the Hospital Survey and Construction Act in providing needed rural hospital, health center, and community clinic facilities and in its policy of local administration are commended. Recommendations for further development of this program include the following:

1. The Hospital Survey and Construction Act should be extended immediately for at least a ten-year period, to provide additional funds to meet the cost of construction for needed facilities in rural areas.

2. Where indicated in rural areas, an appraisal should take place to determine whether an increased percentage of state and/or Federal aid is necessary. Provision should be made to increase appropriations where needed.

3. Hospitals in rural areas should be paid on a realistic, operating, reimbursable basis for the necessary preventive and therapeutic hospital care of patients unable to provide such services from their own resources.

4. In order to avoid duplication of facilities and to encourage the integration of preventive and therapeutic services, health department activities and personnel should be housed within or adjacent to the rural general hospitals.

5. General hospitals in rural areas should be built large enough to ensure efficient and economical operation and the maintenance of a minimum basic medical staff.

6. A co-ordinated hospital program is essential for the equitable distribution to all rural people of health, hospital, medical, and related skills and services.

7. The official public health agency should be responsible for providing mobile facilities where needed (such as dental units, tuberculosis control units, and premature infant and ambulance services).

8. It may be necessary in the most needy rural areas to provide, through tax funds, not only a larger proportion of the construction costs but also funds for maintaining and operating hospital facilities.

Public Health Services.—Rural areas should be completely covered with adequately financed well-staffed city-county and/or multi-county health departments. . . .

Among immediately attainable goals are the following:

1. There should be a safe water supply in every rural home, school, and community.

2. There should be a sanitary privy for every rural family, and an indoor toilet as soon as possible.

3. Existing knowledge on the control of preventable disease should be applied to every rural area.

4. There should be modern health education in every rural school.

5. There should be a program for the training of all types of health personnel needed to staff adequately the local public health units.

Organization of Rural Health Services.—Rural people, in order to enjoy parity of health services with the urban population, must have access to the specialized services which characterize modern medicine. Effective organization and integration of health service is especially important in rural areas. Bearing that in mind, the following needed measures [are recommended]:

1. Organization of group-practice clinics or units at natural trade centers, so that the services of specialists can be made readily available to the majority of the rural population. The dispersion of the rural population is such that these groups will not be able to serve as a substitute for the general practitioner. If, however, general practitioners will associate themselves with such groups and practice in outlying areas, this tendency toward group practice and specialization can be utilized advantageously for rural people, thus providing a quality and scope of service otherwise difficult to realize. This system allows the general practitioner to remain in his important role of family physician.

2. Co-ordinated hospital planning. This would provide a blueprint for facilities into which co-ordinated health services naturally fit.

3. Co-ordination of medical care and public health services. The family doctor and the public health nurse, supplemented by technical skills in such fields as health education, dentistry, nutrition, and sanitation, will be the preventive-medicine team of the future.

4. Development of co-operative health associations. This method can improve the organizational structure. It can provide a broader financial base and planned action. All these benefits will aid in the development of an intelligent and integrated pattern of rural medical care....

Improvement in Rural Living.—A healthy rural America is important to the nation because rural America produces most of the nation's children. Within the next three generations, 80 per cent of the people of America will have come from a farm home. Long-term programs for agriculture that will guarantee the farm family an adequate income are fundamental in making possible a better standard of living. Other essentials are equal opportunities for education and health, improved farm-to-market roads, adequate power electricity, adequate systems of communication, better soil conservation and nutrition, and stabilization of farm income for the purchase of medical care.

Community Planning for Rural Health Services.—A continuous program of community education and community planning is essential if rural people are to realize their health goals. Toward this end the following recommendations are especially directed:

1. Land-grant colleges should be encouraged to undertake research projects and to organize pilot studies in various types of communities, in order to ascertain the amount and kinds of facilities needed and the personnel required for comprehensive health care, including prepayment medical care. These studies should be the basis for establishing future plans....

2. State and local rural health councils should be set up by the people of every state to promote objective study, planning, and organization to improve rural health services.

3. Educational and technical services available in the farm organizations, medical societies, agricultural extension services, public health agencies, and voluntary health organizations can and should be fully utilized by these health councils.

4. This program, if carried out promptly and effectively, will require more educational and technical personnel than is now available. All agencies and groups involved should take immediate steps to employ and train the personnel needed to do this job.

5. The attainment of comprehensive health care in the future lies in broad health and medical education of today's school child. The applied study of nutrition through a balanced school-lunch program should be a part of school education. School teachers will also have to be trained, if this program is to be properly implemented.

6. Health assemblies patterned after the National Health Assembly should be held in every rural state....

B. THE AMERICAN MEDICAL ASSOCIATION *

1. COMMUNITIES should make every effort to attract doctors by providing hospital or clinical facilities and to make community life attractive to them and their families.
2. Wider community participation in securing necessary facilities is a forward step which should be pushed with increasing vigor.
3. Existing and proposed facilities should be coordinated and integrated for an effective and fully utilized program.
4. An intensified educational program is needed to acquaint people with facilities available to them, with university extension services an important medium in this education.
5. Communities must be stimulated to undertake more realistic and objective measurement of health and hospital needs.
6. Tax funds should be used to provide medical care only when it is impossible for an individual to secure such care without such help.
7. Progress has been made in enrolling rural people in prepayment medical care plans but greater efforts should be made in that direction.
8. Medical schools should screen applicants early to eliminate those unqualified to become doctors; should encourage rejectees to prepare for related professions and should incorporate training in rural practice into the curriculum.

FURTHER READINGS

American Medical Association, Council on Rural Health. *National Conference on Rural Health*. Annual conference reports. Chicago: The Association.

American Medical Association, Council on Rural Health. *Programs for the Improvement of Rural Health*. Chicago: The Association, no date. 227 pages.

Johnston, Helen L. *Rural Health Cooperatives*. Bulletin 308, Public Health Service. Washington: U. S. Government Printing Office, 1950. 93 pages. (Includes references).

Mott, Frederick D. and Roemer, Milton I. *Rural Health and Medical Care*. New York: McGraw-Hill, 1948. 608 pages. (Includes references).

Roemer, Milton I. and Wilson, Ethel A. *Organized Health Services in a County of the United States*. Publication No. 197, Public Health Service. Washington: U. S. Government Printing Office, 1952. 91 pages.

United States Department of Agriculture. *Rural Health: Annotated List of Selected References*. Department Library List No. 60. Washington: U. S. Government Printing Office, 1953. 83 pages (processed).

United States Department of Agriculture. *Better Health for Rural America*. Miscellaneous Publication No. 573. Washington: U. S. Government Printing Office, 1945. 34 pages.

* From: "American Medical Association's Rural Health Program," in *Proceedings of the Fifth National Conference on Rural Health*, Chicago: American Medical Association (undated pamphlet). Reprinted from inside front cover (with omissions, including initial paragraphs) by permission of the publishers. (Note: This conference was held on Feb, 3-4, 1950, in Kansas City, Mo.)

CHAPTER X

Public Medical Care

T HE RESPONSIBILITY of the community as a whole for assisting its members in maintaining life and well-being is generally accepted as part of our social order. The circumstances under which the community acts to help meet individual needs, the type and degree of aid, and the definition of the persons considered eligible for community services all vary from one community to another. Medical care is one of the necessities of life which is frequently made available to a greater or lesser degree to some of our community members through the resources of the community as a whole. The trend to extend the availability of medical care services in this way has been accelerated in recent generations. This social movement grows out of the fact that modern medical knowledge and skill make it unnecessary for society to tolerate a substantial part of the human and economic losses due to disease and disability. The further fact that the cost of scientific medical care is beyond the range of many individuals has given added impetus to this movement.

In our society, the community may exercise its responsibility through the activities of voluntary associations or through the functions of various units of government. When medical care is provided by government, or with its direct financial support, it is considered public medical care. A few representative examples of the organized medical care programs sponsored by different units of government are presented in this chapter.

Our public medical care programs date back to the earliest origins of the United States. Today, they provide a large proportion of the total volume of medical care, despite the fact that most public medical care services are available only to limited segments of the community. For example, medical care is supplied to certain groups of people with whom the government has a payroll relationship. For members of the Armed Forces, this means complete medical care for themselves and certain of their dependents. For other employees of government, this may mean emergency medical care services while on the job or a somewhat wider range of occupational health services related to the work situation. Governments assume full medical care responsibility for those designated as wards—Indians, Eskimos and Aleuts; for some of the children who are wards of our courts; and for prisoners. The largest civilian population group eligible for a wide range of public medical care services is that of the veterans. The needy and medically needy constitute the next largest group—and certainly the major proportion of those for whom local and state governments assume the major responsibility.

Some public medical care programs deal with the prevention or treatment of specific conditions or types of illness which have been accepted as community problems by virtue of their wide occurrence, severity, or impact on family or community life. Preventive and treatment services for communicable diseases and for mental illness and other long-term diseases * are included in such programs. Special programs provide services to mothers and children and to handicapped adults. Other programs provide limited services which are intended to benefit the entire population—the clinical aspects of the medical research programs carried out by various units of the Federal government and by some of our states, and even cities, may be considered in this category. The extensive participation of every level of government in the financing of hospital construction, stimulated by the Hospital Survey and Construction Act (1946) and its amendments, has contributed significantly to the provision of medical care services through the development of modern facilities.

Out of the many and varied programs of public medical care, linked by their financial support from tax funds, comes evidence of a dual role of government in medical care. Public agencies have accepted responsibility for meeting medical care needs otherwise unmet—some needs which no other body would meet: a residual function; and other needs which no other body could meet: a leadership function. In many programs both roles have been played.

---

* Because of recent advances in the treatment of tuberculosis and the transitional state which this important field of public medical care is now in, the Editorial Committee considered it inappropriate to include a selection on tuberculosis services in this volume. The new principles of care for the tuberculous, based on the use of the newer chemotherapeutic agents, have not yet been definitively set down in the literature; and older principles are now essentially inapplicable.

68. Programs for the Needy *

For the purposes of this discussion, the term "needy" refers to recipients of public assistance, while the term "medically needy" denotes persons who cannot meet their requirements for medical care although otherwise able to maintain themselves. A useful definition of "medical need" is almost impossible to formulate, since it varies not only with the prevailing economic situation but also with the type of care required; there are very few persons, for example, who can pay the costs of long term hospital care for tuberculosis or other chronic diseases. In actual practice, the determination of medically needy persons eligible for service varies greatly in different localities, depending on such factors as the financial resources of the program, professional pressures, local laws and traditions, and public sentiment.

The present situation with respect to provision of medical care for the needy and medically needy is the result of several hundred years of development. The programs now in operation have evolved from colonial practices based on the Elizabethan poor laws, which placed the responsibility for poor relief on local governments and imposed social and legal penalties on the recipient of relief. As late as 1934, recipients of public assistance were deprived of the right to vote or hold office by the constitutions of fourteen states, while nine states maintained the spirit of the "pauper's oath" through legal provisions regarding applications for public assistance or the penalties for obtaining assistance under false pretense.

Evolution of Services

The evolution of facilities, services, and programs for the medical care of the needy and medically needy followed several independent lines which started at different periods, showed various rates of growth and decline, and tended to become more or less interdependent in different times and places. It is patently impossible to trace their evolution in detail, but a brief description of some of the more important services is necessary to an understanding of the present situation.

One of the earliest and most popular methods of providing physicians' services was the appointment of city or county physicians on a part-time salaried basis. These physicians usually provided home calls and occasionally office care and treatment of needy patients in the hospital. Students of public medical care have found

* From: "Medical Care for the Needy and Medically Needy," by Milton Terris, M.D.; *Annals of the American Academy of Political and Social Science*, Vol. 273 (entitled *Medical Care for Americans*), Jan. 1951, pp. 84-92. Reprinted (with omissions) by permission of the author and publishers. The author is the assistant dean for postgraduate education at the School of Medicine, University of Buffalo, Buffalo, N.Y.

little to recommend this method of providing service, yet it is still used by many local governments.

Public general hospitals have evolved in many instances from the infirmary sections of county workhouses and almshouses. Governmental institutions now provide two-fifths of the total general bed capacity in the country, about equally divided between Federal hospitals and those operated by local or state governments. For the most part, the latter are concentrated in cities with populations of more than 100,000, where they usually furnish services restricted to the needy and medically needy.

Public hospitals also account for 97 per cent of all beds in mental institutions and 87 per cent of the beds in tuberculosis hospitals. The overwhelming majority of the population is medically needy when long-term hospitalization is required; only a very small proportion can afford to pay for private care or meet the full cost of public hospital service.

A considerable amount of care for needy and medically needy patients is provided by voluntary hospitals which may or may not receive reimbursement from public agencies. Recent studies indicate that where such reimbursement is made, it is usually below actual cost; in most instances the payments received from city and county governments are lower than similar payments by state agencies. Lump-sum subsidies to voluntary hospitals are still used in many areas, although there is general agreement that the preferable method is to pay for hospital care at a per diem rate.

The outpatient departments of both voluntary and public general hospitals have come to play a major role in the provision of medical care for needy and medically needy persons in urban centers where these facilities are concentrated. They do not represent a significant resource for persons living in rural areas or in small communities.

Public Health Services

IN THE LAST few decades the rapid development of public health programs has provided an increasing number and variety of personal health services for the needy and medically needy. Traditionally, health department services are preventive in nature and designed for the entire community. Nevertheless, health departments have found it necessary to provide treatment services for adequate control of communicable diseases in general, and tuberculosis and syphilis in particular. Moreover, such preventive services as immunization, prenatal care, and well-child conferences have become basic elements of good medical care, with the result that the dividing line between prevention and treatment has become increasingly difficult to visualize.

The development of various personal health services provided by health departments has occasioned professional demands for limitation of such services to the needy and medically needy. The outcome has varied in different communities. In some, all personal health services provided in health department clinics are limited to these groups; more often there are no regulatory limitations, but the great majority receiving services are needy and medically needy; while in still others, the services are commonly utilized by all economic groups in the community. Certain personal health services carried through on a mass scale, such as sodium fluoride applications for school children and chest X-ray surveys, are provided regardless of economic status. In other programs, such as those furnishing care for crippled children, compromises have often centered around an arbitrary division between diagnosis and treatment, with the former available to all, and the latter restricted to the needy and medically needy.

At the present time, state and local health departments provide a variety of clinic services, such as immunization, tuberculosis, venereal disease, well-child, prenatal, dental, and orthopedic clinics. These services are being expanded to include cancer, cardiac, and mental hygiene clinics, and sometimes hospital services as well. Corrective services are available for school children in many areas, and crippled children's programs provide care for an increasing variety of crippling conditions in addition to orthopedic defects.

Free Service by Physicians

TRADITIONALLY, the medical profession has furnished a considerable amount of free service, with the "sliding scale" of medical fees making it theoretically possible to balance the losses with large fees from wealthy patients. But in 1935 the Bureau of Medical Economics of the American Medical Association pointed out:

The principle has been severely strained by the contemporary evolution of the industrial system, as well as by certain changes within the profession. The greatly increased demands by the indigent sick during the lowest phases of the industrial cycle, which has also often reduced the income of the physician below any reasonable standard of living, has now made this burden unbearable. Moreover, the physician whose practice is established among families with low incomes finds so large a proportion of his patients in the indigent class that his paying patients are too few to enable him to subsist. . . .

FERA and Social Security

THE ENTIRE SYSTEM of medical care for the needy and medically needy—poorly organized, unco-ordinated, relying primarily on local government resources and the charitable services of physicians, voluntary hospitals, and voluntary health and welfare agencies—collapsed under the impact of the depression of the thirties. The Federal Emergency Relief Administration medical care program, organized in July 1933 to fill the gap, was based on the principle that the traditional patient-physician relationship should be preserved. Patients had free choice of practitioner, and payments from Federal funds were made according to state fee schedules adopted by agreement with the organized medical, dental, and nursing professions. The services provided were limited to physician's care in home and office, emergency dental care, bedside nursing service, drugs, and emergency appliances. Because of the limited funds available, hospital care was not included, and sharp restrictions were placed on the services available.

Although it lasted only two and a half years, was uneven in its geographical application, and had many serious deficiencies, the FERA program exercised tremendous influence on the subsequent development of the medical care programs of public welfare departments. It initiated several significant trends which have become intensified in the last fifteen years: (1) the increasingly important role of governmental agencies as purchasers of medical care in contrast with previous tendencies to rely heavily on the free services of physicians, hospitals, and other voluntary agencies; (2) the evolution of more thoroughly organized medical care programs; and (3) the increased participation of state and Federal governments in the financing and development of medical care for the needy.

The Social Security Act of 1935 established the principle of social insurance as a major approach to prevention of dependency. In addition, state and local public assistance was strengthened by provisions for Federal matching of funds for three categories of assistance recipients—the aged, the blind, and dependent children. Federal aid was not made available for needy persons outside these categories or for those residing in public institutions.

An important feature of the Social Security Act was its requirement that in order to receive Federal matching of state funds in the categorical programs, the payment for medical as well as other needs must be by unrestricted money payments to the recipient in order to allow him the fullest possible independence. Unfortunately, this requirement has resulted in considerable administrative difficulty and hindered the development of well-organized medical care programs. In many areas the money payments are so low that increases to meet medical bills are necessarily utilized to provide basic needs of food and shelter, with the result that the practitioner may go unpaid. Large bills present particular problems, since maximum limits on money payments make it impossible to increase them sufficiently to pay for care, even in installments, within a reasonable time. To meet these difficulties, some states decided to forego Federal funds and provide direct "vendor payments" for medical care in the categorical programs to a greater or less extent. In the general assistance program, where there is no question of Federal matching requirements, direct payment to vendors of medical service is the prevailing method.

State and Local Administration

A RECENT STUDY of twenty states by the Bureau of Public Assistance of the Federal Security Agency provides illuminating data on the administration of medical care by state and local welfare agencies. Great variation exists in the extent of state participation in local services. In some states the program is administered directly through state district offices, while in others the state agency may provide a varying amount of assistance and supervision, including formulation of general policies, standards, and procedures, development of medical care manuals and recommended fee schedules, approval of local plans, consultation, and so forth. In still other instances a negligible role is played by the state agency. A contrasting picture is presented by the general assistance programs, which are often financed and administered entirely by local agencies, either counties or the more numerous smaller units.

Very few states or localities employ full-time physicians as administrators of the medical care program. Of the twenty states studied, only five have positions for a full-time medical director, and two of these were vacant at the time of the study. New York State, not included in the study, is outstanding in that a full-time medical director is employed at the state level as well as part-time directors in the counties. Only half the states studied utilize the services of general or technical advisory committees, and local advisory committees are much less frequent.

Generally the assistance recipient has free choice of physician, dentist, or other practitioner, and payment is made on a fee-for-service basis; exceptions occur in those localities which maintain city or county physicians. Payments are usually made at somewhat less than prevailing rates, resulting in some areas in friction with the providers of service. Thus, in several Pennsylvania counties, only a few physicians participate in the medical care program, and some attempt to collect from the patient the difference between the state fee and their usual charge. In Oregon,

In the majority of counties the private practitioners believed that fees were too low. They were accepted by some, however, as a part of the charitable work expected from all physicians. In two counties the low fees and lack of nursing personnel to staff public hospitals had limited hospital care available to recipients.

There are wide divergences among the states studied in the scope and amount of service provided, depending on such factors as the availability of resources furnished by other agencies, the supply of personnel and facilities, and, most important of all, the financial resources of the state. In some, comprehensive services are provided with relatively few restrictions; in others, generally the poorer states, the limitations on service are extreme.

The types of limitation vary. In West Virginia, care is specifically provided only in cases of acute or emergency illness and is limited largely to physicians' services, drugs, and hospitalization. Restrictions on chronic care are frequently made by the states; these may include maximum limits on the number of physician's visits, or review of cases requiring hospital care for periods longer than set maximums. Prior authorization is usually required in the case of dental services, while some states and localities require similar authorization for hospitalization or other types of care. A common regulation is the limitation of drugs to United States Pharmacopeia and National Formulary listings.

Sometimes the theoretical scope of services is wide, but serious restrictions are imposed in practice because of lack of funds. . . .

Present Status of Care

THE PRESENT STATUS of medical care for the needy and medically needy leaves much to be desired. Programs for public assistance recipients vary considerably in the adequacy of service and the quality and continuity of care. Most of the programs are handicapped by the lack of professional supervision of services. Even more important is the chronic insufficiency of funds which results in grossly inadequate medical care in many areas, and in widespread payment at less than prevailing rates, with adverse effects on the quality of care. The oft-repeated statement that "only the very poor and the very rich get good medical care" displays an incredible ignorance of the real situation.

The position of the medically needy is even less favorable than that of the needy. Although they represent a potentially much larger group than the recipients of public assistance, organized measures to cope with their problems are far less developed. In large cities, medically needy persons can avail themselves of the ward and clinic services of public and voluntary hospitals and of the programs of health departments and other agencies. In teaching hospitals, with all the advantages of teamwork medicine, professional supervision of care, and easy availability of specialist, laboratory, and auxiliary services, the care provided is usually of high quality. Yet even here, the situation is not always satisfactory, for too often the overcrowding of clinic and other facilities may result in inadequate service, while insufficient emphasis may be placed on treating the patient as a person or providing continuity of care. These defects are intensified in the ward and clinic services provided by the great bulk of public and voluntary hospitals which do not operate under the stimulus of teaching responsibilities.

Outside large urban centers, facilities for care of the medically needy are relatively meager. Outpatient clinics and public hospitals are rare in rural areas and small urban communities. County physicians may provide a certain amount of service in some areas, public assistance agencies may help "medical care only" cases in others, and health department services may be available for the care of specific diseases or defects. On the whole, however, the organized services are inadequate, and the patient must rely on the good intentions and free services of physicians and voluntary hospitals for necessary care.

In both urban and rural areas, the fact that the medically needy must apply for aid and undergo "means test" investigations constitutes a serious barrier to adequate service. Many persons will delay seeking needed care or do without it altogether because they do not wish to accept charity or submit to the embarrassment of financial investigations.

Lack of Co-ordination

ONE OF THE MAJOR weaknesses of current provisions for medical care of both the needy and the medically needy relates to the wide variety of unco-ordinated programs operated by different agencies. As Dr. Gertrude Sturges pointed out years ago, "Such a scattering of administrative responsibility tends to result in confusion, inefficiency, and waste; duplication, or more frequently, gaps in service; delay in the patient's securing necessary care; and lack of continuity of the patient's care." [1]

A recent study of medical care for the needy and medically needy in New Haven, for example, indicates that service is available from a wide variety of public and private resources, including the city welfare and health departments, the County Commissioners, the State Division of Public Assistance, the State Division of Child Welfare, state tuberculosis sanatoria and mental hospitals, the State Department of Health, the State Department of Education, voluntary hospitals, private physicians and dentists, the Dental Clinic Society, the local chapter of the National Foundation for Infantile Paralysis, the New Haven Visiting Nurse Association, and a number of other agencies. The authors conclude that "the variety of programs should not lead to the rosy conclusion that all the medical needs of all low income or indigent persons are being met adequately. This is far from the case. . . ." [2]

Suggested Improvements

IT HAS BECOME increasingly recognized that improvement of current provisions for medical care of the needy requires effective action along the following lines: (1) increased state and local funds, with Federal matching of medical care costs above the regular maximums and extension of Federal aid to include recipients of general assistance; (2) more adequate professional supervision of services; this may be achieved by the appointment of full-time medical directors, the utilization of departments of health to administer medical care for the needy, or the assignment of health department personnel to welfare departments with establishment of suitable co-ordinating committees; (3) greater emphasis on organization of services to improve the quality and the continuity of care; (4) more extensive use of general advisory committees, with adequate representation of public and professional interests; and (5) greater co-ordination of services provided by various public and private agencies.

An important step has been taken through the Social Security Act Amendments of 1950 which permit Federal matching for vendor payments and assistance to needy persons in public medical institutions. Unfortunately, Congress did not see fit to adopt the recommendation by the Senate Advisory Council on Social Security which would have permitted Federal matching of medical care costs above the regular maximums. Had this recommendation been adopted, the financial base for medical care of the needy would have been greatly strengthened. Nevertheless, since a large proportion of assistance recipients receive less than the maximums,

1. Gertrude Sturges, "Public Medical Service as it is Today at State and Local Levels," *Social Service Review*, Vol. 14 (Sept. 1940), p. 502.
2. Milton I. Roemer and Dorothy R. Granoff, "Medical Services for Needy Persons in New Haven," *Health*, New Haven Department of Health, Vol. 76 (April 1950), pp. 2 ff.

the new provisions make it possible for the states to receive substantial Federal aid for medical care. In addition, state and local funds freed by other amendments liberalizing Federal aid for public assistance may now be available to increase the amount and improve the quality of medical services.

Health Department Programs

OF EQUAL IMPORTANCE is the opportunity for welfare departments to develop some new approaches to effective organization. There is currently a great deal of interest in the possibility of more extensive utilization of state and local health departments in the administration of medical care for the needy. This has already occurred in Maryland, where state and local health departments administer medical care for public assistance recipients and the medically needy. Health departments in some forty other localities, including such centers as Louisville, San Francisco, Denver, Richmond, Philadelphia, Detroit, and Washington, D. C., have assumed major responsibilities for general medical services for the needy and the medically needy.

The use of health departments makes it possible to achieve a much greater coordination of health service programs, particularly of preventive and curative services, and to obtain continuing professional supervision in the interest of a high quality of care. Perhaps the most significant example is the program administered by the Baltimore City Health Department for persons receiving public assistance. The basic centers of this program are the medical care clinics organized in six voluntary and teaching hospitals; these provide every eligible person with a thorough initial physical examination and laboratory work-up, and report the results to the patient's family physician who provides home and office care. The general practitioner is encouraged to refer the patient to the medical care clinic when difficult problems arise on which consultation by specialists is required. The clinic, in turn, can refer patients requiring further study to the specialized outpatient clinics of the hospital with which it is associated. An interesting aspect of this program is the capitation method of payment, whereby the medical care clinics and participating family physicians are paid a specified sum annually for each person assigned, rather than fee-for-service.

It is evident that the Baltimore program is having a salutary effect in raising standards of care. It provides the general practitioner with easily available and competent consultation service, and serves as a very desirable contact with the best clinical practice. The detailed reports which the family doctor receives from the clinic are in themselves a valuable educational tool. In addition, the medical care clinic provides greater continuity of care for the individual patient than is possible in the ordinary hospital outpatient department.

The Baltimore program has been designed to serve an important preventive function. The initial examination of all eligible persons, regardless of their state of health, includes a thorough history and physical examination, chest X-ray, and laboratory tests. This examination clearly provides an excellent means for case finding—for detection of subclinical tuberculosis, syphilis, blood dyscrasias, diabetes, nephritis, heart disease, cancer, and other diseases in which early diagnosis and prompt treatment can have important effects in eliminating disease processes or at least halting their progress and preventing disability....

Prepayment Plans

IN RECENT YEARS public welfare officials have expressed a good deal of interest in the use of prepayment plans for medical care. In the state of Washington, physicians' services are provided through payment by the local assistance agency of $2.50 per month to the medical-society-sponsored county medical service bureau for each person receiving assistance. In Kansas 30 of the 105 counties operate under medical insurance plans; in 1946 the range in cost was from $1.75 per case per month in one county including only physicians' services under prepayment, to $4.25 in another county where physicians' services of all types, drugs, hospitalization, and laboratory fees were included. Such plans simplify the administrative process for the public agency; on the other hand, unless adequate safeguards are taken, they tend to violate the important principle adopted by the American Public Welfare Association that "public funds should be administered by public agencies."

The Broader Framework

THERE IS A GROWING conviction that the problems of medical care for the needy and medically needy cannot be solved in isolation from the general problem of medical care for the whole population. Thus, although the shortages of health personnel and facilities in rural areas are most serious for public assistance recipients and the medically needy, their effects are universally felt by farm people. Similarly, the nation-wide dearth of facilities for chronic disease and rehabilitation is a problem not only for the needy but for almost all sections of the population.

The general dissatisfaction with current methods of providing medical care has resulted in the introduction of a number of measures which would attack the problems of medical care for the needy and medically needy within a broader framework. In addition to the measures designed to meet shortages of personnel and facilities, some proposals would subsidize voluntary prepayment plans to enable them to serve public assistance recipients and the medically needy; these involve an extension of the philosophy of public assistance, with eligibility necessarily determined by a means test. Others would establish national health insurance as a major aspect of the social security program, with eligibility earned through prepayments and with provision for inclusion of public assistance recipients through payments of premiums by official agencies. There is little doubt that the future development of medical care for the needy and medically needy will be largely determined by the action taken on these major legislative proposals.

69. FACILITIES FOR VETERANS *

THE PURPOSE of this paper is to present a historical summary of the Department of Medicine and Surgery of the Veterans Administration; to point out some of its past difficulties; to outline the program of medical care that is now being carried out for the veteran, with particular reference to the basic policies that prevail; to point out some of the problems that confront the Administration, and to describe the quality of medical care that is being provided for the American veteran. . . .

On Aug. 23, 1935 Public Law 312, 74th Congress, was approved. Liberalized eligibility for hospitalization provided that any veteran of any war who was not dishonorably discharged and who was in need of hospitalization and was unable to defray the necessary expenses thereof should be furnished hospitalization in any Veterans Administration facility within the limitation of beds existing in such facility, irrespective of whether disability, disease or defect was caused by military service. An important provision of the law was that the statement under oath of the applicant on such form as may be prescribed by the administrator of Veterans' Affairs would be accepted as sufficient evidence of inability to defray the necessary expenses. This law is essentially the same as that in effect today: the Veterans Administration accepts the oath of the veteran that he is unable to purchase medical and hospital care from his own resources. This is sometimes known as the "pauper's oath," which the average veteran interprets liberally and has no hesitation in signing.

The right of the veteran to receive medical care, regardless of service connection, on his own declaration of inability to pay has been and still is the cause of much criticism from the members of the medical profession, but it should be pointed out that the Veterans Administration is not authorized to investigate the validity of the veteran's statement. Since Congress appears unwilling to restrict this entitlement, the number of available beds remain the only limiting factor on the nonservice-connected cases. . . .

Hospital Construction and Requirements

IT WAS DURING 1943 that the impact of new veterans from World War II was felt in the hospital field. Thus, of the 57,000 hospitalized patients on June 30 of that

* From: "The Medical Care of the Veteran," by Roy R. Kracke, M.D.; *Journal of the American Medical Association* 143:1321-31, Aug. 12, 1950 (No. 15). Reprinted (with omissions, including tables) by permission of the publishers. The author was, until his death in 1950, dean of the School of Medicine of the University of Alabama, Birmingham. (Note: The article from which this selection was taken was originally prepared in cooperation with the Special Medical Advisory Board to the Veterans Administration, of which Dr. C. W. Mayo was chairman and Dr. Kracke, vice-chairman).

year, 45,000 were veterans of World War I and over 5,000 were veterans of World War II; the remainder were veterans of other wars and peacetime service. In that same year the 78th Congress passed Public Law 10, which amended the regulations so as to grant hospitalization to World War II veterans on the same basis as granted to those of World War I: Congress granted a potential load of nearly 20 million veterans the same entitlements as those previously granted to 5 million, and these entitlements included the right of medical care and hospitalization if the veteran was financially unable to pay for it, as stated by his own declaration....

... The discharge of increasing numbers of men from military service in the latter phase of World War II caused a general slowing up of medical and hospital care in the Veterans Administration not only because of overtaxing of physical facilities and the necessity of borrowing facilities from the Army and Navy but also because of the unavailability of personnel, who were heavily engaged in the war effort. Therefore, on June 22, 1944 the Servicemen's Readjustment Act was passed, which labeled the Veterans Administration as an essential war agency and gave it priority, second only to the War and Navy Departments, in securing personnel and equipment to care for disabled veterans. The administrator of Veterans' Affairs was authorized and directed to expedite and complete the construction of additional hospital facilities for war veterans and to enter into agreements and contracts for the use or transfer of Army and Navy hospitals for the use of veterans when they became surplus to the needs of the military services. Also, $500 million was appropriated for the construction of additional hospital facilities....

As early as 1941 the American Legion, having become concerned with the problem of giving good medical care to the veterans, at their Milwaukee Convention urged a reorganization of the Veterans Administration and passed their famous Resolution 528, which was highly critical of the prevailing policies of the Veterans Administration. They strongly reiterated this in 1945. They recommended that an outstanding member of the medical profession head the Department of Medicine and Surgery, that the Department be reorganized and enlarged and, in short, that a new medical director be appointed. In the meantime the demands made on the Department of Medicine and Surgery had reached such proportions that the existing personnel and facilities, even with the aid of men borrowed from the Army and Navy, were not able to do the job properly. This resulted in widespread general dissatisfaction throughout the country, so that the cry for reorganization became more acute than ever. In the resultant reorganization Gen. Omar N. Bradley was appointed administrator of Veterans' Affairs to succeed Brig. Gen. Frank T. Hines....

The Department of Medicine and Surgery Since World War II

GENERAL BRADLEY assumed his duties on Aug. 15, 1945. Prior to that time, while he was still in Europe directing military affairs, he had accepted the post of administrator; while he was still in Germany he called to his headquarters Major General Paul R. Hawley, chief surgeon in the European Theater, and asked him if he would accept the post of medical director. General Hawley in a conference with General Bradley in Wiesbaden, Germany, at which Brig. Gen. Elliott C. Cutler was also present, discussed in detail what new plans might be laid that would give a high type of medical care to the potential load of nearly 20,000,000 veterans from all the wars. At that conference plans were laid for affiliation of a great system of veterans' hospitals with the medical educational forces of the United States. . . . Thus, the idea was born that the backbone of quality of medical care offered to the veteran in the future would be dependent to a large degree on affiliation with teaching hospitals and teaching institutions. . . .

The first step in reorganization was to approach American medicine through the Board of Trustees of the American Medical Association and to enlist the support of American medicine in this program of medical care. The plan for affiliation with medical educational forces envisaged the construction of new hospital facilities near the medical schools of the United States and the utilization of the faculties to aid in the programs of medical care and education. In such institutions the responsibility for hospital operations would be that of the Veterans Administration and the responsibility for the quality of the medical care would be accepted to a large degree by the medical schools. . . .

In addition, the program would develop a situation whereby the Veterans Administration would enlist as many high caliber medical practitioners as possible on full time duty. The professional services of the medical colleges have been utilized by the appointment of consultants for actual service in the program of medical care. These consultants supervise the professional work, carry on the teaching program and make their services available in any other way deemed necessary by the full time members of the staff. There has been appointed a large group of attending physicians and surgeons who, in general, are younger men but who do active service on the medical and surgical wards with residents working full time under their direction. Each affiliated veterans' hospital under this plan is operated by what is known as the Deans Committee, and today such institutions are referred to as "Deans Committee hospitals." In these situations all consultants and attending men are recommended for appointment by the Deans Committee and the appointments made by the Veterans Administration. Thus, there has been developed a tremendous group of part time, high grade medical talent throughout the United States in the capacity of consultants and attending men, whose appointments have been recommended in every instance by Deans Committees of the various medical schools and who are utilized in addition to the gradually enlarging, full time staffs in the various installations.

In order to carry out the foregoing plan it was necessary that all professional personnel be removed from the restrictions of Civil Service. This resulted in the passage by the 79th Congress of Public Law 293, which removed physicians, dentists and nurses from the requirements of Civil Service. Unfortunately, however, it did not remove from Civil Service other auxiliary personnel, such as clinical psychologists, dietitians, physical and occupational therapists, social workers and laboratory and x-ray technicians of various types. After the passage of this law the procurement of physicians, dentists and nurses rose sharply. Many of the new recruits were clearly superior in their professional attainments. One reform that is still needed is the removal of all other auxiliary personnel from the restrictions of Civil Service.

As stated by Dr. Paul B. Magnuson,* now the chief medical director, the objectives of the new program include the following:

1. To attract and retain adequate full time personnel by offering opportunities for professional growth and development and providing salaries commensurate with ability.

2. To secure the services of outstanding medical men to serve as teachers, consultants and attending physicians.

3. To inaugurate a residency training program, by means of which Grade A medical schools would participate in the treatment of patients and the training of the full time staff, and by means of which the critical shortage of medical specialists could be partially overcome.

4. To build new hospitals in urban centers in close proximity to medical schools and medical talent and to attempt to make every VA hospital a teaching hospital.

5. To insure that professional personnel are relieved so far as possible from all nonessential administrative duties and are free to devote their full time and attention to the care and treatment of patients.

6. To develop a research program which would improve therapeutic procedures, provide training materials and make the Department of Medicine and Surgery a professional, alert and progressive medical organization.

The program as outlined has been one of astonishing success. Thus, at this time the Veterans Administration has about twice as many full time physicians, about four and one-half times as many dentists, more than three times as many nurses and seven times as many social workers as it had in 1945. Currently all the full time physicians and dentists are civilian employees of the Veterans Administration. In 1945 large numbers were military officers on detail. Success in the implementation of this program has come about for a variety of reasons: first, the high caliber and professional attainments of the persons who were recruited in the beginning to serve in the Washington Central Office to direct the program; second, the desire on the part of the American people and members of the American medical profession to properly reward the men who served in the various wars and to give them high quality medical care; third, a general dissatisfaction over prevailing policies prior to the reorganization; fourth, the removal of professional personnel from Civil Service, the increase in emoluments for full time personnel and the opportunities for professional advancement and for work in a professional medical atmosphere; fifth, the sudden release of substantial numbers of professional persons from military service at the conclusion of World War II, enabling the Veterans Administration to secure the services of a considerable number of high caliber medical personnel

* Following his tenure of office as medical director of the Veterans Administration, Dr. Magnuson served as Chairman of President Truman's Commission on the Health Needs of the Nation (1951-52). He is professor emeritus of orthopedic surgery at Northwestern University Medical School, Chicago.

at that time, and, sixth, the wholehearted cooperation of the medical educational faculties throughout the country.

The Hospital Construction Program

AFTER THE appointment of General Bradley as administrator in August 1945, it became necessary to greatly enlarge the hospital construction program, which actually already was in effect as a ten year program before he assumed his office. The new administrator made certain changes and revisions so that it became the 1947 Hospital Construction Program.

In the meantime the American Legion Medical Advisory Board recommended a proposed policy with reference to the location of veterans' hospitals. They concurred in the plan that hospitals should be located in urban centers close to the medical schools and the medical centers and in other areas where ample medical talent was available. . . . At the same time, the policy further stated that this should in no way adversely affect the establishment of smaller hospitals in well located communities where less specialized hospital care could be provided. . . .

On Jan. 31, 1950 the Veterans Administration was operating the following number of beds: general medical and surgical, 37,436; neuropsychiatric, 54,589; tuberculosis, 14,187, and domiciliary, 17,946, a total of 124,158.

There is no simple answer to the important question, how many hospital beds should the Veterans Administration operate? . . . It can be stated that, in general, the ex-servicemen's organizations always present powerful arguments for increasing the number of beds. Such organizations as the American Hospital Association, and perhaps also the American Medical Association, have looked with anxiety on additional bed construction in the veterans' hospitals.

Many projections with respect to bed requirements in the future have been made from time to time, but the number of beds that will be operated by the Veterans Administration in the future will depend basically on the wishes of the American people, as indicated through their representatives in the National Congress. Furthermore, projection of estimates of hospital beds for the future cannot be made with any degree of certainty, because it is impossible to predict the many variable factors that enter into bed requirements at any given time. In general, the number of beds that will be required by the Veterans Administration will depend on the number of veterans who seek medical service, on the entitlements conferred on veterans by Congress and on the efficiency with which the beds are operated. For example, the average veterans' hospital bed today does approximately one and one-half times as much work as it did ten years ago. . . .

In a consideration of projected needs for the future, it must be remembered that the tuberculous veteran will probably always receive medical and hospital care at the expense of the government, regardless of service connection, and this is also true of the neuropsychiatric patient. The main issue on projected beds in the future therefore resolves itself around the number of beds to be occupied by general medical and surgical patients. We believe the philosophy of the American people is such that it will always be considered right and proper to offer free medical and hospital service to tuberculous and psychiatric patients in the veterans group regardless of service connection. This fundamental principle has long been accepted by the various states and communities throughout the nation with respect to the nonveteran population. Therefore, the number of projected beds for the future would depend to a large extent on the number of anticipated psychiatric and tuberculous patients. In this important connection the Division of Psychiatry and Neurology of the Veterans Administration, under the direction of Dr. Harvey J. Tompkins, has estimated that the peak neuropsychiatric hospital load expected in 1965 will be 118,600 and the anticipated load in 1975 about 112,000.... The same situation, however, does not prevail in the field of tuberculosis. It is expected that the hospital load of the tuberculous group of patients will increase to a peak in about five years and decline slowly thereafter to about 10,000 in 1975.

A question of considerable importance, and one over which the most controversy develops, is the number of beds that will be required for general medical and surgical purposes in the future. ... About 37,000 beds are now being utilized in veterans' hospitals for these purposes, and it has been estimated that a total of 130,000 beds will be needed in 1975. ...

... A fairly safe and conservative estimate, [therefore,] would be that twenty-five years from now a total of some 260,000 beds will be required by veterans. Indeed, if there is no restriction of hospitalization of the group of veterans with nonservice-connected disabilities and if the entitlements should be liberalized in any way this may run well in excess of 300,000 beds. ...

The Location and Cost of Veterans' Hospitals

VETERANS' HOSPITALS should be located in those areas of the country where the staffing of the institutions will present the least difficulty. Therefore it is necessary that the institutions be located in urban areas where there are large concentrations of physicians and other medical personnel. One of the great mistakes of the Veterans Administration in the past has been the location of institutions in more or less remote areas. This resulted in staffing difficulties to the point where there was serious disintegration in the program of medical care.

Many of the hospitals are being built as teaching hospitals, around medical schools wherever possible, and nearly every medical school in the United States is directly or indirectly concerned in the medical care of the veteran. Great pressures are always brought on the Veterans Administration to place hospitals in undesirable locations. For the most part these pressures have been successfully resisted, although there are rare instances, particularly in the previously established ten year building program, in which an institution has been erected in an undesirable location. ... Furthermore, it is well known that the erection of hospitals of fewer than a certain number of beds is not conducive to efficient operation. Therefore the Veterans Administration has adopted a general policy of building hospitals a certain size:

general medical and surgical hospitals, 500 to 1,000 beds; neuropsychiatry hospitals, 500 to 1,100 beds; tuberculosis hospitals, 350 to 500 beds, and domiciliary homes, 500 to 2,000 beds.

The modern veterans' hospital is constructed along modern and efficient lines. Hospital construction experts have been and continue to be utilized freely in the building of these institutions. . . . Bids are always let on a highly competitive basis. The modern veterans' hospital has within it all physical facilities for the efficient and scientific care of the sick. On the whole these facilities are usually considerably superior to those found in the average nonveteran hospital. The construction costs are practically the same as those for nonveteran hospitals. . . .

Costs of Hospital and Medical Care

WITH RESPECT to hospital per diem cost, the average patient day cost in 1949 was $6.58 in the neuropsychiatry hospitals, $12.72 in the tuberculosis hospitals and $14.22 in the general medical and surgical hospitals.

One of the most reliable indications of the efficiency of any hospital is the length of patient stay. In this important respect the record of the veterans' hospitals has been particularly outstanding in recent years. In the fiscal year 1945 the average general medical and surgical patient was hospitalized thirty-seven days and in the fiscal year 1949 about twenty-nine days. . . . It is certainly true that the over-all efficiency of the Veterans Administration hospitals has been immeasurably increased in recent years so that each hospital unit or each hospital bed appears to be performing about one and one-half times as much work, or servicing about one and one-half times as many patients, as it did a few years ago. It should be pointed out that increased efficiency in any hospital is always accompanied with increased costs of operation. . . .

It costs $1.74 per patient day for all professional services of both full time physicians and consultants for the veteran in the general medical and surgical hospital. When the cost is compared with that for professional care for the nonveteran patient attended by the average practicing physician, it is . . . extremely low and astonishingly so when the high type of medical service is considered. It would appear that the government gets a real bargain in this respect. . . .

Personnel Problems

THERE IS A total of approximately 25,000 professional persons in the medical, dental and nursing groups who actively participate in the care of the veteran. The recruitment of this highly skilled personnel has been astonishingly successful. Several factors are responsible for this, but the chief ones are: an opportunity to render service in an atmosphere of high professional standards; freedom from the restrictions of Civil Service; a compensation scale that is considerably above that existing a few years ago, and, last and perhaps most important, relative freedom from political interference or dictation and freedom from unnecessary burdensome nonmedical detailed work.

Criticism has occasionally been directed at the Veterans Administration for its utilization of so much of the country's professional manpower at a time when shortages are prevalent. It would appear that the use of 4,000 full time physicians and 1,000 full time dentists from the 200,000 physicians and 80,000 dentists in this country should cause no serious concern. It is true that the use of 13,700 nurses produces a sizable deficiency in the civilian nursing group, but it is not excessive because the veteran group comprises about 13 per cent of the entire population and the veterans' nursing group only about 5 per cent of the entire active nursing personnel of the country. . . .

Recruitment of nurses has been satisfactory and few vacancies exist. The same is true in the field of dentistry. However, . . . there are serious shortages in certain categories of specialists, these being notably: anesthesiology, radiology, pathology, orthopedic surgery and psychiatry. The Veterans Administration, however, is training its own personnel in the field of psychiatry. . . .

Specialized Activities

IN ADDITION to the operation of this large system of high grade hospitals in nearly every state of the Union, the Veterans Administration conducts a number of other medical activities designed to give all eligible veterans the best possible medical care in accordance with the highest professional standards. Thus, it conducts a tremendous outpatient medical program in its various hospitals and regional office clinics. The number of patients given outpatient medical examination and treatment by staff and fee-designate physicians in each of the fiscal years 1947, 1948 and 1949 was more than five times greater than the number during the fiscal year 1945. Also, an extensive program in dental care was conducted. . . .

The Veterans Administration has concentrated in special centers the necessary qualified personnel and equipment to give optimum service in the highly specialized branches of medicine such as neurosurgery, paraplegia, plastic surgery, lung surgery, epilepsy, aphasia, mental hygiene and physical medicine rehabilitation. It operates special centers for paraplegic persons alone. Over sixty mental hygiene clinics for veterans have been established, and an equal number serves the veterans on a contract basis, with patients seen by teams consisting of a psychiatrist, clinical psychologist and a social worker in an effort to reduce, if possible, the hospital load of psychiatric cases by preventive measures.

The program in the treatment of tuberculous patients has been outstanding, and the research program in the use of streptomycin has been a noteworthy accomplishment unsurpassed the world over. The Veterans Administration conducts a tuberculosis case register of those discharged from the Armed Services with a diagnosis of tuberculosis and exerts constant efforts to keep them under medical supervision. It conducts an extensive program for 400,000 veterans with syphilis who have had partial or complete treatment while in the Armed Forces, and it keeps in touch with 200,000 such veterans with the cooperation of local health authorities throughout the country.

Its program in the development of prosthetic appliances has been outstanding, and a system has been devised whereby a veteran may secure artificial prosthetic devices or repair services in any part of the country with a minimum of inconvenience and delay. It also conducts a vast program of home medical care, in which the veteran is entitled to consult the physician of his choice in his own home town if he needs treatment for service-connected disability. It has also developed a similar program in the field of dentistry. . . .

The vast outpatient service acts, of course, as the great screening ground for the evaluation of disability and for the admission of patients to the far-flung hospital system of the Veterans Administration. It also serves as a great screening device to prevent the hospitalization of the veteran and treat him on an outpatient basis when possible, thus at the same time rendering incalculable service in the general field of preventive medicine.

In its residency program the Veterans Administration is training as many physicians in psychiatry as all other organizations in the country combined. It has about 50 per cent of all postgraduate students in clinical psychology under the sponsorship of forty-two affiliated universities. It also conducts fifty-five research units in the field of clinical research for the evaluation of streptomycin. Nearly 15,000 patients have been treated in this program with spectacular results. The Veterans Administration operates also three tropical disease clinics for the special study of that particular group of diseases. Another field in which the agency is extremely progressive is in hospital administration. It sponsors a Hospital Managers' Institute, which meets periodically to discuss problems in this field.

Educational and Research Program

ONE OF THE BASIC reasons for the high type of medical care offered in the installations of the Veterans Administration is its vast educational and research program. There are approximately 2,500 residents in postgraduate training in approximately seventy-two hospitals, these residencies incorporating nearly every field of medicine and surgery except pediatrics, obstetrics and gynecology. The Deans Committee hospitals usually have strong residency programs. The impact on postgraduate medical education can be appreciated when it is realized that there are about 15,000 approved residencies in the United States, with the Veterans Administration conducting about 17 per cent of these. About half of the approved residencies in the United States in the field of psychiatry are in the Veterans Administration. Frequently the residents are permitted to leave for detached service in other affiliated institutions in order to have a well-rounded training.

In addition to residencies, the Veterans Administration has developed an approved internship at twelve of its hospitals. These internships for the most part are in straight medicine or straight surgery but are occasionally rotating.... In effect, therefore, the veterans' hospitals in which such programs are conducted are teaching institutions in every sense of the word.

Teaching and educational programs go on constantly in the average veterans' hospital. There are frequent conferences and seminars, staff meetings and group ward rounds. Formal educational programs are in effect in most institutions, with visiting faculty and consultants spending variable amounts of time in ward rounds, consultation on difficult cases, operative procedures and the conduct of numerous seminars and lectures. In addition to this important visiting group there is a well established system of consultation service stemming from the Area Offices....

The educational process also goes on constantly in the field of nursing....

A large number of the physicians employed full time in the Veterans Administration are certified as specialists by their respective boards....

Always a reliable indication of the efficiency of any hospital is its autopsy percentage. In June 1946 the average autopsy percentage in the entire Veterans Administration hospital system was 25.7. The percentage of autopsies now obtained in veterans' hospitals is 67.3, and over forty hospitals accomplish over 75 per cent....

Research activities are constantly encouraged in the agency's hospitals.... In some hospitals there are research facilities specifically designed for that purpose, and there are usually a substantial number of nonmedical personnel, such as biochemists and physicists, participating in these programs. Modern research activities are performed, as indicated by the development of the radioisotope program. There are now twelve established radioisotope projects in veterans' installations, and additional ones are proposed for twenty-five new hospitals. Work with radioisotopes includes not only basic research but clinical and therapeutic application of radioactive isotopes that are useful for such purposes. There is no advance in medicine, however recent it may be, that is not available to the veteran patient. This principle is illustrated by the magnificent clinical research job that has been done with streptomycin in the Division of Tuberculosis. Without question, the most effective evaluation of this new drug on a large scale has been made by the Veterans Administration....

... It has been amply demonstrated that the educational program in a veterans' hospital, by being available to all physicians in the area, has uplifted the general level of medical practice in the entire community. Some hospitals serve as the center for professional educational activities in the entire area. Many are now used for affiliation in programs of nursing education, particularly in the fields of psychiatry and tuberculosis. Since personnel do not always remain with the Veterans Administration but become disseminated throughout the various communities of the country, the nonveteran population benefits from this program and in the years to come will benefit perhaps as much as the veteran population itself.

Auxiliary Medical Services

IN DECEMBER 1945 the chief medical director instituted the plan of giving treatment to the veteran in his home town. The treatment is available only for service-connected disabilities. This program has been carried out through cooperation with local county medical societies and state medical societies over the country. Fee schedules have been established that are satisfactory to both medical societies and the Veterans Administration.

A veteran anywhere in the United States can receive from his home town physician medical treatment for any disability presumed to have developed on a service-connected basis. This has proved popular with the veterans in some sections of the country, and a great deal of home care service is rendered, particularly in the more remote, isolated and rural areas.

Physicians are paid a maximum of $6,000 per year for such services; that is to say, it is not possible for any one physician to collect more than that sum, regardless of the amount of service he may render during the year, and this is also true of any physician serving part time in the Veterans Administration. About 75,000 physicians have indicated a willingness to participate in this program.... In sixteen states osteopaths participate in this program. They have to be graduates of recognized schools of osteopathy and have to adhere to the licensure laws of the states in which they practice.

In addition, in the veterans' outpatient activities throughout the country there are about 1,400 full time physicians and 1,170 part time physicians operating a large system of outpatient clinics. As this program develops further, it is planned to have all outpatient activities in association with the veterans' hospitals, as is the case in any teaching hospital.

The Dental Program

AN IMPORTANT phase of the medical care of the veteran falls within the field of dentistry.... Public Law 242, 1924, was the first law mentioning dental treatment as a specific benefit. In the Executive Order of July 28, 1933 authority was placed in the hands of the veterans' administrator to control dental benefits.

Although the rules and regulations for the establishment of service connection of dental disabilities are extremely complex, it is biologically impossible to separate oral pathologic processes from the patient as an entity, and frequently service connection for treatment of a single tooth, if followed by subsequent degenerative processes involving that tooth and adjacent teeth, will result in bridgework and eventually full dentures—all related to service-connected injury to a single tooth. This means that a dental patient may become a ward for life at a continual increased annual costs for dental treatment. In World War II an effort was made to give soldiers complete dental rehabilitation, particularly those who went overseas, so

READINGS IN MEDICAL CARE

 READINGS IN MEDICAL CARE

that dental claims on the Veterans Administration since World War II have taken a tremendous upsurge. . . .

This method of outpatient treatment operates in every state and is of far greater magnitude both in the number of professional men participating and in dollar cost than is the program of outpatient medical care. Home town participating dentists are recommended by respective state societies, and fee schedules are set at state level. There are inequities between rural and urban areas and between states, but every effort is being made to correct this condition. The ceiling for dental outpatient care is the same for the dentist as for the physician, $6,000 per year, and although there have been abuses in this matter as there have been in consultant fees for services not rendered, it has been the policy to refer disciplinary action to the local dental or medical society, rather than through governmental policing, and the results have been generally satisfactory. . . .

Physical Medicine and Rehabilitation

THERE IS A WELL organized department of physical medicine rehabilitation, headed by a physician, in each veterans' hospital. Many of these physicians are certified by their specialty boards. . . .

The agency conducts the largest program of this kind in the world in its one hundred and thirty-one hospitals and also conducts a rehabilitation hospital at Fort Thomas, Kentucky. The activities of this division include the medical rehabilitation of orthopedic patients as well as the rehabilitation of the 2,400 paraplegic persons who were problems immediately after World War II. Such veterans as require it are not only given the benefit of all possible therapeutic equipment to aid them in their rehabilitation but also may be prescribed appropriate activity with occupational and manual arts therapies of various types. . . . This same division is also responsible for the rehabilitation of the blind, with a special center being established for this group. The rehabilitation program is particularly noteworthy with the tuberculous patients. In addition to the physical medicine rehabilitation service at each tuberculosis hospital there is a special rehabilitation center for tuberculous patients at Oteen, N. C. Also, there are forty-two physical medicine rehabilitation clinics which are operated as a part of the Regional Office outpatient program. The entire program of physical medicine rehabilitation of wounded and maimed veterans has been one of the outstanding accomplishments and achievements of the Veterans Administration since World War II.

Summary and Conclusion

THE AMERICAN people have every right to be proud of the care that has been and is being given to the nearly 20 million veterans of the various wars, and this is particularly true of the high type of medical service that has been maintained since the conclusion of World War II. The accomplishment becomes all the more remarkable when it is considered that the quality of medical service was decidedly improved even though the veteran load increased from less than 5 million to nearly 20 million. This remarkable achievement in mass medical care has never been duplicated here or in any other country. There seems little doubt that the veteran who is entitled to it by law does receive the finest type of medical care in a country where medical science has reached its highest development. For this the American medical profession may justly be proud. . . .

The major factor responsible for the success of the medical program of the Veterans Administration has been the constant adherence to the policy that it remain under the direction and jurisdiction of medical personnel. If this had not been true the entire program would, without doubt, have been a dismal and utter failure. . . . As long as the Department of Medicine and Surgery of the Veterans Administration remains under proper and authoritative medical control this type of superior medical care will always prevail for the veteran. If the time should come, however, when such control is passed to lay, bureaucratic or political hands, that will be the beginning of deterioration of the program of medical care for the veteran.

Therefore it is to the best interest of the American people, the medical profession and the veteran group always to be on the alert to see that this great enterprise of medical care continues under the direction of highly qualified American physicians. . . .

70. HANDICAPPED PERSONS

A. CRIPPLED CHILDREN *

SEVERAL YEARS AGO the teachers of a boy named David noticed that he had a peculiar posture, his walk was like a waddle and he seemed misshapen. A talk with the parents revealed that the parents, too, had been worried, but since there were seven other children to look after on a modest salary, they hadn't done anything. Following the teachers' suggestions, the parents took David to the doctor, who referred him to a public health clinic. There the specialist who examined him found a bad deformity, apparently of long standing. David was now suffering pain and there was pressure on his nervous system and hip joints. Extensive orthopedic care was needed so David went into the hospital under the county Crippled Children's Program.

The parents were eager to help in every way they could. They had hospital insurance and each month were able to help put some of the father's salary toward the other medical expenses.

* From: *The United States Program for Crippled Children*, by the American Parents Committee; New York: The Committee (undated pamphlet). Reprinted (with omissions) from pp. 4-21 by permission of the publishers.

David underwent surgery, a spinal fusion to remove the damaged area, and then later a bone graft. The family hospital insurance ran out long before David was able to leave the hospital. But eventually the long hospitalization was over, the spinal deformity was completely corrected. This year David entered the armed forces, a strong healthy young man ready to serve his country. Without proper medical care, he would have been a cripple with misshapen body and a badly damaged nervous system, perhaps a burden to society.

The treatment and care given David was made possible by the local-state-Federal Crippled Children's Program supported in part by a Federal grant administered by the Children's Bureau in the U. S. Department of Health, Education and Welfare, and in part by state and local taxes. It was put in operation in 1936 by the passage of the Social Security Act. Under it the Congress appropriates each year a certain amount of money to help each of the states take care of children who are crippled or have conditions which lead to crippling, who would not otherwise receive treatment. The states in turn put up money to match and supplant the Federal appropriation.[1] The counties provide buildings, and some personnel. Some counties put up more funds. Consequently the surgery, the treatment, and the care which is given to children like David in certain sections of every state [2] is a partnership arrangement between local, state, and Federal governments.

The purpose of the program is set forth in the Social Security Act, Title V, part 2, Sec. 511 as follows:

For the purpose of enabling each State to extend and improve (especially in rural areas and in areas suffering from severe economic distress) as far as practicable under the conditions in such State, services for locating crippled children and for providing medical, surgical, corrective, and other services and care, and facilities for diagnosis, hospitalization, and aftercare, for children who are crippled or who are suffering from conditions which lead to crippling. . . .

The amount of Federal money for crippled children authorized in the law when first passed in 1936 was $2,850,000 each year. The authorization has since been increased three times, and the amount which Congress is now authorized to appropriate is $15 million annually. Until the fiscal year 1951 the full amount authorized by law was voted by the Congress each year. Since the authorization was increased by the 1950 amendments to the law, however, Congress has never appropriated as much as the amount authorized. For the fiscal year beginning July

1. The Federal appropriation for the Crippled Children's Program is equally divided into Fund A and Fund B. Fund A must be matched dollar for dollar by the states. Out of this fund each state gets a flat grant, then the remainder of Fund A is apportioned on the basis of the number of children in the state. Factors used in allotting Fund B are the financial need of the state to serve crippled children, particularly those in the rural areas, and the number of children in the state. One fourth of Fund B is reserved for grants to states for special projects which will further develop knowledge or techniques needed in some region or which hold promise of being nationally significant.
2. All states and territories of the United States except Arizona participate in the Federally aided Crippled Children's Program. Arizona, however, has a crippled children's program entirely supported by state and local funds.

1954, only $10,800,000 * was appropriated by Congress even though $15 million is authorized by law.

On the other hand the state and local governments are now putting up over six times as much money for crippled children as they did in 1940, and the Federal government is putting up only a little over three times as much. There is a wide range among the states, however, in the amount of money they spend on their crippled children's program. The large amounts being spent by the wealthy states swell the total greatly.[3] There are some states which are appropriating only a small amount over that necessary to match the Federal-aid dollars, and one or two of the states are not putting up enough to draw the full amount of Federal aid due them.

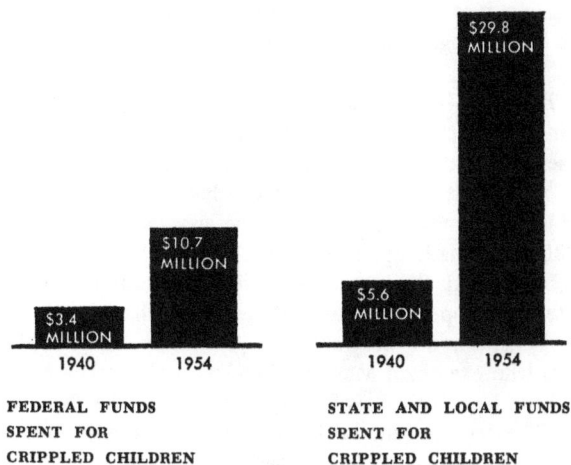

FEDERAL FUNDS SPENT FOR CRIPPLED CHILDREN

STATE AND LOCAL FUNDS SPENT FOR CRIPPLED CHILDREN

FIGURE 29.

More than 250,000 crippled children received treatment through the Federal, state, and local tax dollars allotted to the Crippled Children's Program in 1953. The kinds of programs varied widely from state to state because each state defines the types of crippling conditions it will accept for care. In no state is the program able to take care of all the children whose parents cannot give them adequate care and who need attention from a public agency. Some of these are helped by volunteer organizations, the rest are left to grow up as cripples.

Orthopedically Handicapped Children.—Orthopedically handicapped children get the most attention because this handicap was the first to be handled by the states

* The sum of $15 million was appropriated for the Children's Bureau, however, for the fiscal year 1957-58.

3. In 1940 total planned expenditures for crippled children's services were $9.3 million. Of this amount $3.7 million were from Federal funds, and $5.6 million from state and local funds. By 1954 the total amount had increased to $40.5 million, of which $10.7 million were from Federal funds and $29.8 million from state and local funds. However, approximately 40 per cent of the last named amount was raised and spent in four states.

under the program and one on which great progress has been made. The number of children needing orthopedic care is estimated at one million. In spite of progress made, there is considerable evidence to show that many children are not getting needed surgery or are going without necessary braces.

The greatest need lies in the lack of treatment for children suffering from handicaps other than those classed as orthopedic. Treatment of these other crippling conditions is being given in many of the states but almost always it is on a demonstration basis which takes care of relatively few children and does not cover much of the state geographically.

These other unmet needs of crippled children throughout the country can best be described by some true stories of children who have or have not received treatment, and an estimate of the number of other children with similar handicaps and the inadequacy of the program to meet the total need. . . .

Children with Epilepsy.—Mary was a hopeless case. She was subject to epileptic seizures, and in addition had a degree of cerebral palsy. She did not enter school until she was seven, but after five months in the first grade, she was sent home. She was too much of a problem for the teachers to handle. Mary's mother was frantic. She exhausted her resources trying to find some way Mary could be helped. Finally in the late 1930's, she made application for Mary's admission to the state institution for the feeble-minded. While waiting for the institution to find a place for Mary, she appealed to the Crippled Children's Program which had just begun to operate under the new Federal and state grants.

The doctors who examined Mary in the clinic did not believe she was feeble-minded. They sent Mary to a hospital equipped to make a complete examination and diagnosis. The reports sent back with Mary after her short stay confirmed their original idea that Mary would respond to treatment. So during the next year they tried the various drugs then available that would help most to control her seizures. At the end of that time Mary's application to the state school for the feeble-minded, which had been pending for a whole year, was accepted.

Mary's mother talked to doctors in the Crippled Children's Program. Should she send Mary to the feeble-minded school? The doctors said "No." They thought they should continue to treat Mary and that she should be given another chance at public school. She went and this time, with her seizures under control, she was not "too much" for her teachers. She began to make progress. The progress became greater as the new drugs for epilepsy became available to treat her. In due time she was graduated from high school. Now she is being trained as a physical therapist and will soon enter that profession. Physical therapy, good medical care, and education saved Mary from becoming a statistic, one unit in the population of a state institution for the feeble-minded.

Again let us contrast this story with Melba, who was born about the same time as Mary on a hilly farm on a mud road in a fairly remote section of another state which does not include children with seizures in its Crippled Children's Program. When she was in the second grade she had a severe illness and after recovering began to have seizures. The parents engaged the limited amount of medical advice within their reach for several years but Melba was not helped. The parents felt hopeless and finally adopted an over-protective attitude toward their girl. Like so many other children, Melba has grown up without schooling, subject to ten or twelve seizures a day, and a burden to her aging parents.

Up until about 10 or 15 years ago the drugs available to treat epilepsy were not very effective. Recent research, much of it financed by Congressional appropriations, has been unusually productive and highly effective new drugs for epilepsy have been developed. Neurological specialists say that they can now relieve or completely control symptoms in 80% of their patients, especially if treatment can be started early in childhood. Through proper treatment, most children with epilepsy should be able to attend schools, be graduated, and hold jobs.

Probably in no other field does a dollar of Crippled Children's funds go so far as in the treatment of epilepsy, according to the doctors in charge of the anticonvulsive clinics. They point out that it costs less than $50 a year to see each patient in regularly held clinics. Only about 10% of the patients need hospitalization and then, with the exception of the few very severe cases, the hospitalization is short. The yearly cost of drugs for the patient is around $25. Parents with modest incomes are usually able to buy the necessary drugs and often have hospital insurance to cover the cost of hospitalization. The major cost to the program is to make accessible to the child a clinic where he may be examined and checked and where the right kind of treatment and care can be prescribed by a specialist.

In the light of this knowledge, it is sad to think that fewer than 1,500 of the estimated 400,000 epileptic children in the country receive treatment under the Crippled Children's Program in 1953. How many others were treated privately through the resources of their parents, or through programs of the voluntary agencies is not known, but we know that thousands and thousands are growing up like Melba without benefit of any of the modern discoveries.

Perhaps some of the lag in the treatment of children with epilepsy by state Crippled Children's Programs lies in the unfortunate stigma attached to this condition. Parents do not make their needs known because they want to keep their child's affliction a secret. Doctors know that the proper care of such a child does not end with finding and prescribing the right drug. Someone must persuade the mother that the child will be better off and less likely to have seizures if he is in school learning and playing with other children. Someone must consult with the teacher to assure her that the case is under control, but advise her how to handle the situation if a seizure should occur during school hours. When the child is grown and prepared to earn a living, someone must face the public opinion against the hiring of epileptics and persuade an employer that the patient with seizures under control is capable of competent service on most jobs without risk to himself or his employer. This is the kind of activity to which the Crippled Children's agencies should be giving leadership. . . .

Present Extent of Services.—Government has a definite obligation to its crippled children. Both Federal and state governments have recognized that fact by the money they have appropriated over the past 17 years. Together, they have developed a nation-wide Crippled Children's Program whose only limitation is that it does not go far enough.

To look at the amazing advances made by medical research in the knowledge and techniques for treating crippled children and then to look at the thousands and thousands of children to whom the new knowledge is not available, is a sad picture. The new techniques for treating cleft palate, the new drugs for the control of epileptic seizures, the latest electronic devices for the hard of hearing, the new artificial limbs, the new surgical knowledge for cardiac troubles—these are only some of the many answers science has given to the question of how to help crippled children become normal, self-supporting adults. The rest of society must now see that the knowledge is used for the benefit of all who need it.

In 1953 the Crippled Children's Program provided help for only about 251,000 children in 52 states and territories. The tabulation [that appears below] shows the approximate percentages of funds which went to help children with various crippling conditions. A comparison between these percentages and the estimates on preceding pages indicates what a small number of children, crippled from defects other than those of an orthopedic nature, had any help at all.

TABLE 43.   *The crippling conditions among children who received treatment*

TOTAL NUMBER OF CHILDREN TREATED—251,000

	Percent of all Diagnoses
Congenital malformations, not elsewhere classified	22.4%
Orthopedic other than after-effects of polio	20.8
Poliomyelitis, acute and late effects	16.9
Cerebral palsy	9.7
Cleft palate and harelip	5.0
Effects of accidents, poisonings, and violence, excluding burns	4.0
Burns	2.4
Rheumatic fever, acute	1.9
Arthritis and rheumatism, except rheumatic fever	1.8
Birth injuries, except cerebral palsy and epilepsy, excluding intracranial and spinal birth injuries	1.5
Chronic rheumatic heart diseases	1.1
Deafness and impairment of hearing	1.1
Diseases of nervous system, except mental disorders, excluding cerebral palsy and epilepsy	1.0
Spina bifida and meningocele	1.0
Heart diseases, except congenital malformations, excluding acute rheumatic fever and chronic heart disease	.9
Eye conditions except cataract	.8
Epilepsy	.2
Birth injuries, intracranial and spinal, except cerebral palsy and epilepsy	.2
Diabetes mellitus	.2
Congenital cataract	.1
Other diagnosed conditions, not elsewhere classified	7.0

(Based on estimated data from U. S. Dept. of Health, Education and Welfare.)

It is recognized, of course, that many of the estimated two and a half million crippled children are under the care of private doctors and surgeons engaged and paid for by their families. A smaller number are receiving some help from voluntary agencies. This is as it should be. It was never the purpose of the government to provide for children services which could be financed by their parents. It is recognized, however, that the income of many families is not sufficient to provide the long term treatment and services needed for most crippled children. In many, many parts of the country there are no adequate facilities within reasonable reach. If parents cannot afford the treatment which may be right at hand, or if they cannot afford to send the child to a distant clinic or hospital, that child is doomed to be a cripple for the rest of his life. He may never be able to earn a living and may become a public charge.

It is estimated, for example, that $35 million of tax money is being spent every year to keep only a fraction of those afflicted with epilepsy in our state and Federal institutions. Another $15 million of public money goes for welfare assistance and medical care for another fraction. Since for approximately $75 a year a child's seizures can be controlled so that he can get an education and be self-supporting, it would seem good business for governments to begin spending more money through the Crippled Children's Programs for the diagnosis and treatment of children with epilepsy. They would thereby save the cost of supporting thousands in institutions for the rest of their lives because they had not received treatment.

Money spent for crippled children is an investment in the future of the country. For a small sum a boy like David is made fit to serve the armed forces of his country instead of selling shoe strings on the street corner. A girl like Mary becomes a physical therapist, prepared to help other crippled children, instead of a tax-supported statistic in an institution for the feeble-minded.

A questionnaire answered by directors of the Crippled Children's Program in 42 states revealed great unmet needs in the states.

"We need to extend our services to more kinds of crippled children" and "We need to take what services we have to more parts of the States" were the most universal answers.

About half the states want to begin some treatment for children afflicted with epilepsy; about the same number want to begin treatment for rheumatic fever and other cardiac conditions, or to make their present service in those fields available to more children. The need for braces, for better help in cleft palate cases, and help for the hard of hearing were other widespread needs. Some states revealed waiting lists of as many as 5,000 crippled children who need help. Other states said they do not keep a waiting list record because they do not have funds enough to consider treatment for all who might go on such a list. . . .

B. DISABLED ADULTS *

THE EXPANDED State-Federal program of vocational rehabilitation for the general population now provides the doctor with a new and effective means of helping his

* From: *The Doctor and Vocational Rehabilitation for Civilians,* by the Office of Vocational Rehabilitation, Department of Health, Education and Welfare; Washington: U.S. Government Printing Office, 1947. Reprinted with omissions, including illustrations, from pp. 1-13.

physically or mentally handicapped patients to become self-sustaining, even though they cannot afford to pay for necessary treatment and care.

The 48 States, the District of Columbia, Puerto Rico, Hawaii, and Alaska operate vocational rehabilitation plans which provide public funds to pay for necessary medical and related services for vocationally handicapped persons to the extent of their inability to pay. . . .

Where eligibility and need are established, any type of medical or related care can be provided for the purpose of reducing or eliminating a vocationad handicap.

Services are provided only on prescription. They include medical, psychiatric, and surgical examinations and treatment, hospitalization, convalescent care, dental care, nursing care, physical therapy, occupational therapy, speech therapy, prosthetic appliances, medical supplies, and drugs.

Every applicant for vocational rehabilitation services is required to have a thorough medical examination before any services are provided. This examination usually is performed by his family physician, and the State agency pays for it. The examination also is used as an additional basis for vocational diagnosis.

Physicial restoration is one of the most important services provided through the State Vocational Rehabilitation agencies.

In addition, vocational advice and counseling; any type of training, from on-the-job instruction to a full college course; placement services; and follow-up to assure complete adjustment, are given as indicated.

In each case, the vocational rehabilitation counselor, the doctor or medical consultant, and the applicant for services work as a team to develop a vocational objective and a rehabilitation plan for the individual. All services then are directed toward attainment of the vocational objective, and all are integrated into a rehabilitation plan.

The purpose of the entire program of vocational rehabilitation is to assist the disabled to become self-sustaining men and women.

Who Is Eligible for Rehabilitation Services.—Any person of working age with a physical or mental handicap to employment, or to full employment, can receive educational, advisory, and placement services without cost to himself. Applicants for physical restoration services must demonstrate inability to purchase these services themselves.

Certain additional help is available to the States in the rehabilitation of those who properly constitute a Federal responsibility, in some cases extending to full reimbursement for all costs—such as in the case of merchant seamen disabled in line of duty, and of war disabled civilians.

Veterans may be eligible, as are civilians, but the special legislative provisions for their care and compensation are such that the veteran generally finds it preferable to seek counsel and treatment through the Veterans Administration. If he is ineligible for services through the Veterans Administration, the State-Federal system of vocational rehabilitation is open to him.

Any person of working age is eligible for any necessary physical restoration services if he meets all of the following requirements:

1. He has a physical or mental defect—regardless of origin—which is a substantial employment handicap.

2. It is static, i. e., stationary, stable, or only slowly progressive. (Thus, acute illnesses and emergency cases are ineligible.)

3. It can be removed or substantially reduced by treatment in a reasonable length of time. (Though Federal participation in the cost of hospital care is limited to 90 days for one disability, this does not mean that all treatment must be completed in 90 days.)

4. He is unable to pay the full cost of the services out of his own resources.

5. The necessary services are not available from any other source.

Under these conditions, for example, it will be seen that the State Vocational Rehabilitation agency does not pay for the *treatment* of active tuberculosis. It is not static, treatment is prolonged, the prognosis at any one time is not certain, and arrest depends upon too many uncontrollable factors.

Other rehabilitation services, such as guidance, training and placement, all at the stage deemed most suitable by the doctor, have proved invaluable aids to recovery and freedom from recurrence, and these services are encouraged.

Persons with recent fractures, ordinary pneumonia, and malignant neoplasms are not eligible cases. Postoperative pneumonia, following operation for a distinctly eligible disability, is covered, because it is a recognized complication of surgery for an eligible condition.

The crippling end results of fractures, of radical operations (involving apparent cure) for malignancy, and of other similar conditions, are eligible if they meet the ordinary criteria.

State Purchases Medical Services.—Medical services are purchased by the State. They are rendered by a physician, general practitioner or specialist, duly licensed in his own State, and, in the case of specialists or hospitals, certified by a professionally approved board for specialties or hospitals, where such a physician or hospital is available. Each State establishes its own standards. Physical restoration services are authorized and performed only upon medical prescription.

Services are purchased from existing facilities, public or private.

The physician and hospital are freely chosen by the rehabilitation client from those meeting the above standards, which were established by physicians. The client is urged to exercise free choice for the practical reason that he generally has more faith in his own doctor than in any other and so is likely to follow his prescriptions more closely.

Payment for services is made on the basis of a schedule of maximum fees, worked out between the State Division of Vocational Rehabilitation, its Professional Advisory Committee, and the State Medical Association. The objections to a fee schedule are fully recognized, even to one which is locally agreed upon. Since the clients who receive medical services are, by law, entitled to payment of their bills only to the extent that they are unable to pay their own expenses, compensation cannot exceed the maximum paid by other agencies for similar services.

This represents a distinct professional advance in this particular field, since until a few years ago the Federal law authorized no payment for treatment.

The schedules being used in State agencies represent quite fairly the average fees charged patients of moderate means in average areas.

Although the "top fees" paid for individual services are fixed by local usage, most or all schedules allow substantial exceptions for prolonged and unusual cases, with full freedom for local determination of the reasonable worth of services so unusual as to have no precedent.

It is the feeling of the Office of Vocational Rehabilitation that since the average cost of physical restoration is about $270 over the country, and since, at its completion, the client's income has been raised from an average of $300 to an average of about $1,700, physicians and surgeons deserve fair compensation. This should not be looked upon as a "charity" program, since the increase in income to the client removes him from a state of dependency and puts him on his own feet again.

Millions Need Rehabilitation.—There is a backlog of at least 1,500,000 men and women with physical or mental disabilities which constitute vocational handicaps who need and are eligible for some or all vocational rehabilitation services. Industrial, home, and highway accidents, illness, and congenital causes produce an annual increment of 200,000.

An indication of the extent of the problem is given in the following estimates of the numbers with specific disabilities:

200,000 amputees, requiring prosthetic devices.

30,000—70,000 new amputees per year. . . . 500,000 cases of active tuberculosis, an increasing number scheduled to recover. . . . Of those rehabilitated, 80 percent fewer break down and come back with reactivated tuberculosis.

500,000 epileptics, most of whom can be helped into limited or full employment with proper medical guidance and treatment. Many can resume a normal life in every way after physical restoration services.

225,000—275,000 blind persons, with about 10 percent of this number becoming blind annually. The number of the totally blind is being sharply reduced by advances in medical science and industrial safety measures. . . .

Nearly a quarter of a century of organized effort had been devoted to the rehabilitation of the disabled, by those in the State-Federal program of vocational rehabilitation, before physical restoration was included specifically in the Federal law as an essential of successful rehabilitation.

To the doctor, the physically and mentally handicapped are or have been sick people. They are, or have been, the patients of physicians. And now it is recognized that, before the long, expensive and often unsatisfactory procedure of training these people for jobs is undertaken, there first must be made a determination of whether the handicap can be removed or reduced by appropriate treatment. . . .

The Barden-LaFollette amendments to the National Vocational Rehabilitation Act of 1920, became effective in 1943 as Public Law No. 113, and contained specific authorization for the use of Federal funds, when matched with State funds, for the physical rehabilitation of the disabled as a part of the general plan of vocational rehabilitation. . . .

The Doctor's Contribution.—The first contribution the doctor can make is professional medical guidance, not only of his patient, but of those who must later advise that patient about the choice of a job, who must find the right kind of job for him, and follow him on the job to the point of assured success. The doctor . . . must train the nonmedical rehabilitation worker to think of the medical possibilities inherent in each case.

While the lame, the halt, the sick and the blind have been the wards of medicine for centuries, it was only recently that such developments in the field of vocational rehabilitation as vocational training and education; skill and aptitude testing; individualized job counseling, and selective placement brought new and invaluable resources into being. . . .

Some of the newer resources now make it possible for the doctor to bring the newer developments in medicine into a revitalized kind of rehabilitation. . . .

. . . To individualize medical treatment and the counseling of the disabled, while effecting the placement of millions who now earn little or nothing, and who often are on the welfare rolls, by virtue of a physical handicap which is often curable—that is the doctor's problem in vocational rehabilitation.

In every case which is to receive any services, dependence is placed upon the doctor to discover, through examination and diagnosis the hidden tuberculosis, the latent syphilis, the unsuspected advanced carcinoma, which would not only cause a complete waste of all rehabilitation efforts if overlooked, but would later cost the patient his health or his life. . . .

The job counselor and the vocational educator can, by placing their services at the doctor's disposal, enable him to promise to his patients great hope, even in the most severely handicapped cases, for training and employment in an interesting and remunerative job. Experience shows that this job is a far better paying job than most of the jobs now held by those without medical care for their disabilities, or specific training for the job after the handicap has been lessened or removed.

Medical Guidance Is Essential.—The handicapped man must stand on a platform of physical restoration.

The presence of a physical or mental handicap is not only a medical determination, but it must be established to render the client eligible for *any* rehabilitation service.

After the client is found to have a disability, everything that can be done to get him in shape to work depends upon his physical and mental ability to hold up under the stress and strain of the employment chosen. Without a sound medical diagnosis and medical appraisal of working ability, it would, in most cases, be impossible scientifically to guide, train, and place the client in a job.

It is the counselor who, after getting the best available medical and other advice, works out with the applicant a program beginning with physical appraisal and ending with job placement and follow-up.

The handicapped person meets an experienced conselor, usually at his first visit. This counselor is responsible for assembling and bringing to bear upon the client all of the factors and services that determine his eligibility and feasibility; his ability to absorb training; his medical needs; his skills and aptitudes. Medical diagnosis and medical recommendations for further diagnosis and treatment, determination of physical job limitations and other medical considerations are vital. The counselor arranges to have the client see the doctor for examination and diagnosis, and counsels the client about his job future within the limitations of the medical diagnosis and prognosis, as well as the strictly vocational limitations of natural intelligence and skills.

Most clients come to the vocational rehabilitation agencies after years of struggling against a physical handicap—so many years that it is obvious that something vital has been missing. One missing factor was the lack of authority to furnish curative services. A patient could be taught to weave baskets and sit in a wheel chair, but there was generally no authority to pay for his physical restoration.

Even now, however, there is too long a time-lag between sickness or injury, and the beginning of guidance, curative or remedial services, training, and placement.

Even now, only 3 percent of the States' clients are referred by physicians. . . .

Ideal Steps in Rehabilitation.—While few rehabilitation agencies outside large cities have the staff to render such complete service, an ideal case would go through the following steps in which the doctor's participation is vital:

1. Application for service. Preliminary interview. If other than medical factors are favorable, applicant is referred to the counselor.

2. Discussion of applicant's handicap and work problems and ambitions.

3. Reference by counselor to family physician for general, basic medical examination. On the examination report the doctor is asked for the following opinions:

What are the characteristics of the major disability? (Permanent? Temporary? Stable? Slowly Progressive? Rapidly Progressive? Improving?)

Can it be removed or substantially reduced by treatment? Work capacity (indicated by checks on standard items). Is further diagnostic work recommended? Treatment recommended? What kind; approximately how long?

4. Other data are gathered, including that available through intelligence and aptitude testing; job interests are recorded; family and social relationships noted; if in doubt, the doctor is again consulted by one of the staff, perhaps the medical social worker.

5. Case discussion. The counselor presents the case with his recommendations for handling. The family doctor's report is discussed, with a medical consultant to interpret the report and to see that the plan is kept within the physical capacities of the client and within the medical prescription.

6. The counselor is then authorized to proceed with services. If physical restoration is involved, the doctor chosen by the patient is visited and asked to go ahead with his plan of treatment, and to say when the patient can begin to get

auxiliary services, such as training, job testing, and the beginning of actual supervised work.

7. Follow-up services, including re-referral to the doctor at such intervals as he
may desire.

Naturally, the case is not closed until the client is established in suitable remunerative employment.

Doctor's Report Is Important.—The doctor's report is designed to be a permanent
recording by the doctor of the medical needs and limitations of the patient.

Thus, the rehabilitation agency's strong feeling that the doctor's report must be
complete in every detail is not based upon a desire to be arbitrary or picayunish.
Rehabilitation clients have disabilities which require a clear medical statement on
their limitations and their possibilities. . . .

Lack of thoroughness in measuring the patient's mental ability and aptitude for
the new kind of job will waste time and money, and result in further unemployability.
Lack of a thorough medical diagnosis and prescription is equally serious. For that
reason, the way has been left open for the doctor to ask for more time, even
hospitalization if necessary, for diagnosis. He may have competent consultation
merely by asking for it.

Good medical examinations and good medical care are not cheap. Unless all
of rehabilitation experience is wrong, a good diagnosis is worth what it costs, and
the better the diagnosis, the surer is success in job rehabilitation. . . .

In the larger local offices, there is a medical consultant, selected and employed
locally, by the State. It is his job to see that relationships with doctors and their
professional associations are functioning properly; that the doctor's report is
properly understood by the staff; that the case is handled in both medical and
nonmedical ways in accordance with the doctor's analysis of physical and mental
capacities for the stress and strain of work and daily living.

Medical representation is had at the State office through a State medical consultant, with similar duties but of a State-wide nature.

The fundamental principle underlying the medical consultant's job is not only
a professional review and reinforcement of competent medical opinion, but also a
fiscal one. Every business has a check on the spending of money. Where adequate
medical advice has not been had, this gives the State agency a professional basis
for insisting upon such advice; and where necessary, for asking that the medical
aims be so clarified that one without medical experience, such as an auditor, can
see almost at a glance that a reputable doctor has clearly stated that in his best
professional judgment, not only is the treatment proposed directly designed to fit the
patient into satisfactory rehabilitation, but that the nonmedical plan for the client
is in accord with medical judgment as to his ability to stand the strain of the job. . . .

71. THE MENTALLY ILL *

PUBLIC AUTHORITIES and other thoughtful citizens in every state are seeking more adequate information about the needs of the mentally ill. These may be reduced to two basic questions:

1. At any given time, how many persons within the state will be in need of care in a mental hospital?

2. At any given time how many persons, not requiring institutional care, will be in need of clinical treatment or other mental health services?

... The further we go back into the history of hospitals in this country, the more apparent it becomes that the number of [mentally ill] persons has increased rather steadily since the opening of the first hospital in the United States. The number of mental patients for whom treatment is sought by themselves, their friends, or public authorities has constantly grown. We do not know the cause of this increase, whether it is because of increasing population in general, or because of better diagnosis, or because of changes in general age levels, or because of increasing awareness of available facilities, or because of increasing rates of mental disease. ...

Growth of Hospital Population

BETWEEN 1903 and 1948 the total growth in resident population of all mental hospitals was 406,474 patients. Of this growth, 84 per cent was represented by the growth of state mental hospitals. The hospitalization rate † for state mental hospitals has increased from 159.1 in 1903 to 323.1 in 1948. During that period, resident population of state hospitals increased by an annual average of 7,582. However, the annual increase has been somewhat greater in the past decade, averaging 8,493 per year since 1938.

It will be noted that the number of resident patients in county and city mental hospitals has decreased markedly in recent years. Here is apparent the trend for the states to assume more responsibility for mental patients in public hospitals. This same trend is indicated by the fact that the percentage of total patients in city and county hospitals has steadily declined from a high of 10.9 per cent in 1903 to 3.5 per cent in 1948. For this same period the proportion of patients in state and private hospitals has been relatively constant.

The rate of first admissions to state mental hospitals, between 1937 and 1948, increased from 60.7 to 69.7 per 100,000 of general population. ... The greatest

---

* From: *The Mental Health Programs of the 48 States* (A Report to the National Governors' Conference); Chicago: Council of State Governments, 1950 (Chap. II, pp. 29-44; Chap. X, pp. 201-5). Reprinted (with omissions, including figures and some tables) by permission of the publishers.

† This rate is calculated as the number of resident patients in hospitals per 100,000 of the general population.

[numerical] increase occurred in 1948, when 7,469 more patients were admitted than in the year before. . . .

Some of the influential factors in hospital population growth may be listed briefly as follows:

1. The general population has grown. There are simply more people who could have a mental disease.

2. There are more people in the older age brackets, where the highest incidence of mental disease has always fallen.

3. More hospital accommodations are available for care and treatment of mental patients. In the past, additional accommodations have always meant additional patients because the need for accommodations has been so great.

4. Both the medical profession and the general public know more about mental disease, and have been increasingly willing to utilize mental hospitals. Confidence in the hospitals has grown.

5. The concept of mental disturbance has broadened. Formerly, only the severest types of mental illness were considered for hospitalization, but patients are now drawn from a wider and wider range of disturbed conditions.

6. People live longer, not only in the community but in the hospital. They have a greater average duration of hospital life, partly because of improved standards of general physical accommodation and care that prolong life itself. Some patients, too, remain longer in the hospital because of higher standards of psychiatric care, because of the inability or unwillingness of the community to find places for them, or because of the shortage of social workers for after-care.

7. Urbanization of society is doubtless a factor. Many mentally erratic or disturbed persons, who might be cared for quite well in a farm or small-town environment, may be both helpless and difficult in a crowded urban center. Mentally ill persons, especially the aged and senile, are all too often an unbearable burden in a city apartment. Moreover, the rushing tempo of urban life today is a far cry from the typical living conditions of a century ago. This *may* act to produce more disturbed people; it *does* act to make it more difficult for the disturbed person to get along in the world outside the hospital.

The Makeup of Patient Population

THE ANNUAL INCREASE of first admissions and the annual increment in patient population are considerably lower for state hospitals than they are for "all hospitals." . . . There are specific reasons why the state hospitals can take fewer new patients, and yet have relatively high rate of growth in patient population. The latter, of course, is a matter of patient turnover, and of the specific factors that enter into it: first admissions, readmissions, discharges, deaths, and duration of hospital life.

To begin with, it may be noted that for state hospitals the ratio of first admissions to resident patients falls markedly below that in each of the other types of hospitals for the mentally ill, except the county and city classifications. . . . These differences mean, obviously, that the state, county, and city hospitals have, on the whole, the patients with the longest average hospital stay. The explanation for this may lie partly in the quality of care and treatment, but largely it lies in the diagnostic character of first admissions.

The following table shows selected diagnoses of first admissions to the several types of hospitals, and the percentage of each diagnostic group among total admissions, whether psychotic or non-psychotic, for a recent and probably typical year.

TABLE 44.   *First admissions to hospitals for mental disease in the United States: 1946* [A]

[By Diagnosis and Type of Hospital Control]

Diagnosis	All Hospitals		State Hospitals		County and City Hospitals		Veterans' Hospitals		Private Hospitals	
	No.	%	No.	%	No.	%	No.	%	No.	%
General paresis	6,021	4.1	5,367	6.0	121	4.0	275	1.2	258	0.8
Alcoholic (psychotic)	5,713	3.9	3,932	4.4	94	3.1	912	4.1	755	2.5
Alcoholic (non-psychotic)	9,541	6.6	3,742	4.2	76	2.5	1,424	6.4	4,299	14.1
Cerebral arteriosclerosis	15,665	10.8	13,665	15.3	506	16.8	159	0.7	1,335	4.4
Senile	13,543	9.3	11,345	12.7	791	26.2	52	0.2	1,355	4.4
Involutional	6,888	4.7	3,898	4.4	66	2.2	112	0.5	2,812	9.2
Psychoneurosis	11,677	8.0	2,930	3.3	62	2.1	5,261	23.6	3,424	11.2
Manic-depressive	12,078	8.3	6,951	7.8	188	6.2	820	3.7	4,119	13.5
Dementia praecox	29,753	20.5	16,918	18.9	456	15.1	8,058	36.1	4,321	14.1
Other	34,324	23.8	20,551	23.0	721	21.8	5,241	23.5	7,874	25.8
All patients	145,203	100.0	89,299	100.0	3,018	100.0	22,314	100.0	30,572	100.0

A Adapted from U. S. Bureau of Census, *Patients in Mental Institutions*, 1946, Table VII, p. 18.

From this table the fact appears that the state hospitals receive a majority of the dementia praecox patients (more than half in 1946) and most of the patients (86 per cent) having diseases of the senium i. e., senile psychoses and psychoses with cerebral arteriosclerosis. The proportion of first admissions of dementia praecox cases among total first admissions to state hospitals was 18.9 per cent and the proportion of first admissions with diseases of the senium was 28 per cent. Both of these groups who seek hospitalization, and especially the latter, are increasing in the general population as indicated by the record of first admissions to all psychiatric hospitals in the United States, 1937-1946, and of first admissions as reported by individual states. The increase in admissions with diseases of the senium is related, of course, to the rapid increase in average age of the general population.... [State] hospitals also tend to get a disproportionate share of other long-term or chronic cases, and a smaller share of the short-term patients, such as psychoneurotics and non-psychotic alcoholics.

Duration of Hospital Life

RECENT STUDIES of the duration of hospital life, based on a sufficient number of cases and covering a sufficient span of observation, are not easy to find. To reckon duration backwards—that is, from time of discharge or death—does not give an accurate picture. However, the following figures relating to duration of patients on books in the New York Civil State Hospitals on April 1, 1947, are significant:

In Hospital	Number	Per Cent
Under 1 year	13,415	15.9
1- 4 years	20,460	24.2
5-14 years	27,634	32.7
15-24 years	13,451	15.9
25-34 years	6,338	7.5
35-44 years	2,440	2.9
45 years and over	785	.9
Total	84,523	100.0

The largest number of these patients, 49,083, had dementia praecox—a disease that represents about one fifth of all first admissions, but more than half of all the resident population. . . . Thirty-seven per cent had been in hospital 15 years or more. . . .

However, in terms of the prospects for mental patients admitted to mental hospitals, there is considerable room for optimism. Discharge and recovery rates for patients other than the schizophrenic, the senile and the arteriosclerotic are relatively high. Moreover, the newer therapies are beginning to make headway even with schizophrenia. The Eastern State Hospital of Washington reports that "fifty per cent of the patients are dismissed within one year," and the Western State Hospital that "the percentage of discharged to admissions approaches sixty." While California reports that 40 per cent of the patients admitted at age 60 and over die within a year of hospitalization, the rest of the story is that 40 per cent are eventually discharged. . . . The general fact is that for most mental patients in state hospitals, the eventual chances of improvement and recovery are improving. In the year 1946 there were 89,299 first admissions to state mental hospitals; 116,807 total first and readmissions; and 66,098 discharges.

The condition, or prognosis, on discharge is reported for only those with psychosis on admission. Even so, 47,318 patients were discharged as recovered or as improved, which is 53 per cent of the first admissions in the same year and 40 per cent of the total admissions. A study of readmissions in New York suggested that the differences between the prognoses of "improved," "much improved," and "recovered" meant very little with regard to the likelihood of readmission. In short, it may perhaps be said that the likelihood of getting well, for patients in state mental hospitals, is better than 50-50, and that methods of treatment are improving in efficacy. The chances of improvement or recovery are much better than 50-50 for most diagnostic conditions. . . .

Attacks on the Problem

OBVIOUSLY AN INDISPENSABLE element in any program of care—good, bad, or indifferent—for the mentally ill of a state is the provision of buildings in which that care is to be given. This does not mean that the job can be done merely by getting money with which to erect buildings that are large enough for the number of patients that need care, though indeed it is an achievement when a state does meet this demand. Patients are as various as other human beings. They are alike not in having the same sort of disorder, but merely in that they all are disordered in their mental processes. Some of these patients are young and many are old; some are strong and many are feeble; some are agreeable and tractable no matter how serious their disorder, while others are extremely disturbed and difficult to work with. Clearly then, various kinds of buildings are needed. In addition to housing, there must be provision for the many kinds of services that a patient population (sometimes equal to that of a fair-sized city) may need in the course of a day....

Outpatients

SOMETHING MUST NOW be said about other patients whose condition is not so pitiable as that of many of the hospital cases, but who are in need, and often in very deep need, of treatment. These are a varied lot of people, but alike in at least two regards: first, that they are unwell and unhappy; and second that they are reasonable enough to seek treatment of their own will, or under the advice of friends or professional counselors. Persons of this sort make up about 50 per cent of the patients seen by private physicians, and the cost of treatment is great because it is seldom possible to disentangle the mental webs of individual misery without the expenditure of much time.

It is not possible for the person without financial means to pay for such expensive treatment but his situation is not essentially different from that of the indigent person with gall bladder disease or arthritis. To meet the needs of the unhospitalized patients, a large-scale provision of clinic facilities is needed. This involves space, a moderate amount of equipment, nursing, certainly good social service, clerical help, and psychiatric direction. Nobody knows exactly how large the load will be in any state, for only occasionally, if ever, have the services met the demand. But certainly the effort should be made to provide at least a basic program to meet the minimum demonstrated needs, and the program should be expanded as finances permit. Clinics frequently do not need separate buildings; indeed if an arrangement can be made to hold the mental clinic in the outpatient service of some existing hospital, that arrangement is usually better than to go into a building program. Such outpatient treatment is undoubtedly costly, however, in its salary item.

Extensive consideration should, of course, be given to the existing practices of the state hospitals for the mentally ill with respect to specific care and treatment programs....

Special Categories

IN ADDITION TO THOSE whom we have been discussing—the mentally ill or disturbed —there are a large number of chronic alcoholics, a few drug addicts, a considerable number of epileptics, and a large fraction of mental defectives in any community who also require proper provision in housing and personnel.

Some trends in the thought and feeling of society towards those who cause difficulty may be noted in the current discussion of what to do with the so-called sexual psychopath. More than one kind of person has been thus labeled. . . . There is, to be sure, a group of persons who may be properly called sexual psychopaths, whose behavior in this field is so persistent and at the same time so aberrant that they transgress the rules of society recklessly without regard to consequences and, at times, in such a way as to assure themselves of apprehension and punishment by legal authorities.

For several years we have seen legislation enacted in a number of states placing such persons under medical treatment, the idea being that these men should stay either in a mental hospital or some other institution presided over by psychiatrists until they have somehow recovered from their aggressive condition. In practice this is the equivalent of a long sentence in a pentitentiary, but the wording of the law leads to confusion and causes difficulty for the hospital man who has such persons added to his other burdens—persons who are quite clear in their contact with the environment, decidedly aggressive toward both sexes, and quite ready to impose on the mentally disordered people about them in the hospitals.

Whether the present movement constitutes an advance or a retreat is not important at this point; we are concerned merely with setting forth the fact that here is another group, previously looked after by the penologist, but now in increasing numbers being turned over to the hospital psychiatrist. Not only should proper provision for them be made, but also provision should be made for maximum security, and for employment on whatever basis may be available. Such provision is lacking in ordinary mental hospitals. One of the best illustrations of the sort of provision that should be made, and the kind of management toward which one should aim is in the federal institution at Springfield, Missouri. It is not an institution planned entirely for this group but for all sorts of offenders under sentence in federal prisons and jails, who need medical attention for mental or physical illness.

Almost everywhere in the country it is recognized that alcoholism constitutes a very large medical and social problem. A substantial number of these persons are annually being placed under treatment in mental hospitals of various sorts and in psychiatric services of general hospitals. The actual number admitted to hospitals throws little light on the scope of the problem. Moreover, there is as yet no general agreement concerning effective treatment of alcoholism. There is a strong tendency to keep such people out of prison during the early stage of their difficulty and to get them under medical care. Some of these persons should be treated in an out-patient clinic. A considerable number need to be put to bed in a hospital, for a period varying from three days to several months. . . .

Persons who have convulsive disorders are admittedly a medical problem. Though great numbers of them are useful, cheerful, and self-supporting citizens, a considerable number have to be looked after by state authorities. A few—but only a few—epileptics have very serious mental aberrations and are difficult and sometimes terrifying disturbers of the comfort and safety of their neighbors. Many states make special provisions for them in an institution that studies and caters to their needs. A considerable number of states attempt to provide only for those convulsives who are mentally ill, and who therefore go to the state hospital, or for those who are mentally deficient, and who therefore go to the state training school. Nobody knows how many epileptics there are in the general population, but figures derived from Selective Service Records indicate that this number is surprisingly large.

About the mentally deficient little need be said in the present report. A great number of them do well under the protection of their families. Some school systems provide them with all the book learning that they can absorb and help them to master elementary social prerequisites. But misfortune and difficulties that strike the family of the feeble-minded, quite as often as the family of the mentally alert, make necessary the existence of special institutions for mental deficiency. Moreover, these institutions are needed to care for a great number of persons defective from birth, and those of such low mentality that they cannot even care for their physical needs, much less participate in family activities. . . .

The Financial Problem

NO DISCUSSION of the scope of the problem would be complete without some reference to maintenance expenditures in state hospitals for the mentally ill. The figures run into tremendous amounts, and an analysis turns out to be a grim story. The burden, in many cases, is impoverishing the community, while in others so little has been spent that the standard of care must surely be low. . . .

The costs of hospital care for the mentally ill and of clinical treatment for patients who do not need hospitalization are increasing. So is the cost of all other hospital care. What is, perhaps, the most important question is whether or not full value is secured for the dollar expenditures, and what the consequences are if adequate care and treatment are not given to the mentally ill. . . .

Outpatient Clinics

OUTPATIENT CLINICS during recent years have continued to increase in number and scope and the staff composition of the clinical team has been virtually standardized to include psychiatrist, psychiatric social worker, and clinical psychologist. The functions of the clinic have been extended to include help to former patients of the hospital, the patients about to enter the hospital, to those needing help but not requiring hospitalization (such as psychoneurotics of certain types), to children with behavior problems, and to others.

There has been a tendency in many areas either to separate these several clinical functions from one another, or to separate them from the state hospital, or, in any case, to separate the aftercare clinic from all the others. Part of the reason for such a separation has been the historic isolation of the state mental hospital from the community both geographically and socially. Undoubtedly this separation of clinics and hospitals has done both community and hospital considerable damage. Such separation obviously precludes the building of one of the few possible effective bridges between the hospital and the community. Recently as the state hospital has begun to think of itself as a public psychiatric service, rather than a set of hospital buildings, it has tended to move back toward the community in an attempt to provide a well-rounded program of mental hygiene.

There has also been a trend in some areas to separate former patients into a regular parole clinic. Elsewhere, it has been felt that perhaps this may obstruct the patient's absorption back into the community as a regular member of society. Some hospitals have set up separate clinics for children. In some states, clinics have been conducted by the central authority rather than by the hospitals themselves. Frequently clinics have been conducted by departments other than those concerned with the mental hospitals.

Similarly, mental health clinics have developed extensively under local, public, and private auspices, especially in the larger cities. Nearly all cities over 150,000 in population at present have services of their own. . . . In addition to the usual types of clinics offered by the state (such as traveling clinics, child-guidance clinics and all-purpose clinics) one finds occasionally a special clinic for chronic alcoholics, a clinic for the rehabilitation of veterans, or clinics for schools, emanating most frequently from the department of public instruction. . . .[1]

The service of the rural community presents special problems. It is not adequate merely to authorize an urban clinic to receive cases from other communities or districts of the state, since the distance of the clinic from the patient sharply limits its usefulness. The only answer for the relatively thinly populated rural area seems to be the mobile clinic, and even here it is difficult to achieve much unless the clinic can make community visits at least once a week. Even so, some of the advantages of specialization which characterize the urban clinic will have to be foregone for the sake of general utility.

The following standards have been accepted as guides for the establishment of mental health clinics:

1. There should be at least one all-purpose clinic provided for each 100,000 of the population.

2. Each clinic should have on its staff at least one psychiatrist, one psychologist, and two psychiatric social workers.

1. Recently the National Institute of Mental Health released a significant report on the national clinic program as of 1947. It shows that 471 clinics were in operation at that time. These were sponsored by various types of authorities. For example, health agencies were operating 295, of which mental hospitals sponsored 95. Other categories shown are welfare agencies with 113, education institutions with 49, and judicial agencies with 14. (Mental Health Statistics, Federal Security Agency, Public Health Service, National Institute of Mental Health, March, 1950, Series M H-B50, No. 2, "Availability and Use of Psychiatric Clinics: 1947," by Warren W. Morse and Charles C. Limburg, p. 9.)

3. State mental health authorities should be responsible for traveling clinics in rural areas.
4. Clinics should furnish three broad services:
    a. A community clinic
    b. An auxiliary service to the mental hospital
    c. Mental health education
5. Community support and approval is basic to a successful clinic.

The Clinic and the Hospital

IT HAS OFTEN been argued that by separating the clinics from the hospital service, the clinic loses the stigma which is implied in working under hospital auspices and is thus able to work more freely. Many authorities on the contrary believe that, since the problem is rather to free the hospital of its historic stigma, the clinic is the best means whereby this can be achieved. Another important consideration, however, is that a hospital which is conducting clinic work of high grade with adequate facilities for supervision and training is, in many ways, considerably more attractive to high-grade professional personnel, which the hospital needs in any case. A good clinical program is therefore a help in the solution of the problem.

A number of states provide services which go beyond the mere provision of clinical aid. Such services include correctional institutions, social agencies, public health nursing, youth organizations, and consultation with courts. These services are often purely diagnostic, but beyond the consultation and clinical services, many people are concerned in helping to discover what aspects of community life contribute to mental distress and to help in the correction of these deficiencies in community life. Others are interested in a program of community education, and still others in the provision of psychiatric help in the training of the personnel of other agencies to work with mental health problems and to deal with them more constructively.

Some hospitals permit and encourage medical and other professional personnel from the community to visit the clinical staff conferences of the hospital. Such visits not only give the participants added information and insight regarding psychiatric work and personality problems, but enable them better to cope with human relations problems in their own work.

After-Care Arrangements

IMPROVED METHODS of treatment result in the releasing of more patients from the hospital. They return to their own community or to one that is selected as more suitable for them. All these patients should have after-care services available to them. These patients may be at a convalescent stage in their improvement, on trial visit under various types of arrangements, some of which include the use of outside resources, as indicated in the summary below.

Type of After-Care Program	Number of Hospitals Using Program
Return visits to hospital clinic	126
Hospital social worker calls at home	115
Public social agencies	31
Private social agencies	70
Volunteer workers	81
Other programs	12

An unusual type of extension service has just been reported from England which goes beyond any of the existing services available in this country. The Bexley Hospital, in Kent, states that domiciliary visits have been used successfully. In other words, all the senior physicians of the hospital have been available, when called upon by the general practitioners, to see patients in their own homes. This service frequently short circuits the observation wards, and may well lead to earlier treatment on a voluntary basis. It might be thought of as a mobile individualized clinic service. . . .

A Ten-Point Program for Mental Health *

1. By far the major share of a state's mental health resources must be used for the care and treatment of patients in state hospitals for the mentally ill. Psychiatric treatment with the fullest use of existing knowledge can return many more people to productive and useful lives. Increased appropriations for additional qualified mental health personnel (including psychiatrists, psychologists, social workers, nurses and related personnel) and intensive treatment programs should be provided by the states at their next legislative session to increase the number of patients discharged from state mental hospitals.

2. Training and research in the field of mental health are essential elements of effective mental health programs. The serious accumulation of patients and costs can only be reduced by discovering new knowledge and new methods of treatment and by more adequate training and development of mental health personnel. State legislatures are urged to appropriate specific sums for training and research in addition to the regular appropriations for care and treatment.

3. Ultimate reduction of the population in state mental hospitals can only be achieved by efforts to prevent mental illness. This requires facilities for early identification, for early treatment and for after-care and supervision of those on leave from state hospitals. State governments should take the initiative with both financial and professional assistance in stimulating local and public and private agencies to participate actively in preventive programs.

* From: "A Ten-Point Program on Mental Health," by the National Governors' Conference on Mental Health; *State Government* 27:48, March 1954 (No. 3). Reprinted by permission of the publishers.

4. At present it is estimated that less than 1 percent of total state mental health budgets is expended for research—$4 million out of a total expenditure of about $560 million. Based on a comprehensive survey of state mental health officials, it is recommended that the states should devote a much larger percentage of their total mental health budgets to basic and applied research in the biological and behavioral sciences and to the training of personnel in research methods.

5. Effective training and research programs cannot be achieved without effective organization. A position of director of training and research should be established within the mental health agency in each state to assume responsibility for the coordination of mental health training and research within the state's jurisdiction. A technical advisory committee, composed of scientists and educators in the field of mental health, cooperating with scientists in universities and industry, should be established in each state to advise and assist the mental health agency and other state departments concerned with the coordination of training and research activities.

6. State institutions which are not accredited for residency or as affiliate training centers for psychiatrists, clinical psychologists, social workers, nurses and other professional groups should receive support from Governors and legislatures in their endeavors to raise the level of teaching and supervision in their institutions to secure accreditation.

7. The states should provide stipends for graduate training in the psychiatric field, should adjust salary scales and should provide educational leaves of absence so that state mental hospitals may compete effectively for the limited personnel available to fill treatment, teaching and research positions.

8. One of the important obstacles to adequate evaluation of procedures and therapies is a lack of uniformity in statistical methods in mental hospitals and clinics throughout the country. All states should cooperate with the United States Public Health Service and the American Psychiatric Association in the adoption of uniform terminology for statistical reporting procedures in the field of mental health.

9. Joint action by groups of states may provide one of the most fruitful means of attacking mental illness. This can be partially achieved by periodic regional mental health conferences, regional programs such as that now sponsored by the Southern Regional Education Board, and by active participation in the Interstate Clearinghouse now established through the Council of State Governments by request of the Governors' Conference. The clearinghouse, in cooperation with existing public and private agencies, will provide a medium for exchange of pertinent information among the states, will assist the states in organizing more effective mental health programs, and will help in developing interstate agreements so that groups of states can utilize to the fullest extent existing training and research facilities.

10. State and community mental health organizations should play important roles in educating the public to the problems of mental health and to the methods of improving psychiatric services. The states should encourage and support mental health education in the schools, good relationships between hospitals and surrounding communities, and the provision of adequate community psychiatric services.

These may, in the long run, be most important in determining the mental health of the nation.*

FURTHER READINGS

Over-all Patterns

Christensen, Aaron W., Flook, Evelyn, and Druzina, Georgie B. *Distribution of Health Services in the Structure of State Government, 1950.* Publication No. 184, Public Health Service. Part 3: *Personal Health Services Provided by State Government.* Washington: U. S. Government Printing Office, 1953. 277 pages.

Goldmann, Franz. *Public Medical Care: Principles and Problems.* New York: Columbia University Press, 1945. 226 pages. (Includes references).

Stern, Bernhard J. *Medical Services by Government.* New York: Commonwealth Fund, 1946. 208 pages. (Includes references).

The Needy

American Medical Association, Council on Medical Service. *A Report on Medical Care for the Indigent in Eighteen Selected Communities.* Chicago: The Association, 1955. 170 pages.

American Public Health Association, Subcommittee on Medical Care. *The Maryland Medical Care Program.* New York: The Association, 1948. 151 pages (processed).

American Public Welfare Association. *Role of the State Public Assistance Agency in Medical Care: A Series of Reports.* Chicago: The Association, 1953, 1954, 1955.

Anderson, Odin W. *Administration of Medical Care: Problems and Issues.* Ann Arbor, Mich.: School of Public Health, University of Michigan, 1947. 179 pages.

Anderson, Odin W. *Prepayment of Physicians' Services for Recipients of Public Assistance in the State of Washington: Problems and Issues.* Ann Arbor, Mich.: School of Public Health, University of Michigan, 1949. 62 pages.

Terris, Milton and Kramer, Nathan A. *General Medical Care Programs in Local Health Departments.* New York: American Public Health Association, 1951. 129 pages.

White, Ruth. *Medical Care in Public Assistance, 1946.* Public Assistance Report No. 16, Bureau of Public Assistance, Social Security Administration. Part 2: *Summary Report.* Washington: U. S. Government Printing Office, 1952. 127 pages.

Veterans

American Medical Association, Council on Medical Service. *Veterans Home Town Medical Care Program.* Chicago: The Association, 1949. 17 pages.

Report to the President from the Committee on Veterans' Medical Services. Washington: U. S. Government Printing Office, 1950. 65 pages.

Merchant Seamen

Straus, Robert. *Medical Care for Seamen: The Origin of Public Medical Service in the United States.* New Haven: Yale University Press, 1950. 165 pages. (Includes references).

The Handicapped

Baker, Edith M. and Siegel, Doris. *Medical Social Services for Children in Maternal and Child Health and Crippled Children's Programs.* Publication No. 343, Children's

* This program—signed by the governors of Illinois, Indiana, Kansas, Michigan, Minnesota, New Jersey, Ohio, Oklahoma, Tennessee, and West Virginia—was adopted by the National Governors' Conference on Mental Health on Feb. 9, 1954, in Detroit.

Bureau, Social Security Administration. Washington: U. S. Government Printing Office, 1953. 49 pages.

United States Department of Health, Education, and Welfare, Office of Vocational Rehabilitation. *Comeback*. Administrative Service Series No. 73. Washington: U. S. Government Printing Office, 1951. 137 pages.

United States Department of Health, Education, and Welfare, Office of Vocational Rehabilitation. *Vocational Rehabilitation of Public Assistance and Institutional Cases*. Rehabilitation Service Series No. 269. Washington: U. S. Government Printing Office, 1954. 19 pages.

United States Department of Health, Education, and Welfare, Social Security Administration, Children's Bureau. *The Crippled Children's Program*. Bureau Statistical Series No. 11. Washington: U. S. Government Printing Office, 1953. 17 pages.

United States Department of Health, Education, and Welfare, Social Security Administration, Children's Bureau. *Diagnoses of Children Served in the Crippled Children's Program, 1953*. Bureau Statistical Series No. 29. Washington: U. S. Government Printing Office, 1956. 23 pages.

The Mentally Ill

American Psychiatric Association, Mental Hospital Service. *Standards for Psychiatric Hospitals and Clinics*. Washington: The Association, 1954 (revised). 37 pages.

Department of National Health and Welfare. *Mental Health Services in Canada*. Ottawa, Canada: The Department, 1954. 207 pages (processed).

Deutsch, Albert. *The Mentally Ill in America*. (2nd ed.). New York: Columbia University Press, 1949. 555 pages. (Includes references).

Fuller, Raymond G. *A Study of Administration of State Psychiatric Services*. New York: National Association for Mental Health, 1954. 60 pages. (Includes references).

Kramer, Morton. *Facts Needed to Assess Public Health and Social Problems in the Widespread Use of Tranquilizing Drugs*. Publication No. 486, Public Health Service. Washington: U. S. Government Printing Office, 1956. 31 pages.

Lemkau, Paul V. *Mental Hygiene in Public Health*. (2nd ed.). New York: McGraw-Hill, 1955. 486 pages. (Includes references).

Mental Health in the United States. Vol. 286 of *The Annals*, American Academy of Political and Social Science. Philadelphia: The Academy, March 1953. 254 pages.

Research Council on Problems of Alcohol. *Principles for Public Action on Problem Drinking*. New York: The Council, no date. 13 pages.

Stanton, Alfred H. and Schwartz, Morris S. *The Mental Hospital*. New York: Basic Books, 1954. 492 pages. (Includes references).

CHAPTER XI

Medical Care in Industry

O VER TWO-THIRDS of our labor force of about 60,000,000 workers are industrial workers. Our national economy depends on their health and well-being. There has been increasing recognition of the values to be gained from helping industrial workers maintain their health—and even the health of their families. The acceptance by industry of concern for non-occupational disease and injury in recent years marks a development of great importance. It has been spurred by the inclusion of health and welfare benefits in collective bargaining negotiations between organized labor and industry. These benefits, recognized as part of wages, have come to occupy in labor-management relations as important a place as hours of work, or even as wages themselves.

With a few notable exceptions, early developments in the field of industrial medical care were limited to control of the more obvious industrial hazards, and to provision of limited cash benefits to cover part of the costs of treatment for industrially caused disability. As the costs in lost production due to illness have become apparent, and as the economic advantages of a positive health program have been made clear, employers in large industry have organized in-plant medical services. Under the stimulus and with the cooperation of organized labor, employers have aided in the establishment of broader medical care programs as well. Progress in smaller industries has been much less rapid in general. Since a large part of our labor force works in these smaller plants, this remains a key problem area in industrial medical care. Also persisting as a problem area of major concern is the manner in which workmen's compensation programs are, in general, applied; sufficient emphasis is still not being placed in these programs on the restoration of workers to health and gainful employment.

A. *Methods of Providing Service*

72. DEVELOPMENT OF INDUSTRIAL MEDICINE *

IN ORGANIZING MEDICAL care in the widest sense of the term, industry is confronted with two entirely different problems: (1) the occupational accidents and diseases, and (2) the accidents and diseases not caused by or incidental to employment. In line with modern concepts, extensive preventive activities and health education, as well as provisions for treatment, must be part of the program for the protection of workers in the plants. Community services of this type greatly influence the frequency and the severity of nonoccupational conditions causing absenteeism or impeding the efficiency of the worker.

Various patterns have been developed in establishing and operating medical care programs in industry. Workmen's compensation laws have become the basis for services to workers injured or contracting sickness on the job or in connection with employment. Voluntary action on the part of employers or of both employers and employees has resulted in provisions for workers, or for employees and their family dependents, in case of nonoccupational illness and accident. There is a wide variety in the medical care available at present, dependent on many factors, such as type of work, size of industrial operation, and location.

Workmen's compensation legislation, beginning in the states in 1911 and extended to all states by 1948, led to the development of industrial medicine. It put the responsibility for medical care of the injured upon the employer, who discharged his financial obligations in various ways. Over the years insurance with commercial insurance companies and payment into state funds have become the prevailing methods, while self-insurance has become relatively uncommon.

Originally, injured workers were sent to doctors outside the plant, who as traumatic surgeons became expert in looking after such cases. Many of them became specialists in workmen's compensation medicine, and their practice consisted largely of injured workers. The first pattern of providing service has persisted through the years in many industries; it has been useful to small employers.

As plants grew in size and the rate of accidents increased, many employers found it economical from every angle—promptness of treatment, saving of time and money—to provide in-plant service, with doctors and nurses serving full or part time, depending upon the type of work and the size of the plant. It was soon

* From: "Medical Care in Industry," by William A. Sawyer, M.D.; *Annals of the American Academy of Political and Social Science,* Vol. 273 (entitled *Medical Care for Americans*), Jan. 1951, pp. 151-59. Reprinted (with omissions, including one table) by permission of the author and publishers. The author, who is health consultant for the International Association of Machinists, lives in Rochester, N.Y.

learned that the best treatment was the cheapest. Prompt and adequate care reduced lost time and prevented disabilities. This gave impetus to greater safety
measures, and, in conjunction with safety programs, reduced the toll of accidents.

Because of these efforts there has been a downward trend in the number and
the severity of accidents, but they still represent a costly problem in human lives
and suffering, and in lost wages and production.

Occupational Accidents and Diseases

In 1948, out of 59,400,000 gainfully employed persons in this country, about
1,960,000 suffered disabling injuries while at work, or roughly, 1 out of every
30 workers. The vast majority of these injuries (almost 95 per cent) were minor,
causing loss of work of a day or more, but no permanent ill effect. Of the rest,
however, 16,500 people died from their injuries; 1,800 suffered permanent and
total disability; and 83,700 were injured so severely that they will be disabled to
some extent the rest of their lives. For those permanently injured, and for the
families of those killed, this means not only suffering and grief and a complete
readjustment of their lives, but often economic disaster. Though workmen's compensation payments help with the medical and some of the living expenses, the
families bear the major loss and often undergo hardship and deprivation in reducing
their standards of living.

Industry also loses from these accidents, not only in the services of the
workmen but economically. Cost studies by the National Safety Council estimated
the loss to the national economy for 1948 at $2,650,000,000. This included visible
costs of wage loss, expense of medical care, and overhead cost of compensation
insurance, and the estimated value of damage to equipment, time lost by other
workers, and production slowdowns.

The death and accident rates for 1948 varied greatly in the major industrial
groups, as shown in table 45. . . .

TABLE 45.   *Industrial death and accident rates, 1948*

	Deaths per 100,000 Workers	Injury Frequency Rates per 500 Employees
Trade	14	10.89
Service	15	9.32
Manufacturing	16	10.04
Public Utilities	29	10.72
Transportation	48	17.68
Agriculture	55	unreported
Construction	93	16.51
Mining and Quarrying, Oil and Gas Wells	154	30.46

. . . There is little doubt that systematic efforts to reduce accidents bear results.
For many years the National Safety Council has carried on a program of education
within the industries to reduce the accident rates, and its success has been out-

standing. Among the companies reporting to it (6,700 in 1948, representing 7,000,000 workers), the accident frequency rate declined 58 per cent and the severity rate 50 per cent between 1930 and 1947. This is not representative of industry at large, however. Rieke says that it is an "easily substantiable fact that 70 per cent of industry has the most elementary of safety programs." [1]

As Dublin, Lotka, and Spiegelman point out, industry today is changing so rapidly, and is conducted on such a large scale and at such an increasing tempo, that new hazards arise as old ones are conquered, and it is impossible to know just what is happening. Dust, next to accidents, has been the chief cause of occupational disability and death. The use of chemicals in industry is constantly increasing the hazards of poisoning; yet the number of workmen suffering from industrial poisoning is unknown. The use of carbon monoxide, benzol, lead, mercury, chromium, arsenic, beryllium, radium, X rays, nuclear fission products, and radioactive isotopes makes poisoning a major hazard; but the symptoms of diseases resulting from these things, particularly in the early stages, are so obscure that physicians are often unable to diagnose them. Consequently, many cases are not reported. There is also a lack of uniformity among workmen's compensation board reports which makes it impossible to obtain accurate information. . . .

Many manufacturers of chemicals have established industrial hygiene departments which test new compounds before using or marketing them. This is a wise precaution. In the atomic energy plants where health hazards have been anticipated, proper preventive measures have been taken, with excellent results. More employers are realizing that safe working conditions improve morale and save the cost of unfortunate accidents.

Quality of Service

As FAR BACK as the early 1900's, physicians employed in industry emphasized the unusual opportunity to carry on preventive medicine. Though industry on the whole has viewed medical service chiefly in terms of its economic value and the protection of itself against the excessive costs of caring for the injured as required by workmen's compensation laws, many of the early industrial physicians saw the immense possibilities not only of bringing prompt and adequate relief to the injured, but also of protecting workers from occupational disabilities, guiding them to correct medical care, and educating them in ways of better living and better health.

Enlightened management approved of this. In the industries where management has encouraged him, the physician has seen an ever widening opportunity for preventive medicine. Considering the successful results of his efforts in the far too few places, it is easy to envisage the great benefits that can be derived from extension of preventive medicine to more of the gainfully employed. The caliber of service rendered is usually but the shadow of the top management. If management is enlightened, the attitude of the doctor and the nurse is usually good, and

1. Forrest E. Rieke, "Evolution of Small Plant Health Service as a Private Practice," *Industrial Medicine and Surgery*, July 1950.

the service, as far as it goes, is adequate. The American College of Surgeons, in an effort to raise the quality of service, has given certificates of approval to those industries which meet certain standards.

Nonoccupational Illness

SERIOUS AND COSTLY as are absences from work due to occupational accidents and diseases, they are but a fraction, variously estimated at one-tenth or less, of those caused by nonoccupational disabilities.

Absence rates due to illness are studied carefully by many industrial companies, and every reasonable effort is made to reduce them. One of the interesting facts that comes out of a study of absence due to illness and injuries is that a small percentage of employees accounts for a major part of the absence. In other words, certain individuals are more accident and sickness prone than the majority. These are the ones that a good industrial medical service can help with early diagnosis of their symptoms and proper advice regarding their physical conditions and living habits. This is a real opportunity for prevention.

In an attempt to control absence from work due to illness, many degrees of effort are used, extending all the way from the occasional examination or interview by the physician or nurse to a full-fledged program, such as that of the Hawthorne Works of the Western Electric Company. In a period of five years 13 per cent of the employees were found to be responsible for 50 per cent of the sickness absences during the total service of the 1939 plant population. It was assumed that 87 per cent of the employees did not have an unusual amount of sickness. The five-year follow-up program was based on influencing the record of the 13 per cent. Despite unforeseen wartime complications, the health of this sickness-prone group was improved and the frequency of sickness absence was reduced.

Pre-employment Examination

To THE PHYSICIAN in industry in the early days, it soon became evident that a healthy, able-bodied worker was less likely to have an accident than one who was ailing from some physical defect. This concept led to the pre-employment examination for better job placement, which is a protection to employer and employee alike. Each job calls for certain qualifications: some for special qualities such as above-average manual co-ordination, specific degrees of muscular strength, mental alertness, and good vision. Knowledge of jobs and their environment and knowing supervision are essential to good placement.

If an applicant is not found adequate for the job specified, he is recommended for some less exacting position or referred to his physician for treatment with the hope that he can later qualify. After the condition has been improved by the family doctor, the applicant is often accepted for employment. Not infrequently an applicant with defects is accepted for work with the understanding that within a stated period of time he will see his own physician and receive necessary medical attention. This calls for follow-up examinations and enables the plant medical service to act in the role of expediter in bringing about early remedial attention.

Only a small percentage of applicants are rejected outright for contagious diseases or some degenerative and uncorrectable conditions. The rejection rate during the past war was almost negligible, and over late years it has averaged less than 3 per cent.

Keeping Workers Fit

THE PRELIMINARY examination and follow-up of the new applicant are only a small part of an industrial medical service. It is just as important that everything be done to keep the regular employee on the job as steadily as possible. An employee who is physically fit is a better, more productive, and more efficient worker, less likely to have accidents, and better able to get along with the other workmen. Workers often come to work with minor illnesses or develop them on the job—such as headaches, colds, gastrointestinal upsets, and other discomforting symptoms. These are treated by the medical service to tide the worker over for the day. Diagnosis is expedited by making X rays and laboratory tests so that the employee may get the earliest possible adequate care from his family doctor.

Good eyesight is becoming extremely valuable in our complex industrial production. Proper eye glasses, often with safety lenses, are essential to good production and safe working conditions. Faulty vision is a common defect and must be kept constantly under surveillance. Failing vision in the older employee can be the cause of mistakes and accidents, and this can often be remedied by proper glasses.

Thus, medical programs once instituted and begun on a minimum scale slowly extend their services. In their talking with workers from day to day, both physicians and nurses in the medical service carry on a certain amount of health education—teaching better health habits and care. Specific programs are also developing in this sphere. Nutritionists have been added to some medical departments to consult with employees referred for dietary problems.... Where counseling nutritionists have been added to the medical staff, they have augmented popular knowledge by the printed word and displays, as well as by personal interviews, and have worked toward better-balanced meals in plant cafeterias.

Sustaining Morale

IF EMPLOYEES are paid a sickness allowance when absent from work because of nonoccupational illness, as has been voluntarily done by some industries for many years and is now legally required in four states,* a visiting nurse service is valuable both to employee and to employer. Genuinely friendly visits demonstrate the interest of the company in the employee, and the nurse, an employee herself,

---

* California, New Jersey, New York, and Rhode Island.

forms a liaison between the employee and management. The nurse can determine, from her training, how ill the employee is, whether he is receiving adequate medical care, how long he may be absent, and whether the company can do anything to facilitate his recovery.

The industrial physician finds, just as does the private physcian, that a surprisingly large percentage of the visits to the medical service in which the patient complains about one or more physical discomforts—headache, gastrointestinal upsets, and so forth—lead to discovery of some personal problem confronting him. Sometimes the doctor or nurse can only encourage and comfort by listening; the mere opportunity of having understanding listeners is in itself a partial cure. It is human to have fears and "gripes"; in the impersonal atmosphere of high-pressure industry, it is a relief valve for all to have someone to whom employees, including management, can go with the assurance that their well-being is the important thing. Much of the effort in the medical service is directed in the last analysis toward good employee relations and adjustment to jobs.

Thus, the doctor who at first confined himself to traumatic problems found that if his professional training was to be of the greatest benefit, he must be mindful of the "whole man"—not only the detection of disease, but the maintenance of good health; not only the organic structure, but the emotional and social aspect of the worker as well.

Types of Programs

A VERY SMALL number of industrial companies, chiefly those with a large labor force, have extended their services by providing their employees with comprehensive medical care for nonoccupational as well as occupational diseases and accidents, and a few have included also the family dependents of the worker. In some instances all the costs are borne by the company, and in others a varying proportion of the costs is met through voluntary prepayment plans to which the workers contribute.

Examples of various types of organization are the Endicott-Johnson Company in Johnson City, New York; the American Cast Iron Pipe Company in Birmingham, Alabama; the Tennessee Coal, Iron and Railroad Company in Fairfield, Alabama; the Homestake Mining Company in the Blackhills District, South Dakota; and the Standard Oil Company of Louisiana in Baton Rouge. The programs at these companies are noteworthy for the inclusion of all essential services, especially hospitalization and specialist services. In some instances the hospitals are owned by the company, and in others hospital and clinic facilities within the community are utilized. . . .

Achievements of Industrial Medicine

THE REAL achievement of industrial medicine is its effect on the health and happiness of the workers whom it has served. In 1948, Dr. C. O. Sappington surveyed for the Industrial Hygiene Foundation 278 industries with medical services and gathered convincing evidence of its value. He lists under economic benefits the prompt treatment of injuries which has ensured the prevention of infection and other complications, and the early control and prevention of disability. He finds that in-plant service is much more economical than referral of workers to outside agencies and that it gives better control of medical, hospital, and workmen's compensation expenses. Good medical care is more economical than high compensation rates, which can be translated in terms of dollars and cents if need be, and has long been the contention of good insurance carriers. That a healthy worker is more productive and less prone to accident, he feels, has been demonstrated many times.

Among the professional benefits, Dr. Sappington brings out the irrefutable fact that proper health supervision provides a very unusual opportunity for case-finding, in which early disease may be discovered before disability occurs, and when disease can more easily be cured. Industrial medical care is a direct approach to health maintenance, resulting in uniformly high standards of treatment and efficiency. It is a check on placement, transfer, exposure, accident proneness, and absenteeism, with emphasis on prevention.

Among the many social benefits, Dr. Sappington finds that contentment and stability among employees are promoted, and this means better industrial and public relations. Industrial medical care is an aid to proper job adjustment, and promotes "take-home" health standards. It preserves industry's greatest asset—people. "The human body has no spare parts." It solves many petty personal problems and overcomes emotional difficulties.

Another possible yardstick by which the achievements of industrial medicine can be measured is the status it has gained within the medical profession. Organized medicine has been slow to recognize industrial medicine as a specialty. Many thought it departed too far from the time-honored orthodoxy of private practice and smacked somewhat of "contract practice." Industrial physicians formed their own organization in 1914—The American Association of Industrial Physicians and Surgeons—which has continued its leadership ever since. Shortly after, the National Industrial Conference Board formed a small kindred organization of Physicians in Industry. These two groups did more than any others to advance the ideals and standards of physicians in industry in the early years.

Recognition of Industrial Medicine

IT IS AN ACHIEVEMENT that medical service in industry has reached a point of importance where surveys of its quantity and quality are made, and attempts by professional groups are made to raise its standards. In addition to the above, the Industrial Hygiene Division of the United States Public Health Service has endeavored to influence its development, the first survey being in 1919. Through state labor departments and workmen's compensation boards, efforts at standardization have been made and the industrial hygiene division of state health departments have played an increasingly important role in helping industrial companies to develop various types of service.

In 1937 the American Medical Association officially recognized industrial medicine by establishing the Council on Industrial Health, which is doing much to further the values in this specialty. Efforts are being made to establish industrial medicine under the American Examining Boards for specialty rating. To accomplish this, it is necessary to have in our medical schools and schools of public health, departments of industrial medicine with fellowships and the equivalent of residencies in hospitals. Already there has been some accomplishment in providing both under-graduate and postgraduate instruction in our medical schools in co-operation with some of the larger industries. This is a requisite of recognition and a means of providing well-trained personnel.

In World War II a great deal of emphasis was placed on the value of medical service in the war industries. A splendid record of achievement was made in con-trolling the health of those exposed to hazards in munitions work. Also, a notable accomplishment took place in those projects having to do with the development of the atomic bomb.

Through the years there has been some union recognition of pre-employment examinations, whereas in the beginning there was almost complete refusal to approve such procedures. A notable example of union approval was the early establishment by the International Ladies Garment Workers' Union of its Union Health Center, which has grown into an admirable example of how unions can provide medical service at low cost. . . . Lately, the United Mine Workers * have set up a high quality of medical service. Sufficient time has not elapsed to estimate its success. Any recognition of the principle of such medical service by unions is a step forward.

Inadequate Coverage

WHILE THERE HAVE been distinct achievements by industrial medicine since it came into being, there have also been shortcomings. For one thing, it has not been sufficiently accepted. It is somewhat like the democratic form of government. Even though it has succeeded in some places, not enough have embraced it. Unfortunately, on-the-job medical service has not been provided widely enough. In attempting to consider the extent of it, we are faced with insufficient factual information. It has been estimated that not more than 10 to 15 per cent of the 60 million gainfully employed in all occupations receive such service. To many engaged in such service, this seems an overly generous estimate; but it does point out the inadequacy of coverage. Limited surveys have been made, but they have never covered more than 2 million employees.

Most of the industrial medical services are concentrated in the manufacturing industries. In the other major employment groups there are few medical pro-grams. . . .

Many employers believe that a worker's health is his own responsibility. Especially among proprietors of small plants there is a reticence about being in-volved in the difficulties of setting up, or participating in, a medical care program,

* See Selection No. 76A in this chapter, beginning on page 521, for a description of the medical care program of the United Mine Workers.

and a fear of its cost. A lack of understanding of its efficacy in making for a better working force is doubtless a big reason why there is so little service available in small units. It is a safe guess that not 5 per cent of the companies with fewer than 500 employees have any such service.

There are no complete factual data on the subject available. A few plants with under 500 employees have done an outstanding job, but there were 266,000 firms of that size listed in 1948. In that year 52 per cent of the manufacturing establishments in the country employed fewer than 10 workers, which is an important reason why service has not been extended more widely. Accident frequency is much higher in small factories than in large. It has been said by state labor departments, state health departments, and insurance inspectors that there is a woeful lack of response on the part of small employers, especially to recommendations regarding certain accident and health hazards. Few, if any, industrial communities have developed medical care programs designed to meet the needs of small plants.

The lack of properly trained personnel in industrial medicine, as in other spheres of activity, is outstanding. The failure of some employers and some unions and part of organized medicine to see the full implications of a truly preventive program in our industries is indeed discouraging.

Need, Prospect, and Methods

THE NEED FOR ADEQUATE medical care in industry, small as well as large, is overwhelming.

How to break through the indifference, the ignorance, and the fears is one of the imponderables. That some progress has been made is scant comfort when vision and initiative are lacking in so many quarters and there is so little of the will to give industrial medicine a trial.... What of the future?

Industrial medical service might be approached through one of several ways:

1. It can continue to be an employer provision, as it is now for the most part, and as it began.

2. It can be on an insurance basis as a voluntary measure or as a governmental requirement.

3. It can be financed by a tax on the product, as in the plan of the United Mine Workers, or by joint contributions of employers and employees, as in the International Ladies Garment Workers Union.

4. It can never be provided adequately by private practitioners, although it has been hoped that they could play a larger part in providing service for the smaller businesses. At all times, it must be remembered that any plan should be based on teamwork, participated in by all of the medical profession, general practitioners and specialists, by nurses, technicians, social workers, voluntary and official public health agencies, hospitals, social welfare groups, and any other organized and trained personnel which can contribute to the physical, mental, and social well-being of those who are gainfully employed.

73. PROVISIONS FOR IN-PLANT CARE *

THERE HAS BEEN too great a tendency for industrial hygiene physicians and engineers to gather at official conferences, association assemblies, and annual banquets of medical directors, and discourse at great length on what they are doing to protect the health of workers while in reality their programs fall far short of these objectives. Sometimes the impression is quite evident that these mutual admiration contests are a sort of defense mechanism for what is being left undone.

In too many plant medical departments, the primary and often the sole function is to provide reparative service for injuries, and the medical department owes its existence to the fact that the plant is a self-insurer. Although it can be shown that a medical department can usually provide more efficient treatment of injuries, it should not limit its activities to "finger-wrapping," either on a literal or figurative basis. Within certain limits, it can prove its greater value by expending its activities to include the prevention of disease as well as the treatment of injuries....

Preplacement Physical Examinations

THE PURPOSE of a preplacement physical examination should be to determine in what capacity the prospective employee can be utilized most efficiently without detriment to himself or his fellow workers. The emphasis should be on spreading employment to as many workers as possible rather than on exclusion. In the past, physical requirements have often been too exacting. Even in times of peace, this has resulted in many undue hardships and has been partially responsible for coolness, if not open opposition, on the part of organized labor toward industrial medical services....

Physical standards should be based on the requirements of the job involved. For example, most persons free of mental disorders, active pulmonary tuberculosis, or severe visual defects are capable of performing clerical duties. The loss of a lower extremity, or the presence of hernia, moderate degree of heart disease, or diabetes mellitus under adquate control need not be a bar to employment. In sedentary occupations, in general, the usual requirements are likely to be far less exacting than for the more strenuous jobs.

The unreasonable attitude toward arterial hypertension is a case in point. In the past there has been too great a tendency to set arbitrary standards. All persons

* From: "Medical Services," by O. F. Hedley, M.D.; Chap. IV (pp. 43-65) in *Manual of Industrial Hygiene and Medical Service in War Industries* (William M. Gafafer, ed.), Philadelphia: W. B. Saunders, 1943. Reprinted (with omissions, including initial paragraphs) by permission of the publishers. The author was, at the time of his death in 1952, medical director of the Public Health Office, Mutual Security Agency, Washington, D.C.

with arterial blood pressure over 150 millimeters of mercury systolic pressure, or over 90 millimeters of mercury diastolic have often been declared ineligible for employment at a given plant, even though there was no evidence of cardiac insufficiency or other organic changes due to arterial hypertension. Save in infrequent instances, such as the jobs of crane operators, locomotive engineers, or other special occupations, most persons with moderate degrees of arterial hypertension should be regarded as employable. Similarly, most persons with inactive pulmonary tuberculosis, heart disease without cardiac insufficiency, diabetes mellitus, bronchial asthma, orthopedic defects, and many other conditions are fit for most jobs. *If the applicant is not fit for the job for which employment is sought, efforts should be made in the direction of job placement.*

Workers exposed to toxic substances such as TNT, DNT, tetryl, fulminate of mercury, or lead azide should be subject to more rigid requirements than other workers. Efforts should be made to eliminate habitual users of alcohol, mouth breathers, those with marked dental defects, and particularly persons showing any indication of anemia, liver or kidney diseases, or chronic respiratory diseases. Persons undergoing treatment for syphilis should not be employed in toxic operations. Persons with skin diseases should not be exposed to substances known to cause occupational dermatoses.

Because a liberal policy is advocated in the matter of spreading employment, this should not be interpreted as condoning laxity or slipshod preemployment physical examinations. There is probably no other criterion as reliable in determining the efficiency of a medical department as the thoroughness with which it performs these examinations....

One of the criticisms directed at preemployment physical examinations by organized labor is that applicants are not informed concerning causes for rejection or about physical defects which should be corrected. In the mind of labor such an examination is quite one-sided. This criticism is not without merit. Regardless of the desirability for speed in examining large numbers of applicants, the physician should take the time personally to inform the rejected applicant of the cause for his rejection. Accepted applicants should be informed of physical defects, particularly if they may be corrected. The physician, if possible, should inform them concerning the more serious defects with a view to facilitating corrective measures, while employees can be informed of less important defects by the nurses who should exert influence toward having them corrected....

Plant physicians by their manner and their interest in prospective employees' welfare during the preplacement examination have an opportunity to gain the workers' confidence. If the worker looks upon the physician as an interested friend, if he feels that the medical department is a "neutral zone" in which his confidences will be respected, he will avail himself of the opportunity to discuss his health problems with the plant physician. This will redound to the greater efficiency of the medical department which can only attain its greatest usefulness by winning the confidence of both management and labor.

Periodic Physical Examinations

UNDER NORMAL CONDITIONS each employee should have a health audit, preferably once a year. Some plants limit these examinations to employees past the age of 40. Other plants find that by examining workers returning from illness, approximately 80 per cent of their employees are examined during the course of the year. These examinations are used in lieu of examinations at stated periods. This plan has the advantage of examining an employee at a time when he is more likely to be interested in his health than simply by appointment. The remaining 20 per cent who have not been absent on account of illness are examined by appointment. . . .

This discussion is particularly applicable to the explosives industry, either manufacturing or the filling and assembly of projectiles, bombs, or their components. Other war industries have workers who are exposed to lead, mercury, silica, benzene, solvent vapors, metallic fumes, dermatitis producers, and other substances whose control should include physical examinations of exposed persons at periodic intervals. It should be emphasized that the physical examination should be used in conjunction with engineering methods of control, never in lieu of a proper working environment. In the prevention of occupational disease the physician and the engineer must work side by side to attain the proper results.

To prevent occupational disease the plant physician should have a working knowledge of the industrial processes involved, the number of workers exposed, and the degree of exposure. He should inform himself with regard to the maximum permissible concentrations and know under what circumstances and in what places the maximum allowable concentrations may be exceeded. He should make frequent inspections of the workrooms and of the change houses, and should determine the adequacy and efficiency of the shower baths. It is essential that he have a thorough insight into the clinical manifestations of occupational diseases to which workers under his supervision may become exposed. He should know the prodromal as well as the full-blown manifestations of these conditions. . . .

Other Examinations of Employees

BECAUSE OF THE shortage of physicians and the pressure of production, it is doubtful if it is feasible to examine physically every employee who has been absent from work on account of illness. He should be required to obtain a clearance through the medical department, and the nurse should obtain a record of the cause of illness. He should be examined by a physician if the illness is over a designated number of days' duration (usually three or seven days), if he is still having a fever, if the illness has apparently been due to a communicable disease, or if he appears too weak to resume work.

The objection may be raised that this leaves too much to the discretion of a nurse. As a matter of fact, it would be almost impossible to have a physician examine each employee who has been absent in a plant covering many acres or square miles, and which is operating three shifts a day. In times of emergency, more responsibility should be given the nurses.

One of the chief practical values of sick absenteeism records is that they enable the plant physicians to examine employees with poor attendance records to determine the causes of absenteeism with a view of correcting them. Here the industrial hygiene nurse or the visiting nurse can be of considerable assistance in determining the validity of alleged causes of absenteeism.

This raises the point about the attitude of the medical department to malingering, either due to feigned illnesses or injuries, or attempts to exaggerate existing injuries. Insofar as possible the medical department should assume the role of neutral arbiter. It should not exist primarily for the purpose of serving as a sort of truant system; neither should it condone flagrant malingering. It has a responsibility both to the employee and to the firm.

Many concerns have the policy of physically examining employees on transfer or promotion. Where the transfers involve changes in exposure to a deleterious substance, or there is a history of injury on the previous job, such a physical examination would seem indicated. . . .

The purpose of the medical department is to serve the plant and the employees. It will be requested by the workers for examination and advice concerning many conditions not directly due to their occupations. Unless such requests become unreasonable or tend to conflict too greatly with the private practice of medicine, efforts should be made to comply with such requests. . . .

Supervisors not infrequently request that a worker be examined either to detect communicable disease or to determine his fitness for work. Such examinations should be performed, but every effort should be made to respect the right of the employee with regard to professional confidences.

It is the practice of some industrial establishments to examine a person at the time of discharge to determine if he has developed an injury or occupational disease while working for them. Such a practice has merit in instances where persons are exposed to dust or toxic chemical substances, or where there is a history of injury. . . .

Records

THE RECORDS OF THE medical department should be retained in the medical department and kept in such a manner that the confidence of the employee is respected. Statements to other departments should be couched in general phrases, and except for injuries and occupational diseases, diagnostic expressions should not be included in oral or written communications to other departments or persons.

A cumulative health record should be maintained on each employee. This should include the history and physical examination obtained on employment, laboratory studies including X-ray findings, and the results of periodic physical examinations. . . . For the sake of convenience and in event the records are subpoenaed for court action, it is desirable that they be kept in a folder in such a manner as to insure against parts of the record being lost. . . .

The Small Plant

AMONG THE MANY unsolved problems in industrial medicine is that of furnishing adequate protection for the employees of small plants. Plants with less than a thousand employees are often unable to supply adequate medical facilities at a cost which they regard as within their means. Certainly few of them can afford to employ a full-time physician; in some of the smaller plants it is not even feasible to employ a nurse on a full-time basis.

Ideally, it would be advantageous for a number of these plants to obtain the services of a physician, each paying a prorated amount.... Industrial hygiene clinics, offered as a suggestion, are only available in a few places.

It is doubtful if any plan could be developed which would be universally applicable to this group of plants.... The following suggestions are made with a hope that some of them may serve as a guide in solving this problem:

1. Combine resources where possible.
2. Utilize industrial hygiene clinics of good repute.
3. Seek advice of the State division of industrial hygiene in planning program, and in identifying and controlling occupational hazards.
4. Obtain the services of a visiting nurse if plant is too small to justify a full-time nursing program.
5. Even though the physician is part-time he should develop an interest in the preventive aspects of industrial medicine and in employee welfare. To this end the employment of physicians on an "on call" fee basis should be discouraged....

74. THE PREPAYMENT PRINCIPLE *

DURING THE PAST 35 years, the increasing interest in industrial medicine has been paralleled by the growing interest in voluntary prepaid medicine....

In Tacoma, Washington, a plan of prepaid medical care for industry was started by the County Medical Society in June, 1917. This plan is actuarially sound, as its long record of successful operation testifies. It is a "service"-type plan in which, by agreement, certain medical services are rendered to policyholders. This is in contrast to the "indemnity" or "fixed-payment" policies widely advocated by many present prepay medical care plans.

One of the commonly accepted viewpoints of industrial practice is that it must carefully refrain from personal medical services other than those of a temporary

* From: "Successful Prepaid Medicine in Industry: A Complete Industrial Medical Program," by Charles M. McGill, M.D., and Sherman S. Pinto, M.D.; *Industrial Medicine and Surgery* 21:438-39, Sept. 1952 (No. 9). Reprinted (with omissions) by permission of the authors and publishers. The authors are, respectively, the medical director of the Tacoma Smelter, American Smelting and Refining Company, Tacoma, Wash.; and the medical director of the American Smelting and Refining Company, Denver, Colo.

type. However, . . . the nation's pioneer medical society-sponsored, competitive, service-type health insurance plan . . . provides complete, continuing medical care for an industrial group.

As stated, this plan, the Pierce County Industrial Medical Bureau, has been in effect since 1917. Since 1931 similar health insurance plans sponsored by medical societies have been inaugurated in 21 other counties in Washington State, and all are inter-related with a cooperative group sponsored by the State medical association. This is the best answer yet made available by the medical associations for the socialistic-minded who clamor for control of our medical practice. It is of importance to us primarily as it affects industry and industrial medical practice. This Tacoma plan provides complete medical care for over 700 industrial groups, covering more than 22,000 men and 8,000 women employees (plus a catastrophic coverage for other members of the family numbering in excess of 11,000). This is the bulk of our employed population in a community of about 200,000.

The only industry having a full-time physician is the one I * serve. This group of 1,200 in a basic non-ferrous smelter and refinery has been insured under this Medical Bureau since 1939. Before that time medical coverage was obtained through a private contract. Some 95% of the 200 eligible county physicians are members of this non-profit Medical Bureau, and are available to provide service to all our employees. These doctor-members elect a board of directors each year, and this board employs an executive secretary to supervise the 16 employees administering the plan. Since the physicians control and run the plan themselves, they are the ones who suffer if it is mishandled. In effect, they underwrite any operating deficit by means of a percentage reduction in their basic fee schedule.

The plant with which I am associated is about five miles from the center of town, where the majority of the physicians have their offices. The Medical Bureau is eager to give our employees the most convenient medical care possible. This is done through an arrangement with the smelter which allows the physician to provide such medical care in the plant dispensary, employee's home, or hospital as the physician or patient feels is indicated. The smelter physician, then, can see an employee for either occupational or non-occupational conditions and can follow the diagnosis with such treatment as is necessary. It should be emphasized again that these employees have a free choice of physicians and are not restricted to the physician at the smelter. From experience we know the majority of these employees visit our dispensary, even though many of them concurrently or later go to their own family doctor. Such visits permit medical counseling in the truest sense of the word.

Plans such as this give a tremendous advantage to the industrial physician in his control of occupational diseases, and greatly expand his activities and opportunities in the field of public health and preventive medicine. The routine daily services of an adequately equipped and easily accessible plant dispensary, available to employees on company time, encourage early and continuous medical care without regard to the etiology of the condition. The services are not limited to

---

* I.e., Dr. McGill.

emergency non-occupational treatments or to plant-developed injuries or illness. The workmen visit the dispensary for any reason they wish, including regular medical treatments requested by their private doctors, or to discuss any matter of personal, family, or plant health. This greatly expands the areas of discussion for the doctor and employees at the health and safety committee meetings, and permits a greater utilization of the local public health facilities for the workman and his family. They can be referred to any general or special practitioner at their own or the industrial physician's request. Everything is prepaid. Diagnostic and preventive services are thus readily available without difficulty or without the intervention of any third person. The Medical Bureau pays in full to its physician members, on a fee schedule basis, the medical bills for direct services on anything coming under the provisions of the health policy.

Needless to say, there are minor limitations of the prepaid responsibilties. These include venereal disease except diagnosis, dental services, psychiatric services except diagnosis, criminally acquired injuries, congenital defects (e. g., harelip); [only] three (no more) months' hospital care for any one condition, or one year's therapy for any one condition, [are covered.] This latter limitation, however, is not too serious in Washington where the State welfare department provides full health services for all persons determined by it to be medically indigent. All other medical and surgical services are covered. This is full office, home, or hospital care. No salary limitation is applied to any industrial group.

The doctors are reimbursed for specific services on a definite point schedule basis, e. g., an appendectomy is 150 units; a gastrectomy 325 units; a colostomy 150 units; and bilateral hernia repair 160 units. To deter excessive or unnecessary office-call scheduling by the physician or patient, a monthly case average system is used. Under this arrangement, the physician is paid the same basic fee per patient seen each month regardless of the number of office calls made. Hospital costs to the extent of $400,000 were paid out last year. Although the Bureau owns and operates its own 61-bed hospital and is now expanding to twice this capacity, free choice of any of several recognized local hospitals exists. Any deficit of monthly income to total monthly bills is adjusted, after hospital bills and fixed charges are paid, by proportionally decreasing the physician's own point fees. At that, over 54 per cent of gross income, or about one-half million dollars, was paid out to member physicians last year. This is a substantial part of their income. Administration expenses were only 4 per cent, a low figure and much below usual level.

This Medical Bureau also administers the local veterans medical program and our State social welfare medical program for all categories. The plan continues to recruit industrial groups and, as evidence of its service to the community, rarely if ever do any of these groups relinquish their coverage. In fact, many groups have had continuous Bureau coverage for over 20 years.

The basic disadvantage of the plan is that it does not directly encourage preventive medicine. However, under its provisions the industrial physician or any member physician is able to do anything indicated for preventive or definitive medical care. What more ideal program could any industrial physician want? It makes more office practice of a minor nature but eliminates the money barrier to any health service that is indicated, and offers unlimited opportunity for conservation of workers' health.

These services are all provided for a basic premium of $3.40 per month for men and $3.90 per month for women, as, of course, women's special health problems are covered, excluding pregnancy, with the exception of the family coverage.

This prepaid plan greatly facilitates our medical program and in our experience has decreased the loss of time from work until it is now half the national average. This plan is further expanded by a Family Coverage Plan available for hospital and catastrophic expense illness, but not for the low-cost office and home calls. Over 65 per cent of our eligible plant families are included.

Although of less importance to our plant services, those retired at the age of 65 may continue their coverage by payment of an additional $2.50 per month, a total of $5.90. This fulfills the recommendations of the Commission on Chronic Illness for the older persons and eliminates their dependence on any socialistic-sponsored plan for the senior citizen.

Our program is effective and successful because it is locally administered and controlled, because it is competitive, because it is sponsored by the medical society, and because it is a prepaid "service"-type health insurance. It supplements an all-inclusive industrial medical program in which the fullest aspect of preventive and industrial in-plant medical service complements definitive care. It keeps men at work, decreases lost time and labor turnover, and, by permitting early and complete medical care, keeps more men at work more days—the objective of all of us practicing industrial medicine.

75. ORGANIZED LABOR'S ATTITUDE *

A MAJOR TURNING point in the history of medical-care insurance [1] for industrial workers occurred in 1950. In the late 1940's, signs of imminent change were abundant, but there was much speculation about what would develop. However, the patterns established in 1950 make possible a clearer picture of the future in this field.

1. In this article medical-care insurance refers to planned methods for budgeting and paying the cost of medical care by pooling the economic hazards of sickness, injury, and maternity and the financial resources of a group of individuals. It includes hospitalization, physician services, and services from other professional health personnel and facilities. It excludes planned methods for compensating the loss of earning due to disability for nonoccupational causes, frequently called temporary disability insurance or weekly sickness and accident benefits. The term health insurance is avoided in this article because it is commonly applied to these two types of programs together or separately. . . .

* From: "Medical-Care Insurance for Industrial Workers," by Walter J. Lear, M.D.; *Monthly Labor Review* 73:251-57, Sept. 1951 (No. 3). Reprinted with omissions. The author is associate medical director of the Health Insurance Plan of Greater New York.

The beginnings of medical-care insurance in this country were made to meet the needs of specific industries or groups of workers. This trend was definitely limited. In the past decade, industrial workers have obtained medical-care insurance coverage from programs sponsored and controlled by interests other than management and labor—principally the health professions and the private insurance companies. In this way, management and labor have accepted, although at times reluctantly, existing patterns of health and medical services.

Introduction of health programs under collective bargaining has provided a major opportunity for significant changes of many kinds. By the end of 1950, the primary effect of these changes had been to extend the coverage of existing plans to more workers and to help shift a greater part of the direct costs of medical-care insurance to the employer. Like other industrial medical-care insurance programs, collective-bargaining programs have, with few exceptions, utilized Blue Cross, medical society, and insurance company plans.

With reasonable progress in answering the special problems of workers as well as the general questions raised by a more enlightened public, these three principal types of medical-care insurance can be expected to cover the largest proportion of the employed population with hospitalization and in-hospital physician services. Nevertheless, these programs cannot be expected to give much help to the solution of major problems in the organization of medical-care insurance or the quality of medical care. Rather, they are more closely identified with the old and continuing drive for economic security—the strivings of the gainfully employed to cushion financial pressures in an industrialized society.

Developments Prior to 1950

INDUSTRIAL WORKERS benefited from some of the earliest forerunners of present-day medical-care insurance plans. These were the mutual-benefit associations, first started in the 1860's and 1870's, which spread rapidly to a wide variety of industries and businesses.

Some of these mutual-benefit associations were initiated, administered, and financed by management; some, by the workers; and some, jointly. Their principal function was the payment of cash benefits to the member when he was sick and to his family when he died. Medical-care benefits, when provided, were almost always limited to cash payments.

At about the same time, the lumber, mining, oil, and railroad industries were expanding into new areas. Frequently isolated, they found it useful to provide their employees with rather complete medical services. In some instances, extensive medical staffs and facilities were organized, and in a few, hospitals were built which continue in operation today. The enactment of State workmen's compensation laws in the early 1900's further stimulated the development of medical-service plans.

Benefit programs were important in the early development of labor unions. They were financed by the union members and generally provided cash benefits similar to those of the mutual-benefit associations. Only in a few notable cases did labor unions add medical services of some type to their benefit activities.

Whether sponsored by management, by the workers, or jointly, industrial medical-service plans proved to be definitely limited in both number and enrollment. . . .

Enrollment in industrial medical-service plans, however, represents a fraction of medical-care insurance coverage of industrial workers. By the late 1940's, the Blue Cross, medical society, and insurance company plans were well established. All these plans, at least initially, sought mass enrollments from groups to which coverage could be sold with relative ease and which represented in terms of health an average or better cross section of people. Since industrial workers meet both of these requirements, it is not surprising that the bulk of the membership in these plans was drawn from employed groups and their families.

A development with perhaps the greatest potentialities was the inclusion of health and welfare plans in labor-management agreements. The first agreement with an employee benefits clause was negotiated in 1926 and provided weekly sickness benefits. This type of clause, however, was infrequent up to World War II and the concomitant wage stabilization programs, which limited wage increases but permitted reasonable employee benefits. In that period of control, medical-care benefits were first included in employee benefit programs under collective bargaining. The obligation to bargain on such programs was an issue in a number of cases heard by the National War Labor Board and subsequently taken through the courts. Decisions in these cases established health, welfare, and pension plans as proper subjects for collective bargaining.

The inclusion of employee benefit programs in collective-bargaining agreements became widespread in 1949. This trend was greatly accelerated by the conclusions of the President's Fact Finding Board in the Steel Industry Dispute and by the inclusion of the recommended insurance programs in the subsequent agreements between the large steel companies and the United Steelworkers of America (CIO). . . .

Types and Extent of Insurance, 1950

THE MEDICAL-CARE insurance plans covering most industrial workers are the same three types that are generally available to the public—Blue Cross, medical society, and commercial group insurance.

Blue Cross hospitalization insurance is provided throughout the United States by about 85 autonomous nonprofit organizations, sponsored by the local hospitals and approved by a national coordinating body, the Blue Cross Commission of the American Hospital Association. Their ideal is to provide service benefits—hospitalization in ward or semiprivate rooms at no cost beyond the premiums for a period which will include almost all acute illness. This ideal is approximated by some of the Blue Cross plans, notably Michigan Hospital Service, which provides 120 days of hospital service. On the other hand, some Blue Cross plans provide cash benefits only. . . .

Insurance against some of the costs of physician services is available throughout the country from plans sponsored by State or local medical societies. About 80 autonomous plans of this type are in operation, and most of them are nonprofit. Almost all of these plans are closely associated with Blue Cross plans either through single boards of directors, identical executive staffs, or joint operating agreements. Many belong to the Blue Shield association, originally a subsidiary of the American Medical Association but recently given independent status. The American Medical Association retains the mechanism for professional approval of these and all other plans which prepay the costs of physician services.

These medical-society plans are usually limited to surgery, although some also cover other physician services in the hospital. Over half of them provide (1) service benefits to subscribers having annual incomes of less than a stated amount, and (2) cash indemnities, according to a fee schedule, to those with higher incomes. About a third provide cash benefits only. . . .

A large number of insurance companies now sell group-insurance policies which provide one or more of the following cash benefits: hospital expense, surgical expense, and medical expense. Hospital room and board reimbursements are generally $4 to $8 a day for 31 days. An additional amount is allowed for so-called "extras," such as laboratory tests, anesthesia, and operating room fees. Allowances for extras cannot exceed a set total, usually ranging from 5 to 10 times the daily rate. Reimbursements for surgeons' charges are made according to a fee schedule with a maximum generally set at $150 or occasionally at $225. Other physician services are covered by the medical expense plans. These usually exclude the first few visits provided during an illness. . . .

An outstanding feature of these three principal types of medical-care insurance is that they give the plan member free choice of participating physicians and hospitals. This generally means most physicians and hospitals within the area covered by the plan. . . .

In a study of employee benefit programs in 12 metropolitan areas, made in 1948 and 1949 by the Research Council for Economic Security, over 6,800 firms, 34.7 percent of the sample, returned questionnaires. These employed almost 2.5 million employees—27.4 percent of the nonagricultural employment in the 12 areas. According to this study, 42 percent of the firms reporting, which employed 35 percent of the workers, utilized local Blue Cross plans. Another 33 percent of the firms, with about the same percentage of workers had group hospital-expense coverage underwritten by insurance companies. In about 52 percent of the firms with hospitalization plans, this benefit was financed solely by the worker, and in about 20 percent it was financed solely by the employer. The remainder were jointly financed.

It was also disclosed that about 12 percent of the reporting firms, with about 13 percent of the employees, utilized local nonprofit plans for surgical insurance— primarily Blue Shield plans. Group surgical-expense insurance was reported by 32 percent of the firms, which employed about the same percentage of workers. In the firms with surgical plans, about 33 percent were financed solely by the worker, while about 26 percent were wholly employer-financed.

Some 9 percent of the firms in this study had group medical-expense insurance, and another 4 percent had other types of coverage for nonsurgical physician services. Together these firms employed about 8 percent of the workers covered. The workers paid for the entire cost in 25 percent of the firms with this benefit, and the employer alone financed it in the case of 38 percent of the firms. . . .

Collective-Bargaining Plans.—Employee benefit programs under collective bargaining also differ widely in the types and amount of benefits and the methods of financing and administration. Despite the differences, most of these programs have a very significant similarity in that they use existing voluntary medical-care insurance. Existing plans present the fewest problems to both union and management leaders who are busy with many other activities and are often inexperienced in medical-care administration. In fact, many unions, as a protection, insist on writing into the collective-bargaining contract the detailed descriptions of the benefits available from their local Blue Cross or medical-society plans or the benefits that a particular insurance company has agreed to provide for the money available.

Exceptions to the general pattern of using existing plans are few but nevertheless quite significant.

Collective-bargaining plans are financed by the employer alone or jointly with the workers. The employer's contribution is calculated most often on a percentage-of-payroll or cents-per-hour formula. In some instances, it is based on a specified sum per unit of production or per employee per week or month. Administration is by the employer or by various types of joint labor-management arrangements, such as formal tripartite trust funds. . . .

Among the benefits furnished by the long-established welfare programs of the International Ladies' Garment Workers' Union (AFL) are cash payments for hospitalization and ambulatory medical services. The hospital benefits, self-insured as are the other insurance benefits of the union, are currently $5 a day for 75 days in a calendar year. The medical services are provided by the union's well-known health centers. Because the administration of these programs is, to a large extent, the responsibility of many separate union-managed welfare funds, the amounts of benefits vary somewhat from local union to local union. Generally these funds are now financed entirely by employer contributions, set at about 4 percent of the payroll. . . .

In the precedent-making 5-year contract between the General Motors Corporation and the United Automobile Workers (CIO), the company pays half the cost of local Blue Cross and Blue Shield coverage for the worker and his family. In addition, the company pays the entire cost of cash-indemnity insurance for physician services to the employee during hospitalization for nonsurgical reasons; the maximum benefit is $5 a day for 70 days.

A health and welfare fund covers the over-the-road truckdrivers in 22 Central, Midwest, and Southern States who belong to the Brotherhood of Teamsters, Chauffeurs, Warehousemen and Helpers (AFL). Included in the group-insurance "package" purchased by this jointly directed fund are hospitalization and surgical benefits. Hospital expenses are reimbursed up to $10 per day for not more than

31 days per disability with a $200 maximum for "incidental" hospital charges; the schedule for surgical reimbursement has a maximum of $300. The fund is financed by an employer contribution of $1 a week per worker.

A survey by the Bureau of Labor Statistics of the U. S. Department of Labor reports that as of mid-1950 health and welfare programs under collective bargaining covered over 7 million workers. They exist in practically all branches of industry as well as in most of the major AFL, CIO, and independent unions. Although there is a wide variety of benefit combinations, hospitalization and surgical insurances have become a frequent item in the health and welfare package. About 80 percent of workers who have employee benefits and for whom information was available have hospital insurance, and about 72 percent of these workers have surgical insurance, medical insurance, or both. The employer is the sole source of funds for 65 percent of the workers with hospitalization coverage and for 72 percent of the workers with surgical and medical coverage. The other programs are jointly financed by the employer and the workers.*

Future Problems and Prospects

As MANAGEMENT and labor acquire greater familiarity and experience with medical care insurance, they will undoubtedly raise some significant questions. The way in which these questions are answered will profoundly influence the ultimate role of present voluntary plans in providing medical-care insurance to industrial workers.

The questions, which have their origin in problems of the worker as such, primarily concern the continuity of coverage. For example, what happens when a worker changes from one establishment to another? Some current developments give a partial answer. For establishments which are part of one company, insurance companies and also Blue Cross plans in a few recent instances have made available uniform Nation-wide programs for group contracts. In industries composed of many relatively small firms concentrated in one or a few geographic areas, industry-wide funds have provided continuity of coverage despite a high degree of mobility of the workers within the industry. However, many situations still remain under which a worker changing jobs must accept one or more disadvantages in relation to his medical-care insurance coverage.

Periods of temporary unemployment create a second phase of the same problem. Some industries have seasonal slumps when a considerable number of workers are laid off for as long as 3 to 6 months. Then work stoppages may arise from collective-bargaining disagreements. Aside from unemployment during major eco-

---

* In a talk delivered before the National Industrial Health Conference, in Philadelphia in 1956, Bradshaw Mintener, an Assistant Secretary of Health, Education, and Welfare, reported that at the end of 1954 "some 31,000,000 employees were covered for hospitalization under employee health and welfare plans. This represents nearly 60 per cent of all employees. Approximately 53 per cent of all employees had surgical coverage and 33 per cent had some type of financial protection against the cost of physicians' services in medical cases...." ("Meeting the Health Needs of the Nation," in *Industrial Health: Its Contribution to the Health of a Nation*," New York: Occupational Health Institute, 1956, p. 27.)

nomic depressions, experience has shown that during occasional recessions many, if not all, industries lay off a smaller or larger number of employees. A partial answer to this phase of the problem is given by some of the plans, principally those of the Blue Cross type. These allow the worker to continue payment of his own premiums during periods of unemployment. However, at such times the worker himself is financially handicapped. Although it is important for him to be protected against the additional economic burden of illness, he finds it difficult to pay the premiums, particularly if the insurance is of the relatively expensive type which covers his family and provides a fairly wide range of benefits. Some of the funds covering workers in irregular or seasonal employment recognize this problem by furnishing the health benefits to their workers who have been unemployed for as much as 4 months, or who have worked a minimum amount of time during the year, e. g., 6 months, or who continue to pay their own contribution into the fund.

A third aspect of the same problem is continuance of coverage for the worker who must retire from employment because of old age or permanent disability. Among the sources of money which have been suggested for the premiums of these various types of unemployed workers are private or Government subsidy, industry, unions, and State unemployment insurance programs.

Other questions that informed management and labor will want answered concern the plans themselves. These are the same questions that leaders of the health professions and other students of the subject ask: Are the people getting their money's worth from these plans? Do the plans really meet the needs? Are they providing and promoting a high quality of medical care? . . .

Exemplifying the criticism by many union leaders of the major alternatives for insuring the costs of physician services is the following excerpt from a recent address by Harry Becker, director of the Social Security Department, United Automobile Workers (CIO):

Even though collective bargaining is beginning to make sufficient funds available for medical care financed on the basis of the insurance principle, a satisfactory mechanism for the provision of medical benefits and services has still to be developed. . . . In no instance have the insurance companies assumed the social responsibility of working out with organized medicine a medical-insurance program that will assure covered workers that their insurance benefits will meet the full cost to them of covered medical or surgical items when such services are provided by their physician. . . .

Although most Blue Shield plans provide that families with incomes below a given figure will be guaranteed protection against medical expense for covered medical or surgical procedures, the income ceilings are generally so low that they exclude most workers. The Blue Shield plans, however, have a potentiality for flexibility and development, because of their sponsorship by State medical societies, that does not exist for the insurance companies. So far this potentiality has not been realized.[2]

There is general recognition that the more comprehensive the range of benefits, the more effective the plan. However, comprehensive benefits would require a

2. Becker, Harry: "The U.A.W.-C.I.O. and the Problem of Medical Care," *Amer. Jour. of Public Health* 41:1112-1117 (Sept. 1951).

considerable increase in premiums for the principle types of medical-care insurance which utilize the fee-for-service and solo-practice patterns of physician care. Of course, this does not apply to the medical-service plans in which physicians practice as a group and are paid on a salary basis. In these plans, comprehensive services are available within reasonable costs.

Another important consideration affecting the quality of care relates to the way that industrial medical-care insurance programs can be integrated with the other health services that the worker and his family are receiving from private physicians and voluntary and governmental agencies. There follow some pertinent remarks on this subject by Dr. E. Richard Weinerman ... and Dr. Herbert K. Abrams ... :

The first principle to be recognized is that preventive and therapeutic service are—or should be—inseparable, and that both can be furthered through the provisions of collective-bargaining agreements. While preventive health and safety measures have occasionally been included [in collective-bargaining agreements] this aspect of health protection is usually subordinated to the provision of the more dramatic hospital-care benefits. Nursing services, sanitation, case-finding, and other basic elements of good preventive medicine are rarely provided. Moreover, medical services for occupational illness and injury under compensation laws have not been coordinated with the newer arrangements for the care of non-occupational cases....

The recent experience of labor groups in California demonstrates that labor health funds *can* satisfy more of the basic elements of good medical-care planning than is now true of most union plans. These include:

(1) Nonprofit financing.
(2) Service rather than cash benefits.
(3) Coordination of preventive and curative services.
(4) Comprehensive scope of medical care.
(5) Family coverage.
(6) Coordination of professional personnel in modern medical facilities.
(7) "Consumer" voice in policy making.[3]

A unique example of a medical-care plan which was developed under collective bargaining and includes all seven "basic elements of good medical-care planning" listed by Drs. Weinerman and Abrams is the Labor Health Institute in St. Louis. However, for many administrative and sociologic reasons this type of plan is difficult to organize and operate, and in many States during the past few years has been illegal to establish.

State temporary disability insurance programs in four States and serious consideration of such laws by many State legislatures make possible one type of governmental medical-care insurance system for industrial workers. In fact, the State of California has already taken an important step in this direction by adding a hospital-expense benefit of $8 a day, up to 12 days, to its temporary disability insurance program....

The future of present medical-care insurance programs for industrial workers,

3. Weinerman, E. Richard and Abrams, Herbert K.: "New Patterns in Industrial Health and Medical Care Programs in California," *Amer. Jour. of Public Health* 41:703-11 (June 1951).

if any Federal or State governmental medical-care insurance programs were enacted, would depend on the provisions of the enabling legislation. Some of the possible results are suggested by existing situations in related benefit programs as well as by several of the legislative proposals themselves. A governmental program, as in some of the State disability-insurance programs, might permit the substitution of the privately operated programs if they met certain requirements, such as those specifying the extent of benefits and amount of premium. Or, the privately operated program might be adapted, as is done under many pension plans, to provide benefits supplemental to those of a governmental program. In any event, it would seem likely that plans which operated their own facilities and had their own professional staffs would be able to continue their activities in the same way as would other hospitals or clinics.

Labor and management support of industrial medical-care insurance programs is growing more widespread and active. For example, Earl O. Shreve, past president of the Chamber of Commerce of the United States, has said: ". . . Employers have come to realize that—apart from conditions on the job—the general health of their employees is a matter of concern to them. The good health of the workers is essential for high production . . . Closely related to the matter of maintaining the health of employees is the problem of aiding them to meet their health bills. Insurance is perhaps the best means of distributing the costs of serious illness over groups of people and over periods of time." [4]

Such support makes it likely that growing numbers of workers, whether members of unions or not, will, in the next few years, be covered by voluntary insurance programs for hospitalization, surgery, and some other physician services. This support will also help to prevent such plans from becoming casualties of future labor-management disputes or of economy efforts during less prosperous times.

The principal types of voluntary medical-care insurance plans now in operation appear to be both adequate and flexible enough to meet most of the current stipulations of management and labor. In the absence of new factors, it can be expected that the trend to use these existing plans will continue. As at present, they will be financed only occasionally by the workers alone, often jointly by the employer and the workers, and, with increasing frequency, by the employer alone.

4. Shreve, Earl O.: "The Employer and His Workers' Health," *Amer. Economic Security* 6:41, 43 (June 1949). The demand for medical care insurance on the part of labor is now evident even in those local unions whose national leadership does not actively encourage such programs. It is interesting, however, that almost all of the major unions continue to be emphatic in their support of national health insurance. They describe their collective bargaining activities as one side of a two-way drive towards social security. They believe that the Congress will in the near future continue to legislate only a minimum social security program and that the rest they must get through collective bargaining. . . .

76. THE COLLECTIVE BARGAINING APPROACH

A. THE UNITED MINE WORKERS *

THE MEDICAL CARE program of the UMWA Welfare and Retirement Fund is extended to approximately one and one-half million potential beneficiaries consisting mostly of miners and the dependent members of their families. They are located in the mining areas of 24 states and the Territory of Alaska. The program has been in operation for thirty-two and one-half months as of July 1, 1952. The services provided are as follows:

1. Hospital care for such time as necessary.
2. Medical care in the hospitals.
3. Specialists' services outside the hospital as necessary.
4. Rehabilitation services under the management of physicians at special centers.
5. Drugs administered to hospital inpatients.
6. Certain expensive drugs requiring long continuing use outside the hospital.
7. Physical examinations in connection with applications for prescribed cash benefits.
8. Home and office care for severely handicapped patients following discharge from special rehabilitation centers.

The following services are not provided:

1. Available services which the patient may be entitled to receive from an agency of the government, such as treatment for tuberculosis or mental disease in a state or county hospital, or from a private organization in the case of tuberculosis, infantile paralysis, cancer, etc.
2. Services for which the employer or some other party is legally responsible, such as medical service in compensation cases, etc.
3. Long-term treatment for mental illness.
4. Tonsil and adenoid removal.
5. Dentistry.

An experiment in providing home and office care to a limited number of beneficiaries on a free-choice-of-physician fee-for-service basis was tried for about eight months. It was unsatisfactory in every respect and therefore discontinued.

During the 12-month period ending June 30, 1952, 2,154,882 days of hospital and medical care were provided for 215,372 beneficiaries. Expenditures for all medical care benefits amounted to $49,996,517.88. Of these benefits, 85.6 per

* From: "United Mine Workers of America Welfare and Retirement Fund Medical Care Program," by Warren F. Draper, M.D.; *American Journal of Public Health* 43:757-62, June 1953 (Part I, No. 6). Reprinted (with omissions) by permission of the author and publishers. The author is the executive medical officer of the Welfare and Retirement Fund, United Mine Workers of America, Washington, D.C.

cent were received by working or retired miners and their families; 4.1 per cent
by widows and orphans of deceased miners, and 10.3 per cent by disabled beneficiaries.*

Some 2,100 hospitals all told have cared for our patients, and some 8,000
physicians have received payment for services rendered.

Of the combined cost of hospital and physician services about two-thirds was
for hospitals and one-third for physicians.

Responsibility for the development and operation of the medical program rests
squarely in medical hands. This is a principle that the medical profession has
always staunchly advocated and is quite the antithesis of much of the experience
elsewhere. In other words, our medical program is as good or as bad as we doctors
in the fund, our medical advisers, and the physicians who care for our patients
succeed in making it. If our combined efforts are not successful in fulfilling our
objective of providing a good quality of hospital and medical care at fair and just
cost, we alone will be to blame.

The medical program is administered through 10 area offices, each responsible
for the activities within a specified area. Together, they cover the coal mining regions.
Each area office is in charge of a physician who is an experienced medical care administrator. He works under the general direction and supervision of the executive
medical officer of the fund at the Washington headquarters office. . . .

. . . The medical administrators are generally recognized as outstanding in their
field. All were occupying positions of large responsibility prior to joining the fund.
Many possess the certificate of the American Board of Preventive Medicine and
Public Health; the applications of others are pending.

An administrative officer in each area office assumes the responsibility of management and operation under general medical direction. All possess special qualifications as to professional education, training, and experience. Most have university
degrees.

There is provision for a public health nurse on the staff of each area office.
They are highly trained women with postgraduate education who have occupied
positions such as director of public health nursing in a state department of health,
nurse officer in the Commissioned Corps of the United States Public Health Service,
territorial supervisor of a large national life insurance company, etc. Their duties
are broad in scope with especial attention to the development of cooperative
relationships with official and voluntary groups and organizations for the purpose
of extending their services to the mining population.

All area officers employ one or two consultants in rehabilitation to follow up
on the rehabilitation phases of the program. The balance of the personnel is engaged in lesser administrative duties and in clerical work.

* For the year ending June 30, 1957, the Fund provided hospital and medical benefits for
215,702 beneficiaries, including 1,631,144 days of hospital care and 885,944 specialist consultations in doctors' offices and outpatient clinics for diagnostic and treatment purposes. Expenditures for all medical care benefits amounted to $59,584,594 for the year, of which $389,944 was
for services to widows and orphans of deceased miners. (*Annual Report of the UMWA Welfare
and Retirement Fund for 1957*, Washington: The Fund, 1957.)

The medical headquarters of the fund in Washington consists of the executive medical officer and two associate physicians, a dentist whose duty is to work with official health agencies toward the extension of public health dental services to mining areas, an administrative officer, a hospital consultant, and a rehabilitation consultant. The rest of the persons employed serve under the direction of the supervisors mentioned. . . .

Hospital Services.—The fund has neither owned nor operated hospitals up to the present time. Existing hospitals have been used according to convenience of location and their willingness and ability to provide a satisfactory quality of service on an acceptable cost basis.

Representatives of the area offices visit the hospitals from time to time and arrange with them individually for services and terms. Only hospitals with which arrangements have been made may be used by beneficiaries at fund expense. Exception may be made in case of dire emergency. The bills are sent to the area offices for certification as to charges for services rendered. From there they are transmitted to the Washington office for review, auditing, and payment.

Beneficiaries are provided with identification forms acceptable to the hospitals and physicians who are authorized to care for them.

When a beneficiary is afflicted with an illness or injury of an exceptionally serious or baffling nature which cannot be adequately cared for locally, the area office may arrange for his care at the nearest medical facility that can provide the service that the case requires.

Not all of the local hospitals are satisfactory either as to service or to cost. Unsatisfactory services, however, may be preferable to none at all and may be purchased in the interest of the patient if nothing better is available. Even when the charges are exorbitant, they are paid if other means of caring for the patient are impracticable. The area offices have devoted much patience, time, and effort to improving the conditions of substandard hospitals as far as possible. They have at times been forced to adopt heroic measures against exploitation through poor service and exorbitant charges. Considerable numbers of patients have been transported by ambulance for distances of from 30 to more than 100 miles when occasion required. Such action constitutes a hardship and heavy expense to all concerned, but it has almost invariably resulted in improved conditions and fairer charges in the end.

Hospital Construction.—Certain mining areas, especially in Kentucky, Virginia, and West Virginia, have been woefully lacking in hospital and medical care throughout the history of the industry. Much of the service that the miner has received has been of inferior quality, although the money he has paid through the years has been sufficient to provide the best. The chances for improvement were found by the fund's medical staff to be nil in these communities because competent well qualified physicians sufficient to meet the needs could not be induced to practice in areas in which neither hospital nor other facilities were available. As there were no indications that the deplorable conditions of the past would not extend indefinitely into the future, the fund had no other recourse than to arrange for the establishment of new hospitals in some of the areas in which most desperate need existed. Therefore, there have been created the Memorial Hospital Association of Kentucky, the Memorial Hospital Association of Virginia, and the Memorial Hospital Association of West Virginia. These associations are nonprofit corporations organized in accordance with the laws of the respective states. They are responsible for constructing, equipping and operating new hospitals at or near Harlan, Pikeville, Hazard, Middlesboro, Whitesburg, and Wheelright in the State of Kentucky; at Wise in the State of Virginia, and at Beckley, Logan, and Williamson in the State of West Virginia.

Views as to the methods of staffing and operation that will insure the highest type of hospital and medical service possible under the conditions that exist, either have been or will be sought from physicians in the areas concerned, from their state and local medical societies, from the Medical Advisory Committee of the fund, and from other sources from which useful knowledge and experience are obtainable. Final decision as to the plans to be adopted will be reached only after thorough consideration of all the data and experience that can be gathered.

Each Memorial Hospital Association consists of a Board of Directors composed of four employees of the UMWA Welfare and Retirement Fund. Legal and fiscal services are provided by the legal counsel and the comptroller of the fund. The membership of each of the three boards is the same. A medical administrator and a deputy medical administrator are appointed by the Board of Directors of each association. They are responsible to the Board of Directors for carrying out the duties which the board assigns. The medical administrator and the deputy medical administrator of each association are the same.

Money for the Memorial Hospital Projects is provided by the UMWA Welfare and Retirement Fund through loans made in accordance with agreements between the Board of Trustees and the Board of Directors of each hospital association. . . .

While the primary purpose of the Memorial Hospitals is to provide good hospital care and facilities that would not otherwise be available to fund beneficiaries, they may also provide services to other members of the community to the extent that services may not be needed by beneficiaries of the fund.*

Physicians' Services.—Payments are made by the fund for the services of physicians as follows:

1. Medical care of beneficiaries during their period of hospitalization.

2. Diagnostic services of specialists to whom patients are referred by their attending physician.

3. Follow-up care in the home and office prescribed by physicians at the special rehabilitation centers for severely handicapped beneficiaries for such time as necessary after discharge from the center.

4. Physical examinations required in connection with applications for prescribed cash benefits from the fund.

* All ten Memorial Hospitals were completed and in operation by 1956.

Any physician may receive payment from the fund for services rendered its beneficiaries under the following conditions:

1. He must be in good professional repute.

2. He must indicate his desire or willingness to provide treatment to fund beneficiaries at a charge that is reasonable for the type of patients treated under the conditions that exist.

3. He must abide by the regulations of the fund in regard to the submission of clinical records and data required for payment of services rendered. These are kept to a minimum. No physician has been critical of the paper work required.

The large majority of physicians who care for our patients are able, conscientious men. They participate wholeheartedly in the medical program of the fund, and render the best service of which they are capable at rates which are acceptable both to them and to the fund.

We are studying a method of payment to physicians on a time basis which may be more satisfactory to all concerned. This may be conducive to a better quality of medical care, ease of administration, early referrals, and utilization of group practice.

Among the physicians who serve our patients are a number of the leading men of the country in the various specialties of medicine. They have assured us again and again that, busy though they are, they are eager to receive our patients because "they are such nice people, so appreciative of what is done for them, and often present such a challenge to all the ingenuity and skill that we possess." It is a heart-warming experience indeed when a miner who has gone through untold agonies writes to the fund and says, "Doctor X is the finest man I ever saw" or "He took the time to explain and tell me what to do."

In the field of rehabilitation alone, thousands of crippled miners have been restored to usefulness and to re-employment. The arduous, costly task of restoring men with crushed limbs and backs in the terrible toll of the coal mines is one of the finest chapters in the history of medicine. The physicians and members of their staffs in their devoted and selfless treatment of these men are bringing new knowledge of inestimable value to medical science.

While we are deeply and sincerely appreciative of the cooperation of the majority of the physicians who have served our patients and the excellent service they have rendered at what we believe to be fair and just cost, there is another side of the picture which in fairness must be mentioned.

In a program as extensive as ours we have experienced also some of the most tragic practices and conditions that can be imagined. Some continue at the present time, although steps that I shall mention are on the way to curb them. There are physicians who, though licensed, are not competent to provide the quality of service that the present day requires. There are others who perform work which they know they are incapable of doing properly. There are still others who render needless and ill-advised services. There are some who are able to maintain a monopoly in medical practice in certain areas and whose charges are far in excess of those of equal competence elsewhere. There are those who are interested only in the maximum payments that can be extracted. There are those who will take advantage of an emergency situation to charge for surgery on a coal miner the amount that might be charged his wealthiest patient.

The physicians of the fund have done much to improve the standard of practice in many of the mining areas by bringing eminent consultants to remote coal mining areas where they see problem patients, review clinical records, suggest corrections, and in general improve the quality of local practice. They have provided incentive for better service by referring patients to medical centers. They have received assistance and cooperation from liaison committees in the state and local medical societies.

While it will no doubt be possible to continue to make improvements by various means that may be used, they will not be adequate, nor do we feel that the total responsibility should rightfully be placed upon us. We have, therefore, presented the facts to the appropriate bodies of the American Medical Association, which has evinced a keen interest and determination to gather further information and take such steps or actions as are necessary to improve the quality of medical and hospital care in coal mine areas.

Toward this end, a survey team was appointed by the American Medical Association to visit some of the areas and submit its findings and recommendations. This was followed by a conference in one of the mining areas initiated by the AMA. Invitations were issued to the presidents and other representatives of the five state medical societies concerned, to the health commissioners of those states, to representatives of the medical schools of the state universities, and to physicians of the UMWA Welfare and Retirement Fund. Some 70 of these persons were present at the conference which lasted two days.

Many rcommendations were submitted for study and final action by the conference at a later meeting. Those approved will be presented for implementation by the various agencies concerned. The recommendations that are finally adopted and the manner in which they are carried out may have a strong bearing upon the future course of our program.

I believe that the best conception of the medical care program of the UMWA Welfare and Retirement Fund, and the direction in which it is headed, is expressed in the words of John L. Lewis, the man who made it possible. In an address to the Forty-First Convention of the United Mine Workers Constitutional Convention held in October, he stated as follows:

"This plan of the United Mine Workers is not socialized medicine. This plan contemplates the purchase of the services of the medical profession and establishes the best possible service at a fair and just cost. That is free enterprise. That is not socialized medicine. And in this work, more and more as the days go by, the eminent figures in the American medical world are coming to understand more and more the value of this great arrangement in our industry and more and more are extending their cooperation and their helpfulness to make it the most successful of any plan in the country."

B. LABOR HEALTH INSTITUTE *

THE LABOR HEALTH Institute, located in St. Louis, Missouri, is a nonprofit organization devoted to preventing illness and curing its members when they become ill. The Institute was established by a union through collective bargaining with management in November 1945. At that time the organization covered only 2,500 members in the shops under contract with the union. At present there are nearly 8,000, membership having been extended to cover any other union groups which include the LHI clause in their contracts with management. Associate members are also accepted on an enrollment fee and regular dues basis, which entitles them to receive medical care at a reduced fee-for-service basis.

The first contracts called for the companies to pay an amount equal to 3½ per cent of the worker's wages to the LHI. For this amount, the workers themselves were given complete health and sick care on the basis of need. After two years' experience, the union and the companies realized that the workers' families should be included in the program because the health of the family has a direct bearing upon the health and efficiency of the worker. New contracts call for a 5-per cent contribution by the management to provide health and medical care not only for the worker but his family as well.

The pivot of the entire program is the physical examination. Special emphasis is made to get every member into the LHI for a physical to determine his present state of health and to correct any major or minor disorders or diseases before they become serious. Media utilized to instruct the members are the official newspaper of the sponsoring union, company bulletin boards, shop meetings, and labor-management committees.

Physical Facilities.—The Institute occupies two floors of the Publicity Building. The clinic includes a spacious, well-lighted, attractive waiting room, modern examining rooms, a surgery department equipped for minor surgery, three dental offices, a complete X-ray room, laboratory, physiotherapy department, eye examination room, basal metabolism machine, electrocardiograph and other equipment necessary for complete diagnosis and treatment outside a hospital. By having the LHI physicians under one roof, members may see as many specialists as necessary in a single visit to the health center.

Coverage.—Medical personnel includes physicians, dentists, medical social workers, nurses, laboratory technicians, X-ray technicians, physiotherapist, pharmacist, medical librarian, and clerical personnel. All except the physicians and dentists are employed full time. General medical service is given at the health center, in the home or hospital. Specialist services include surgery, gynecology, obstetrics,

* From: "Labor Health Institute Medical Care Program," by Elmer Richman, M.D.; *Industrial Hygiene Newsletter* (Division of Industrial Hygiene, Public Health Service) 9:8, 10, Jan. 1949 (No. 1). Reprinted (with omissions) by permission of the author. The author, formerly medical director of the Labor Health Institute in St. Louis (1944-51), is now practicing internal medicine in Clayton, Mo.

pediatrics, eye-ear-nose-throat, urology, allergy, internal medicine, dermatology, orthopedics, neuro-psychiatry, cardiology, gastroenterology, arthritis, and certain consultative services not available at the health center. These services are given without cost to the members.

The following dental care also is given without cost to the members: dental examination and diagnosis, including X-ray, prophylaxis and gum treatment; extractions; and emergency work. Restorative dentistry, including bridges, fillings and false teeth, is provided the members at low fees, approximating the cost of the materials used.

A registered pharmacist is on duty full time to fill prescriptions at low cost. The LHI pharmacy also carries drugs and sundries at low prices.

Hospitalization is provided under Blue Cross. The LHI pays initiation fees and membership dues and arranges for the members to get into the hospital.

Counseling service is provided at home, in the hospital and the health center. In addition to these services, the medical social worker acts as liaison between the LHI and the community agencies and institutions.

Personnel.—Physicians are selected for their skill and knowledge and also for their understanding and appreciation of the workers' problems. They have private practices and represent all of the hospitals and medical schools of the city. Obviously, to secure the best doctors possible, salaries are made attractive and schedules are arranged to fit in with the heaviest load at the health center. Since most of the members have to obtain their medical care after work, the doctors' schedules are concentrated between the hours of 3:30 and 6:30 in the afternoons. There are morning clinics, however, and certain doctors are on call on assigned nights to handle inquiries, home visits, and emergencies for LHI members. They also see LHI members in their private offices, if the need arises, during the morning hours before the doctors arrive at the health center. . . .

The Labor Health Institute is based on the recognition of the fact that health is man's greatest asset. In its short existence the LHI has proven on a small scale that service and not money to pay for service is the answer to the health needs of large groups of people. Regardless of the method of paying for medical care, no plan will work if there is a continuous struggle between the premium and the benefit. It will only work if the best available service is brought to the people when they need it, where they need it and for as long as they need it.

B. *Workmen's Compensation*

77. GROWTH OF THE COMPENSATION CONCEPT *

No COMPENSATION law ever developed spontaneously. The constant stress of social, economic, and labor problems in Europe gradually, though very slowly, molded the various influences and philosophic opinions. This resulted in a more intelligent and widespread understanding of the principle of compulsory workmen's insurance particularly in Germany during the Bismarckian era. Previously the status of the injured workman in relation to his master or employer was considered to be purely a personal one.

By virtue of the doctrines or rules established under the so-called master and servant relations, the employee was placed at a decided disadvantage. The doctrines or rules are as follows: first, the contributing negligence rule was so construed that the employee was considered negligent if he accepted employment when the risk was so great that a person of ordinary prudence would not take it; second, the fellow-servant rule, in which one who enters the service of another takes upon himself the ordinary risks of the negligent acts of his fellow-servants in the course of his employment; third, the doctrine of assumption of risk was interpreted that an employee accepted employment with his eyes open and therefore assumed the incidental risks. In addition to these three doctrines, the injured servant was obstructed in the processes of recovery of compensation by what might be considered acts of God or by the necessity of proof of the employer's liability through personal negligence. With the rapid growth of industry and the intricacy of corporate structure the personal relationship between master and servant became so remote as to obliterate any chance to prove personal negligence. Furthermore, it was impossible for an uninformed workman to determine the hazardous nature of the occupation before accepting employment, and, finally, the complexity of growing mass production so obscured the identity of a fellow-servant that these rules became obsolete to the point of absurdity. Recovery through common law while not only doubtful was exceedingly slow and expensive. Attempts of European countries to fix liability, and the subsequent narrow laws that were passed, met with the usual accompaniment of opposition from the parties most affected.

Switzerland in 1881 was the first country to declare that for accidents in certain employments the employer was to be liable without any proof of fault.

The rise in strength of the Socialistic Party in Germany after the Franco-

* From: *Medical Service in Industry and Workmen's Compensation Laws,* by the American College of Surgeons (Gaylord R. Hess, ed.); Chicago: The College, (revised) 1946 (Chaps. VIII and IX, pp. 62-71). Reprinted (with omissions, including tables and figures) by permission of the publishers.

Prussian War led Bismarck to adopt the German Industrial Insurance Act of 1884, which is considered to be the first modern compensation law embodying the compulsory insurance principle. In this modern version of workmen's compensation the obsolete personal and employer liability status was abandoned and industry was saddled with the responsibility of compensating its injured employees as a part of its operating expense. An injured employee who has lost an extremity or suffered the loss of wages through a disabling injury should be compensated and this cost passed on to the consumer just as would be the cost of the wear and breakage of machinery and tools and of used raw material.

England adopted the new compensation principle in 1897, but in 1906 it greatly amplified its statutory provisions. The laws of England were not nearly as thorough and elaborate as the earlier compensation laws of Germany but it is upon the laws of these two countries that most of the subsequent laws of other countries have been patterned.

The United States was one of the last countries to adopt the compensation principle. In 1908 a federal act provided limited benefits for designated classes of public employees of the United States.... As was to be expected, the United States also had its opposition to the introduction of workmen's compensation laws and questions as to their constitutionality arose.... Although United States Supreme Court rulings upholding workmen's compensation laws have removed the general doubt as to constitutionality, some states have taken the precaution to provide for such enactments in their Constitution.

Wisconsin, on May 3, 1911, was the first state whose compensation laws became effective. Washington, on March 14, 1911, was the first state to enact a permanent compensation law which, however, did not become effective until October 1, 1911....

Need for More Uniformity

LACKING CENTRAL correlation through the federal government it was inevitable that state laws followed during the rush for enactments from 1911 to 1915 that were lacking in the desired uniformity. The underlying principle was to provide compensation for all injured workers whose injuries arose out of and in the course of employment, yet its stated expression and administration in the various states is so divergent that it does not always serve the best interests of the employer, the employee, and the public. Inadequate or ambiguous compensation laws and varying interpretations by individuals and occasionally by biased groups keep the scene changing and render laws not only uncertain but even unjust in some instances.

Practically all states have made amendments to their original compensation laws. The recent tendency is to liberalize these laws in favor of the employee in regard to medical service and compensation and particularly to provide for occupational diseases. In this connection several states have again appointed commissions for the purpose of studying and recommending compensation legislation. These investigations have been followed by the enactment of occupational disease laws in a number of these states.... Undoubtedly within the next few years all of the industrial states will have compensation laws which include occupational diseases.

The medical profession was not consulted in the formulation of the earlier compensation laws but medical advice is now being sought more freely in connection with such contemplated legislation. It is hoped that the medical profession, the federal administration, and other recognized authorities will continue to extend a more active advisory and guiding influence, since local peculiarities and problems are no longer sufficient excuses to withhold the application of proven principles in obtaining desirable and uniform workmen's compensation laws.

Injured Worker Bears Large Proportion of Injury Cost

OF GREATER economic and social importance than the distribution of compensation between different types of disability is the extent to which compensation actually compensates for the loss of wages. When an employee sustains a disabling injury, how far does the compensation he receives offset his loss in earnings? The following are some of the reasons why the injured worker bears the burden of considerable economic loss:

1. The rates of compensation in the different states vary from 50 to 70 per cent of the average weekly wage.

2. There are so-called "waiting periods" of one week in the majority of the states during which no compensation is paid unless the disability is sufficiently serious to compel the worker to remain away from work for more than 14 to 28 days. One state requires a two-weeks' "waiting period," another ten days.

3. There is a maximum weekly compensation limitation, the amount of which may be only a relatively small per cent of his regular weekly wages.

4. In permanent total disabilities, the subsequent earning power of the worker may be either partially or completely impaired for the rest of his life. The employee unfortunate enough to become permanently disabled by injury in the state where he bears the greatest per cent of the burden of loss, often becomes an object of charity since the period and amount of compensation do not always cover the entire time and need of disability.

5. In fatal cases, dependent survivors may receive, for example, the equivalent of the average earnings which the deceased worker would have received over a period of four or five years. Obviously, the average employee at the period of his death may have had an expectancy of considerably more than those four or five years of gainful employment.

On the other hand, employers are occasionally held responsible for workers' disabilities and deaths that had no causal relationship to employment.

Industry, too, has grown so that the numerous industrial organizations that individually operate plans in more than one state are subjected to compensation laws that vary not only in their coverage and phraseology, but also in their interpretation and administration. This situation should arouse enough public interest to urge the enactment of workmen's compensation laws that are uniform, just, and certain in their action. The United States Supreme Court has ruled that those engaged as longshoremen and harbor workers should not be governed by divergent state workmen's compensation laws, but should receive uniform treatment through legislation by Congress.

Administrative Organization [1]

REALIZING that a definite organization was essential for the most efficient administration of the statutes, most states have provided a commission or board to administer and supervise the compensation laws.... These commissions may consist of one or more commissioners, usually appointed by the governor, who in turn may appoint a number of deputy commissioners or referees and other assistants as is the case in large industrial states. A number of industrial commissioners have at their discretion appointed medical advisers to assist them in an advisory capacity, but not until the occupational disease situation threatened further serious confusion were there definite provisions made in the statutes of the compensation laws for the appointment of medical boards to assist in compensation administration....

In a number of states the compensation commission is a part of or closely correlated with the departments of labor and industry....

Types of Insurance Systems

INSURANCE may be provided through a state fund, through mutual or stock insurance companies, or by self-insurance, subject to general supervision by the commission. While many of the larger industrial organizations are self insured, the bulk of the compensation insurance is carried by stock and mutual insurance companies....

The securing of insurance ordinarily does not discharge the employer's liability for compensation except when insured in the state funds. Some states permit subcontracting and substitute benefit schemes, but the employer is still held liable as fixed by the acts. The amount of compensation in the substitute benefit plan must be equal to that in the act and approval by the commission is required. Where employees contribute to such schemes, additional benefits must be commensurate therewith. In states not making such specifications, however, some employers have taken advantage of this opportunity and arranged for the workers to bear some of the compensation costs. For this reason several states make it a misdemeanor to

1. It is impossible to give an accurate generalized summary of the various state compensation laws due to their differences of expression and administration. Furthermore, the compensation laws are subject to amendments at each legislative session, in which case a single amendment would render a detailed presentation obsolete. Reference should be made to the statute and court rulings of the state involved for full information concerning phraseology and interpretation of any given subject. Consideration is herein largely confined to principles and fundamentals of the laws up to 1945....

collect from the wages of employes any portion of the insurance premium or to withhold sums collected for medical purposes.

In most states compensation insurance rates are approved or adjusted by the superintendent of insurance or by some other designated state authority. In a few states the approval of rates is vested in the workmen's compensation commission.

The present accepted schedule of insurance rates in the United States permits insurance companies to deduct approximately 40 per cent out of every dollar collected for workmen's compensation insurance. This 40 per cent is subdivided as follows: acquisition cost, 17.5 per cent; claim adjustments, 8 per cent; auditing of payrolls, 2 per cent; inspection, 2.5 per cent; taxes, 2.5 per cent; and general or administrative expense, 7.5 per cent. Actually more than the 40 per cent deduction from the insurance dollar is permissible. An increase in deduction, over the usual rate, is commonly made to offset the special tax requirements that may exist in the various states, and to that extent the increase is allowed. The state taxes on insurance premiums range from 2 to 4 per cent. . . .

78. THE LEGAL FRAMEWORK *

WORKMEN'S COMPENSATION legislation has been enacted by all of the States, as well as Alaska, Hawaii, and Puerto Rico. Federal laws cover Government employees and longshoremen and harbor workers. The Federal act covering longshoremen and harbor workers has also been made applicable to private employees in the District of Columbia. However, because of coverage limitations and the adoption by about half of the States of an "elective" rather than a compulsory system of workmen's compensation, many workers are still unprotected by these laws.

In States which have an elective law, employers may refuse to operate under the compensation act if they prefer to risk an injured worker's suit for damages. Although most employers elect to come under the act, some do not. In the latter case the employees may be unable to obtain compensation unless they sue for damages. Workers are also deprived of protection in a number of States because of numerical limitations on required coverage and in others due to the fact that the law applies only to certain "hazardous" industries. Agricultural and domestic workers are usually excluded from coverage. Also there is no Federal workmen's compensation law to protect railroad workers and seamen engaged in interstate commerce. . . .

---

* From: *State Workmen's Compensation Laws as of September 1950* (Bulletin No. 125, Bureau of Labor Standards, U.S. Department of Labor); Washington: U.S. Government Printing Office, 1950 (pp. 1-9, 33-36). Reprinted with omissions, including tables and initial paragraphs.

Types of Laws

COMPENSATION LAWS may be classified as compulsory or elective. A compulsory statute is one which requires every employer within the scope of the compensation law to accept the act and pay the compensation specified. An elective act is one in which the employer has the option of either accepting or rejecting the act, but in case he rejects it he loses the customary common law defenses—assumed risk of the employment, negligence of fellow servants, and contributory negligence.

No compensation law covers all employments. Usually agriculture, domestic service, casual employment, and in some laws nonhazardous employments, are exempted from the provisions of the act. In most States, however, such employments may come under the provisions of the law through the voluntary acceptance of the employer. Such coverage is called voluntary because as a rule the employer loses no rights or defenses if he does not accept. Thus, in operation a compensation law may be either compulsory or elective as to certain employments and voluntary as to others. . . .

Persons and Employments Covered

BECAUSE OF WIDE variations in the coverage patterns of the laws, it has never been possible to measure accurately the extent of coverage. It has been noted that no law covers all employments. Under some laws the coverage is limited to so-called "hazardous" employments; often employers having fewer than a specified number of employees are exempted; and many of the laws are "elective," permitting employers to choose to stay outside the coverage. Other curtailments of coverage are caused by the specific exclusion of a designated industry or employment, and by the conflict of State and Federal authority, especially in relation to interstate transportation and to maritime operations.

The largest population group deprived of workmen's compensation protection by the "specific exclusion" clause is that of farm employment. Other specific exclusions usually found in the laws are applicable to domestic servants, casual workers, and employees of charitable institutions.

Two of the major groups outside the coverage of the compensation laws are interstate railroad workers and maritime employees. Railroad employees engaged in interstate commerce are covered by the Federal Employers' Liability Act. Maritime workers are subject to the Jones Act, under which the provisions of the Federal liability act are applicable to seamen. . . .

Injuries and Diseases Covered

COMPENSATION LAWS are limited not only to persons and employments included, but also as to injuries covered. In some States injuries due to the employee's intoxication, willful misconduct, or gross negligence are excluded. The limitation of the coverage of injuries may be by definitions or lists, or both. The usual definition of a compensable injury is one "arising out of and in the course of employment." Under most of the early laws, only "accidental" injuries were covered. Some laws omitted the word "accidental" but specifically excluded occupational diseases. Under several laws, however, the terms "injury" or "personal injury" have come to include, by definition or court interpretation, occupational diseases. An increasing number of the States have changed the specific exclusion of occupational diseases to specific or general inclusion. An occupational disease is usually held to be an injury of gradual or slow development, by comparison with the sudden effect of an accident. However, in States not covering occupational diseases, the courts sometimes attribute a sudden or "accidental" origin to an injury known to physicians as a disease. States are ending this confusion by expressly bringing occupational diseases under the workmen's compensation laws.

It is now generally recognized that occupational diseases should be compensated, and some provision for this is made in 41 States, Alaska, the District of Columbia, Hawaii, and Puerto Rico. Such protection is also given to employees covered by the Federal Employees' Compensation Act and the Longshoremen's and Harbor Workers' Act. Some of the laws list the diseases that are included, while others cover all occupational diseases. An outstanding development in this field in recent years has been the increasing use of general coverage. . . .

Rehabilitation

A SPECIFIC PROVISION regarding the rehabilitation of the injured worker is contained in 18 of the workmen's compensation acts (Arizona, Arkansas, District of Columbia, Florida, Minnesota, Mississippi, New Jersey, New York, North Carolina, North Dakota, Ohio, Oregon, Rhode Island, Utah, West Virginia, Wisconsin, and United States Civil Employees' Act and Longshoremen's Act). In most of these acts the provision pertains to special maintenance and other compensation to facilitate the vocation rehabilitation of the worker. The Arizona law gives the Commission broad authority to provide such awards as may be necessary for the promotion of vocational rehabilitation. Under the Wisconsin law, provision is made for the payment of full compensation for a maximum period of 40 weeks during rehabilitation training. In addition, the actual and necessary costs of maintenance and travel are paid for a maximum period of 40 weeks, if the training is elsewhere than at place of residence. For amputees, there is no limit on the number of weeks for which full compensation is paid while training in the use of artificial members. In the other laws providing special maintenance or other compensation for rehabilitation, there is a maximum limit on the amount of compensation or period of weeks or both.*. . .

In addition to any special rehabilitation benefits and services provided under the workmen's compensation law, an injured worker may also be eligible for the

---

* See Selection No. 79B in this chapter for fuller discussion of the rehabilitation aspects of workmen's compensation.

services provided by the State-Federal program of vocational rehabilitation. This program is operated in all the States, the District of Columbia, Hawaii, and Puerto Rico by the State divisions of vocational rehabilitation. The services rendered include medical care, counsel and guidance in selecting the right job, and training for and placement on the right job. In addition, the medical treatment, transportation, maintenance, occupational tools and equipment, and training supplies are provided without cost where the client's inability to pay has been established.

Medical Benefits

IN ALL THE COMPENSATION acts medical aid is required to be furnished to injured employees. In the early legislation the provision for medical aid was narrowly restricted as to the monetary cost, the period of treatment, or both. In the later development of the acts such absolute restrictions have been changed in many cases either by providing for unlimited benefits or by authorizing benefits in addition to the initial maximum upon the approval of the administrative authority. Forty-five acts require the employer to furnish artificial limbs and other appliances.* ...

79. MEDICAL CARE SERVICES

A. PATTERN OF BENEFITS †

EQUAL IN IMPORTANCE to the compensation payments which an injured worker may receive are the medical services to which he is entitled under the workmen's compensation law. The speed of recovery for the injured worker, the degree of his disability, and his restoration to maximum earning capacity are dependent on the effectiveness of the medical-aid provisions of the workmen's compensation law.

All the compensation acts contain some provision for medical aid to be furnished to injured workers. In the early legislation, the provision for medical aid was narrowly restricted as to the monetary amount, the period of treatment, or both. In the later development of the acts and particularly in recent years, the trend has been toward granting unlimited medical benefits. In July 1953, full medical aid was being provided by 36 of the 54 State, Territorial, and Federal compensation laws. Seventeen of 36 laws specifically provide that medical aid must be furnished without limit as to time or amount. The administrative agency, in the other 19

* See Selection No. 79A, immediately following in this chapter, for specific data on provisions for medical benefits in State workmen's compensation systems.

† From: "Medical Services," by Bruce A. Greene; in *Workmen's Compensation in the United States* (Bulletin No. 1149, U.S. Department of Labor), Washington: U.S. Government Printing Office, 1954 (pp. 25-28). Reprinted with omissions. The author is a workmen's compensation consultant for the Bureau of Labor Standards, Department of Labor, Washington, D.C.

TABLE 46. *Statutory provisions relating to medical benefits* [A]

FULL BENEFITS

Jurisdiction	By statute	By administrative authority	Jurisdiction	By statute	By administrative authority
Arizona	(B)	(B)	New Jersey	....	Dx
Arkansas [C]	....	Dx	New Mexico	....	Dx
California	x	....	New York	x	....
Connecticut	x	....	North Carolina [C]	....	Dx
Delaware	....	Dx	North Dakota	x	....
District of Columbia	x	....	Ohio	....	x
Florida	....	Dx	Oklahoma	....	Dx
Hawaii	x	....	Oregon	....	Dx
Idaho	x	....	Puerto Rico	x	....
Illinois [C]	x	....	Rhode Island	....	Dx
Indiana	....	Dx	South Carolina	....	Dx
Maine [C]	....	Dx	Utah [E]	....	Dx
Maryland	....	x	Washington	x	....
Massachusetts	x	....	Wisconsin	x	....
Minnesota	x	....	Wyoming	....	Dx
Mississippi	x	....			
Missouri	....	Dx	United States:		
Nebraska	x	....	Civil employees	x	....
New Hampshire	....	Dx	Longshoremen	x	....

LIMITED BENEFITS

Jurisdiction	Period	Amount	Jurisdiction	Period	Amount
Alabama	90 days	$500	Montana	12 mos.	1,500
Alaska	2 yrs.	....	Nevada [C]	6 mos.[I]	....
Colorado	6 mos.	1,000	Pennsylvania	90 days	J $225
Georgia	10 wks.[F]	F 500	South Dakota	20 wks.	K 300
Iowa	....	G 1,500	Tennessee	1 yr.	1,500
Kansas	120 days [H]	1,500	Texas	4 wks.[I]	....
Kentucky	....	2,500	Vermont [C]	180 days [M]	L 2,500
Louisiana	....	1,000	Virginia	60 days [I]	....
Michigan	6 mos.[I]	....	West Virginia	....	M 1,600

[A] Data include 1953 legislation up to June 1, 1953, insofar as available.

[B] Full medical aid, in the judgment of the Arizona Industrial Commission, is authorized through a combination of the medical care and rehabilitation provisions of the law. Medical benefits for occupational diseases are payable for total disability, maximum $500, and for partial disability due to listed disease, $250.

[C] In case of silicosis or asbestosis, reduced benefits.

[D] After an initial period or amount, the administrative agency may extend the time or amount indefinitely.

[E] In case of occupational diseases, reduced benefits.

[F] Period may be extended for additional time and amount not exceeding $250.

[G] $1,000 maximum for hospital service and supplies and $500 for medical and surgical services. Commission may authorize an additional $1,000.

[H] In case of occupational diseases, may be extended an additional 90 days.

[I] May be extended for specified limited period of time.

[J] Hospital services also allowed for 90 days, maximum $225.

[K] Also hospital benefits not to exceed $700.

[L] Also hospital charges, 180 days but amount expended for services and supplies shall not exceed $2,500.

[M] Additional $800 may be authorized. $800 may also be paid for vocational rehabilitation. No allowance for medical treatment for silicosis.

laws, is authorized to give unlimited medical aid. (See accompanying table.) The remaining 18 laws impose limitations on the cost of the medical aid or on the period of time during which such aid shall be rendered, or both. All but a few of the medical-aid provisions include the furnishing of artificial appliances wherever necessary.

The efforts to remove any limitations on medical aid are usually related to the experience that adequate medical aid is economical. Most employers and insurance carriers generally recognize that the best medical care reduces their costs by lessening the period during which such care is needed, and in many cases, lessening the degree of permanent disability suffered by the worker. Even in the States with limitations on medical benefits, it is not uncommon for the employer or insurance carrier to provide medical care over and beyond the legal requirements.

Several organizations and conferences have adopted recommendations for medical-benefit provisions. The National Conferences on Labor Legislation have repeatedly recommended unlimited medical benefits as the desirable standard for State laws. The medical committee of the International Association of Industrial Accident Boards and Commissions (IAIABC), in its 1949 convention report, stated:

> Your committee agrees that, in the case of the injured workmen, medical aid should not be restricted by legal limitations and costs; that disability resulting from industrial accident or disease should be the responsibility of industry so long as it continues and medical aid should be furnished on this basis.

A recommendation in support of full medical aid was made in 1952 by a Subcommittee on Industrial Relations of the American College of Surgeons, headed by Dr. Alexander P. Aitken, of Boston. This committee agreed that "the need for full medical care, including rehabilitation, under competent supervision is recognized."

Choice of Physician or Surgeon.—The medical-aid provisions of workmen's compensation laws involve the problem of the method in selecting the physician or surgeon to attend the injured worker. Various methods are provided for under the laws. A survey of the provisions for selection of attending physicians made by the statistical committee of the IAIABC in 1949 showed that, in most States, the law provides for the choice to be made directly by the employer or insurance carrier. In a few States, the selection is made by the worker from a panel made up by the employer or carrier. In about one-fourth of the States, the worker has some form of "free choice" but only a few of these authorize unlimited "free choice." In actual practice, it is quite common for employers or insurance carriers to forego their legal rights and allow the worker his choice of a physician.

The National Conferences on Labor Legislation have always recommended that the worker be given the choice of physician. In reporting upon this problem to the 1949 convention, the IAIABC medical committee stated:

> Unrestricted free choice as so often advocated is not compatible with the best of care —most people choose their physician or surgeon because of a friend's advice, a liking for

his personality, an admiration of his office or equipage, or a report on his charges, if not for his availability and location alone. Thus, the man most skilled in pediatrics may be chosen to treat a fracture—or the man who directed the last family confinement called to treat a spinal-cord injury. The best cannot be thus obtained!

On the other hand, the family physician, the trusted friend of the claimant, can frequently attain results in cases within his competence far beyond those of his more skilled but unknown brother.

Free initial choice retains all of these advantages and, if under advice by a competent, skilled, and unbiased medical officer of the commission, can lead by consultation and reference to the best of surgical care.

Your committee, as that of last year, believes that the trend is in this direction—that the physician of free initial choice, in conference with a skilled, unbiased medical officer of the commission, can best arrange for the most advanced and adequate medical care. In order to properly accomplish this, the law should place control of medical aid in the compensation authority, and free initial choice be allowed by ruling of the commission.

Supervision of Medical Aid.—Supervision of the medical-aid features of workmen's compensation laws includes the duties of ascertaining whether the injured worker is receiving adequate medical care, checking on the promptness and completeness of reports required from attending physicians, regulating charges for medical services, and evaluating medical reports and testimony in relation to the cause and extent of disability. The degree of supervision exercised over these matters varies widely among the States. Lack of medical staff is given by compensation officials as one of the main reasons for failure to provide more adequate supervision. Less than half of the State workmen's compensation agencies have medical personnel and in many of these States, only part-time medical staff is available.

The control provisions of some of the workmen's compensation laws are meager and ineffective. The Utah workmen's compensation act is an example of a law which gives *effective* controls to the Industrial Commission. This law reads in part as follows:

All physicians and surgeons attending injured employees shall comply with all the rules and regulations, including the schedule of fees for their services, adopted by the commission, and shall make reports to the commission at any and all times required by it as to the condition or treatment of any injured employee, or as to any other matters concerning cases in which they are employed. Any physician or surgeon who refuses or neglects to make any report required by this section is guilty of a misdemeanor, and shall be punished by a fine of not more than $500 for such offense.

In supervising medical care, compensation officials state that one of the main points to guard is that the injured worker is treated by a physician, surgeon, or specialist whose competence to treat the type of injury sustained has been determined by recognized medical organizations. Inexpert medical care often proves expensive and may have a very harmful effect on the rehabilitation of the injured worker. For example, improperly handled amputations can leave too long or too short a stump for effective use of an artificial appliance. In some instances, the choice of physician who treats the injured worker has been determined not by his excellence as a surgeon, but by his skill as a medical witness. Under proper supervision, such practices do not exist.

Medical Aid and Rehabilitation.*—Medical aid includes not only the primary medical or surgical care, but also the rehabilitative, convalescent, or post-operative care. This phase of medical treatment is developing rapidly as the result of World War II experience in returning injured servicemen to their line of military duty.

Very few of the workmen's compensation laws contain any specific provision for the physical rehabilitation of injured workers. However, the medical-aid provisions of many of these laws are interpreted to include such treatment. . . .

Improvement of Medical Services.—The IAIABC medical committee, in its 1951 and 1952 convention reports, reiterated the recommendations made as the result of the study of medical services conducted by the committee in 1949. It submitted as a basis for working out the details of problems in cooperation with workmen's compensation administrators and members of the medical profession and its organizations, the following recommended principles:

1. A recognition of the necessity for more adequately trained and skilled medical and surgical care of injured workers.

2. A recognition that medical aid to injured workers should not be limited by cost or other legal prohibition.

3. A recognition that the goal of medical aid in compensation cases is prompt recovery, minimum residual disability, maximum physical restoration, and preparation of the injured worker for resumption of gainful employment.

4. A recognition that the law should place direction of medical aid in the compensation administrative authority.

5. A recognition that rehabilitation must begin with first aid and continue throughout the period of disability; that, in order for a physician to carry out his responsibility under workmen's compensation medical practice, it is basic for him to consider the total medical problem, including preparation for the injured worker's return to work; that the physician, therefore, must bring to bear on these problems all of the skills and disciplines that science and society can offer and utilize all community resources in the accomplishment of such objectives. [Paraphrased from item 5 of Basic Principles for the Rehabilitation of the Injured Worker, in a report of the Subcommittee on Industrial Relations of the American College of Surgeons.] †

6. A recognition of the necessity for close association and cooperation between the compensation administrative agency and the State, Provincial,‡ and local medical groups for the purpose of (a) procuring and giving the medical attention recog-

* See selection immediately following (No. 79B) for fuller discussion of the rehabilitation aspects of workmen's compensation.
† Brackets in original text.
‡ In Canada.

nized in item 3; and (b) securing written reports and advice necessary for the rehabilitative agency's case records.

7. A recognition of the need for more expertly trained and better informed physicians in traumatic surgery, occupational medicine, and physical medicine, to be achieved by (a) undergraduate specialized courses in medical schools and colleges; and (b) postgraduate review by seminars, meetings, and bulletins.

An adequate and successful workmen's compensation system depends materially on the extent to which these recommended principles are carried out.

B. PROVISIONS FOR REHABILITATION *

WHEN WORKMEN'S compensation legislation set out to provide medical care and replace lost income for injured workers, it embarked on a course that could not be complete without a third goal—the rehabilitation of the worker to optimal family, social, and economic life. This goal is potentially the most significant improvement in the concept of workmen's compensation.

The original legislation was based on an essentially static concept of disability. The medical care of the day was relatively limited. When first aid and medical treatment had been rendered there was little to do but accept the residual incapacity as it stood. The medical care required by statute usually ended after the initial healing period and the program thereafter dealt primarily with cash payments. Compensation for permanent partial disabilities was based on indemnities fixed by statute for specified losses. It was assumed, moreover, that the "loss of both hands, or both arms, or both feet, or both legs, or both eyes, or of any two hereof shall, in the absence of conclusive proof to the contrary, constitute permanent total disability." Where further treatment held no promise, the tendency to establish fixed liabilities for fixed losses was both humane and practical.

The rise of rehabilitation, however, has introduced infinitely improved means of regaining lost health and overcoming loss of function. It has narrowed the area of permanent disability so that today it scarcely has any valid meaning except to the extent that rehabilitation is unsuccessful or not feasible. Certainly it has shattered the notion of *presumptive* permanent and total disability. It has opened the prospect of improved methods of evaluating disability which would overcome some of the deep-seated deficiencies of the system. Rehabilitation cannot, of course, be the sole objective of workmen's compensation, although such assertions are sometimes loosely made. But it offers a set of services essential to the proper functioning of workmen's compensation legislation; the availability of these services to injured workmen is supported by compelling reasons of social and economic policy.

Nature and Effectiveness of Rehabilitation.—In part, rehabilitation is an outgrowth of workmen's compensation experience. Compensation administrators soon recognized the incompleteness of the legislation and gave the movement for vocational

* From: "Rehabilitation," by Jerome Pollack; in *Workmen's Compensation in the United States* (Bulletin No. 1149, U.S. Department of Labor), Washington: U.S. Government Printing Office, 1954 (pp. 40-45). Reprinted with omissions. The author is program consultant in the Social Security Department of the United Automobile Workers of America, Detroit.

rehabilitation "its most direct and substantial support." [1] Their efforts paved the way, when the First World War came, for the first national legislation for rehabilitation of veterans. The war enlarged the need for rehabilitation and stimulated awareness of its potentialities. Rehabilitation centers began to be established. Legislation followed, providing a financial base and establishing organized programs of rehabilitation successively for veterans, the industrially disabled, and the general population. There emerged the modern concept of rehabilitation made possible by great advances in the general practice of medicine, in orthopedic surgery, physical medicine, and other medical specialties; and by the pioneering of specialized institutions for the care of the disabled, which had served such groups as handicapped children, the ruptured and crippled, the deaf, and the blind, and which had stimulated, concentrated, and coordinated efforts to overcome disability.

Modern rehabilitation has been defined as "the restoration of the handicapped to the fullest physical, mental, social, vocational, and economic usefulness of which they are capable." Its practice has developed in two segments: *medical,* aimed at maximum recovery of health and the fullest possible restoration of lost function; and *vocational,* to promote an optimal economic adjustment, through vocational counseling and training, transitional employment, and placement services. Currently the *psycho-social* elements of evaluation, social service, personal counseling, psychometrics, recreation, and psychiatric service are recognized as a third coordinate segment. Each segment is a composite of many disciplines. In severe cases, the necessary medical specialists may include: "A general surgeon, an orthopedic surgeon, a neurosurgeon, a plastic surgeon, an internist, a urologist, a roentgenologist, a doctor of physical medicine, a psychiatrist, and sometimes others . . . indispensable for the proper handling of a single case . . ." [2] And before rehabilitation is completed, many nonmedical specialists may have to be called upon. Integration of the diverse disciplines, services, and facilities toward a single goal is the crucial administrative problem. The goal is total rehabilitation. The process cannot stop with the best artificial appliance and its most skillful use if the worker is unable to cope with his social environment or his employment. Proper rehabilitation thus necessitates the availability, where needed, of all the component services and of the institutions which house and coordinate their work.

Of its effectiveness there is hardly room for question. The will to live revealed by many persons despite the most severe afflictions, their courage and resourcefulness, combined with the new ways to achieve restoration, inspires the common designation of "miracles." Many accounts could be cited which recall Biblical passages. A history of the Institute for the Crippled and Disabled is appropriately entitled "Take Up Thy Bed and Walk." Dr. Howard Rusk has given an inspiring account of the rehabilitation of 500 paraplegics [3] under the program sponsored by the United

[1] Federal Grants for Vocational Rehabilitation. By Mary E. MacDonald. Chicago, University of Chicago Press, 1944 (p. 11).

[2] Rehabilitation of the Disabled. Washington, United Mine Workers of America Welfare and Retirement Fund, [1950?] (p. 10).

[3] Hope for paraplegics is in itself a startling innovation. "Until the last 10 years," as Dr. Rusk has pointed out, "paraplegics had been no problem because the mortality rate was 90 percent the first year. There were 400 paraplegics in World War I. Only two are living today . . .

Mine Workers. These were

... the toughest cases that anybody ever saw, bar none. You always like to tell about your worst case, but there were many as bad as this one:

This man was 40 years old and his back was broken 20 years before. How he survived that length of time I don't know. When he was found ... he ... had not seen a doctor in 3½ years. There was not even a wagon road to his house and he was carried down in a sling between two bed poles by friends. The man had 11 bed sores from the size of a plate to the size of a dollar; stones in both kidneys and his bladder, and his lower extremities were almost up under his chin.

You might ask, is it worth fooling with a person like that? He thought it was. He wanted to live. And we felt we had an obligation. It took 26 surgical procedures and 13 months before we could even start to train this individual. ... We trained that man to walk, swing through a gait on crutches in 90 days, and in control of automatic bladder and automatic bowel. And during the last 3 months of his stay in the institute he ran for sheriff in his county ... and he has been the sheriff there for more than 3 years.

New ways of rehabilitation hold promise of still newer ways and broader applications. Rehabilitation is being extended to mental illness, heart disease, epilepsy, blindness and aging. Its horizons are expanding and the hope it holds for tomorrow makes it all the more important to perfect the institutional arrangements to bring rehabilitation to the disabled.

Provision for Medical Rehabilitation.—From the beginning, workmen's compensation legislation accepted, at least in part, a responsibility for restoring health which often extended into medical rehabilitation as it then existed. True, restrictions on the total cost or duration of care were the rule. Nevertheless, more than a third of the laws enacted by the end of 1919 defined medical care to include such items as "crutches and apparatus," "artificial limbs," "mechanical appliances," and the like and it is probable that other States also furnished them under the general provision that "all necessary" or "reasonable" services, medicines, and supplies were to be provided.

Although medical rehabilitation was partly anticipated, it was largely an unforeseen development requiring a greater emphasis on medical care, a broader scope of services, and possibly a reexamination of the arrangements for medical care.

Progress toward adequate medical care, however, has been slow. One authority poses the problem as follows: "Those laws which should have restored the disabled worker to gainful employment failed to provide even adequate medical care by the statutory limitation of the cost and duration of such care. It should be obvious that no true rehabilitation can possibly be afforded if medical benefits are to be so restricted." [4] Such restrictions still exist in as many as 17 States. The practice is

---

In this war it was a different story. We had 2,500 and they didn't die because you could control their infection and we knew about the management of their bed sores." (*In* Application of Rehabilitation to Workmen's Compensation, Medical Aspects of Workmen's Compensation, Commerce and Industry Association of New York, Inc., 1953, p. 62.)

[4] Rehabilitation in Workmen's Compensation. By Dr. Alexander P. Aitken. (*In* Workmen's Compensation Problems, U. S. Department of Labor, Bureau of Labor Standards, 1953. Bull. 167, p. 212.)

sometimes more enlightened than the legislation, but this does not establish a satisfactory financial base for medical rehabilitation.

Modern rehabilitation involves the total medical practice as it affects the injured. It begins with the attending physician—and even with the medical school. In order for the physician to carry out his responsibility as defined by the American College of Surgeons, "... it is essential for him to recognize the total medical problem of the patient in addition to his injury, as well as his personal problems. The physician must bring to bear on these problems all the skills and disciplines that science and society can offer, and utilize all community resources which can assist him in the accomplishment of these objectives." [5]

The community resources bearing closest on medical rehabilitation are the community hospital and the rehabilitation center. The President's Commission on the Health Needs of the Nation has underscored the need for establishing departments of physical medicine and rehabilitation in general hospitals. The Commission concluded that the average community hospital of 200 beds could profitably assign perhaps 20 percent of its beds for rehabilitation and convalescent care. However, only 19 of 1,600 general hospitals replying to a questionnaire by the Commission on Chronic Illness had any bed allocation for rehabilitation services; and very few of these actually offered comprehensive service. The President's Commission found, moreover, that: "All told, there are less than a dozen comprehensive rehabilitation centers in existence ..." and that they meet only a small fraction of the need. To make the miracles of medical rehabilitation a reality for most of the Nation's disabled workmen, a great expansion in hospital and center facilities is obviously needed.

Provision for Vocational Rehabilitation.—A few States were prompt to amend their laws to bring vocational rehabilitation within the scope of the compensation system. Massachusetts was the first to establish, in 1918, "a division for the training and instruction of persons whose capacity to earn a living has in any way been destroyed or impaired through industrial accident." The following year California, North Dakota, and Oregon adopted similar measures. Oregon's compensation law set a high standard:

One purpose of this act is to restore the injured person as soon as possible to a condition of self-support and maintenance as an able-bodied workman, and final settlement shall not be made in any case until the commission is satisfied that such restoration is probably as complete as can be made ... the commission is authorized to expend money from the accident fund to accomplish this purpose in each case and the amounts so spent shall not be charged against the compensation allowed by this act to the injured workman ... [6]

But rehabilitation was also developing in a broader direction. Support was growing for the idea that it should be made available to all of the disabled regard-

[5] Ibid., p. 207.
[6] Workmen's Compensation Law of 1913, Ch. 112, sec. 23 (as amended by Ch. 288, acts of 1919).

less of the origin of disability. This idea was embodied in the Federal Vocational Rehabilitation Act of 1920 which provided for technical and financial assistance from the Federal Government for State-operated vocational rehabilitation programs serving the general population. There had been some resistance to the inclusion of vocational rehabilitation under workmen's compensation; within that framework, rehabilitation faced uncertain financing and restrictive standards of eligibility. The Federal-State program, on the other hand, was readily accepted as the means of providing vocational rehabilitation for the occupationally disabled, and the drive to bring rehabilitation under workmen's compensation generally abated.

As a result, only 17 States have made any statutory provision whatsoever under their workmen's compensation laws to provide, promote, or facilitate rehabilitation. Fifteen States facilitate rehabilitation by providing limited maintenance allowances during its course; a few among them, probably five, finance or help pay for rehabilitation services as a direct part of workmen's compensation. Four States and Puerto Rico directly operate rehabilitation facilities for injured workers under the workmen's compensation program.

There thus exist in America today two basic patterns in providing rehabilitation services for injured workers: in a few States the services are directly provided by the workmen's compensation agency; overwhelmingly they are furnished through cooperation with the Federal-State program.

The few States which directly operate rehabilitation facilities under workmen's compensation—Ohio, Oregon, Rhode Island, and Washington—offer potentially the most complete integration of the two programs. There are evident benefits in centers concentrating on traumatic disabilities; there is greater specialization; the cases tend to be relatively recent in origin and can be processed before despair patterns become confirmed. The patients generally retain employment ties that may be reactivated and have a job orientation that is often helpful. The rehabilitation is financed as a workmen's compensation cost. To the injured worker it comes as an insured right without any means test or any implication of public assistance. Such centers have been performing excellent services for the injured employees under their jurisdiction.

The success of workmen's-compensation-operated centers, however, requires an administrative agency with considerable authority, empowered not only to establish the necessary facilities and provide the services, but also with clear authority to refer cases for rehabilitation. Such agencies are the exception rather than the rule in present American compensation practice. The fact that so few States have taken this course during four decades does not inspire much hope for a major trend for the direct provision of rehabilitation services under workmen's compensation.

A plan of rehabilitation geared to State, local government, and community centers offers a number of advantages. Community centers tend to be broader in scope than centers dealing exclusively with work injuries. They represent an investment in services and facilities available also to the worker's family and to the worker injured off the job. Community centers can make for fuller utilization of scarce resources by avoiding the duplication of personnel and facilities performing the same functions for different population categories. Local arrangements, moreover, can bring rehabilitation closer to the workers' communities—an important factor in inducing workers to accept rehabilitation. Such arrangements can provide for better integration of rehabilitation with the sources of medical education, medical service, placement agencies, and other community services.

Considering its vast responsibilities and chronically limited budgets, the Federal-State program has achieved remarkable results, especially since the Barden-LaFollette Act of 1943 broadened its scope to embrace the full range of rehabilitation including medical and psychiatric services. Nevertheless, examination of the volume of rehabilitation of injured workers, the delays in securing service, the weaknesses in the referral system, the shortages of personnel, the inadequate financing, and other serious shortcomings, revives the question as to whether it was proper for workmen's compensation to have transferred, largely or entirely, the responsibility for rehabilitation to another program without at least sharing in the cost and without taking definitive responsibility for following its cases through to complete rehabilitation. The question persists whether the responsibility to purchase or provide rehabilitation services must not be made an integral part of workmen's compensation, just as medical care is.

The volume of rehabilitation is critically inadequate. The Labor Department and the Office of Vocational Rehabilitation have estimated that at least 200,000 of the nearly 2,000,000 workers injured each year could benefit from rehabilitation. By this standard of eligibility, "only 3 percent of the injured workers in the United States are receiving the type of service needed." [7] About 6,000 injured workers annually receive rehabilitation services under the Federal-State program, but each year fully twice as many sustain serious permanent disabilities and are in acute need of rehabilitation. Most of the rehabilitation is received, not by those currently becoming disabled, but by a portion of the vast, and growing, backlog of persons needing rehabilitation.

Authorities are unanimous in stressing the crucial importance of promptness. Nevertheless, the Task Force on the Handicapped has made public the fact that, while the Rehabilitation Center of the Liberty Mutual Insurance Co. in Boston reported an average lag of 6.4 months from injury to admission, under the Federal-State program it had taken 7 *years* on the average for occupationally disabled workers to find their way to the rehabilitation agencies in 1951. [8]

The tendency has been to approach the matter of referrals superficially. The problem is far too deeply rooted to be overcome by merely urging more prompt action or even through improvements in the mechanics for referral. One important cause of delay is built into some of the statutes; rehabilitation is not authorized until the worker qualifies by becoming entitled to an award for major permanent disability. Claim settlement procedures which require the worker to maximize his disability

[7] See Report of Rehabilitation Committee to 1950 Annual Convention of the IAIABC. (*In* Workmen's Compensation Problems, U. S. Department of Labor, Bureau of Labor Standards, 1950. Bull. 142, p. 173.)

[8] See Report of the Task Force on the Handicapped to the Chairman. Washington, Office of Defense Mobilization, Manpower Policy Committee, 1952 (p. 31).

in order to secure fair compensation also interfere with rehabilitation—and this is one of the deep-seated evils of present compensation practice that may prove exceedingly difficult to overcome.

Far greater access to facilities is needed. Injured workers usually must travel to the large urban centers at considerable hardship and expense. In most States, travel and maintenance expenses are not provided under the compensation law and, indeed, the regular cash benefits themselves are insufficient for this purpose.

Rehabilitation is not grossly underfinanced but, partly as a consequence, seriously understaffed. . . .

Trends and Developments.—Two of the more significant attempts to extend rehabilitation for injured workers have come from a labor union and an insurance company. The union is the United Mine Workers, which concluded that "the problems which the severely disabled face in making a recovery are created in great measure by the present inadequacies of our workmen's compensation, relief, and rehabilitation programs." The union's Welfare and Retirement Fund set out to supplement and coordinate the rehabilitation of disabled miners in conjunction with the Federal-State and other public and community agencies. The signal contribution made by this program has been to demonstrate the effectiveness of rehabilitation and to improve screening and referral procedures for its members. Other unions are now studying the possibility of promoting rehabilitation through collective bargaining.

The insurance company is Liberty Mutual, one of the major insurers of workmen's compensation liabilities. It observed the slow progress in bringing modern rehabilitation to injured workers. It was concerned with the rising cost of workmen's compensation and saw rehabilitation as one constructive method for controlling cost. Since 1943 it has operated a center in Boston which has produced excellent results, having derived many of the advantages of a program closely integrated in the workmen's compensation process. Its contribution is the demonstration that rehabilitation pays. The savings in reduced medical and compensation costs are difficult to measure by rigorous standards, although many specific cases can be cited in which very substantial amounts were saved. . . .

Sweeping changes are needed to modernize the Nation's workmen's compensation laws. There is probably no better place to start than with the establishment of a definitive program of rehabilitation for occupationally disabled workers. Rehabilitation should be as firmly established under workmen's compensation as the responsibility for medical care. Whether the services should be directly provided by the workmen's compensation board or purchased from community centers is not the basic issue. The need is for the assumption of responsibility for comprehensive rehabilitation and for a vast expansion in its availability. The medical care provisions should be broadened to cover the cost of medical restoration in full. The administrative agency should be given clear authority to make rehabilitation services and income-maintenance benefits available to all who need them. The administrative reforms which are urgently needed in workmen's compensation generally—in the direction of a clinical rather than a forensic system—can most logically and appropriately begin with rehabilitation. Once rehabilitation becomes a definitive part of workmen's compensation, further improvements will become possible, such as the revision of the much-criticized disability rating system. This is the most promising prospect for workmen's compensation as it stands today.

C. Disability Insurance

80. THE PHYSICIAN'S ROLE *

MOST SOCIAL legislation of the past has contributed directly or indirectly to improved health. Compulsory sickness disability insurance constitutes a new form of social legislation which has almost unlimited potentials in fostering the development of modern preventive medicine. A reasonably good estimate of these potentials can be made from a study of present practices and trends, and from analogy with other types of social legislation, particularly workmen's compensation laws.

It has been repeatedly demonstrated that once the principle of a new type of social legislation has been accepted, pressures in the direction of extending and liberalizing the laws develop very quickly. It would be most surprising if sickness disability laws should prove to be an exception to this rule; in fact, the effects of such pressures have already become manifest in California. All physicians, whether they be in private practice, in public health positions or engaged in industrial medicine, should be alert to the possibilities created by sickness disability insurance laws for furthering the ends of preventive medicine. Since these laws directly concern all physicians, the profession should take an active interest in their formulation and administration.

The Role of the Private Physician

Medical Examinations.—All sickness disability insurance laws now in effect require certification of disability by a physician before a claimant may collect benefits. It is almost certain that a similar provision will be incorporated in all future laws of this type. This means that every individual covered by the law who wishes to take advantage of its protection presumably will be seen by a physician. The

* From: "Sickness Disability Insurance and Preventive Medicine," by Leonard J. Goldwater, M.D.; *American Medical Association Archives of Industrial Hygiene and Occupational Medicine* 2:682-89, Dec. 1950 (No. 6). Reprinted (with omissions, including initial paragraphs) by permission of the author and publishers. The author is professor of occupational and administrative medicine at the School of Public Health and Administrative Medicine, Columbia University, New York.

present legal pattern provides that sickness benefits are payable for nonoccupational disabilities the duration of which is longer than one week, so that a physician will not necessarily be consulted in all cases of minor illness of short duration. Nevertheless, the certification requirement will surely result in the utilization of a physician's services in many instances in which a doctor would not otherwise have been seen.

The mere fact that contact with a physician must be established for the purpose of certification does not necessarily mean that anything related to preventive medicine will be accomplished, but the opportunity is there if the doctor or the patient wishes to take advantage of it. In addition to the examination necessary for certification, the physician might suggest a complete medical check-up for the patient and for members of the patient's family, and he also has a favorable occasion to present something in the way of health education.

Epidemiological Observations.—In communities which are largely industrial, practicing physicians, through the operation of a disability benefits law, may be presented with opportunities for detecting the presence of unhealthful working conditions. Records of the frequency and the nature of illness among employees in commercial and industrial establishments might provide the earliest evidence of general or specific health hazards.

Most individuals whose disabilities will call for certification will not be suffering from illnesses which must be reported to the public health authorities. The practicing physician may therefore be the only one who has information on the incidence of many diseases. The lack of reliable morbidity statistics has been a serious handicap to public health departments and to industrial physicians in developing preventive programs. Disability benefit laws can provide private physicians with opportunities to fill some of the gaps. Communicable and other reportable diseases will naturally be reported to the health authorities, but the operation of a sickness benefit law may result in many of these cases being seen (and reported) earlier. It may also result in more such cases being seen by physicians.

Opportunities for detecting "sickness prone" workers will be presented to practicing physicians; thus those individuals will be indicated who may be in greatest need of preventive or constructive medicine.

Early Diagnosis and Early Treatment.— ... The basic features in any modern program of preventive medicine are early diagnosis and early treatment. Since disability claims are recognized after the first week of disability, there exists an incentive for an insured patient to see a doctor not later than one week after the onset of disability. In terms of a chronic ailment this might be considered early diagnosis. Obviously the term "early" is a relative one. In the case of lobar pneumonia or an internal hemorrhage, diagnosis at the end of a week would be "late."

Ordinarily, treatment is instituted promptly on the establishment of a diagnosis. In fact, treatment often precedes diagnosis. The probability of a favorable therapeutic effect is greatest in the early stages of most diseases. Thus the prevention of complications and of disability, two of the important objectives of preventive medicine, are most likely to be achieved when diagnosis is made and treatment instituted early in the course of a disease. Opportunities for this are enhanced under sickness disability insurance laws and are most likely to be utilized when the patient is able to pay for the necessary diagnostic and therapeutic service.

Evaluation of Disability.—It can be reasonably asserted that premature return to work and unwarranted prolongation of a period of sickness disability are both inimical to the physical and mental well-being of an employed person. In order to avoid potential harm to a patient, as well as unpleasant disputes with the patient or his employer, physicians will be called on to exercise judgment and firmness in deciding when a period of disability is terminated. The decision may require familiarity with working conditions beyond the ken of many medical practitioners. In such cases, a conversation with the employer, or a plant physician may be indicated. Increasingly, the private physician must orient his thinking toward the patient in relation to the patient's job if effective preventive medicine is to be practiced. . . .

The Department of Public Health

Control of Communicable Diseases.—The operation of sickness disability insurance laws may be expected to result in the detection of an increased number of cases of communicable disease. In some instances, as has already been mentioned, detection and reporting may occur earlier than would otherwise be the case. This places the health officer in a favorable position to take action directed toward preventing the spread of disease. Arrangements can and should be made whereby reports of disability due to communicable disease are transmitted promptly from the agency which administers the sickness disability fund to the appropriate public health official. Under such a plan, any tardiness on the part of physicians in reporting infectious cases to the health department would not delay the institution of proper control measures. A check on complete reporting would also be provided.

Morbidity Statistics on Noncommunicable Diseases.—The operation of sickness disability insurance laws may be found to provide the richest source yet known of information on general morbidity experience, particularly as related to industry and occupation. Such information is badly needed by health departments, since without it there can be no intelligent planning for the control of many forms of illness. While reporting is a function of the practicing physician, recording and statistical analysis are responsibilities of the health department. Unfortunately, the diagnoses given in the disability certificates may not always be entirely accurate, owing to the fact that a diagnosis must be given. It is obvious that a physician cannot always be expected to establish a diagnosis on the strength of a single examination. Despite this possible shortcoming, there is little doubt that the disability reports will contain a wealth of information which can be used to great advantage by public health departments. Utilization of the reports will of course depend on a suitable working arrangement with the agency responsible for the administration of the disability benefit law.

Diagnostic Services.—The general acceptance of the principle that early diagnosis is an essential part of preventive medicine has led an increasing number of public health departments to expand their diagnostic services. The availability of such services to practicing physicians for use in determining disability in patients who cannot afford to pay for expensive diagnostic tests would facilitate early diagnosis and enhance accuracy of diagnosis. The advantages in terms of preventive medicine are readily apparent.

Grants-in-Aid to Physicians.—The expenditure of funds for finding cases of illness has long been recognized as a proper function of public health agencies. With the present shift of emphasis from communicable to noncommunicable diseases a parallel shift in expenditures must follow. Sickness disability insurance laws create an opportunity for public health departments to enlist the aid of large numbers of physicians as "deputy health officers" in the field of case finding. It has been pointed out that disability benefits are not likely to provide sufficient funds so that individual beneficiaries can shoulder the full costs of all diagnostic tests or the costs of a comprehensive medical examination. As an alternative to the provision of diagnostic services by health departments, properly regulated subsidies to individual physicians might be used to enable them to give applicants for disability certificates the benefit of the best type of medical examination. This, in turn, would form the basis for a case-finding program which could scarcely be duplicated in extent or in effectiveness. Carried a step further, subsidies to physicians and hospitals might be granted to help defray the costs of early treatment in cases where financial considerations might be responsible for a delay. Activities of this type on the part of a health department can be justified if early treatment is accepted as an essential part of a program of preventive medicine.

The Industrial Physician

IN COMMERCIAL and industrial establishments where a plant physician is employed, the physician will often be the first one to become aware of disabling illness among the employees. This places him in a strategic position to institute measures directed toward early diagnosis and early treatment and may also bring to light other opportunities for practicing preventive medicine.

Diagnosis and Treatment.—Ordinarily it is not the responsibility of the industrial physician to provide diagnosis and treatment in cases of disabling nonoccupational illness. Nevertheless, in the case of some individuals who are eligible for sickness disability payments the industrial physician may be in a position to direct the patient into the best channels for receiving the required medical services. Since the employee will not be totally devoid of income during the period of disability, the advice of the industrial physician has some likelihood of being followed, particularly if diagnostic services, or aid in obtaining them, are available. Furthermore, recommendations as to periods of convalescence can be expected to be carried out, thus minimizing the possibility of relapses or of premature return to work, dangers which exist when the disabled individual is without income during the period of disability.

Supplementary Benefits.—While sickness disability laws provide limited cash benefits during periods of illness, they make no provision for defraying the costs of medical services. There is, however, a growing tendency for employed persons to secure some form of hospitalization or medical care insurance as individuals or groups, often through collective-bargaining agreements. The industrial physician who is familiar with the advantages and shortcomings of the various forms of health insurance can advise the employer and the employee on the type most advantageous to the persons concerned. When cash benefits are available through sickness disability insurance, a "service" type of hospital or medical-care insurance is more appealing to the insured worker. The well-informed industrial physician is in a position to guide the employer and the employee in the selection of that combination of insurance plans which will provide the greatest benefits, thus contributing to preventive medicine through the availability of early and adequate medical care.

Absenteeism and Experience Ratings.—There are strong indications that experience ratings, based on sickness absenteeism, will be a factor in calculating employers' payments into the sickness disability insurance fund in some of the states. This obviously lends support to industrial physicians who wish to strengthen their occupational health program. Since industrial medicine is primarily preventive medicine, and since preventive medicine can be expected to reduce sickness absenteeism, sickness disability insurance laws which provide for experience ratings provide the industrial physician with a very effective argument when it comes to seeking adequate support from the employer. . . .

Payments to Physicians.—Sickness disability laws as they exist today make no provision for paying physicians for certifying disability. The disabled employee receiving the limited benefits allowed under the law is in a poor position to pay any more than is required for the certification. This fee is actually an additional tax on the employee, since without a doctor's certificate he cannot collect his benefits. No one will deny that the physician is entitled to a fee for examining a patient and filling out a disability certificate. In view of the fact that a physician's certificate is essential in the administration of the law, it seems appropriate to have the doctor's fee paid by the agency which administers the law. A reasonably adequate fee paid from such a source would serve as an incentive for the certifying physician to exploit fully his opportunities for practicing preventive medicine. A complete medical evaluation, not restricted to determining presence or absence of disability, would undoubtedly lead in many instances to the detection of incipient diseases at a time when preventive procedures could be most profitably employed. . . .

FURTHER READINGS

Medical Care Services

American Dental Association, Council on Dental Health. *Group Dental Health Care Programs*. Chicago: The Association, 1955. 98 pages. (Includes references).

American Foundation of Occupational Health. *Medical Services in Industry*. Chicago: The Foundation, 1952. 45 pages.

American Medical Association. *A Survey of Union Health Centers*. Chicago: The Association, 1954 (revised). 46 pages.

American Medical Association. *Guiding Principles for Evaluating Management and Union Health Centers*. Chicago: The Association, 1955. 14 pages. (Includes references).

Baisden, Richard N. and Hutchinson, John. *Health Insurance: Group Coverage in Industry*. Berkeley, Calif.: Institute of Industrial Relations, University of California, 1956. 76 pages. (Includes references).

Dunning, James M. *Dental Service at the St. Louis Labor Health Institute*. St. Louis: The Labor Health Institute, 1955. 10 pages. (Includes references).

Goldmann, Franz and Graham, Evarts A. *The Quality of Medical Care Provided at the Labor Health Institute, St. Louis, Missouri*. St. Louis: The Labor Health Institute, 1954. 11 pages.

Klem, Margaret C. and McKiever, Margaret F. *Small Plant Health and Medical Programs*. Publication No. 215, Public Health Service. Washington: U. S. Government Printing Office, 1952. 213 pages.

Lear, Walter J. *Small Plant Health Programs: A Bibliography*. Bibliography Series No. 3, Public Health Service. Washington: U. S. Government Printing Office, 1951. 28 pages.

National Industrial Conference Board. *Company Medical and Health Programs*. Studies in Personnel Policy, No. 96. New York: The Board, 1948. 72 pages.

Slavick, Fred. *Distribution of Medical Care Costs and Benefits under Four Collectively Bargained Insurance Plans*. Ithaca, N. Y.: New York State School of Industrial and Labor Relations, Cornell University, 1956. Bulletin 37. 39 pages.

United States Department of Labor, Bureau of Labor Statistics. *Health, Insurance, and Pension Plans in Union Contracts*. Bureau Bulletin No. 1187. Washington: U. S. Government Printing Office, 1955. 8 pages.

United States Department of Labor, Bureau of Labor Statistics. *Older Workers under Collective Bargaining*. Part 2: *Health and Insurance Plans; Pension Plans*. Bureau Bulletin No. 1199-2. Washington: U. S. Government Printing Office, 1956. 27 pages.

Workmen's Compensation

American Medical Association. *Medical Relations in Workmen's Compensation*. Chicago: The Association, 1955. 10 pages.

Dawson, Marshall. *Problems of Workmen's Compensation Administration*. Bulletin 672, Bureau of Labor Statistics. Washington: U. S. Government Printing Office, 1940. 229 pages. (Includes references).

Somers, Herman Miles and Somers, Anne Ramsey. *Workmen's Compensation: Prevention, Insurance, and Rehabilitation of Occupational Disability*. New York: John Wiley and Sons, 1954. 341 pages. (Includes references).

United States Department of Labor, Bureau of Labor Standards. *Proceedings of the National Conference on Workmen's Compensation and Rehabilitation*. Bureau Bulletin 122. Washington: U. S. Government Printing Office, 1950. 119 pages.

United States Department of Labor, Bureau of Labor Standards. *Workmen's Compensation Problems.* Bureau Bulletin 186. Washington: U. S. Government Printing Office, 1956. 230 pages.

Disability Insurance

Sinai, Nathan. *Disability Compensation.* Research Series No. 5, Bureau of Public Health Economics, School of Public Health, University of Michigan. Ann Arbor, Mich.: School of Public Health, University of Michigan, 1949. 126 pages.

United States Department of Labor, Bureau of Employment Security. *Temporary Disability Insurance: Problems in Formulating a Program Administered by a State Employment Security Agency.* Washington: U. S. Government Printing Office, 1953 (revised). 66 pages.

CHAPTER XII

Medical Care Insurance

EARLIER CHAPTERS have emphasized the unpredictability for the individual of illness, and therefore of the costs of medical care. The significance of economic factors in restricting the distribution of medical care resources and services has also been pointed out. Social efforts to resolve many of the problems implicit in these facts have centered, to a large extent, around various applications of the insurance method.

Essentially, medical care insurance is a method of pooling risks and resources based on the fact that the total risk for a large group, and therefore the extent of necessary resources, is predictable. Those who view the risk in financial terms alone—as the risk of economic loss associated with illness—generally view resources in the same terms—that is, as cash benefits to recompense "the loser" or, more recently, benefits in the form of a fully or partially paid-up service. It is also possible to recognize the risk as illness itself, and the resources as those which may be made available to promote, restore and maintain health. Herein lies the basis for some of the fundamental differences among the various applications of the insurance method in the medical-care field.

Regardless of these differences, medical-care insurance has made some of the costs of illness, injury and maternity more predictable and less burdensome for a great many individuals. It has facilitated access to all of the services covered by insurance by removing part of the cost barrier. And, as a manifestation of the fact that insurance can serve not only as a financial protection but also as the financial foundation for bringing together necessary resources, it has demonstrated its capacity to influence the organization of medical services. The first part of this chapter provides a picture of the development, nature, extent and problems of the voluntary medical-care insurance movement.

The risk of illness and its costs is only one of the major risks growing out of our highly industrialized urban society with its money economy. We depend upon our earnings for our living. Few of us can make for ourselves even the more essential of the things we need in order to live; we buy them instead with our income. The continuity of that income, for most families, is threatened by a series of risks which, like the risk of illness, are ordinarily beyond their direct and individual control. These risks include:

> unemployment resulting from lack of available work;
> unemployment due to disability;
> premature death of the wage earner;
> old age (as defined by the variable standards of the labor market).

Protection against the results—which are often disastrous for society as a whole as well as the individual—of any or all of these occurrences is therefore developed by group participation in the protective machinery.

Social efforts to help the individual and his family achieve protection against these risks have taken several forms. Early developments in life insurance and in the endeavors of craft-sponsored mutual benefit associations, which involved the pooling of funds to provide specified benefits to the wage-earner's family in the event of his death or incapacity—these gave rise to many of the extensive activities of today's insurance industry and provided the basis for many of our contemporary benefit or protective associations, fraternal orders and lodges, and other similar organizations.

Recognition of the fact that the community as a whole could be badly hurt by the inability or failure of individuals and families to protect themselves against the economic risks of modern society has led gradually to development of the concept of social security, and to creation of a system of social insurance, especially in the more highly industrialized areas of the world. The community as a whole has participated in this system through the mechanism of government. Such participation has been widely proposed—and just as widely assailed—for a system of medical-care insurance in the United States. The debate over the nature and extent of the government's role has dominated discussion of medical-care problems in this country for many years. The second half of this chapter presents a description of the movement favoring a national approach to health insurance with government sponsorship, and some of the main arguments for and against this approach.

A. *Voluntary Medical Care Insurance*

81. VOLUNTARY PLANS: TYPES AND OBJECTIVES *

INSURANCE AGAINST the economic hazards of sickness, injury, and maternity is a method of pooling risks and resources to budget and pay the cost of medical care, compensate for loss of earnings due to disability, or fulfill both these functions. According to its principal objectives it may be "medical care insurance," "disability insurance," or a combination of both. The widely used generic term "health insurance" lends itself to misinterpretation and therefore should be replaced by the specific terminology whenever feasible.

By proper application of the principle of insurance, the costs incident to sickness, injury, and maternity can be made predictable, budgetable, and less burdensome for the individual. Moreover, access to available services can be facilitated, as the purchasing power of all those who are insured is increased.

To be insurable a hazard must be (1) accidental (a loss must be neither necessary nor impossible), (2) sporadic, (3) expected neither too frequently nor too rarely, and (4) statistically measurable and computable, or at least, estimable. Even if only some of these elements are present, the principle of insurance can be applied successfully. The same rules govern establishment and operation of plans insuring people against the economic hazards of sickness, injury, and maternity.

Like any other form of insurance, medical care insurance rests on the mathematical theory of probabilities, originally designed to determine the chances of the game of dice and later, with full development, widely applied to life contingencies and social problems. The "magic of averages," so frequently mentioned in popular writings on this field, is anything but a mystery.

The probable frequency and severity of many types of illness can be fairly well measured and predicted for large groups of people and over periods of time—unless all calculations are temporarily upset by severe epidemics. The services required to meet the needs of a large group of people can be defined in terms of averages, and the type and number of needed personnel and institutional facilities can be determined accordingly. This knowledge renders it possible to estimate, with a reasonable degree of accuracy, the average amount of money each member of a group has to pay in order to obtain protection against certain costs of medical care.

* From: *Voluntary Medical Care Insurance in the United States*, by Franz Goldmann, M.D.; New York: Columbia University Press, 1948 (Chap. I, "The Principle of Medical Care Insurance," pp. 6-10; and Chap. II, "Trends of Development in the United States," pp. 51-52). Reprinted (with omissions, including initial paragraphs) by permission of the author and publishers. The author is associate professor of medical care at the School of Public Health, Harvard University, Boston.

To achieve effective pooling of risks and resources, two requirements must be met. Many people must band together under a single plan, and each member of the group must make small regular prepayments into a common fund. Thus the risks are shared and the costs are spread over groups of people and periods of time. Large size of the group and sufficient prepayments are essential to both the establishment and the successful operation of a medical care insurance plan. Even a large group may be composed of persons constituting unfavorable risks because of their poor health conditions. Adverse selection of risks can best be avoided by inclusion of many and varied groups representing a cross section of the population and by acceptance of subscribers regardless of income. The greater the number of persons covered by the plan and the more diverse the occupational and economic groups represented in the membership, the better the chances of spreading the risks, increasing the income from prepayments, keeping the rates within reasonable limits, providing for broad scope of service, and paying adequate compensation to the participating members of the professions and the hospitals.

Medical care insurance is distinguished by several characteristics. It is a modern form of social action substituting solidarity for individual effort and certainty for uncertainty. It is organized self-help to remove, or reduce, the financial burden which may arise from sickness, injury, or maternity. People can budget and pay for the cost of medical care when they are healthy and earning. They can obtain service to prevent illness and disability and receive treatment when they are sick.

The members of the plan pay for their own care; they don't "get something for nothing." They are entitled to any or all of the benefits covered by their prepayments without investigation into their economic conditions and without obligation to repay the costs. Equal advantages are offered to all who are eligible, regardless of their social and economic status. Hence the popular appeal of insurance plans.

Because it is a device for pooling risks and resources, medical care insurance is limited in applicability. It is unsuited to cope with such catastrophes as widespread and severe epidemics. It cannot meet all the needs arising out of serious and prolonged sickness, such as mental illness and tuberculosis, as the incidence and severity of such conditions are hard to predict, the probability of future losses is difficult to measure owing to the unusually great variability of costs, and the expenditures involved are very high. The method is feasible only for people able to make regular contributions. Even under the most favorable employment and income conditions, there are certain to be persons who have to depend upon public aid for maintenance and, also, self-supporting individuals and families with many children who cannot make more than a token payment, if any, toward the cost of adequate medical care insurance. In periods of slackening business and low incomes, not to mention severe economic crises, the number and proportion of such people is bound to increase substantially. Finally, difficulties in organizing groups and collecting contributions may prevent effective operation of an insurance program in thinly settled areas.

Funds obtained through prepayments under an insurance plan may be used to provide the participants with cash benefits, services, or both. . . .

The relative merits of cash indemnity and service plans are still debated, although both have a record of more than one hundred years. . . .

The existing [voluntary medical-care insurance] organizations may be classified in various ways. They may be divided into nonprofit plans and plans operated for profit. They may be grouped according to the type of administrative control, such as control by medical societies, consumer cooperatives, private groups of physicians, or community organizations, or according to the socioeconomic groups covered by distinguishing industrial and rural plans. Useful as this approach may be, it does not bring out the very facts that determine the ultimate value of a plan applying the principle of insurance.

If the classification is to serve the measurement and appraisal of medical care insurance plans, it must take into account the basic policies followed in providing for benefits. Applying this principle, one may classify the existing plans in two broad categories, one comprising cash indemnity plans and the other one service plans. Each category may be subdivided according to the type of care provided, for example, hospitalization, physicians' service, or professional as well as hospital service. Organizations furnishing professional services may be grouped according to the pattern chosen for practice, such as individual and group practice. In each subdivision, nonprofit plans must be distinguished from plans operated for profit. The following is a systematic classification of medical care insurance plans.

A. Cash Indemnity Plans

1. Plans indemnifying for hospital expenses only
2. Plans indemnifying for professional expenses only
   (1) surgical expense indemnity plans
   (2) medical (nonsurgical) expense indemnity plans
   (3) plans indemnifying for surgical and nonsurgical expenses
3. Plans indemnifying for hospital and professional expenses

B. Service Plans

1. Plans providing for hospitalization only
   (1) free choice plans, organized to provide service by a number of participating hospitals
   (2) single hospital plans, organized to provide service by one hospital
2. Plans providing for physicians' service only
   (1) individual practice plans
   (2) group practice plans
3. Plans providing for hospitalization and professional services
   (1) individual practice plans
   (2) group practice plans . . .

82. BLUE CROSS AND BLUE SHIELD *

Prepayment for Hospital Care

A BLUE CROSS PLAN is a nonprofit corporation organized under community and professional sponsorship and approved by the American Hospital Association for the purpose of enabling the public to defray the cost of hospital care on a prepayment, group basis. Benefits are in terms of hospital service rather than cash indemnity and are guaranteed by the participating hospitals through contractual arrangements between the hospitals and the Plan. There is an agreement between the subscriber and the Plan, listing benefits to which the subscriber is entitled. When a subscriber has occasion to be hospitalized, he may choose any member hospital of his Plan, subject to his attending physician's referral. (The determination of the necessity for hospitalization remains with the physician.) Upon admittance to the hospital he presents his Blue Cross identification card and no further credit reference is ordinarily required by the hospital. Upon discharge he is billed by the hospital for only such special services as may not be included in his Blue Cross contract, his eligibility for care having been confirmed by the Plan during his stay.

Out of its subscription income the Plan pays its hospitals for the services rendered to its subscribers. These payments are made on a basis previously determined by mutual agreement and approved by the proper regulatory bodies of the state in which the Plan operates.

In addition to the service contract benefits available to subscribers in member hospitals of each Plan, the Plans also make provisions for cases where the subscriber has to be hospitalized elsewhere, as while traveling or while in temporary residence in another area. In such cases the Plan frequently reimburses the subscriber a fixed cash amount per day of hospitalization. Many Plans, however, are participating in a reciprocal program (which will be described later), enabling them to provide service benefits "out-of-area." Thus, the subscribers of any one Blue Cross Plan are protected to a substantial degree regardless of where they may be at the time of hospitalization. This coverage extends to any accredited hospital in the world.

Organization of Blue Cross Plans.—Blue Cross Plans are sponsored locally by the hospitals, the medical profession, and the general public. In most cases the principal initiative in the formation of a Plan has been the county or state hospital association,

* From: "Voluntary, Non-Profit, Hospital and Medical Care Prepayment," by Paul R. Hawley, M.D.; Chap. XVI (pp. 245-68) in *Administrative Medicine* (Haven Emerson, M.D., ed.), Baltimore: Williams and Wilkins Co., 1951 (revised). Reprinted (with omissions, including tables and initial paragraphs) by permission of the author and publishers. The author is the director of the American College of Surgeons, Chicago.

which is only natural. However, it is evident that no Plan can succeed without the approval and support of the medical profession and of the public at large. Initial working capital has often been provided not only by the hospitals but also by local community chests, business and civic organizations, foundations, and individual civic leaders. Initial capital is usually repaid within a very short time out of Plan income.

Blue Cross Plans are controlled by their Boards of Directors (sometimes called Trustees). The Board appoints the executive director and decides all major policies. The method of election or appointment of Board members varies in different localities. In fact, there is so much variation in this respect that generalizations are difficult to make. A few remarks, however, may be pertinent. In a majority of the Plans the entire Board is elected by the members of the corporation. In such Plans the extent to which the member hospitals influence the election of Board members depends upon the representation of the hospitals in the corporation. This varies considerably but in many cases each member hospital has a representative in the corporation. In other instances, the local hospital association elects a certain number of representatives from the hospital field to the Board. In a smaller number of Plans, each member hospital has the right to appoint its own representative on the board.

In one Plan the entire Board is appointed by the member hospitals.

Regarding the extent to which the medical profession controls the election or appointment of Board members, in about one-half of the Plans there is no official control of appointments by the profession. In about one-third of the Plans the local medical society has definite authority to appoint a certain number of Board members. In about a dozen Plans the medical society does not have specific powers of appointment but the doctors are represented by voting members in the corporation. In no Plan is the entire Board appointed by the doctors.

The above paragraphs, however, are by no means to be taken as an indication of the proportional representation of hospitals and doctors on the Plan Boards as they actually exist. The medical profession is represented on virtually every Board to some extent and in the case of about half of the Plans to the extent of 20 per cent or more of the Board membership. Hospital representatives are in the majority in about two-thirds of the Plans.

Representatives of the general public are present to the extent of 20 per cent or more on the Boards of the great majority of the Plans. This means people not directly or officially connected with hospitals or the medical profession. However, the proportion of "public" representation may actually be considerably greater than the above would indicate, because many Boards include hospital trustees who are civic leaders in other fields as well, and may very well consider themselves representatives of the community rather than of the particular hospital with which they are associated, or of hospitals in general. Board members who are hospital administrators, on the other hand, may naturally be expected to have the interests of the hospital primarily at heart.

Direct representation of the subscribers themselves, as such, is a recent development. It may take any one of several forms. . . .

Regarding control of the Plans in general, hospital representatives appear to play a dominant role in most cases as far as official representation is concerned. However, it may not be too much to say that when civic-minded hospital trustees (that is, trustees who will vote on matters of Plan policy in terms of their conception of the public interest rather than of the interests of their hospitals) are added to those Board members who are *officially* representatives of the public, control of the Plans in most cases is dominated by the people who think of themselves as acting in the public interest rather than in the special interests of the hospitals or of any other special group.

Enrollment Methods and Service.—Blue Cross enrollment has been primarily conducted among groups of people working for a common employer. The group insurance principle, with insistence upon a minimum percentage of enrollment within each group, minimizes adverse selection of risk and makes possible maximum extension of benefits. It also helps to put the Plan into an actuarial position whereby it can carry non-group subscribers and other poorer risks, thus carrying out the social purpose of Blue Cross Plans in extending coverage eventually to the largest possible cross section of the entire population.

The minimum percentage of enrollment required within each group varies in inverse ratio to the size of the group.

Besides groups united by a common employer, groups suitable for enrollment may be those with some other common economic interest, such as the membership of a trade union, a professional society, or a trade association.

The minimum size of an eligible group varies among the Plans but the tendency is to extend eligibility to smaller and smaller groups—sometimes as few as two or three persons. In general, 100 per cent enrollment is required in groups of 10 or less, with the percentage decreasing to about 40 or 50 per cent in groups of 25 or more.

Ordinarily contact is first made with the employer to secure his sponsorship and if possible his co-operation in the collection of subscription charges—preferably by payroll deduction, which of course minimizes clerical expense to the Plan. Enrollment opportunity is then presented to the employees through literature and through personal presentation by Plan representatives, and a deadline for initial enrollment is set. After the initial enrollment, arrangements are made for enrollment of new employees, and old employees who did not join at the time of the initial enrollment are usually given an opportunity to join at stated intervals, ordinarily semiannually or annually.

Payroll deduction is the preferred method for collecting subscription dues. The employer assumes the task of collection by deducting the subscription from the employees' pay checks and remitting the total amount monthly to the Plan.

When deduction is not obtainable, or in groups that are of such nature that they do not have a common employer, a group leader or group treasurer is chosen by the subscribers and voluntarily assumes responsibility for collecting from each individual and submitting the total to the Plan at stated intervals. The group leader receives no compensation other than reimbursement for postage, stationery, etc.

When a subscriber leaves an employed group he is permitted to continue his membership on a direct-payment basis, usually at a slight extra charge. The term "conversion" is used to indicate the change from group membership to direct-pay membership, or vice versa. . . .

Developments in Nongroup Enrollment.—In order to fulfill one of the social purposes of Blue Cross and reach the widest possible segment of the population, rather than enrolling only preferred risks, most Plans offer enrollment to persons who are not members of employed groups. . . . The most effective method of doing this which has so far been devised is to throw open enrollment at periodic intervals to all persons in a community who are self-employed or unemployed. To guard against too much adverse selection, a minimum percentage of this section of the population is required, and the enrollment period is limited usually to one or two weeks at intervals of once or twice a year. The campaign is carried on through the active co-operation of civic organizations such as the local chamber of commerce, the men's and women's service organizations and clubs, and individual civic leaders.

The hospital utilization rate for persons enrolled on a community basis is higher than that for employed groups. One reason for this is that more people in elderly age-brackets are allowed to enroll. Another possible reason is that unemployed people are sometimes unemployed because of the very fact that their health is not good. When enrollment is offered to persons in a large group, such as an entire community and if group enrollment requirements are low or are not applied, the normal tendency is to enroll a high percentage of poor actuarial risks. Those most likely to need hospital care will be the first to enroll, while those in the best of health will be the last. . . .

Enrollment of farmers and others living in sparsely populated areas present a special problem. Such people are not as hospital-conscious as are urban dwellers, and therefore a special effort in public education must be made. Employed groups are small and few. The scattered population makes difficult the billing and collection of subscription dues.

Blue Cross Plans have used two principal methods in enrolling the farm population. One is to consider each family as part of the town or village and to offer enrollment on a community basis as described above. The other is to consider the farmers as a special economic group and to offer enrollment through their own organizations, such as the farm bureaus, the granges, the Farmers Home Administration (formerly the Farm Security Administration), farmers' unions, co-operatives, and others. Co-operation on the part of the farm bureaus and their federations has been particularly effective. In a number of states, the farm bureau federations have assigned special workers to promote enrollment of their workers.

Blue Cross Plans in several midwestern states have encouraged the formation of independent, self-governing county health associations. Working in co-operation with the farm organizations, these associations offer enrollment to all farm families. The subscribers' councils previously mentioned have served as effective enrollment agencies in some Plan areas, notably in Kansas and Ohio. . . .

In addition to enrollment through employed groups, communities, and farm

organizations, an increasing number of Blue Cross Plans are now offering enrollment on a direct basis. This means that applications are accepted by mail or over
the counter from individuals wishing to subscribe. When this was first tried by
several Plans about ten years ago, the same contracts were offered as to group
subscribers. It was found that a greatly disproportionate number of applicants
were people who knew that they were in need of hospitalization. The utilization
rate in one large Plan, which enrolled a large number of such individuals, went so
high as to endanger the Plan's stability. Accordingly the Plan had to cancel many
of these contracts. Since then all Plans have placed restrictions on this type of
enrollment in order to keep the loss ratio from getting too much out of line. Restrictions at the time of acceptance of an application may include medical examination, statement as to former illnesses (with denial of benefits for hospitalization due
to pre-existing conditions), age limitation (usually 65 years), and others. Maternity
care is often excluded from the benefits. The subscription rate is usually higher than
for group enrollment. No recent survey has been made to determine the extent
of this type of enrollment. However, it is known to be on the increase in certain
areas.

Benefits.—Blue Cross Plans provide hospital service benefits. In general, "hospital
services" means those services which routinely appear on the hospital bill, as
contrasted to services which appear on the doctor's bill. For the most part, the
distinction is clear-cut, but in the case of certain specialties there has been a great
deal of controversy. These specialties include radiology, pathology, anesthesiology,
and physical therapy. In the vast majority of hospitals these services appear on the
patient's hospital bill, and the public has naturally come to look upon them as
functions of the hospital. However, physicians specializing in these fields have insisted that they are medical services and that they should not be included among
the benefits of a hospital service plan. . . . The great majority of hospitals own their
own x-ray equipment, and pay their staff radiologist on a percentage or on a salary
basis. The same is generally true for hospital pathologists and physical therapists.
In many hospitals, anesthesia service is performed by nurse anesthetists employed
by the hospitals; in others by physicians employed on a full- or part-time salary
basis. Thus the hospital assumes a degree of responsibility for these services, and all
these are charged for on the patient's hospital bill.

The recent rapid growth of medical-surgical service plans offered in conjunction
with Blue Cross Plans is tending to resolve this controversy, with the inclusion of
the above services as benefits under the medical plan rather than the hospital plan.
Another solution has been to continue to offer these services under the Blue Cross
Plan but to designate them specifically as "medical" services.

The member hospitals of the Blue Cross Plans contract with the Plans to
furnish certain services to subscribers, in return for which they are paid by the
Plan according to a contractual arrangement. The hospitals guarantee service to the
subscriber. . . . This distinguishes Blue Cross from commercial insurance.

The term *service-benefits* means that the subscriber receives benefits in terms
of hospital service to the extent of his contract and is billed by the hospital only

for such services as are not covered under the contract. This is in contrast to cash indemnity insurance, under which the policy-holder pays the whole hospital bill and then files a claim with the insurance company for cash reimbursement in the amount specified under his policy.

The service-benefit principle of Blue Cross works to the advantage of the subscriber in several ways. First, his Blue Cross card serves as an adequate credit reference upon admission to the hospital. Second, he need not lay out cash for the whole hospital bill and then file claim with the insurer, as in the case of an indemnity policy. Third, his benefits are usually more liberal than under indemnity, since certain hospital services are provided regardless of cost. Blue Cross Plans frequently pay bills of several hundred dollars (sometimes thousands of dollars) for single cases. Such Blue Cross benefits as oxygen and penicillin in large amounts often run into hundreds of dollars on a single case.

Under the Blue Cross service-benefit contracts, hospital care is available to subscribers in member hospitals to the extent that it is needed, without being restricted to a limited number of dollars per day. This is important because no one individual can foresee when he will need care or what it will cost. The additional fact that 35 per cent of all hospital cases are for six days or less (hospitalization expense is ordinarily highest during the first few days) makes most indemnity schedules inadequate to cover the bulk of such expense.

Blue Cross Plans originate under local sponsorship, and the benefits and subscription rates are designed to suit the requirements of the particular locality of each Plan. In general, benefits are available for most types of illness or injury except those covered by workmen's compensation laws. The specific benefits offered by any given Plan, however, are determined largely by availability of the types of hospital accommodations in the Plan's area, and by the demand for such accommodations on the part of the subscribers and potential subscribers.

Another factor governing the extent of benefits offered is the income level of the particular Plan area....

The general tendency of Blue Cross Plans has been to offer more and more liberal benefits as the Plan expands in size—aiming toward as complete a coverage of the hospital bill as is at any time actuarially feasible.

All Blue Cross Plans provide for room and board, general nursing care, use of the operating room, laboratory service, routine medications and dressings, and use of the delivery room. Beyond these basic services, Plans provide for various other special services. The tabulation below indicates several types of such services covered and the number of Plans providing them in whole or part:

Special diets	83
Emergency room (in accidents)	81
Anesthesia	73
Basal metabolism tests	71
Oxygen therapy	68
X-ray	61
Electrocardiogram	54
Physical therapy	49
Pathology	46

Obstetrical care is provided by all Plans under family contracts, normally with a waiting period of from eight to twelve months. Some plans restrict the length of stay and others the extent of coverage on maternity cases.

Full benefits are provided for a period which varies among the Plans but which averages from twenty-one to thirty days per contract year. Nearly all the Plans provide partial benefits for an additional period, averaging about 50 per cent of full benefits for an additional ninety days.

Regarding the extent to which the average Blue Cross subscriber's hospital bill is covered by his Blue Cross benefits, adequate data on which to base a national figure are not available. However, a recent survey of a small number of Plans showed that when the subscribers to those Plans used the room accommodation specified in their contracts, from 77 to 95 per cent of the average bill was paid by Blue Cross.

Subscriber certificates generally fall into three classifications: one person, two persons, and family. There is a trend toward a two-rate structure, with elimination of the two-person certificate. . . .

The *family certificate* usually covers the subscriber, his wife, and all dependent children under the age of 18. In all of the Plans, dependents are entitled to the same benefits as the subscriber, although in a few Plans dependents must make a small daily payment to the hospital when hospitalized; the amount is usually one dollar per day.

About one-third of the Plans offer a *sponsored dependent certificate.* "Sponsored dependents" are dependents who live with the subscriber but who are persons other than his spouse or children. The subscription rate is usually the same as that for a single person.

Inter-Plan Reciprocity.—The term "reciprocity" has been used somewhat ambiguously to refer to two separate and distinct sets of working agreements which exist among Blue Cross Plans.

The first of these is the *Inter-Plan Transfer Agreement,* in which virtually all Plans participate and which operates as follows: Each Plan accepts the applications of paid-up subscribers of other Blue Cross Plans who establish residence in its area, without regard to local enrollment requirements. Credit is given for the length of time such subscribers have been enrolled in their original Plan, toward meeting any waiting period requirements for benefits in the new Plan. In addition, local employed groups which are branches of organizations with headquarters outside a particular Plan's area are accepted for membership by that Plan, even though smaller in number than regular minimum group requirements, provided that enrollment of home office employees is proceeding or has been affected by another Blue Cross Plan.

The second agreement involves *reciprocity of service benefits* to subscribers of Plans who are hospitalized outside the area served by their own Plan. Under this agreement, for example, if a subscriber of the New York City Blue Cross Plan is hospitalized in Chicago, he is treated temporarily as though he were a member of the Chicago Blue Cross Plan, and receives the same benefits in the Chicago hospital as would normally be provided a local member of the Chicago Plan. The Chicago Plan would pay for this care, and bill the New York Plan for it. Under the program, known as the Inter-Plan Service Benefit Bank, the "Host" Plan pays the local hospital for such care, and is reimbursed through the Bank. The "Home" Plan, to which the patient belongs, is billed by the Bank on a formula based upon the cost of care in its own area. . . .

Blue Cross Subscription Rates.—As indicated previously, subscription rates vary considerably among the individual Blue Cross Plans because of the variation in the cost of hospital service in different areas and because of other factors. . . .

Space does not permit a detailed account of the numerous factors affecting the determination of a particular rate. However, a few of the most common will be briefly mentioned. As a base for a rate structure, the Blue Cross Commission estimated several years ago that approximately eight per cent of the population was hospitalized for acute illnesses in the course of a year, and that the average hospital stay was from ten to twelve days. This means that the average person spent from .8 of a day to one day in the hospital each year. On this basis, the Commission recommended that Blue Cross subscription rates be high enough to cover every subscriber for one day's care per year, plus an additional amount for administration and reserves. For family agreements, the recommendation was for a rate high enough to cover three days' care per year. (Current percentage of population hospitalized and average length of stay are somewhat different from the above figures, but the latter will serve as an illustration of the theory.) To illustrate, suppose that a Plan proposes to pay its member hospitals an average of $6 for care of its subscribers or their dependents. Suppose also that $1.50 is to be added for administration and reserves. The annual subscription rate for a single subscriber would be $7.50. The rates for two-person certificates and for families would be correspondingly greater.

The above rule of thumb should not be used indiscriminately. It is merely a starting point from which to build a rate structure. The utilization of Blue Cross benefits by subscribers varies considerably not only among the different Plan areas, but also according to the type of group enrolled, as pointed out earlier. Not only the costs of hospital service, but also the costs of administering a Blue Cross Plan, vary in different areas. Another factor affecting rate determination is the per cent of income which a Plan aims to allocate to contingency reserve. Changing economic conditions must also be considered. Many Plans, founded during the depression of the 1930's, have had to raise their subscription rates substantially as a result of the current inflation. All of these elements must be balanced against one another whenever a particular rate is under consideration.

Reimbursement to Hospitals.—Payment by Plans to member hospitals for services furnished to Blue Cross subscribers must fulfill two requirements: (1) it must be adequate to reimburse the hospitals for the expense they have incurred; (2) it must be reasonable, bearing in mind the responsibility of the Plan to its subscribers.

There are three basic methods of payment in current use: (1) a uniform rate to all hospitals or to groups of similar hospitals; (2) differing payments based on each hospital's *charges* for service; (3) differing payments based on each hospital's service *costs*.

When there is a uniform rate, it is usually graded so that the payment is higher for the first few days of the hospital stay than for subsequent days. This is because the first few days of a stay are usually the most expensive. . . .

When a payment is made on the basis of the established charges of a hospital, a few Plans pay 100 per cent of such charges, but it is more usual for a Plan to pay slightly less than 100 per cent, on the basis that Blue Cross saves the hospital collection losses on Blue Cross patients, and also that many Blue Cross patients would have been charity cases had they not subscribed to the Plan.

Payment on the basis of hospital costs presents particular difficulties of administration. For one thing, the accounting methods used by hospitals vary greatly, even within the same locality, so that it is often difficult for a Plan to set up a system of payment which will be equally fair to all of its member hospitals. Another trouble, now that Blue Cross patients constitute such a large percentage of all general hospital patients, is that payment on a cost basis tends to penalize those hospitals whose operation is most efficient and economical.

Recognizing the difficulties involved in setting up a fair system of hospital reimbursement, the Council on Administrative Practice of the American Hospital Association formulated, in 1946, a set of principles for the guidance of hospitals and Plans. A few highlights of this set of principles are: (a) "Hospitals should not expect to receive rates of payment from Blue Cross Plans for basic services provided to subscribers in excess of the cost of such services, cost to include an allowance for depreciation of buildings and equipment and allowances for other contingencies . . ." nor in excess of "100 per cent of the average gross earnings at established rates for all private patients occupying similar accommodations in the hospital." (b) The basis and rates of payment should in all cases be negotiated between representatives of the Plan and representatives of the hospitals, both groups having at hand the facts (financial and service data) necessary for enlightened decisions. (c) Both groups, as public service agencies, should bear in mind the needs of each other. . . .

Plan Growth and Financial Data.—The growth in enrollment of Blue Cross Plans in the United States and Canada has proceeded at a rate during the past ten years that is little short of phenomenal. On July 1, 1938 total enrollment was 1,949,294; as of September 30, 1949, it has reached 35,110,593! This is more than 22 per cent of the entire population.* . . .

* See table 47, in this chapter, p. 593, for information on estimated number of persons with Blue Cross coverage for 1953. In 1956, according to a Blue Cross Commission report, 54 million persons were enrolled in Blue Cross plans throughout the country, and more than $1 billion was paid by the plans to their more than 6,000 member hospitals for the more than 53 million patient-days of care they provided to Blue Cross subscribers during the year. (*Blue Cross Report to the Nation,* Chicago: Blue Cross Commission of the American Hospital Association, 1957, pp. 2, 5).

During the same period, the number of Plans has increased from 40 to 90. This latter trend, however, has been offset to some degree by mergers of two or more Plans and by the Blue Cross Commission's policy of encouraging the formation of state-wide Plans when granting first approval to a hospital service plan. Most of the newer Plans are state-wide; where they are not, it is because local legal, or other considerations make a state-wide Plan impracticable. For instance, in Georgia there is a statute limiting a Plan's area of operation to a circle of a 50 mile radius from its headquarters city.

Blue Cross Plans are now in operation in all but one (Nevada) of the 48 states, in the District of Columbia, in 8 Canadian provinces, and in the Territory of Puerto Rico.

There is considerable variation among the Plans in respect to proportional allocation of the income dollar. However, the over-all average distribution, for the first nine months of 1949, was as follows: Paid to hospitals for care of subscribers: 85.12 per cent; administrative expenses: 8.85 per cent; retained for reserves: 6.03 per cent. . . .

Attitude of Organized Labor.—The role of Blue Cross and Blue Shield in relation to labor is increasingly important. Many welfare or group insurance plans negotiated as part of collective bargaining agreements include provision for Blue Cross or Blue Shield benefits, or both. . . .

Blue Cross coverage is endorsed by outstanding trade union leaders in the AFL and CIO, and Blue Cross benefits are an integral part of plans included in the collective bargaining agreements in the building trades, automobile industry, hotel and restaurant industry, furniture, electrical products, machine tool, rubber, and other industries throughout the United States.

Many Blue Cross Plans have labor representatives on their boards of directors or advisory committees.

The participation of labor in providing Blue Cross and Blue Shield protection is also directly related to the question of Federal "health insurance." Until very recently, almost all trade union leaders have said that they were for Federal "health insurance" because they could not see any other way of providing their members with necessary benefits. But, increasingly, there is a recognition that Government standards are usually minimum standards, while voluntary plans, negotiated as part of collective bargaining agreements, offer the union leader an immediate opportunity to provide his members with better than minimum standards. . . .

Prepayment Plans for Medical-Surgical Care

THE FIRST STATE-WIDE medical care prepayment plan was the California Physicians' Service, established by the California Medical Association in 1939. Complete physician's service was offered at a subscription rate of $1.70 per month. There was also a more limited contract available. Enrollment was limited to employed persons earning less than $3,000 per year. Physicians were reimbursed on a "unit" basis, the unit having a par value of $2.50 (the fee for an office visit), with other services being valued at multiples of this unit. Experience in the early years, however, was unfavorable, as demand for services far exceeded expectations, and the effect was to devalue the unit. So, beginning in 1941, all contracts were modified. This resulted in much more favorable experience, and the unit value now approximates par.

In 1934 the House of Delegates of the American Medical Association adopted a set of 10 principles for the guidance of medical service prepayment plans. Some of the more important of these principles were: all features of medical service should be under the control of the medical profession; no third party must be permitted to come between the patient and his physician in any medical relation; the patient must have absolute freedom to choose any participating physician; the confidential nature of the patient-physician relationship must be preserved; medical service should be paid for by the patient in accordance with his income status and in a manner that is mutually satisfactory.

In 1938 a resolution was adopted endorsing "the principle that in any plan or arrangement for the provision of medical services, the benefits shall be paid in cash directly to the individual member."

During the next few years, a number of state medical societies developed their own voluntary prepayment plans. Service benefits were usually offered to subscribers within certain income limits; benefits in terms of indemnity were also offered. . . .

In [1943] the A.M.A. established a Council on Medical Service and Public Relations. . . .

The Council formulated a preliminary set of "Standards of Acceptance for Medical Care Plans." Plans which meet these standards are granted the privilege of using the "seal of acceptance" of the Council on Medical Service. Some of these standards are: approval by the local state or county medical associations; responsibility of the medical profession for the medical services included in the benefits; free choice of physician; maintenance of the confidential patient-physician relationship; maximum benefits consistent with sound financial operation; benefits may be in terms of either cash indemnity or service units; sound enrollment and administrative practices; acceptance of Plans by the Council is ordinarily for "a period of two years or until revoked."

In December, 1945 the House of Delegates had instructed the A.M.A. Trustees and the Council "to proceed as promptly as possible with the development of a specific national health program, with emphasis on the nation-wide organization of locally administered prepayment medical plans sponsored by medical societies." In 1946 there was established a new central co-ordinating organization known as Associated Medical Care Plans, Inc.

Medical-Surgical Plans Affiliated with Blue Cross Plans.—An overwhelming majority of the enrollment in successful nonprofit medical care plans has been carried on in connection with Blue Cross hospital service plan enrollment. This has been logical, since in most areas the Blue Cross Plans were already established and were willing to make available their administrative experience to the medical plans. The degree of co-ordination, however, between local Blue Cross Plans and their corresponding medical care plans varies considerably. The most common arrangement at present is for the two plans to have separate governing boards (and separate corporations) but to have a single executive director and administrative staff. Such an arrangement eliminates duplication of effort in enrollment and administration, and usually works out quite successfully. An even better arrangement is complete integration, with one corporation, one governing board, one executive, and one staff. This exists in only a few areas so far; its extension is hampered possibly by these factors: (1) fear on the part both of the doctors and of the hospital people that the other group wants to control such a plan; (2) the fact that in most areas the Blue Cross Plan was there first, and the medical plan is often not yet sufficiently well developed to command an equal share of public acceptance; (3) the fact that a number of states require by law that medical and hospital prepayment must be provided by separate corporations.

In some areas there is partial administrative co-ordination between medical and hospital plans, with separate corporations, boards, and executive directors, but with the hospital Plan performing certain (not all) administrative services for the medical plan. In such cases the medical plan reimburses the hospital plan for its staff service, usually on the basis of a percentage of income, arrived at by mutual agreement.

In January 1950, 79 of the 90 Blue Cross Plans were co-ordinated in one way or another with companion non-profit medical-surgical plans, in 44 states, the District of Columbia, Puerto Rico, and five Canadian provinces. . . .

Establishment of Blue Shield.—As mentioned above, Associated Medical Care Plans, Inc., was founded in 1946 under the auspices of the American Medical Association, to serve as a central co-ordinating agency for voluntary nonprofit medical care prepayment plans. In general, its role in relation to the medical care plans is analogous to that played by the Blue Cross Commission in relation to the hospital service plans.

Associated Medical Care Plans, Inc. (governed by the Blue Shield Commission) as originally organized was officially related to the American Medical Association because its original constitution provided that three members of the Commission must be appointed by A.M.A.'s Council on Medical Service. . . . In June 1949 the A.M.A. House of Delegates approved a complete separation of A.M.C.P. from the A.M.A. on the ground that A.M.C.P. had matured to the point where it could function more efficiently as an autonomous trade organization. The remaining commissioners are elected by the Plans themselves, by districts, in a manner similar to the election of the Blue Cross Commissioners.

To be eligible for full membership in A.M.C.P., a medical care plan must meet the standards of acceptance of the Council on Medical Service, referred to above, must be nonprofit, and must be in actual operation. . . . The activities of the central organization are financed, as are those of the Blue Cross Commission, by dues from the individual Plans prorated according to each Plan's enrollment.

As of September 30, 1949, there were 64 Blue Shield (A.M.C.P.) Plans with a total enrollment of 11,302,233, in 37 states, the District of Columbia, two territories (Hawaii and Puerto Rico), and two Canadian Provinces (Manitoba and British Columbia). About half of these Plans are state-wide, the remainder covering smaller geographic areas. The September 30, 1949 enrollment represents 86 per cent of the 13,138,790 total enrollment in all nonprofit medical care plans.* ...

As for distribution of the income dollar, the Blue Shield Commission issued a report as of September 30, 1949, covering the Blue Shield Plans and 10 other nonprofit medical plans. The combined average for all these plans was: paid in medical or surgical benefits: 80.88 per cent; administrative expenses: 13.19 per cent; added to reserves: 5.93 per cent.

Blue Shield Benefits.—Under a straight service-benefit contract, the subscriber is entitled to such surgical (or medical) services as are included in the contract and as he may require, and he receives no bill from the physician. The physician accepts from the Plan, as full payment, the fees for various operative or other procedures as established under his contract with the Plan.

Under a straight indemnity contract, the subscriber receives cash or credit in predetermined amounts toward the physician's fee. The physician is free to charge the patient fees in excess of these amounts.

In point of fact, the most typical Blue Shield contract is one which is a combination of service and indemnity. That is, a subscriber whose annual income is below a certain amount (say, for instance, $3,000) receives service benefits, but a subscriber with a larger income receives only specified credits toward the doctor's total bill.

The *service-benefit contract* is generally the most favorable one to the subscriber, since he knows he is fully protected. One practical advantage to the doctor is that prepayment serves to cut down his collection losses. However, subscription rates must be kept down to a level generally acceptable to the public, and this may mean that the Plan's income per subscriber will be insufficient to reimburse the participating doctors adequately. Another problem with service benefits is that it is often both difficult and awkward for the doctor (or the patient himself at times) to determine whether the patient's income is over or under the specified limit.

An *indemnity contract* eliminates these difficulties for the physician, and is generally to his advantage, since it puts a floor under his charges without establishing a ceiling. It is, moreover, simpler to administer. The subscriber, however, has no definite assurance of what proportion of the doctor's fee will be covered.

As far as enrollment is concerned, a relatively small number of subscribers have straight service contracts, a considerably larger number have indemnity, and a still larger number (about one-half of the grand total) have a combination of the two. No matter what the form of contract, however, subscription rates must be adjusted from time to time to meet changing economic conditions such as

* See table 47 in this chapter, p. 593, for information on the estimated number of persons with Blue Shield coverage in 1953. An estimate of the number of persons with Blue Shield coverage as of Dec. 31, 1956, may be found in *The Extent of Voluntary Health Insurance Coverage in the United States,* New York: The Health Insurance Council, 1957, p. 13.

the rising inflation of the past several years. A contract which may seem fair one year may become quite unfair a couple of years later.

Since surgical procedures are usually more costly than medical therapy (not only in themselves but also because they ordinarily require hospitalization of the patient), it is only natural that the medical care prepayment plans have emphasized coverage for surgeon's fees. However, there is a steadily growing tendency to include coverage for nonsurgical treatment, not only in the hospital but in the office and home as well.

It is customary to list, on the subscriber's contract, a number of the most common operative procedures, with the amount covered for each operation. Obstetrical care is usually included. Surgical care contracts for the most part bear subscription rates about the same as or slightly less than corresponding Blue Cross hospital service contracts. Regarding the trend toward more and more comprehensive coverage, it might be noted that a Plan will sometimes start out with a surgical contract, then offer a supplementary contract or rider to cover nonsurgical physicians' services, and finally combine the two into a comprehensive contract.

Virtually all Blue Shield enrollment is carried on in conjunction with Blue Cross or other hospital service plans' enrollment. Usually, in fact, it is the Blue Cross staff personnel which sells Blue Shield. It is offered either to previously enrolled Blue Cross groups, or to non-enrolled groups in a combination "package" along with Blue Cross coverage. The advantages of co-ordination with Blue Cross, from the standpoint of economical and efficient administration, have already been pointed out in connection with medical care plans generally.

Plan-Physician Agreements and Payments to Physicians.—Agreements between Blue Shield Plans and their participating physicians are characterized by three main features. First, the doctor agrees to abide by the rules and regulations of the Plan corporation. Second, when there is a service-benefit contract, the doctor agrees to accept the Plan's payment as full reimbursement for his services to a subscriber. Third, in most cases he agrees to accept *pro rata* payments from the Plan in the event the Plan cannot pay the full value of the service unit or of the indemnity; in this respect the doctor guarantees or underwrites the Plan, just as Blue Cross member hospitals underwrite the Blue Cross Plans.

Some Plans which are on a straight indemnity basis require no guarantee on the part of the physicians; they merely pay the same indemnities to all physicians, in or out of their areas.

In the vast majority of Plans, payment is made directly by the Plan to the physician. Where it is not, the claim report form usually provides for assignment by the patient to the doctor.

Legal Status of Blue Shield Plans.—In general, the legal status of Blue Shield Plans is similar to that of Blue Cross Plans. Most of them are organized either under special enabling legislation or under the general laws. The first legislation authorizing medical care prepayment by nonprofit plans was passed in several states in 1939. Similar legislation has since been passed in a number of other states, in several of which the law permits one plan to issue both hospital and medical service contracts.

In most states the medical plans, as well as the Blue Cross Plans, are subject to supervision by the Insurance Commissioner. The degree or extent of such supervision varies greatly among the states.

. . . Where the law provides for separate medical care plans, the provisions follow the pattern of the hospital service plan law of the same state, except for sections dealing specifically with medical service. With a few exceptions, the medical plans are exempt from state and local taxation.

Control and Administration of Medical Care Plans.—Where hospital and medical service prepayment is offered by a single corporation, the personnel of the board of directors, or trustees, is usually divided equally between the medical profession, hospital representatives, and the general public. In the more numerous cases where the medical care plan is a separate corporation, the doctors usually have majority representation on the board. A recent Blue Shield survey showed that the average composition of all Blue Shield boards was two-thirds doctors and one-third laymen.

The administration of medical plans is of much the same character as that of Blue Cross Plans. Enrollment, billing, and maintenance of subscriber records are usually handled for both plans by the same staff personnel. There is usually one executive director (virtually always a layman) for both plans. Most medical plans have a professional committee or a medical director, to review claims and arbitrate cases where there is a question as to the propriety of the fee.

After a participating physician has treated a subscriber, he sends the plan a bill or report of service. The plan checks the patient's status as a paid-up subscriber, records the service performed, and sends a check to the physician. . . .

83. Commercial Insurance *

The purpose of the present article is to describe the health protection offered by insurance companies through policies covering individuals or family groups.

In order to obtain reliable data, the Insurance Department of the Chamber of Commerce of the United States sent a carefully prepared, special questionnaire to all companies replying to its regular 1950 survey of numbers covered by such policies. This special survey was undertaken at the behest of the Brookings Insti-

* From: "Benefits and Costs of Individual and Family Health Insurance Policies," by Benjamin B. Kendrick and A. L. Kirkpatrick; *American Economic Security* 8:17-32, Jan.-Feb. 1951 (No. 1). Reprinted (with omissions, including figures and initial paragraphs) by permission of the publishers. The authors are, respectively, research associate, Life Insurance Association of America, New York; and manager of the insurance department of the United States Chamber of Commerce, Washington, D.C.

tution for use in connection with the large-scale health study now in progress at Brookings.

Responses were received from 120 organizations out of some 500 which issue individual or family health policies. These responses, supplemented to some extent by other information, furnished a representative cross section of insurance company activities in the field. Cooperating with the Chamber's Insurance Department, the Life Insurance Association of America tabulated and analyzed the data. . . .

Policy Provisions on Hospital-Expense Benefits

AT PRESENT, about nine million workers have primary or "personal" hospitalization protection through individual and family policies, and in addition there are over six million wives, children, and others whose hospital expenses are defrayable through dependents' provisions in family contracts.* These figures include both those protected by separate hospitalization policies and those protected through the incorporation of hospital benefits in a basic loss-of-income contract.

In general, the same distinctions as to occupational, "commercial," noncancellable, fraternal, and industrial policies [that apply to] loss-of-income contracts, apply to hospital policies or provisions as well. They also apply to the surgical and medical provisions, considered further along, which usually are a part of the same policy providing the hospital benefits.

The two most important features concerning hospital benefits are the daily benefit rate and the maximum number of days for which the daily rate will be paid. Here, there may be a distinction between the rate and duration for personal coverage and a somewhat lesser rate and/or duration applying to dependents. Also, a few companies, following a common Blue Cross practice, issue policies providing a full daily rate for an initial period, with a reduced rate for a further period applying to extended hospital stays.

In addition to what may be called "room and board" hospital benefits, policies normally offer some reimbursement for miscellaneous hospital expenses. Another aspect to be noted is the varying reimbursement practices as to hospital confinements for childbirth, both for female policyholders and for the wives of male policyholders who have dependents' coverage.

The daily hospital "room and board" benefit rate in policies currently being issued ranges from a low of about $3 to as high as $22. However, as yet only a few large companies issue policies with daily rates above $15. Within these limits, a few companies apply a lower range to dependents than is applied to personal coverage.

The daily rates provided in the most popular policies vary from $4 for personal coverage and $3 for dependents up to $10 for each. The unweighted average daily

* See, for more recent estimates of the number of persons covered by hospital-expense policies written by private insurance companies, table 47 in this chapter, p. 593; and *The Extent of Voluntary Health Insurance Coverage in the United States,* New York: The Health Insurance Council, 1957, p. 13.

rate among the policies most frequently bought in the different companies is $6.25 for personal coverage and $5.35 for dependents. Weighted averages would be at least slightly higher than these figures.

Leaving supplementary benefit periods at reduced rates out of account for the moment, the maximum benefit durations offered by replying companies range from about 30 to 365 days for personal and dependents' coverage. Quite a number of companies offer only one standard duration provision of, say, 90 days.

Most companies report either 90 or 100 days as their most popular benefit duration. However, because many of the remaining companies find a 30-day provision most in demand, an unweighted average of the reports yields a figure of 75 days of hospitalization during which the full daily benefit rate is payable. A weighted average would be little if any higher. It may be noted that no company reports a "most popular" figure for dependents differing from that reported for personal coverage.

None of the larger companies and only a handful of other companies offer policies providing supplementary benefit durations at reduced daily rates. For those that do, the maximum supplementary duration in the most popular policies averages 85 extra days. During the supplementary period, one-half the regular daily benefit is normally payable.

The term "miscellaneous hospital expenses" ordinarily includes such items, among others, as charges for operating room and anaesthesia, laboratory fees, and the cost of drugs. A few companies issue policies providing hospital benefits which do not contain any provision for payments to meet these expenses. At the other extreme, a few other companies issue policies which reimburse for them without limit. But the common practice is for such reimbursement to be limited by a specified sum. The lowest limit reported is $15, while only a scattering of companies offer reimbursement above about $150.

Unweighted averages of the reimbursement provisions which the reporting companies find most popular yield figures of $70 for personal coverage and $65 for dependents. Weighted figures would be about the same.

Approximately half the replying companies stated that all such policies which they issue provide hospital benefits for childbirth. The remaining replies were about evenly divided between companies whose policies uniformly do not provide benefits for childbirth and companies whose policies vary. In general, the replies suggest that about three-quarters of the adult females having hospital expense protection are covered with respect to childbirth—a conclusion applicable to both personal and dependents' coverage.

Policy Provisions On Surgical-Expense Benefits

SURGICAL-EXPENSE benefits began to be generally offered by insurance companies within a few years after hospital-expense benefits started to achieve popularity. At present, over five million persons have primary protection against surgical expense through individual and family policies, with some four million others protected as dependents.* The chief feature with respect to surgical benefits is the schedule of operations contained in the policy, listing the amount payable by the company with respect to various surgical procedures. These schedules are ordinarily quite complete, but, should the policyholder or dependent undergo an unlisted operation, the company usually pays an equitable amount in reimbursement for the surgeon's fee.

To obtain information on surgical schedules, companies were asked to furnish data on the top schedule benefit in policies offering surgical protection and on the benefits with respect to two common operations, appendectomy and tonsillectomy-adenoidectomy. Companies were also asked to state the extent to which surgical schedules include obstetrical benefits.

The top surgical benefit may be as high as $500 in the surgical schedules of policies currently being issued by reporting companies. However, only a few companies go above $400, while $100 is about the lowest top benefit. For dependents' coverage, only a few companies go above $300 as the top surgical benefit.

With respect to the top benefit in the most frequently purchased policies, unweighted averages of the separate company reports yield figures of $163 for personal and $147 for dependents' coverage. However, for a group of the largest companies, averages of $192 and $183, respectively, represent the top benefit in the most popular policies.

For appendectomies, policies being issued by reporting companies provide benefits ranging from about $50 or $75 up to about $250, although a few companies go as high as $400. In policies reported as most popular, the average amounts paid are $108 for personal coverage and $92 for dependents. Among the largest companies the corresponding figures are $125 and $113, respectively.

For tonsillectomy-adenoidectomies, current policies of reporting companies offer benefits ranging from $10 to $20 at the bottom up to $100 or more at the top, with figures for dependents' coverage a shade lower. The average benefit in the most popular policies is $29 for personal coverage and $27 for dependents. For a group of the largest companies the comparable figures are $39 and $36, respectively.

More than half of the reporting companies state that none of the surgical schedules which they issue cover obstetrical procedures. However, about a third of the remaining companies state that all of their surgical schedules include such procedures. All in all, it appears that somewhat over one-third of the policies being issued provide obstetrical protection. There are no clear differences here in the practices of larger and smaller companies or as between personal and dependents' coverage.

---

* See, for more recent estimates of the number of persons covered by surgical-expense policies written by private insurance companies, *The Extent of Voluntary Health Insurance Coverage in the United States,* New York: The Health Insurance Council, 1957, p. 13; and table 47 in this chapter, p. 593 (combined estimate of the number of persons covered under either surgical or medical policies).

Policy Provisions on Medical-Expense Benefits

ONLY IN THE last few years have insurance companies and Blue Shield plans begun to offer general medical benefits. At present, the experimental phase of this development is just ending, and a broad expansion of general medical coverage appears to be commencing. At present, over two million individuals have protection against general medical expense through individual and family policies, of whom about two-thirds have personal coverage, with the remainder protected as dependents.*

The term "general medical expense" as used with respect to insurance policies means the cost of doctors' treatments. Three types of treatment, or visit, may be distinguished: The doctor may visit the patient at a hospital (suggesting a relatively serious condition); the doctor may call at the patient's home; or the patient may visit the doctor's office.

While policies protecting against medical expense may be on a so-called "blanket-limit" basis, most policies are on a so-called *"per diem"* basis. The blanket-limit basis, as the phrase suggests, involves the setting of a maximum expense amount for which the company will reimburse, with a deductible amount usually provided also. Under the more popular *per diem* basis, a reimbursement limit is set with respect to each call, subject to the possible elimination of an initial number of calls from benefit considerations. Commonly, *per diem*-basis policies also contain an over-all reimbursement limit. The following three paragraphs relate entirely to *per diem*-basis provisions, there not being sufficient data on blanket-limit policies for further comment.

Reporting companies limit reimbursement for the cost of doctors' hospital visits to from $2 to $5 for each visit under *per diem* policies, with only one visit a day ordinarily taken into account. Most companies do not offer a choice on reimbursement limit, generally providing a flat $3 a visit for both personal and dependents' coverage. A large proportion of the companies do not provide any elimination of an initial number of hospital calls, this being particularly notable with respect to accidents. Other companies eliminate the first two or three visits.

Benefits for home calls average a shade higher than for hospital calls. While $3 a visit is the most common provision, a number of companies offer $4 and $5 provisions, particularly for personal coverage. Usually benefits are not paid for the first two or three home calls.

For visits to the doctor's office, benefits are a bit lower than for home or hospital calls. Most reporting companies provide either $2 or $3 a visit, with the $2 provision somewhat more popular. There is almost always an elimination of the first two or three office visits, with the elimination provision sometimes omitted in case of accident. . . .

* See, for more recent estimates of the number of persons covered by medical-expense policies written by private insurance companies, the sources cited in the preceding footnote.

84. Comprehensive Service Benefits *

Organization

THE HEALTH INSURANCE Plan of Greater New York is a community-sponsored, voluntary medical care plan incorporated under the New York State Insurance Law as a nonprofit agency. It is not intended to be merely another medical insurance company. Its purpose is to provide comprehensive medical services to workers and their families through medical teams which assume full responsibility for medical care of the group in return for distribution of the premium income in the form of capitation payments. It was hoped that in this manner comprehensive medical care —preventive, early diagnostic and curative—could be provided on a sound financial and actuarial basis and without any restrictions or supplementary charges.

The Board of Directors of the Health Insurance Plan includes the mayor and high officials of the municipal government, the heads of two of the largest banks, important leaders of private industry, representatives of the Congress of Industrial Organizations and the American Federation of Labor and eight physicians selected for their professional or administrative experience, two of whom are the administrative heads of medical schools (Columbia University College of Physicians and Surgeons and Long Island College of Medicine). The determination of professional eligibility of participating medical groups and of standards for their professional services is the responsibility of a Medical Control Board comprised of medical members of the Board of Directors and representatives of the participating medical groups, the New York Academy of Medicine and two of the larger county medical societies (New York and Kings). Matters which concern the relationship of participating physicians to the Health Insurance Plan and its subscribers are cleared through a Joint Conference Committee consisting of four physicians who are elected by the participating groups, one from each major borough of the city, and four members of the Board of Directors, two of whom are physicians. The medical department of the plan is assisted by a division maintaining liaison between the physicians and the subscribers to facilitate the work of the medical groups. A Division of Research and Statistics constantly studies the utilization of services.

Insurance Costs

IN ORDER to enable the lower paid workers to subscribe to the plan, the employer is required to pay half the premium. Unless the employer paid at least half, the

* From: "Health Insurance Plan of Greater New York: The First Three Years," by George Baehr, M.D.; *Journal of the American Medical Association* 143:637-40, June 17, 1950 (No. 7). Reprinted (with omissions, including initial paragraph) by permission of the author and publishers. The author is a special medical consultant for the Health Insurance Plan of Greater New York and was, until recently, its president and medical director.

lowest paid workers could not afford the high annual premium required to provide comprehensive care of high quality for them and their families. Workers with low incomes also require an incentive to join, for few can appreciate the value of complete medical coverage until they begin to use the service.

Enrollment in the plan is open to groups of twenty-five or more persons having a common employer, if at least 75 per cent join; also to employed groups of ten to twenty-five persons if 90 per cent agree to join and include their dependents. Most subscribers to the plan have been enrolled in family units. . . .

For employed groups which have the so-called "family contract," the basic premium rate for a member without dependents is $17 a year with an equal contribution by the employer, making a total of $34 a year.* Couples pay double and families of any size pay three times the single rate, the employer in each instance contributing an equal amount. . . . A family of fourteen pays the same premium as a family of three, which of course reduces the average return per enrollee to the plan. Payment to the medical groups for their services is not affected by the family size, for they are remunerated on a per capita basis. . . .

New York state law enacted in 1946 authorizes the City of New York to pay half the premiums for its employees who desire to enroll and for all dependent members of their families. Now in its fourth year of operation, the Health Insurance Plan is providing comprehensive medical care to more than 235,000 persons in their homes, at physicians' offices, at medical centers and in hospitals.† In addition to employees of the City of New York, the insured include the employees of the United Nations and of one hundred and fifty-one other business and industrial firms, labor unions and social welfare agencies within the city.

Medical Groups

THE PROFESSIONAL services are provided through twenty-eight medical groups situated in various parts of the city, each group having twenty-five or more members. The twenty-eight groups comprise 845 physicians, of whom 334 are general practitioners and 511 are internists, pediatricians and other specialists.‡ The subscribers therefore have a wide selection of medical groups and of family physicians. To maintain a high level of service to subscribers and to open the plan to other physicians who desire to participate, additional medical groups are activated from time to time as enrolment increases. In all groups, the chief of each of the twelve basic specialties must hold a certificate from an American specialty board or an appointment as attending or associate attending physician on the staff of a hospital approved by the respective specialty board for resident training in his specialty, or he must have equivalent qualifications.

---

* The present premium rate for a *family group of three or more persons* is $64.08 per year for the employed member and a like amount for his employer, or a total of $128.16.

† Plan members (including dependents) numbered close to 500,000 in 1956.

‡ There were 32 medical groups in the Plan in 1956, comprising approximately 1,000 physicians—both general practitioners and specialists.

The subscribers are entitled to general medical care, specialist and surgical care, preventive services, maternity and pediatric care, all diagnostic laboratory procedures, roentgen examinations and roentgen therapy, radium and radon treatment, physical therapy, administration of blood and plasma, and psychiatric advice and guidance but not prolonged treatment. They are also entitled to visiting nurse services in their homes and to ambulance transportation. No additional charge is made for any service except for night calls between 10 P.M. and 7 A.M., for which a fee of $2 may be collected by the medical group. Many of the groups ignore this unless there is abuse. All types of illness and disability are covered, including preexisting conditions. There are no physical examinations for admission and no age limits or waiting periods. The cost of hospitalization is covered by a separate Blue Cross or commercial hospital insurance contract, which all subscribers must carry.

Not included are treatment for drug addiction, acute alcoholism or chronic conditions, such as mental disease and tuberculosis, which require care in an institution other than a general hospital. Drugs, dentistry, prosthetic appliances, eyeglasses and purely cosmetic surgical measures are not covered. For exceptional procedures such as brain surgery, fenestration surgery for deafness and operations for congenital heart disease, the groups reinsure themselves through a special reserve fund, which engages some of the best surgeons in the city for the care of these patients and thereby relieves the groups of this unusual and unpredictable responsibility and expense. The cost of radium and radon is also paid from this central fund.

When a subscriber enrolls, he selects one of the several medical groups serving the county or area in which he lives. He then selects one of the general physicians in the medical group as his personal or family physician, who in turn arranges for all necessary specialist or laboratory services.

The medical groups are individually organized as partnerships and are completely autonomous, except that they must possess the physical facilities and meet the organizational pattern and professional requirements of the Health Insurance Plan's Medical Board. The required physical standards vary with the number of subscribers enrolled in the groups; there are three categories, less than 5,000, and 10,000 and above 10,000. Three medical groups are serving more than 20,000 subscribers each, and one group serves about 26,000.

Income to Physicians from the Plan

UNDER THE PRESENT capitation rates, the plan is making monthly payments to its medical groups at a rate of over $5,520,000 a year for the care of its 235,000 subscribers, many of whom previously paid little or nothing for their medical care.* Although still in its early promotional stage of development, costs of central administration are already down to less than 12 per cent; an additional 4 per cent of gross premium income is set aside for the legal reserve required by the State Insur-

* In 1955 the amount paid by the Plan to its affiliated medical groups totaled more than $12.5 million.

ance Department, and a similar amount is being withheld temporarily to cover indemnity for illnesses and accidents to subscribers away from home, for other possible contingencies and for amortization of the generous loans which were made at the outset by several philanthropic foundations to assist in establishment of the program.

A medical group on reaching its objective of 20,000 subscribers has a gross income of $460,000 a year, more if better paid workers among the enrolled employees join in the future at the higher premium rate. The medical groups, in accordance with their partnership arrangements, remunerate their members by an annual salary, after defraying their operational costs. In addition, almost all the groups have accumulated reserve funds during the past year with which they intend to improve their medical center and extend the scope of their services.

After all operating costs of a group are defrayed, the average net income of its physicians for full time service is at least $10,000 a year.[1] Since younger physicians of the medical group who are on probation and are not yet partners receive less and senior members substantially more, it is believed that this is reasonably adequate compensation for medical services rendered to persons of moderate income, many of whom formerly received free care at clinics and hospitals or were treated by physicians at reduced fees or as charity cases. One large group pays young physicians a starting salary of $7,500; when they become junior partners, after a year of trial, they receive $10,000; senior partners are remunerated at the rate of $17,000 to $18,000 for full time service. In addition to their income from the Health Insurance Plan, the physicians affiliated with the groups derive additional income from noninsured patients and from services rendered in compensation cases of veterans and workmen. . . .

Only one medical group is partly manned by full time physicians and specialists who do not engage in private practice. In all other medical groups, most of the participating physicians give part time to the plan and almost all engage in a variable amount of individual private practice.

Organization and Efficiency of Groups

EACH MEDICAL group operates through a central administrative office and laboratory with a variable amount of office space for members of its staff. Eight groups have their basic clinical and laboratory services located in a complete health center, although many of the general physicians and some of the specialists in six of the eight (all but the New York University and Montefiore units) continue to see insured patients in private offices because these are located nearer the homes of their enrolled subscribers. In the remaining groups, the requirement of a complete health center to house the offices of the entire staff was waived temporarily because of low enrollment in the early days and because of the postwar shortages and high costs of building materials. All medical groups will now be required to meet the

---

[1] Full time service is defined as forty hours a week. This leaves sufficient time for additional private practice and for hospital or other extracurricular work.

terms of their contract in regard to the establishment of a complete health center as soon as their subscriber enrollment reaches 10,000.*

From the previous experiences of older groups in other parts of the country, it was estimated that twelve and a half full time physicians or an equivalent proportion of physicians on part time would be able to provide the medical services required by 10,000 persons, or one physician per 800 subscribers. This number has seemed to be adequate for most of the insured groups. Differences in the age-sex composition of a given group's enrollment, as well as the extra work necessary shortly after a new enrollment because of the backlog of previously unmet medical needs, are important factors in determining the required number of physicians, as is also the judicious use of auxiliary personnel, visiting nurses and optometrists to relieve the physicians of unnecessary labor.

It is already obvious that the caliber of work of the various medical groups is not uniform. The medical and research divisions of the Health Insurance Plan have recently completed a special survey of the staff operations and clinical services rendered by each of the twenty-six medical groups in operation before January 1 [1950], which revealed differences in performance. Four groups maintain the highest standards of service, nine other groups are not far behind, and there are gradations among the others. The groups are comprised of physicians and specialists who represent a good cross section of the reputable members of the medical profession of the city. It is our belief that a plan such as this, if it is to have broad application, should not depend too largely on medical groups at teaching hospitals, except that their professional work may be used to measure the performance of other groups. It must also be able to take an average sample of the physicians and specialists in the community and, by welding them together into a coherent medical group and gradually indoctrinating them with the ideals of modern preventive and curative medicine, enable them to provide medical care of better quality and of far broader social significance than they could as unsupervised physicians, practicing medicine in relative isolation.

The survey has disclosed deficiencies in all groups which would have gone undetected in ordinary private practice. Without any pressure from the Health Insurance Plan, revelation of these shortcomings to each medical group by the physician making the survey usually results in correction. The most effective means at the disposal of the Health Insurance Plan for elevating the standards of medical practice by all groups is to use the experiences of each group as yardsticks for measuring the performance of the others. . . .

A recent study of 1,015 consecutive obstetric deliveries during the period July 1, 1948 to June 30, 1949 revealed no maternal deaths. Surgical intervention (cesarian section) was required in 2.7 per cent of the deliveries, compared with 4.7 per cent for the city of New York generally; the neonatal mortality was 9 per 1,000 live births, compared with 20 per 1,000 for the city as a whole during this twelve month period. This favorable experience occurred in spite of the fact that under the Health Insurance Plan the proportion of primiparas and multiparas

---

* Most of the medical groups were housed in health centers in 1957.

35 to 39 years of age was twice that reported for the city of New York, the proportion of multiparas over 40 was double and of primiparas over 40 was four times that for the city. In a similar manner, the experience of the plan in a variety of other clinical fields, such as preventive medicine, pediatric services and cancer detection, is being used as a yardstick for measuring the general adequacy of its medical services and for determining their costs.

Fears that the availability of unlimited medical services would be abused by subscribers have proved to be unfounded. In fact, continued education of subscribers is required in some instances to encourage more adequate utilization of the available services, especially among trades whose workers are generally of a low educational level.

Approximately 500,000 physician services (exclusive of those of radiologists and pathologists), from a home or office visit to a major operation, have been required per 100,000 subscribers per year. This is less than was anticipated. Of these, about 56 per cent have been rendered by general physicians and 44 per cent by specialists. The combined services of the general physicians, internists and pediatricians accounted for 69 per cent of all services. It is particularly interesting that the recently completed survey revealed little evidence of excessive referral of patients to specialists. Several medical groups, among them the one with the largest enrollment, require all children to be cared for by pediatricians from the time of birth to 12 years of age and relieve the general physicians of this responsibility. In all groups, 98 per cent of all deliveries are performed by obstetricians.

Home calls constitute 12 per cent of all services. About 79 per cent of the medical services are rendered in the health centers of the groups or in the doctors' offices. Despite the Blue Cross incentive to hospitalization, laboratory services for hospitalized patients being paid in New York City by the Blue Cross and not by the Health Insurance Plan, one of the most surprising experiences has been that only 8.9 per cent of the total number of medical services have been rendered in hospitals. These statistics include every preoperative and postoperative visit to a hospitalized patient as well as the operative service itself, but not the services of radiologists or pathologists at either the group center or the hospital. The fact that 91 per cent of all medical services under a comprehensive prepayment plan are rendered outside of hospitals is a demonstration of the inadequacy of limited insurance coverage restricted solely to hospitalizable illness. It is an unanswerable argument in favor of coverage for comprehensive medical care.

In line with their present emphasis on preventive care, twenty-three of the medical groups of the Health Insurance Plan distribute informational bulletins to their subscribers periodically. These contain preventive information appropriate to the season and also advice on how to obtain the maximum benefit from the service. Through this means, more adequate utilization by subscribers of the groups' facilities for disease prevention and early diagnosis is being stimulated. Some groups are offering educational lectures to their enrolled subscribers. . . .

85. Extent of Coverage

*A. A 1951 REPORT ***

THE BASIC FACTS concerning the extent to which the American people were enrolled in voluntary medical-care insurance plans at the end of 1950 are illustrated in figure 30. It shows that out of our population of 150 million people, an estimated 75 million have insurance against some part of the costs of medical care, while another 75 million have not yet been reached by voluntary medical-care insurance. In considering this diagram two factors should be kept clearly in mind: One, among the group shown as having medical-care insurance of any type are included those with partial or limited protection; and two, among the group with no insurance protection are included the recipients of public assistance, a certain number of veterans, and other individuals with some public resources for medical care available to them, as well as an unknown number of persons of economic status such that they may not feel a need for insurance.

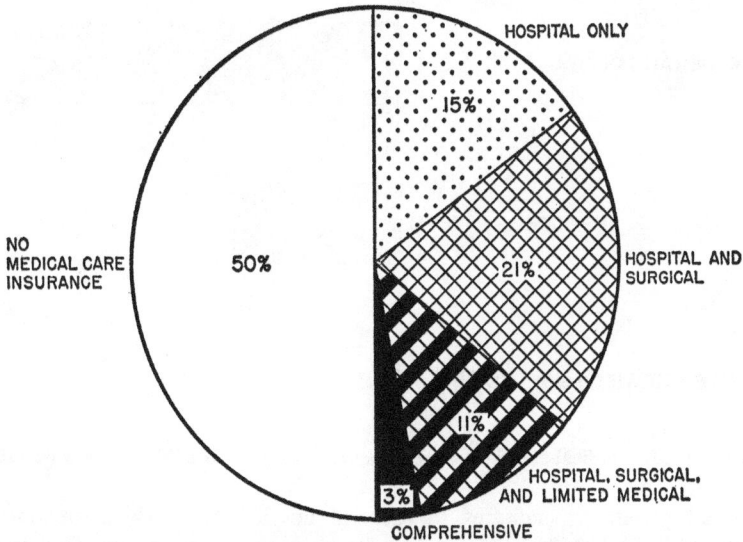

FIGURE 30. How many people have any medical care insurance?

According to figure 30, hospital insurance alone is held by 15 per cent of the total population, or approximately 23 million persons. An additional 21 per cent of the population, or 31 million people, have some degree of protection against

* From: *Health Insurance Plans in the United States* (Report No. 359 of the U.S. Senate Committee on Labor and Public Welfare), 82nd Cong., 1st Sess.; Washington: U.S. Government Printing Office, 1951 (Part I, pp. 1-10). Reprinted with omissions, including initial paragraphs and some figures.

the costs of both hospital and surgical care. Another 17 million persons, representing 11 per cent of the country's population, have hospital, surgical, and limited medical insurance—all in varying amounts. And finally, less than 3 per cent of the population, composed of between 3 and 4 million persons, have comprehensive medical care insurance, including hospital, surgical, and relatively complete medical insurance.

There has been a striking increase in the last 10 years in the number of people in the United States who have been reached by voluntary insurance, especially group insurance, against some part of the costs of medical care. The numbers who had some protection against the costs of hospital care, for example, rose from less than 6 million in 1939 to an estimated 75 million at the end of 1950.

The benefits of medical-care insurance are in largest amount for the costs of hospital care and, next, for the costs of physicians' services. Insurance benefits for general hospital care amounted to $530 million in 1949, while benefits for physicians' services totaled $225 million. Almost none of the insurance in force relates to the costs of dental care, nursing, drugs or medical supplies outside the hospital. The amount of insurance benefits spent for each class of services is illustrated in figure 31.

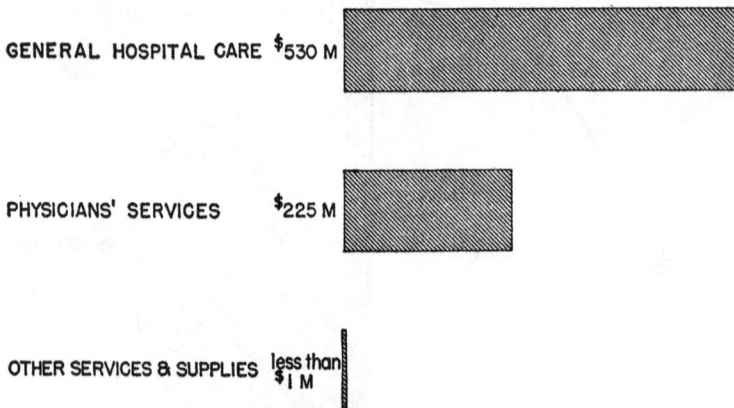

GENERAL HOSPITAL CARE $530 M

PHYSICIANS' SERVICES $225 M

OTHER SERVICES & SUPPLIES less than $1 M

FIGURE 31. Medical-care insurance benefits amounted to $755 million in 1949.

Of all private expenditures for general hospital care, which amounted to $2,027 million in 1949, insurance benefits paid about one-fourth. This was the most widely insured item. Of total private expenditures for physicians' services, which totaled $2,267 million, insurance paid one-tenth. Expenditures for dental care, nursing care, one-third of the costs of drugs and medical supplies outside the hospital,* together with the net costs of insurance amounted to approximately $2,056 million in 1949. Insurance benefits for such items were negligible. These facts are illustrated in figure 32.

* Items, that is, sometimes not considered "insurable."

Medical-care insurance at present is provided by three large groups of organizations: (a) the nonprofit Blue Cross-Blue Shield plans; (b) the casualty, life, and other insurance companies; (c) a number of organizations independent of the first two groups, including industrial and labor-union plans, consumer cooperatives, programs under the auspices of private medical groups, some medical societies, community organizations, and others.

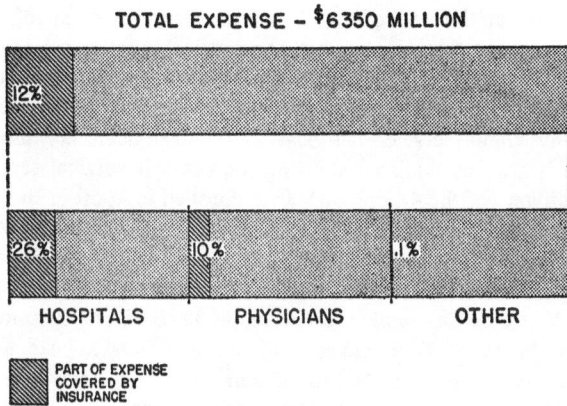

TOTAL EXPENSE – $6350 MILLION

12%

26% 10% .1%

HOSPITALS   PHYSICIANS   OTHER

PART OF EXPENSE
COVERED BY
INSURANCE

Figure 32. Insurance benefits covered 12% of private medical care expense in 1949.

The approximate number of people reached in 1950 by the three main groups of organizations providing medical-care insurance and some measure of the average financial protection afforded by insurance are as follows:

(a) More than 4 million persons at the end of 1950 had medical-care insurance through "independent" organizations, of whom over 3 million were insured for comprehensive benefits. For those people enrolled in comprehensive plans more than 80 per cent of the costs of services rendered by both physicians and general hospitals were paid for by their insurance in 1949, the latest year for which financial estimates are available. Protection against the costs of dental and nursing services were occasionally included. In all, these plans paid about $78 million in benefits in that year, of which $35 million was for general hospital care and $43 million for physicians' services.

(b) Seventy-five million persons (including the four million above) had at the end of 1950 some form of insurance against the costs of hospital care. About half of these 75 million were insured through the 84 nonprofit Blue Cross plans, a majority of which contract with hospitals to provide most of their services in semi-private accommodations with a minimum of additional charges to the enrollee. Blue Cross plans appear on the average to have paid from 70 to 80 per cent of the average hospital bills of their subscribers in 1949. In all, Blue Cross plans paid

$303 million in hospital-care benefits in that year. About 34 million people at the end of 1950 held policies issued by the insurance companies, 20 million under group policies, and 14 million under individual insurance, under which cash indemnities are paid to the policyholder to apply against his hospital bill. In 1949, insurance companies appear to have paid from 45 to 55 per cent of the average hospital bills of their policyholders, whether under individual or group enrollment. In all, insurance companies are estimated to have paid $192 million in hospital benefits in that year.

(c) Forty-eight million persons (who are also included in the seventy-five million above) had at the end of 1950 insurance against some of the costs of physicians' services, mostly surgery and non-surgical physicians' services in the hospital. For these enrollees the total benefits—whether for surgical insurance only or for surgical and limited medical insurance—are compared to total expenditures for all physicians' services, surgical and nonsurgical, because data on a Nation-wide basis are not available showing the costs of surgical services only.

About 18 million (of the 48 million) were enrolled in 1950 in the 66 nonprofit Blue Shield and similar plans. These plans provide cash indemnities to their over-income subscribers and what may be called service benefits to their under-income subscribers. It has been estimated that from 67 to 75 per cent of Blue Shield members receive cash indemnities, while the remaining 33 to 25 per cent are eligible for service benefits. In 1949, Blue Shield and similar plans appear to have paid about 45 per cent of the average total physicians' charges of their subscribers, with total benefits payments for the cost of physicians' services of $79 million.[1]

About 30 million people at the end of 1950 held insurance company policies (21.5 million group and over 8 million individual) against the cost of surgical and, in some instances, limited medical services by physicians. In general, such policies paid policyholders cash indemnities to apply against their physicians' bills. Like Blue Shield, insurance companies had, in some areas and applying to about 640,000 policyholders in 1949, agreements with physicians to accept, on behalf of under-income policyholders, their fees as full payment for the insured items. In 1949, group and individual insurance written by insurance companies appear to have paid 46 per cent of the average total of physicians' bills for those policyholders having both surgical and limited medical insurance. These policyholders accounted for about one-fifth of the total number of people in 1949 having protection through insurance companies against the costs of either surgical or medical services. For group and individual policyholders with surgical insurance alone, about 29 and 22 per cent, respectively, of the average total bills (for surgical and nonsurgical services combined) was paid. Total benefits paid by insurance companies for physicians' services amounted to $103 million in 1949.

The above percentages represent the proportion of the Nation-wide average private expenditure for broad classes of care (hospital and physicians' services) which is paid through voluntary medical-care insurance. They should not be con-

[1] Amounts paid for hospital care under some Blue Shield plans have been subtracted from total benefits paid by Blue Shield to reach this figure because the benefits appear under Blue Cross.

fused with that proportion of the individual's hospital bill or surgical bill for a particular illness which is paid by his insurance plan. . . .

Figure 33 illustrates the average dollar amount of insurance benefits for hospital and physicians' services paid in 1949 on behalf of those enrolled in the various types of insurance organizations. The chart also shows the national average per capita private expenditure for general hospital care ($13.70) and for all physicians' services ($15.35) against which the average insurance benefits may be measured.

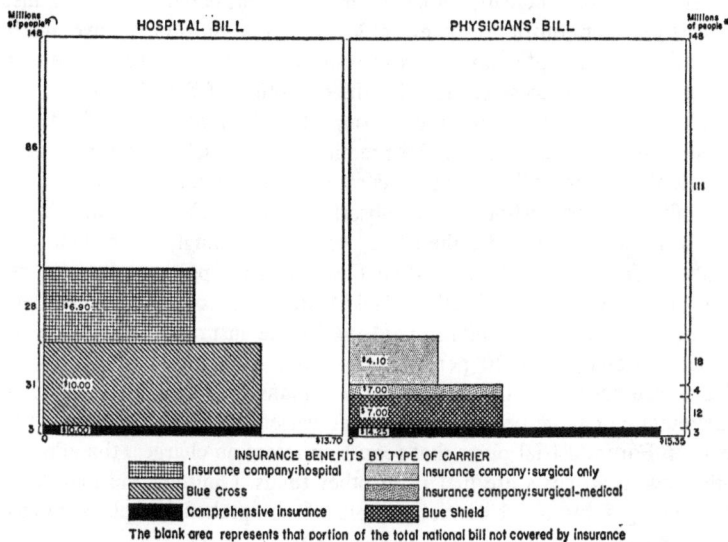

*As of midpoint 1949.

FIGURE 33. Insurance benefits in 1949 were less than the average annual bill per person of $13.70 for general hospital care and $15.35 for physicians' services.

It should be recognized that the percentages given above are average figures for all the types of insurance, and that in some individual cases the insurance benefits may pay the entire hospital or physician's bill; conversely, except in the few truly comprehensive plans in which all services are provided on a contractual service basis, the benefits may, in many cases, amount to a portion of the bill only, leaving a substantial amount for the insured person to pay in addition. It was impossible to obtain during the course of this study data showing with any precision the number of persons having some form of medical-care insurance, who, after insurance benefits have been paid, still have a serious financial problem in meeting their medical bills.

It is also true that the greatest number of subscribers carry insurance which does not provide benefits paying all medical-care costs. Such partial insurance, limited either in the range of services included or in the dollar amount of the benefits, carries a somewhat lower premium than more nearly complete protection, which may be available but which such subscribers may or may not wish to have or be able to afford. In the case of hospital benefits, the proportion of the bill covered depends not only upon the scope of benefits provided by the insurance, but also, in part, upon the accommodations selected by, and available to, the patient. Similarly, the proportion of the physician's bill covered also depends upon the charges of the particular physician selected.

Very few people have any insurance against such costs of dental care, and, except in the hospital, against such costs of nursing, X-rays, laboratory or other diagnostic tests, drugs or medical supplies as may be considered potentially insurable. These costs together constitute somewhat less than one-third of the average family's medical bill. A number of comprehensive insurance plans have been able to include protection for some of these items, with the exception of dental care.

There is considerable variation among the different types of medical-care insurance plans in the amount of the premium paid which goes for what may be called "retention charges," i. e., administrative costs, reserves, taxes, and, in some plans, profits. The proportion of the subscriber's or member's dollar which comes back in benefits or dividends, therefore, varies accordingly. For their combined group and individual enrollment, Blue Cross plans report an average retention charge of 15 per cent in 1949. Blue Shield states that its average retention charge was 21 per cent of the premiums paid, while the insurance companies estimate their retention charges at 20 per cent for group insurance and 45 per cent for individual insurance. For the comprehensive plans it is difficult to state a single average retention charge because of the wide variety of these programs with differing benefits. For industrial plans that report no retention charges, the administrative and other overhead costs are met from other funds. Omitting the industrial plans, retention charges for a substantial sample of comprehensive plans ranged from 20 to 7 per cent in 1949.

In other words, from 55 to 93 cents of the subscriber's dollar comes back in benefits and dividends, depending upon the particular plan to which he belongs and whether he is insured as an individual or as a member of a group.

Broadly speaking, voluntary medical-care insurance is most common among people easily accessible to group insurance and less common among those difficult to reach by the group method. Certain factors influence the ease or difficulty with which a person may be included by group or individual enrollment in voluntary plans. . . .

The bulk of existing medical-care insurance is for hospital care, surgery and in-hospital physicians' services. It does not attempt to cover, for the most part, protracted illness (hospitalized or nonhospitalized) such as chronic disease, nor does it meet the medical expense of preventive care and physicians' care for short-term nonhospitalized illnesses, or for illnesses in their early stages.

This emphasis upon hospitalization, surgery, and in-hospital physicians' services as noted above furnishes an incentive to physicians and patients alike to increase to an extent greater than medically necessary the performance of surgical procedures or the use of hospital-bed facilities, and, therefore, the need for hospital construction. It also does little to encourage preventive medicine, early diagnosis or treatment. A different pattern is set by those comprehensive plans that stress preventive medicine and the provision of services outside of the hospital.

It is self-evident that the mechanism of insurance substitutes a recurring periodic charge for medical bills of uncertain amounts, that insurance of even limited scope tends to reduce—in differing degrees—the burden of large medical bills, but that under the present pattern of medical-care insurance there remains an additional financial problem for those with insurance who have a serious illness requiring nursing services, expensive diagnostic services and a protracted period of hospitalization.

Measures to improve the kind and quality of medical services have been included in very few voluntary insurance plans, except those providing comprehensive services through medical group practice units.

The growth of comprehensive insurance has been restricted by difficulties of initial financing and organization, by the frequent opposition of organized medicine, and by restrictive laws enacted in more than half of the States, usually at the instance of physicians and medical societies. . . .

B. A 1954 REPORT *

IN JULY 1953 there were over 87 million people, or 57 per cent of the population of the United States, enrolled in voluntary health insurance and protected against part of the costs of hospital services, and over 74 million people, or 48 per cent of the population protected against part of the cost of surgical and other physicians' services. These figures were derived from house to house interviews of a representative national sample of 2,809 families, comprising 8,846 individuals, subdivided by age, sex, income, family size, rural-urban, occupation and region. Thus it has been possible for the first time to project, with a high degree of validity, the extent of enrollment in voluntary health insurance in the United States.

Total enrollments of over 87 million in hospital insurance and over 74 million in surgical and other medical services did not take place suddenly, to be sure, but expansion since 1940 has been phenomenal. In 1940, approximately 9 per cent of the population was enrolled in hospital insurance as against 57 per cent today. Four per cent of the population was covered by surgical insurance compared with 48 per cent today. That there has been great demand is self-evident. Who are the people enrolled and where are they? What is the enrollment by income, occupation, region, and rural-urban characteristics? If the present expansion is to continue unabated, to what segments of the population must voluntary health insurance be made available? This report will document facts which have heretofore

* From: *National Family Survey of Medical Costs and Voluntary Health Insurance: A Preliminary Report,* by Odin W. Anderson; New York: Health Information Foundation, 1954 (Part I, "Extent of Voluntary Health Insurance as of July 1953," pp. 11-17, 20). Reprinted (with omissions) by permission of the publishers. The author is the research director of the Health Information Foundation, New York. (A more extensive discussion of this section of the 1953 survey conducted by the Health Information Foundation is provided in pp. 12-20, 97-98, and 100 of the volume entitled *Family Medical Costs and Voluntary Health Insurance: A Nationwide Survey,* cited in the acknowledgment note for Selection No. 14C, in Chap. III).

been expressed mostly as opinion, and it is now possible to answer the foregoing questions in some detail.

National and Regional Enrollment.—Over one-half of the population in the United States is enrolled in some type of hospital insurance, divided almost equally between Blue Cross and private insurance companies. Almost one-half of the population is enrolled in surgical or other medical insurance of which about five million, or 3 per cent, are covered by substantially complete physicians' services. In surgical or medical insurance, private insurance companies' enrollment exceeds that of Blue Cross and Blue Shield.

Some duplication of enrollment is evident in that slightly over 10 per cent of the people who carry hospital insurance have more than one hospital policy and slightly more than 10 per cent of the people who have surgical or medical coverage have more than one policy. Sometimes persons are covered for the same service by more than one policy in order to bring their protection into line with prevailing costs. Other times it may be that people are protected in excess of prevailing costs which leads to over-insurance. (See table 47.)

The total number of people enrolled in insurance is, of course, a basic indication of sheer volume, but the degree of protection afforded should also be known in order to evaluate what the coverage means. Lacking any standards as to "adequate" coverage in terms of range of services, it would be difficult to assess the coverage even if the nature of the services provided or indemnified were known. For those who believe that services provided on a prepayment basis should be substantially complete, the adequacy of the coverage is, of course, very low because there are relatively few people with complete coverage today. For those who believe that services provided on a prepayment basis should cover hospital care and in-hospital physicians' services only, the adequacy of the present coverage would be judged in a more favorable light.

The enrollment by regions in the United States shows some variation. A higher percentage of the population is enrolled in the Northeast and North Central areas than in the South and West. When these data are broken down by type of insurer, enrollment in private hospital insurance is double that of Blue Cross in the South and West, whereas Blue Cross has somewhat more than private insurance company enrollment in the Northeast and a slight edge in the North Central region. For surgical and other medical insurance, private insurance companies have twice the enrollment in the South and West over Blue Cross and Blue Shield, and also have a slight excess in the North Central region, but are behind in the Northeast.

Enrollment by Work Status and Occupation.—The main earners in the families who are employed either by private employers or by government, and therefore largely on a group enrollment basis, have generally a larger percentage of people enrolled than do the self-employed. When enrollment is broken down by occupation there is a range of 33 per cent to 90 per cent of people in specified industries enrolled in some type of insurance. Those employed in agriculture, forestry and fisheries have the lowest proportion enrolled, and people employed in mining and manufacturing have a very high proportion enrolled.

TABLE 47. *Estimated number of persons having voluntary health insurance by kind of insurer*

Type of Protection and Kind of Insurer A	Percentage of Persons in Sample With Coverage	Estimated Number in Civilian Non-Institutional Population B
Total, with some protection	58 per cent	89.5 millions
HOSPITAL		
Net total, after eliminating duplication	57	87.4 C
Blue Cross	27	41.1
Group private	17	26.2
Individual private	11	17.1
Independent and other	6	10.0
Insurer unknown	*	.6
SURGICAL OR MEDICAL		
Net total, after eliminating duplication	48	74.5 D, E
Blue Shield and Blue Cross	19	29.1
Group private	17	25.9
Individual private	10	14.7
Independent and other	7	10.5
Insurer unknown	*	.2
OTHER		
Dread disease	4	6.0
Major medical expense	(F)	.4

* Less than one-half of one per cent.

A In classifying insurers the definitions were those used in the *Report of the President's Commission on the Health Needs of the Nation*, Vol. 4 (U.S.G.P.O. Washington, 1953). See Table No. 11.5, especially footnote p. 336.

B The civilian non-institutional population for July, 1953 is estimated at 154.6 million.

C Since a good many individuals (7.5 million) were covered by more than one kind of insurer for hospital expenses, this net total is less than the sum of the totals for the different kinds of insurers. The net total of 87.4 million represents the number of persons with hospital expense protection, eliminating duplication by two or more *different kinds* of insurers. Another 1.6 million persons have two or more plans or policies with the *same kind of insurer* covering hospital expenses, but this kind of duplication does not appear in the totals for the different kinds of insurers which show *number of persons* covered by *one or more* group private, individual private, etc., hospital policies.

D These figures include 4.9 million persons who belong to plans which provide substantially complete medical service; the remainder are covered only for surgical fees or for limited medical service.

E This net total of 74.5 million represents the number of persons with surgical or medical expense protection, after eliminating duplication of such coverage by two or more *different kinds* of insurers for 6.2 million persons.

Another 2.9 million persons have two or more plans or policies with the *same kind* of insurer, but this kind of duplication does not appear in the totals for the different kinds of insurers.

F Less than one-half of one percent (about .3 percent) were covered by major medical expense protection.

READINGS IN MEDICAL CARE

The self-employed and people employed in very small groups are a particular problem facing health insurance plans today. The relatively low enrollment of people in this segment of the population is not necessarily a measure of the unavailability of health insurance to them, but it certainly indicates that they are not availing themselves of insurance for one reason or another. The unavoidably high cost of acquisition, waiting periods, and the limitations on benefits to prevent self-selection are common problems to be faced in the enrolling of self-employed groups, in contrast to enrollment of employed groups. Thus, it is necessary for voluntary health insurance to devise means whereby people without a common employer or in very small groups can be grouped in order to be enrolled with as low an acquisition cost, as few limitations in benefits, and the same premiums as those now experienced by large employed groups. . . .

Enrollment by Family Income.—One hears a great deal about protection against costs of personal health services for the "middle" income group, since it is often said that the poor and the well-to-do obtain good medical care without insurance, but the family in the middle needs some method of pooling costs. Also, one hears that voluntary health insurance is designed for "low" income as well as for "middle" income.

For the purpose of meeting costs of personal health services, it is difficult to determine "low", "middle" and "high" income, because they do not necessarily correspond to even statistical divisions but must be related to ability to pay for an accepted standard of living as well as for unpredictable costs of personal health services. Thus, no definitions are proposed here, but the per cent of enrollment in some type of insurance by family income will be presented. For families under $3,000, 41 per cent have some type of health insurance; between $3,000 and $5,000, the proportion increases to 71 per cent; $5,000 and over, 80 per cent. (See table 48.) It is apparent that there is quite a break between the family income under and over $3,000. It is reasonable to assume that the group under $3,000 contains more old people and farmers than the groups over $3,000.

TABLE 48. *Percentage of families with voluntary health insurance by income group*

Annual Family Income [A]	All Families	Percentage of Families With Some Coverage
Total, all families	2,809	63 percent
under $3,000	958	41
$3,000 — $4,999	912	71
$5,000 and over	920	80
Income unknown	19	B

[A] This breakdown by family income shows roughly the lowest third with family income under $3,000, the middle third with family income $3,000 to $4,999, and the highest third with family income $5,000 and over.

[B] Percentages not computed for groups of less than 50 families.

The median income in families with some insurance is approximately $4,500, which means that half of these families earn more than $4,500 and half earn less. The median income for families without some protection is $2,700. The median income of all families is $3,900. Approximately 20 per cent of the families in the United States earn less than $2,000 annually, and approximately 30 per cent of these families have some type of coverage. Since five to six million people at any one time receive public assistance, they are part of the 20 million under $2,000 a year income or approximately 25 per cent of this income group, and they are not able to purchase health insurance.

Enrollment by Age of Family Head.—The proportion of families enrolled by age of male family head shows relatively small differences until after age 65, at which point there is a sharp drop from near 70 per cent to 50 per cent and after age 75, a further drop to 35 per cent.

Families with female heads have an appreciably smaller percentage enrolled in some type of insurance, but also show a distinct drop after age 65. On an average, 66 per cent of the families with male heads are enrolled in some type of health insurance and 48 per cent of the families with female heads.

Enrollment by Rural-Urban Areas.—Rural areas have less enrollment in voluntary health insurance than urban areas. As measured by families, 70 per cent of urban families have some type of insurance and 45 per cent of rural-farm families. For hospital insurance alone, 63 per cent of the individuals in urban areas carry hospital insurance, and 38 per cent in rural-farm areas. The differences in urban and rural areas are a reflection of the opportunity of voluntary health insurance to enroll employed groups in urban areas and the difficulties of creating groups for insurance purposes in rural areas. Farmers do have access to health insurance policies on an individual basis, but as discussed previously, health insurance sold on an individual basis costs more and has more limitations in benefits than group contracts. The chief problem is one of creating groups for health insurance purposes.

Other Considerations in Enrollment.—The overwhelming proportion of families, 80 per cent, enrolled in some type of health insurance obtained their policies through their place of work or some other group. Nine per cent of the families held policies which had been obtained while members of a group, but had retained their policies on an individual basis after leaving the group. Finally, 32 per cent of the families were carrying policies which had been obtained as individuals, and not through a group. It will be noted that these percentages add up to more than 100 per cent because some families had more than one kind of policy. Again, it is necessary to underscore the need for creating groups among individuals who are not in employed groups if health insurance is to enroll a larger proportion of the population.

86. The Role of Voluntary Plans

A. DIFFERENCES OF OPINION *

THERE ARE differences of opinion on a number of important points concerning medical-care insurance. Some of the differences reflect the divergent points of view of some of the providers of insurance, as contrasted with the views of some representatives of people who purchase it. Differences also appear to spring from differing social philosophies. Some of the points of difference are:

1. What is the purpose of medical-care insurance? Some believe that the sole desirable purpose is financial protection against the costs of "catastrophic illness." Others take the view that insurance is the desirable method of paying for all or most medical services, as against the system of post-payment by consumers on a fee-for-service basis. There are those who would limit medical-care insurance strictly to a financial arrangement, and others who believe that insurance should be looked upon as a means for influencing favorably the availability of preventive medicine, early diagnosis and treatment in case of illness, the quality of the services provided, and the improvement of medical facilities both quantitatively and qualitatively.

2. What items of medical service is it desirable and possible to pay for in whole or in part by insurance? From the experience of both comprehensive and limited plans, it is evident that the insurability of many items of service varies with the form of medical and administrative organization of the plan providing the insurance. If insurance against the costs of certain items is possible only through major changes in the pattern of medical practice, are the benefits to be gained large enough to justify disturbances and controversies that may accompany such changes? Here sharp differences of opinion are found.

3. Who should be insured? Do, for example, people of the highest economic status really need or desire insurance and, if not, at what income level should the line be drawn? Or is any income limit desirable? Other issues relate to insuring those persons in the lower economic groups who can pay little or none of the insurance costs. Therefore, if insurance is to be utilized for these groups, at least a part of its costs must be met by other public and private sources, including employer contributions under group enrollment.

4. How should the payment of insurance costs be distributed? Here appears a contrast between the positions of private and social insurance. On the one hand, the position of private insurance is that the premium for the individual or group insured should be related more or less directly to the expected cost of insuring that individual or group; on the other hand, the position of social insurance is that costs

* From: *Health Insurance Plans in the United States* (Report No. 359 of the U. S. Senate Committee on Labor and Public Welfare), 82nd Cong., 1st Sess.; Washington: U.S. Government Printing Office, 1951 (Part I, pp. 10-12). Reprinted with omissions, including initial paragraphs.

should be distributed so far as possible over the whole society or community and be borne by individuals largely in proportion to their ability to pay. A middle ground is also found, combining some elements of both of the above viewpoints.

5. How far should governmental action go in extending medical-care insurance? There are those who believe that insurance legally required of the whole self-supporting population, or of the larger part thereof, is the only way whereby the benefits of such insurance can become available promptly and economically to the majority of the population; and who believe that such action should and can be so designed as to maintain medical efficiency and freedom and democratic methods of administration. On the other side are those who believe that a widespread legal requirement of medical-care insurance is unnecessary, because voluntary plans will meet all or most of the needs that should be met; and who believe serious evils for medical practice and American freedom would result from such legally required insurance. Between these two groups are others who believe that voluntary plans alone will not cover all the needs and who favor governmental aid to voluntary plans, under various terms and conditions.

6. How much of the national product (or of a family's income) do we wish to use for the support of doctors, dentists, nurses, hospitals, and other health services and facilities? To put it bluntly, how many doctors, etc., having what standard of living, do we think it worth our while to support?

7. Finally, there is no general agreement as to whether the Nation is spending, through insurance or otherwise, enough on medical services to assure the best health for all its people. There are no accepted and absolute standards by which this can be judged. If we examine expenditures for general hospital and physicians' services, we find that in some comprehensive insurance plans, where liberal use of these services is encouraged for both preventive and curative purposes, annual expenditures for physicians' and general hospital services, range from $22 to $38 per capita. This may be compared with an expenditure of approximately $30 per capita for the same services for the population as a whole in 1949. . . .

B. MAJOR PROBLEM AREAS *

THE ISSUE of "compulsory vs. voluntary insurance" is one that involves mainly the question of future growth. It is agreed generally that volition is preferable to compulsion as a means toward any end in the United States. The question therefore is whether the voluntary movement has in it the elements of reasonably rapid growth or, stated more precisely, whether by voluntary action as many as 90 or 100 million of the population can be drawn into a system of prepaid services.

* Reprinted by permission of the publishers and the Commonwealth Fund from Nathan Sinai, Odin W. Anderson, and Melvin L. Dollar, *Health Insurance in the United States;* Cambridge, Mass.: Harvard University Press, 1946. (The excerpt reprinted, with omissions, is from Chap. VI, "Problems Before Voluntary Plans," and Chap. VII, "The Health Insurance Movement Continues," pp. 69-106). Drs. Sinai and Anderson are, respectively, the director of the Bureau of Public Health Economics of the School of Public Health, University of Michigan, Ann Arbor, and the research director of the Health Information Foundation, New York; Mr. Dollar was formerly executive director of Group Health Association, Washington, D.C.

The question does not lend itself to any "yes or no" answer based on hazy opinion. Such an answer might have been permissible a decade ago but in the intervening years a body of experience has accumulated and at least the outlines of problems have sharpened. The problems are many and they could be considered in finely divided categories, but for the sake of clarity they are presented in a broader classification, under the following heads: 1) enrollment of geographic and occupational groups; 2) enrollment of income groups; 3) extension of benefits to low income groups; 4) centralization and coordination or merging of plans; 5) availability of service facilities; and 6) unemployment and maintenance of membership. Within these problems are others, and all combine to form a complex total. . . .

ENROLLMENT OF INCOME GROUPS

THE PROBLEM of coverage not only involves geography and types of occupations; it is also related to the income groups in the population to whom the hospital and medical plans must be sold. A different set of problems is associated with each group. No attempt is made to give a precise definition of these income groups, but for the sake of simplicity they are divided into four classes—the upper, middle, and lower income groups, and the indigent. Actually many variables other than money income enter into the determination of the income group to which the individual belongs. Size of family, cost of living, individual responsibilities, and many other factors are combined in various proportions to determine the economic status of the individual family. For the purposes at hand extremely generalized definitions of income groups in terms of ability to pay for medical care are used. In considering the definitions one important fact should be kept in mind: income groups are not divided by sharp lines. In any graphic presentation incomes from low to high comprise a shading process; an income classification, for example, between $2,000 and $3,000 shows the greatest concentration toward the lower figure.

The *upper income* group can be dismissed from this discussion with the statement that it constitutes that segment of the population to whom the economic burden of illness offers no acute problem. Its resources are such that it is able to meet the costs of adequate medical care without financial assistance. The percentage of the population that has the good fortune to be in this income bracket is so small as to be of little significance in any computation regarding the medical needs of the population.

The *middle income* group falls below the level of complete medical self-support. This group, especially in its upper portion, is able financially to meet the costs of its ordinary medical needs, but it is unable with its limited resources to meet the costs of serious and prolonged illness without suffering hardship. However, through the device of insurance, the group can afford to finance relatively complete medical service. It is in the middle income group that the insurance movement has found its most fertile field for development and, to date, promotion of the plans has been directed almost entirely toward it. No attempt has been made to promote the program in the upper income group because of the objections of the medical profession and because health insurance with limited benefits lacks appeal for this group.

The income limits of the participants in the program have been controlled more or less automatically since health insurance has been offered for the most part to selected groups of wage earners whose employment fits into the enrollment and collection schemes of the plans. It is to be expected that the management of the insurance plans will continue to utilize their present mechanisms of enrollment until such time as all industrial groups that can readily be reached have been enrolled. As the plans approach the saturation point within the industrial groups, plan management likely will turn its attention to devising methods of operation that will make the insurance available to groups outside of industry. This process of expansion is illustrated by the Blue Cross plan of Michigan, which has expanded its membership to include a relatively high percentage of all industrial groups in the state and is making an effort to extend its services to rural groups.

There are a number of difficult problems involved in the achievement of full health insurance coverage of the middle income group under a comprehensive voluntary plan. For instance, there is to date no plan that offers complete health care, including hospitalization, physicians' and surgeons' care, nursing, dentistry, drugs, and other health services. If such a plan were offered the subscription rate would of necessity be much larger than the rate for the limited service plans now operating. Furthermore, there are many areas in the United States where there is no health insurance plan in operation and in the areas now having plans there are many persons in the middle income group who are ineligible for membership.

While the present success in enrolling the middle income group in hospital plans would seem to augur well for the future of voluntary insurance, experience indicates that a significant proportion of this group likely will never take advantage of health insurance protection. The introduction of a comprehensive contract would doubtless increase the number choosing to remain outside the plan since the increased costs of the insurance would be a serious obstacle to its sale. In addition to the problem of acquiring membership there remains the problem of retaining in membership persons who, because they have received no benefits, have real or imagined grievances, or for some other reason are likely to drop out of the program. Thus, even to approximate complete coverage and to maintain it would require a continuous educational program and sales campaign.

The effects of increased costs for insurance are demonstrated in part by the slow growth of the more expensive medical society insurance plans as compared with the less costly hospital plans.... It is realized, of course, that there are many factors which have influenced the development of these plans, yet their experience would seem to indicate that at the premium rates that are charged, there is a resistant market for this insurance. Consequently, it is reasonable to assume that there would be greater sales resistance to a more costly comprehensive plan.

In addition to the inherent sales problems, the medical society plans have introduced an artificial barrier to the attainment of a high percentage of membership among the middle income group. The majority of the plans set an upper income limit above which persons either are not eligible for membership or are eligible only for limited benefits. Such limitations are established on the theory that persons whose income is higher than the limit established by the society are able to meet the costs of medical care. In giving service to people above that level the physicians feel that they should not be bound by contracts which set their fees. This restrictive clause has acted as a serious deterrent in the growth of the medical plans.

The plans that offer to the higher income group only limited payment to be applied toward the cost of a given medical service are little more than cash indemnity plans, since the patient remains responsible for the charges beyond the amount covered by the insurance.

Management in industry has frequently balked at dividing their employees according to income groups. It is their feeling that any benefits offered to one group of their employees should be available to all since such a division makes for strained employee relationships. Furthermore, since the income of employees in many industries fluctuates, the application of income limitations necessitates a great deal of clerical work to determine the eligibility of the individual for the insurance.

As has been pointed out, each of the arbitrary income groupings on which this discussion is based represents the whole income range. The composition of the *low income* group can best be described, perhaps, in terms of some of the occupational groups which make up a major part of it. Included in this category are semi-skilled and unskilled factory workers, laborers, domestic help, a high proportion of clerical workers, and farmers.

In general the people included in the low income group are able out of their own resources to meet the cost of most of the daily essentials of life; however, they find it difficult to meet the full cost of their day-to-day medical needs. Serious and prolonged sickness is beyond their means. This group, more than any other, is in need of an insurance program that will enable it to carry or participate in carrying the economic burden of medical care. Unfortunately, the price of a complete medical service, even under an insurance plan, would be beyond the means of the people living on this low economic plane.

The leaders in the health insurance movement are alert to the special needs of this group and are putting forth considerable effort in an attempt to find a solution. Many concede the necessity for some form of subsidy to lighten the cost of the program to this group. Others have suggested plans that would substitute limited health services at a smaller premium for those unable to pay for full insurance protection. This approach is more feasible in hospital insurance than in medical care insurance. The hospital plans have found it possible to modify their rates somewhat for the benefit of the low income groups by offering a ward contract. This is a satisfactory means of reducing the cost of the protection since it offers the participant adequate hospital care. If the patient's condition necessitates a private or semi-private room the accommodation ordinarily is substituted, the patient being billed only for the difference in cost between the two types of rooms.

The medical care program offers little opportunity for similar adjustments in rates since the quality and quantity of medical services can be reduced, in most cases, only at the expense of the patient's welfare. Although none of the plans has suggested compromise in quality of care, many have attempted to meet the need of the lower income group through a limitation in the quantity or type of care. This has been done through limiting contracts to certain specified services, such as surgical contracts only and various combinations of home, office, and hospital care and through deductible clauses which assess the subscriber the cost of the first visit or of the first two in any given illness. While it must be agreed that a quarter-loaf is better than nothing, such compromises fall short of the objective of a complete medical service for all the population. Medical services not covered under the insurance contract must be met from some source or neglected to the detriment of the individual's health.

In the past the practice generally has been to provide treatment for the low income group at the expense of the physician. Through its charity the medical profession has developed a noble tradition and much credit must be given to physicians for their contributions and their idealism. However, the burden of providing adequate medical care for all members of the low income group is of a weight far beyond the ability of the medical profession to bear. No insurance plan for the low income group should be drawn up at the expense of the medical practitioner. That is, the practitioner should not be asked to accept lower fees under an insurance contract sold at a lower rate as a means of meeting the medical needs of the low income group. When charity is defined through a contractual arrangement it ceases to evoke a sympathetic response on the part of the physician and is replaced by resentment. Under such an arrangement the physician can only feel that he is under compulsion to give charity. Such an attitude on the part of the physician is not conducive to the establishment of the sympathetic physician-patient relation which the medical profession insists is so important in therapy. Without the reasoned support of the participating physicians no insurance plan can hope for continued success—a fact demonstrated too often in the plans controlled by the physicians themselves.

EXTENSION OF BENEFITS TO LOW INCOME GROUPS

IN THE ATTEMPT to devise a program that will provide adequate health services and at the same time make it possible for those in the low income group to pay for the protection offered, the voluntary insurance plans find themselves in a dilemma. The dilemma arises from the uniform charge to all the subscribers. Obviously what is purchasable by a family with an annual income of $3,000 is beyond the means of a comparable family with an annual income of $1,500.

Adjustment of Rates.—A number of devices have been suggested to overcome the difficulty. One that may be questioned—not in theory but on the basis of widespread applicability—is the adoption of a scheme of payment based upon income. In effect this would mean that the middle income group would voluntarily provide a subsidy for the lower income group.

Another suggestion is that a flat rate be charged for each contract, whether it be for a single person or for a family. At present approximately half the subscriptions are for single contracts and, in general, the cost of the family contract is approximately double that of the single contract. If a flat rate were introduced the theoretical effect would be to decrease the cost of the family contract by 25 per cent, the difference being made up by an increase of 50 per cent for the single contract.

In considering the application of this device certain unknowns call for consideration, at least. The first one is the assumption that all the single contracts would be continued at the higher rate. Consideration should also be given to the fact that a considerable portion of the subscribers holding single contracts are family breadwinners who have chosen the cheaper contract. The adoption of the flat rate scheme would mean that the single contract subscriber would become a family contract subscriber.

Employer Participation.—A more satisfactory and hopeful solution of the problem is to be noted in the growing emphasis that many of the plans place upon the participation of employers in the payment for health insurance for their employees. Some of the hospital and medical plans report that an appreciable number of employers pay the entire costs of the contracts and that a growing number contribute a portion. In the immediate past such payments were made at little cost to employers because of the extremely high taxes on profits and the privilege of deducting the payments as a cost of operation. At the same time the labor unions in their conferences with employers on wages have stressed the item of protection against the costs of sickness.

The future extent and degree of employer participation will be an important determining factor in the ability of the plans to meet the needs of the low income population that can be reached through their employment. For the low income group not so engaged other methods must be devised.

Government Subsidy.—The health problem of the indigent portion of the population is frankly acknowledged by most leaders in the voluntary health insurance movement to be a matter of concern to governmental agencies. It has been said, also, that the "medically indigent" are a government responsibility. Thus it is suggested that a portion of the low income and all of the no-income groups have their health needs supplied within the framework of the voluntary plans and that the costs be paid by government agencies. Under this arrangement the insurance organization relieves the welfare agency of the function it has performed in making arrangements for payment on an individual basis for medical cases among its clients. One advantage of this arrangement to the recipient of public aid is that as a patient his identity as a welfare client is lost and the stigma attached to his status need not affect his relationship with the medical personnel who handle the case.

The concept that government subsidy is limited to the disbursal of funds is an illusion. Few government officials—local, state, or national—would agree that their responsibility would be met unless they assured the public that funds were being expended properly. Such assurance would call for a body of rules and regulations regarding the quantity and quality of services, the costs, and the methods of administration.

Government subsidy would also raise the question of the form of payment—whether by lump sum or by fees—for each of the services rendered. Although there are instances of lump-sum contracts between government agencies and organizations representing those who render the services, the fact remains that there is an aversion to the assignment of public funds to private agencies for expenditure. Here again there is the issue of public control of such funds by rules and regulations.

Finally, there is the issue raised by the existence of multiple voluntary health insurance plans as well as the limited services included in the plans. In general the group of the population that needs government subsidy also needs comprehensive services. In order to provide these services the majority of existing medical plans would need to include many services now excluded. And because of the autonomy of the plans, contracts to provide services would need to be drawn with hospital plans, medical plans, and, ultimately, with dental, nursing, and other plans. Thus, government would be placed in the position of integrating the plans and, perforce, settling many of the issues that now serve to obstruct integration or amalgamation. Certain of these issues will be discussed in connection with factors that encourage and others that limit the growth of the voluntary insurance plans.

CENTRALIZATION AND COORDINATION OF PLANS

MOST OF THE HEALTH insurance plans have grown up as more or less independent units limited in their operation to restricted areas. Because the plans have not been generally available to all communities, their growth in membership has been greatly retarded. Through the consolidation of existing plans and the formation of statewide plans, this failing could be corrected and the potential membership could be increased greatly. Where a statewide plan exists the individual community does not have to await the establishment of an entirely new plan but can readily be brought into the program by a simple extension of the existing organization. The leaders in the movement, especially the leaders of the Blue Cross hospital plan, are alive to the possibilities inherent in such consolidations and are making considerable effort toward the accomplishment of this end.

The larger membership resulting from amalgamations would put the plans in a financial position to carry out a program of expansion which would not be possible for the small individual plans. It has been the general experience that in acquiring membership in new areas and especially in areas with small populations, the insurance organizations suffer initial losses. The smaller plans without large reserves would be unable to absorb such losses while waiting for the new groups to become self-supporting. The reserves of the larger plans would also permit experimentation with new methods of enrollment and techniques of actuarial control. Such experimentation might spell financial ruin to a smaller plan. Thus, unless the numerous small plans now in operation join their efforts, it is likely that the possible growth of the voluntary health insurance plans will proceed at an unnecessarily slow pace.

The advantages mentioned with regard to a statewide plan would be multiplied in the formation of an interstate or nationwide plan. It is pointed out, however, that the formation of a national organization is not in itself a solution to the problem of achieving uniform coverage. This results from the fact that a nationwide program would have to work within the limitations of the laws of each state, which would make for some variation in the operation of the plans in various states. The situation might be altered through efforts to obtain uniform laws in all the states; however, the legal difficulties involved in such an action are apparent. The National Association of Insurance Commissioners is working on this problem.

Until recently any discussion of a nationwide voluntary medical plan including even the limited services provided by the existing plans would have been largely academic. The possibility of this type of development was extremely remote because of the lack of any adequate mechanism to effect it. Unlike the Blue Cross plans, the medical plans had no central agency to function as a clearing house of information and to arrange for inter-plan or interstate agreements. Such an agency was created by the American Medical Association in February, 1946. The success of the agency will depend upon the strategy and wisdom applied in developing a national plan and the willingness of state and local medical societies to compromise their differences of opinion.

In those states where more than one plan is operated by local medical societies there is a tendency to resist consolidation. The strong individualism that characterizes the profession is reflected in the relationships between the local components of their own organization. Hence the county societies are reluctant to surrender the control of their insurance plans to the state organizations or their right to reject any state plan.

The leaders in the hospital insurance movement have shown a much keener interest in forming larger units of organization than have leaders in the medical field. There are several factors which may contribute to this difference in attitude. Since the hospital association is not based on the close-knit local and county units that typify the medical organization, the problem of local determination does not deter formation of larger units of organization. Furthermore, the hospitals are promoting insurance plans because they have found that they provide a worthwhile service both to the public and to the hospitals and consequently are willing to encourage the growth of the plans. Another important consideration is the fact that the management of the hospital plans for the most part is in the hands of competent business executives who are permitted a fairly wide latitude in developing their programs. As businessmen these executives recognize the soundness of the formation of larger units of operation and are not moved by philosophical considerations regarding local determination. . . .

In spite of opposing interests among their own groups, the leaders in the voluntary hospital insurance movement are leaning more and more toward consolidation of plans as a means of meeting the challenge of making health care available to all the population. However, there is a step short of actual consolidation that is being encouraged, especially by the older hospital plans. This step is the coordination of existing plans through the adoption of a subscriber contract that is uniform in its benefits and through the development of reciprocal arrangements permitting subscribers who move from one state to another to transfer their Blue Cross membership from one plan to another.

The unification of the administration of hospital and medical plans operating in the same area represents another aspect of the movement toward coordination. Under such a unified program the governing boards of the medical and hospital plans retain their autonomy in the determination of policies. Essentially this plan provides for the sharing of a common administrative staff, office, and sales force. The arrangement makes for economy of operation by eliminating duplication of public contacts, collection procedures, and record keeping. It encourages the sale of a more complete health service since the public is served by only one agent who endeavors to sell a combination hospital and medical insurance plan.

Almost all the medical plans have some sort of cooperative arrangement with Blue Cross hospital plans. . . .

The joint administration of hospital and medical plans poses a delicate problem, even though there is little disagreement with regard to the advantages of joint operation. The issue centers around the degree to which Blue Cross plans should manage the affairs of medical plans. Since Blue Cross plans were in the field first and therefore had administrative organizations already operating, it was a natural development that Blue Cross plans should assist in the administration of medical plans. It would have been just as logical for medical plans to perform these services for Blue Cross, had medical plans occupied the field first.

The stronger position of the Blue Cross plans has excited some adverse comment in medical publications. . . .

The uniform benefits resulting from the coordination of health insurance plans makes possible the establishment of standards that should protect the interests of the subscriber. Such standards have not been practical in the past because of the wide variation in benefits and in combination of benefits. As a result the public has been faced with such puzzling problems as the choice of a plan offering 21 days of full hospitalization costs plus half costs for 60 days or one offering 30 days of full hospitalization costs. In the establishment of uniform benefits the determination of such technical points will be made by experts, and the public should profit from their decisions.

Among the advantages of the coordination of the plans are the increased coverage made possible through a division of territory, the division of overhead expense, the simplification of membership exchange, and the sharing of actuarial experience. Perhaps the greatest advantage to the plans is the development of a unified organization directed toward a common goal. One of the most significant aspects of the movement toward coordination is the fact that it lays the groundwork for complete amalgamation of the plans in the future. The development of uniform plans and of reciprocal arrangements makes the next step, amalgamation, a simpler one to take.

Obviously unless the Blue Cross plans and the medical society plans can settle the differences that arise between them the voluntary health insurance movement will suffer. As mentioned previously, joint administration of the two plans is a means of encouraging their expansion unless too many disagreements over the degree of cooperation arise.

One of the most important current controversies is over the problem of furnishing the services of medical specialties. The hospital insurance plans, through their service contracts which usually include among their benefits x-ray, laboratory, physiotherapy, and pathology services, find themselves inadvertently drawn into a quarrel of long standing between the hospitals and the medical profession. The trend is toward a concentration in the hospitals of expensive diagnostic and therapeutic equipment and the technical personnel to operate these departments. As a result the hospitals have encountered considerable opposition from the medical profession. The medical profession maintains that the hospital in offering these services is actually entering the practice of medicine, a forbidden field. The physician contends that these services should be performed by or under the supervision of a doctor of medicine who should be compensated for his services in the same manner as are other members of the profession. . . .

While the hospital insurance plans do not enter directly into the disagreement between the hospital and the medical profession, they are brought into the controversy through the fact that their contracts often provide for these services in the hospital. Actually, hospital insurance, through offering certain limited medical services, is in a sense entering the field of medical insurance. Since the profession has taken a strong stand on the principle of medical control of medical services, vigorous protests, including the withdrawal of the approval of a Blue Cross plan, have resulted.

The problem of medical specialties in relation to hospital insurance plans has been brought to a sharp focus through the proposal of a uniform contract for all Blue Cross plans which includes the services under question to be rendered in the hospital. The American Medical Association in 1943 took issue with this proposed contract and requested the American Hospital Association to withhold approval. The American Hospital Association, rejecting the plea of the American Medical Association, officially approved the inclusion within the Blue Cross benefits of all services customarily furnished by hospitals.

In spite of the strong feeling regarding the issue, the organized medical profession in many states, recognizing the functional relationship between the hospital and the disputed diagnostic and therapeutic services, has tried to reach compromises with respect to hospital insurance that cover these services. At the same time medical organizations have sought to erect safeguards to protect the interests of the profession. . . . In spite of compromise, . . . the issue has not yet been resolved and the inclusion of these services remains a point of conflict between the medical profession and the hospitals. In view of the fact that the practice of including diagnostic and therapeutic services in their contracts has become customary in many of the hospital insurance plans, there seems little likelihood that any change will be made until such time as medical plans are introduced that will cover these items of medical costs.

An outgrowth of the controversy between the hospital and medical plans is evident in the attempts of some hospital plans, notably in Washington and Oregon, to sell medical indemnity contracts as well as hospital service contracts, whereby the subscriber is reimbursed in cash for stipulated medical services rendered to him by the physician. The physician has no connection with the plan since the hospital plan acts in the same capacity as do commercial insurers. In order to strengthen their contracts so as to have more sales appeal, the hospital plans feel impelled to sell medical and surgical indemnity if the medical societies refuse to organize their own plans in the same territories. . . .

Perhaps a more elusive factor that may limit the expansion of plans is the domination and control of the boards of directors by hospital officials and physicians. It is the contention in some quarters that when there is not adequate representation, amounting perhaps to actual control, on the boards of directors by the subscribers, the voluntary plans must be considered simply another insurance company and popular interest will be weak. It is said further that health plans, being of paramount concern to the community, should be controlled by the community. On the other hand, plans organized and operated on the cooperative principle have not shown any real expansion.

AVAILABILITY OF HEALTH FACILITIES

THE EXISTENCE in a community of some hospitals which for one reason or another are non-participants in the hospital plan may result in a dilemma for the subscriber. However, most Blue Cross plans are providing for this contingency by paying the non-participating hospital an arbitrary per-diem rate if a subscriber chooses such a hospital. The subscriber does run the risk of having to pay the hospital an extra charge for bed, board, and nursing care over and above that paid by the Blue Cross plans, a situation that would not arise in the participating hospitals.

A more serious problem presents itself in connection with the medical plan since the subscriber may find, when medical services are needed, that the physician of his choice is not in the plan. Thus he must decide whether to utilize the insurance or retain the services of his chosen physician. A survey of some of the medical plans reveals that the percentage of eligible physicians participating varies from 40 to 100, most of the plans concentrating around 75 per cent. It is seen, then, that an appreciable number of physicians practicing in areas where plans are operating are not participating in the plans.

One of the knottiest problems with which voluntary health insurance must deal in its program of expansion is the lack of adequate hospital facilities and medical personnel in certain areas of the country. In areas where the economic level is high there are usually hospitals, physicians, dentists, and auxiliary personnel adequate to meet the current effective demand. By contrast, in those sections of the country where the economic level is low and in those that are sparsely populated, health facilities are insufficient and widely scattered. This mal-distribution may be expected to continue as long as the receipt of medical care is dependent wholly upon the ability of the individual to pay for it when needed.

If, in the near future, a health insurance program should expand to cover a high percentage of the population, it would be expected that in some areas the demand for services would far exceed the capacity of the existing facilities and personnel. For instance, in Georgia there are 1,106 people per physician as contrasted with the state of New York where there are 496 per physician. Georgia has but 1.9 general hospital beds per 1,000 population whereas New York State has 4.9 beds per 1,000 population. Obviously, if through a health insurance program the demand for care in the state of Georgia were to increase to the level of the existing demand in the state of New York, the medical personnel and hospital facilities in Georgia would be far from sufficient to meet the demand.

These differences in availability of services are most important considerations in the determination of the benefits that can be offered by an insurance plan. It does little good to offer hospital care to people living in an area where there are no hospitals, and antepartum care would mean little to the woman who lives many miles from the nearest doctor and has no means of transportation. In planning a comprehensive health service careful consideration must be given to the problem of making facilities and personnel available. In the areas of low income and sparse population it is obvious that health insurance plans cannot be sold to the public unless medical facilities and personnel are available to fulfill the terms of the contract. On the other hand, it will be difficult to get physicians to go into those areas until they can be assured an adequate income and adequate medical facilities with which to work. This situation poses a problem which any health insurance plan, whether compulsory or voluntary, must solve if it is to achieve total population coverage. Hospital officials and physicians are very much aware of this situation and are supporting proposals for grants-in-aid to states and local communities for the construction of hospitals and health centers where such facilities are at present non-existent or inadequate.

UNEMPLOYMENT AND MAINTENANCE OF MEMBERSHIP

As THE INSURANCE plans now operate, one of their great weaknesses is the fact that the continuation of insurance protection depends upon the continuation of employment. In some of the plans the subscriber loses his insurance contract upon cessation of employment. Continuation of insurance protection is provided for by some of the plans through carrying the unemployed individual as a single subscriber. This means, however, that the unemployed must continue to pay premiums on the insurance. The financial situation of the majority of workers is such that after their income has been terminated, they find themselves unable to continue payment. Thus, at the time when it is most needed the worker finds himself without health protection.

The problem of unemployment is, of course, much more difficult among certain occupational groups than among others. . . . Unless the insurance program can be so adjusted as to protect the worker during these periods it will fall short of its objective.

From some quarters has come the suggestion that the subscriber premium be increased in order to provide a reserve fund that could be used to carry the unemployed worker in active insurance status for a limited period of time during unemployment. The proposal would seem to have merit and careful study should be made to determine its feasibility. However, there are some difficulties that can be foreseen in the establishment and operation of such a plan. Doubtless those workers employed in occupations that are fairly stable would raise some objection to paying an excessive rate in order to furnish protection to other workers whose tenure of position is less certain. There would also be the problem of ascertaining whether the worker was unemployed by his own choice or whether it was a matter beyond his control. Those paying premiums regularly would most certainly object to carrying the insurance risk of individuals who deliberately choose periods of unemployment. Furthermore, workers in trades where periodic unemployment is inherent presumably earn a sufficient income during their employment period to make up for the loss of time between jobs. Whether workers in such employment should be given the benefits of health insurance without charge during these recurring periods would doubtless be questioned.

In the health insurance plan now in operation in the state of Connecticut an attempt is being made to meet the problem of the unemployed. The plan makes provision for the continuation of membership during unemployment on payment of half of the usual premium. The payment is made directly to the plan by the unemployed worker and may be continued subject to certain restrictions for a period of six months. After six months, the subscriber must resume payment of the full premium if he wishes to continue his membership. In order to protect the plan against abuses of malingering on the part of the unemployed, the subscriber, as a condition of continued membership, is required during unemployment to apply to the United States Employment Service at regular intervals and accept any job for which he is qualified that may be offered to him. . . .

While it is possible that a scheme may be devised that will enable the plans to carry the load of unemployed members during normal periods, it is unlikely that a plan would be able to carry the load of heavy and prolonged unemployment among their membership should a general depression occur. Thus at a time when the public's need for the protection of health insurance would be at its height the insurance plan would be unable to fulfill its function. In fact, with the wholesale loss of membership that would likely accompany a general depression, it is probable that many plans would find it extremely difficult to continue operation. Since there is no assurance that depressions will not continue to occur periodically, it must be recognized that great fluctuations in plan memberships and consequent loss of health protection to unemployed subscribers are inherent in a health program based on insurance alone with current payments intended to provide for only current needs.

Viewing the health insurance development as a whole, certain significant features become apparent. Whatever may be the differences between plans, all have one characteristic in common: an easy form of payment for the medical services offered. This feature, combined with the evidence obtained from public polls and the still better evidence of the response to the plans themselves, indicates what is the primary public interest in health insurance.

The other significant aspect involves the trend that marks the development of the plans. With only minor exceptions those now offered to the public are of a limited type. The limitations present many variables, such as geography, type of services, and age groups served. The trend, however, is toward the reduction of limitations and this trend may be interpreted either as a response to public demand or as a growing recognition of public need.

The observer of incidents or events in health insurance over a short time might conclude that the movement is a chaotic one. But observing the whole over a period of more than a decade, the episodes fit into a rather orderly pattern. Prepayment is linked to the problem of security in earning a living; comprehensive services are joined to the problem of distributing the abundance of service. This pattern of purposes does not change; it is the same whether it is expressed by a Blue Cross plan, a medical society plan, or a compulsory health insurance bill.

The evolution of official professional attitudes toward health insurance presents some impressive changes. The principle was opposed, then its local application was approved, then the approval was expanded to a statewide program and now to an interstate or national health plan under professional control. At the same time consideration is being given to the ways and means of including comprehensive services. Again, the pattern of action conforms.

It is a phenomenon of social movements that, periodically, a redefinition of tangible issues is indicated. The reason lies in the tendency to continue a form of shadow-boxing with issues that have already been settled. Twelve years ago prepayment was an issue. Five years ago prepayment for comprehensive service was an issue. One year ago prepayment for comprehensive service on a nationwide basis was an issue. None of these is an issue today; endorsement, both professional and lay, has been given to a comprehensive national health program financed by pooled funds.

The chief issue in the United States today involves the organization and administration of a national health program. There is before the professions and the public the essential task of applying the principle of health insurance in a way that will produce the most satisfactory results. More and more it is becoming apparent that the period of broad generalities—broad recommendations, broad endorsements, or broad rejections—has come to an end. . . .

There are many examples of attention to satellite rather than central problems. The one that excites much of the current discussion is the issue of compulsory versus voluntary insurance. Yet the trend in the voluntary plans is toward compulsory or quasi-compulsory devices to increase the number of subscribers. Aside from the various procedures that comprise the usual sales pressures, more attention is being given to contributions by employers and to contributions by governmental agencies for low income groups. To say that these forms of compulsion are the normal and acceptable accompaniments of a voluntary program is only to say that there are "good" compulsions. Or to propose, as an alternative to compulsory health insurance, that all employers be required to provide protection for their employees against the costs of hospital and medical services through established voluntary plans, changes the whole basis of the issue.

Whether the voluntary plans alone are the future answer to problems of health insurance in the United States depends first of all upon the answer to the question: Will they be given the opportunity to work out the solutions? The opportunity involves time, in terms of years, plus another factor, that of unquestionable evidence that each year that passes produces tangible progress in terms of better organization and wider coverage. Nor will it be permissible to base a judgment concerning the medical plans and their future upon the accomplishments of the Blue Cross hospital plans. And, by the same token, no valid judgment concerning the probable accomplishments of the Blue Cross movement can be based upon the attainments of a few of the plans while the others lag. In short, the evidence must involve a widespread pattern of progress where the hopes for the future are supported by the accomplishments of the immediate past. If the future holds the answer, the present is the logical time to consider some of the problems, the solution of which will be used to measure progress from year to year.

JUDGMENT OF THE voluntary plans will depend first upon the degree to which medical statesmanship replaces the strategy and tactics of defensive warfare. That the medical plans organized by the medical societies face complex problems is true. But not the least of the problems is the forthright support of the medical profession itself. . . .

Another test the voluntary plans will meet relates to the adoption and application of specific medical policies. In their very nature the plans involve the professions and the public. The time is past when any program that involves two groups is to be dominated completely by one, in this case either by the profession or the public. Upon matters that concern the technical aspects of medical service the profession is in a strong position by reason of its technical knowledge. But this knowledge does not automatically confer the rights of decision upon all the social, economic, and administrative questions that are an important part of any plan.

Still another issue whose outcome may be an indication of progress is the relation between hospital plans and medical plans. The present antagonism is the outcome of any attempt by one group to dominate or, what amounts to the same thing, of any suspicion that one group desires to dominate. Nothing will so affect the future of the plans as the continuation of this distrust; that it exists is unquestionable. Throughout the country there are too many hospital and medical plans with completely divided authorities and, here and there, what is worse, medical plans that offer hospital services in competition with existing hospital plans and hospital plans that offer medical coverage either because of friction with a medical plan or because the profession has refused to organize a medical plan.

The obstacles to coordination become enormous when, as in Illinois, the medical society is charged by the Blue Cross plans with an action that "sidesteps the real need for medical participation." The controversy arose over the society's decision to sponsor a surgical-obstetrical insurance plan underwritten by a group of insurance companies.

Of the same character is the disagreement over what are hospital services and what are medical services. The friction engendered here is evident particularly with reference to x-ray services. . . . Whatever the merits of the argument and however heated the issue, it should be recognized that the public has little interest in the exact lines of demarcation. If the public were asked to express an opinion it probably would be, "We don't care how the matter is settled, provided that it is settled."

THE GROWTH of the voluntary plans, especially the Blue Cross, during the past five years, has been rapid. The answer to the question: Will the expansion continue? is another test the voluntary plans must meet within the next few years. There are a number of possible lines of further development. The first is the extension of the medical plans that offer surgery and obstetrics to the point where their medical services cover approximately the same number of people as are covered by the Blue Cross plans operating in the same areas. The statements that medical plans are more complex than hospital plans and that more experience is needed, as reasons for their slower growth, may be questioned in view of the experience that has accumulated in such plans as those operating in Michigan and elsewhere.

An equally important method of expansion will be the extension of both the medical and hospital plans to cover the population of states, exclusive of the rural residents. . . .

While the enrollment of larger numbers of people over more territory and in both types of plan is one important means of growth, there is another. As the plans extend to cover more people they must also expand to provide more services. In the hospital plans extension and expansion have taken place at the same time. Therefore, for these plans the problems are not too complex. The medical plans, having experienced little expansion, face the most acute problems. . . .

BENEFITS AND QUALITY OF SERVICE RENDERED

ANOTHER MATTER deserves attention because of its bearing upon the future of voluntary plans. Although the American Medical Association gave its first endorsement to cash indemnity programs, later it approved the service plans operated under the direction and control of medical societies. In the proposed national plan approval is given either to cash or to service benefits and recently there has appeared a tendency on the part of some local societies and one national physicians' organization to support cash indemnity and oppose service plans. It is doubtful that the public will give hearty support to a program where, as described previously, the degree of protection is unknown until illness occurs; the patient visits a physician for treatment and is then told what the costs of the service will be. . . . Calling for attention [also] is the matter of payment for services which raises the question of adequate controls. It is one of the unfortunate results of misunderstanding that control devices are interpreted as attacks upon integrity. Yet, without some control of the minority—be it a minority among physicians, hospitals, or other personnel or agencies—the economic solvency of any plan is endangered.

On the subject of the quality of services there have been many loose and confusing utterances. Too often quality is presented and discussed as though it were a single element instead of one of the most complex compounds. Because of the meager knowledge that exists and because of the lack of specific standards of measurement the fallacy of direct comparisons between countries or between areas in the United States is apparent. No comparison will be productive except, ultimately, the comparison between what service is rendered and what service should be rendered.

The preceding pages present some of the problems of organization and of expansion whose solution will determine the future of voluntary health insurance. Whether voluntary health insurance will be given the opportunity to work out the solution depends on the rapidity with which difficulties are faced and overcome. . . .

B. *The Role of Government*

87. PHILOSOPHY OF SOCIAL SECURITY *

Making a Living and Making Money

TODAY WE DO not make a living. We buy it. We make money, and that money mostly determines the kinds of houses we live in, the food we eat and the clothes we wear, the security and independence we look to in hard times, sickness, and old age. . . .

In the towns and cities, money is the means of existence from day to day.

The home of a pioneer family was a little world in itself. Members of the family were their own farm and factory workers, butchers, bakers, and barbers; policemen and firemen; often their own doctors and nurses; and sometimes their own teachers as well.

As one of these occupations after another has gone out from under a family's roof, it has become possible for us to have more goods and services than a family can produce for itself. But most of a family's chance to have them depends on its ability to buy a living. . . .

As we have shifted from a land economy to a money economy, the work of children and old age has lost much of its economic importance to a family. So also has the work of women in the home. . . .

During our lifetime it has become increasingly difficult for a family to pull together and go into business for itself in one way or another.

For years there was good land to the westward to be had for the taking. Homesteading was an outlet for the sturdy and ambitious. In the towns, family shops and businesses were carried on with relatively small amounts of capital.

There is no more free land on which a living can be made. A farmer needs machines as well as skill and grit if he is to compete in the market. In the towns

* From: *Why Social Security?* by the Social Security Administration, Department of Health Education, and Welfare (Publication No. 15); Washington: U.S. Government Printing Office, 1951 (rev. ed.). Reprinted with omissions, including initial paragraphs.

and cities, modern methods of production and merchandising have greatly increased the experience and capital needed to go into business and stay in business.

Individual enterprise, which often meant family enterprise, now plays a minor part in the earning of our national income. Including the farmers, less than one gainfully occupied person in five works for himself. As a people, we no longer work as individuals or families, but as employees.

Now the livelihood of most families depends largely or wholly on the wages of a breadwinner who works for someone else. His job is likely to depend, in turn, on the general state of business or on other circumstances over which he himself has little or no control. If he loses his job or is too sick to work or becomes disabled by age or illness, his wages stop. . . .

As far as we can look back, men and women have lost one way of earning a living and have had to find others. Groups of workers, like the hand weavers, have seen their work taken away by new inventions or by changes in customs and fashions. But only in recent decades has so large a part of the population faced the risk of having income cut off for a longer or shorter time during which they have little or no other way of making a living.

Only recently have we realized that at any time, even in a good year, an industrialized country has a large group of people who want work and need work but cannot get a job for which they are fitted. The Oxford Dictionary says that the word "unemployment" did not enter the English language till 1888. "Unemployable" appeared only a year earlier. . . .

Over a year, many more families are affected by unemployment than are represented in the figure for any one month. In ordinary times, most workers who lose their jobs will find others or be called back to the old ones before many weeks have gone by. The "unemployed" are not a special group of people who are too shiftless or incompetent to hold jobs. At one time or another, they include many of our ablest workers.

When the breadwinners are out of work, their loss of earnings affects not only themselves and their families but also the community. When a factory shuts down, its neighborhood and city suffer. Everyone who has been selling goods or services to those wage earners is likely to be affected—storekeepers, landlords, barbers, owners of movie houses, and, in turn, the workers whom these people employ and the workers who produce the goods they sell.

Serious unemployment spreads like an epidemic of sickness. When large numbers of people in one part of the country are without earnings, families on farms and in towns hundreds of miles away may find their living less secure.

It was not until machines had knit our lives closely together in industry and trade that unemployment could weigh down families throughout a community or a nation. We have become interdependent on the well-being of one another. That interdependence makes it necessary for us to insure that no common hazard should cut down or cut short the livelihood of numbers of our people.

Risks to Family Independence

UNEMPLOYMENT is only one of the common risks to earning capacity and family independence. The other chief ones are old age and death of the breadwinner and the costs and losses of sickness and prolonged disability.

At any time except when there is mass unemployment, sickness and disability and death before one's time together constitute the greatest cause of poverty and dependency in the United States.

The security of life itself has never increased as rapidly at any time as in the past 60 years. . . .

Though our success in saving life has been spectacular, millions of our people suffer from ailments and defects that modern medicine can prevent or cure or at least check, so that the patient can live a useful and comfortable life. The appalling number of young men who were found physically or mentally unfit to serve in World War II shows that disease and defects are widespread even at the ages when health and vigor should be greatest.

On an average day, some 8,000,000 of our people are incapacitated by sickness to such an extent that they cannot go about their ordinary business—school, home duties, job, or whatever it is. Of these, some 4,000,000 or more are persons who would be in the labor force except for their disability. . . .

When the breadwinner's job is in a factory or office, there is little or nothing that members of the family can do to replace him there if he must take time out. If he becomes disabled, some other member of the family who otherwise might help support the family may have to stay home to care for him. The losses and costs of sickness and disability force many families to ask for public medical care. Often they must also ask for public assistance in money to help them pay the rent and buy food.

Costs of relief, loss of manpower, and lowered efficiency of half-sick people on the job are some of the bills that the whole Nation pays because we have not yet done all we can to prevent and remedy sickness and disability.

On any day, millions of people who would like to be and should be at work are without jobs or are incapacitated by temporary sickness. Their own losses in wages run to billions of dollars a year, and costs of the medical care they need is an additional staggering amount. Other millions of people who have been or would be workers are incapacitated by old age or long-continued disability.

We can prevent some of the interruptions of earnings that are due to temporary sickness or to unemployment and some of the permanent losses that come with continued disability, premature aging, or death before one's time. We can do away with much physical and mental suffering and discouragement by assuring timely and adequate medical care for all who need it. Insofar as we can stabilize high levels of employment, we can avoid the disaster that hit or threatened most workers in the 1930's and can cut down losses that confront thousands upon thousands of workers even in good years.

But doctors are the first to declare that they still stand helpless before many kinds of illness. Changes in industry are a sign of a progressive people. In a free economy, some people will always be thrown out of work for a shorter or longer time as such changes occur. Try as we may, sickness and disability, unemployment, old age, and death of the breadwinner will continue as risks to the earning capacity of most workers or to family security in an industrialized nation.

What we can do is to assure, in the national interest and the interest of the families concerned, that people will have some means of livelihood when earnings are interrupted or stop.

We have shown great ingenuity in making machines and scientific discoveries. Our very success has bound us together, so that the well-being and independence of families hinge on the judgment, skill, and good luck of many people besides themselves. As we have become interdependent, it is increasingly necessary to national welfare and security to adapt our common life so that all our people can benefit from our progress.

Family Security and Social Security

THE WORDS "social security" have become popular in the last 15 years. Actually the right and duty of a community to protect its members are as old as the records of men. Primitive tribes have rules and customs to assure the safety of all.

Even pioneer American families, of course, relied on each other for help in trouble and emergencies. Barn raisings and corn huskings, which have lasted down to our times, are a survival of years when a household asked the neighbors' help in an emergency, knowing it would give its help when its turn came.

But communities did not rely wholly upon the willingness of people to help each other. They did not rely wholly even on the willingness of families to support their own members. The common law of England, for example, lays down the duties husband and wives owe to family support.

As conditions have changed we have found many of the older family laws oppressive, such as the laws which restricted the right of a woman to her earnings, or her right to hold or will property, or to make decisions about her children. Those laws, however, were intended for the protection of families in the circumstances which existed when the laws were made. They held a family together as an economic unit. . . .

Since a living was made in families, it was through families that a community made and enforced its security measures.

Many of these measures remain with us today. The security of children, wives, and aged parents does not depend on the willingness of their family to support them. In most jurisdictions it is written into our laws and enforced daily in our courts. It is a form of social security, because as a society we see to it that members of a family give this support when they can, whether they wish to or not.

Most families do wish to do all they can to assure their independence. They try to save for a "rainy day." That expression recalls the time when people stored wood in the shed and food in the pantry and cellar for the seasons when it would be hard or impossible to go outside to fetch them. Why do they not store money in the bank now for the time when sickness or unemployment or old age stops earnings? . . .

There is no doubt that American families, by and large, want to save and do save when they have a fair margin of income over the requirements of a decent living. Even in good years, however, many family incomes are too low to meet the losses and costs if the breadwinner is out of a job for any considerable time because of unemployment or illness or if others in the home have serious or prolonged sickness. One such catastrophe may wipe out savings of past years and leave debts.

Still less can most families build up through individual savings alone a sufficient bulwark to withstand, without losing their financial independence, the long-continued or permanent loss of income that comes when the breadwinner must stop work because of disability or old age or when he dies leaving others who have depended on him for their support.

It is essential to the Nation as a whole, as well as to the families directly concerned, that people should have a steady income sufficient to meet their basic needs.

It is part of our national standard of living, part of the heritage we claim for ourselves as a healthy, progressive, and prosperous people, that even low-income families should have things our grandparents may have done without, such as running water, adequate heat in winter, electricity, a radio, an occasional movie, greater variety in diet and clothing. Many workers have to have a car to get to and from their jobs. The families that now save little—those with low and moderate incomes—make up a large share of the markets on which our economy depends. Their spending is necessary to hold up the fabric of trade and industry and agriculture on which the living of the Nation depends.

When a large part of the population cuts down spending, that fabric sags, and workers, farmers, and others feel the weight of hard times. That is what happened in the early years of the depression when fear and necessity made people stop buying.

When trade and industry brought people together in towns and cities, it no longer was safe for each house to have its own well. The safety of the whole town made it necessary to have a town water supply.

The safety of all of us now depends also on regular earning and spending to keep factory wheels turning and goods moving across store counters. Unless many people are buying what others are producing and selling, earnings are less, jobs are fewer, and all of us have less chance to earn. The well-being of families depends on the ability of other families to buy.

Family security, once dependent on work done at home, has followed the work of the family out of the home. Social security is no longer home-made.

Community Protective Action

LONG BEFORE we began to talk about social security, local communities and States began to take steps to safeguard life, health, and livelihood. As cities grew up we banded together to pay for certain kinds of protection that no one family can provide for itself. We established police and fire departments, for example. We made fire laws governing the kinds of buildings that people may build in safety to themselves and their neighbors. We organized public health departments. We set up traffic regulations to protect safety of life on the highways and streets.

We also took steps to aid helpless people who need a kind of care or an amount of protection that many families cannot provide for themselves. As our increasing scientific knowledge showed the need and the way, we built hospitals for the mentally sick and for people with tuberculosis. We made laws and opened clinics and special schools for crippled children.

At first these measures to help unfortunate people dealt chiefly with those who might be dangerous to others, such as mental patients and people sick with communicable diseases. More recently we realized that it is public economy as well as kindness to get care to sick people, since often they can recover enough to earn a living for themselves. It is cheaper to cure them when possible than to care for them for years in institutions.

About 50 years ago we began to realize that security in health and life must follow people out of their homes and into the factories. States passed laws to promote health and safety in work—laws governing hours of work, night work, dangerous work, and the like. These are conditions which workers no longer can control for themselves as they could to a large extent when they worked at home. . . .

And some 40 years ago we began to take steps toward assuring not only health and safety in work but also the money to which working families must look in order to buy their living. . . .

In 1911, two States passed laws to give small money allowances to needy mothers, so that they could keep their children at home rather than put them in an institution. By the beginning of 1935, 45 States, Alaska, Hawaii, and the District of Columbia had laws on their books to aid needy widows with children and occasionally other needy mothers.

Other laws looked to the earnings of adults. . . .

By 1911 a majority of the States had passed laws establishing minimum wages for employees on public works.

In 1911 the State of Washington passed a workmen's compensation act. In the next ten years similar laws were enacted by more than 40 other States. These laws provide money and medical care for workers who suffer work-connected injuries and they provide compensation to the families of workers who are killed. They require employers to insure their employees. Under them the costs of industrial accidents, and to some extent the costs of sickness due to work, have become a part of the running costs of industry. . . .

Starting in the 1920's, many States took steps to provide some security for another large group of their people—the old people who were in need and who probably would never be able to earn their own living again. . . .

Mothers' aid and old-age allowances and other types of public assistance are not "pensions" in the sense in which we generally use that word. Widowed mothers and old people do not get assistance just because they are widowed or have reached a certain age. They have to show that they are in need.

This kind of assistance is a modern way of meeting an old responsibility. It recognizes the duty of government to provide basic security for people who cannot earn it for themselves, and it is a just and orderly way of meeting that responsibility.

It is a better method than those which States and towns and counties long had used, such as giving baskets of food or tons of coal, or building orphanages and almshouses. It gives needy people a greater chance to choose how they will live. It provides them with what all of us now need to keep our freedom and self-respect —money to provide the necessities of life. . . .

One social historian has called measures like these "social inventions." They are ways we have invented to fit our social life to the changes brought by mechanical and scientific inventions.

One major social invention was put into use for the first time in the United States when Wisconsin passed its unemployment compensation law in 1932. This law, like the workmen's compensation laws, was a form of social insurance.

As workmen's compensation protects workers against the losses and costs of accidents to life and limb, so unemployment insurance protects them against part of the wage loss they suffer from the accident of having no job. It is not charity or relief. It helps to prevent need for relief. Like other kinds of social insurance, it spreads the cost of losses among large numbers of people and over a period of time, so that not all the burden falls on the workers who are out of jobs.

By the beginning of the 1930's, many people were talking about our need for social insurance, not only against unemployment but also against other widespread economic risks of workers and their families.

Social insurance is a form of savings. It is designed to enable people to meet the unusual demands for which most of us, low and moderate-income people, cannot hope to save enough individually—disability that strikes at an early age, more than average costs and losses from sickness or unemployment, death of the breadwinner on whom others depend, and so on.

If all families met only *average* costs and losses from all such causes, all but those with very low incomes could meet them individually. But the losses come unevenly and unpredictably and in some homes, repeatedly. Saving through social insurance spreads the risk and the costs over the whole group of people who are subject to them and gives individual families far greater protection than they can secure alone.

Under social insurance, workers or employers or both, and sometimes also the Government, lay aside small regular contributions to build up the insurance funds from which benefits are paid to insured workers or their families when the worker's earnings are lost by reason of one of the causes covered by the insurance system. The contributions made by or on behalf of individuals while they are earning thus meet part of the wage loss that some of the covered group will suffer in any year and that practically all will suffer at some time during their lives. They are like the premiums that people pay for fire insurance or insurance on their car, in which the costs of the misfortune of those who have a fire or an accident are spread over the whole insured group and over a period of time and so are not a crushing catastrophe for the unlucky ones.

Social insurance benefits are intended to provide a basic minimum security which families will supplement in other ways, by other insurance, home ownership, bank accounts, and so on. The insurance benefits replace part of the worker's wage loss when he cannot earn, and thus help him and his community by supplying some money to help him and his family pay the rent, grocery bills, and other essential expenses. The assurance of small regular amounts when a man cannot earn encourages rather than discourages thrift by making savings more worthwhile and by keeping misfortunes from wiping out the savings of past years. The benefit for which an insured worker qualifies is paid to him regardless of any other resources he or his family may have.

Social insurance in this and other countries is geared to employment covered by the insurance system. Some people will not have been able to earn insurance rights because they have worked in noncovered jobs or have not held covered jobs long enough to qualify. Others may meet with a series or combination of misfortunes that uses up their insurance rights or requires more compensation than the system can afford to provide out of the contributions workers can readily pay. Still others may suffer wage losses or other economic catastrophes from causes the system does not cover.

For these and other reasons, the United States and most other industrial nations have established public assistance to complement their social insurance system. While social insurance benefits are paid as a consequence of past covered employment, public assistance payments are made to people because they are in present need. In the interest of the Nation as a whole, as well as of the needy person, they are intended to see that no one lacks the means of subsistence.

Social insurance and public assistance are the financial foundation of a social security program. In this country and others, such a program also includes public services to promote health, thrift, and other aspects of the economic, social, and individual well-being of the Nation's people.

Our Social Security Program

BEGINNING WITH THE Social Security Act of 1935, our national program of social security has grown out of the changes in American life and our past experience in fighting insecurity.

Through that program the Federal Government has added its resources to those of the States to enable the States to provide more effective money assistance and services to needy people and to strengthen community services for public health and for the health and welfare of children and mothers. These are programs that have enabled all States to do better what many or most of them had already undertaken to some extent. To these have been added other services of the Federal Government and the States to promote general security and well-being.

In social insurance we have broken new ground to serve old needs. We have provided ways through which workers and employers and government collaborate to enable families to keep their independence when circumstances beyond their control cut short or cut off their capacity to earn.

What we want today is what Americans have always wanted and worked for. The colonists and frontiersmen wanted independence and opportunity for themselves and their children. They wanted to make their own living and to take an active share in the life of their times. All that has changed today is the way we take to get these things. Our security is the security of the whole people.

88. Proposals for National Health Insurance: 1910-1950 *

THE AGITATION for and against the adoption of a compulsory system of medical care insurance in the United States began shortly before World War I. It is the purpose of this article to trace the main events and developments of issues during these forty years, dividing the time into three broad periods. The first period, 1910-20, reached the legislative stage in several states, but no bills were passed. Action for compulsory medical care insurance appeared to be ill-prepared and hasty, and subsided abruptly as soon as unexpected opposition mustered its forces effectively. The second period, 1921-33, was a quiet one devoted to study of basic facts and problems only superficially comprehended in the first period. The third period, beginning in 1933, has been characterized by action similar to that of the first period, but on a much broader base of support and opposition, and in a profoundly different social, political, and economic context.

First Period, 1910-20

DURING THE FIRST period the American Association for Labor Legislation (AALL) was the chief group calling attention to the problem of medical care insurance and making concrete suggestions for its solution. The AALL was organized in 1906 by a handful of prominent economists. By 1913 it had over 3,300 members consisting of economists, lawyers, political scientists, historians, and members of other fields concerned with social problems. It passed out of existence in 1942.

It is important to note that the AALL was dedicated to the improvement of various phases of society within the contemporary economic and social structure and ideology. The organization was primarily interested in the effects of industrialization as seen in industrial accidents, occupational diseases, and general working condi-

* From: "Compulsory Medical Care Insurance in the United States," by Odin W. Anderson; *Annals of the American Academy of Political and Social Science*, Vol. 273 (entitled *Medical Care for Americans*), Jan. 1951, pp. 106-13. Reprinted by permission of the author and publishers. The author is the research director of the Health Information Foundation, New York.

tions. Workmen's compensation was greatly emphasized and pushed as the prime method of reducing industrial accidents and diseases and protecting the earning power of the workers. In this regard the AALL was very effective, because workmen's compensation laws were enacted in thirty states by 1915. The AALL was thus flushed with a seemingly easy victory and was looking over the social scene for some other problem to attack.

Medical care insurance was selected as the next logical step for action. Workmen's compensation protected the workers against the economic loss of accidents and illness arising out of employment, while medical care insurance was designed to cover workers for illnesses and accidents not related to employment.

In 1912 the AALL established a Committee on Social Insurance, the first of its kind in the United States, which in the next few years carried the main burden of medical care insurance study and activity. Three of the members of the committee were also members of the Social Insurance Committee established by the American Medical Association (AMA) in 1915. They were Alexander Lambert, I. M. Rubinow, and later S. S. Goldwater, all physicians. As will be seen, these cross connections had interesting results.

At the seventh annual meeting of the AALL held in Washington, D. C. in December 1913, Joseph P. Chamberlain delivered the first paper on medical care insurance, recommending a compulsory system for state and Federal consideration.

In 1914 a subcommittee of the Committee on Social Insurance was appointed to draft a bill in preparation for an active campaign in the states and in Congress. By the end of 1915 a model bill was drafted to be introduced in several state legislatures in January 1916. At the same time it was reported that the AMA had appointed a committee to co-operate with the Committee on Social Insurance "in putting the finishing touches on the medical sections of the bill." Also, several other important organizations appointed committees early in 1916 to study the proposal of the AALL. The Secretary of the AALL optimistically wrote in the annual report: "The opportunity now appears good for a big educational campaign for the conservation of health, with fair prospects for legislative commissions to investigate in 1916 and for compulsory health insurance legislation in this country in 1917."

So far so good for the protagonists, but opposition emerged very rapidly after the AALL had unstrategically exposed itself completely. It was naïvely assumed that a reform which they thought should be deemed good by everyone would triumph on its own merits.

As long as medical care insurance was discussed without relation to specific and concrete actions, the potential opponents apparently were not aware of its implications. However, when ten state commissions were established to study the subject and make recommendations, and bills were introduced in sixteen state legislatures, the proponents were surprised at the opposition's vehemence and gathering strength. Within the AALL itself, Frederick L. Hoffman, statistician for the Prudential Insurance Company of America, resigned from the Committee on Social Insurance in 1916 when it endorsed compulsory medical care insurance. He and I. M. Rubinow became opposing symbols of the controversy. They were inveterate traveling lecturers; both used words effectively, and both had a following.

By 1918 the movement had reached its peak as represented by activities of state commissions in the state legislatures. The most intense activity was found in California and New York. At this point the seemingly favorable attitude of organized medicine turned into vigorous opposition. Simultaneously, pharmaceutical companies, accident and health insurance companies, companies selling industrial insurance, and healing cults proved to be too much for the proponents of compulsory medical care insurance. Furthermore (and this was a dismaying discovery for the AALL), Samuel Gompers, president of the American Federation of Labor, was very outspoken in his denunciation of government-operated social insurance schemes. Numerous state federations of labor supported the AALL proposal, particularly in New York State, but their support came too late and Gompers' prestige was too great.

It appears to be coincidental that the prominent physicians in the American Medical Association were able to have a committee established in 1915 to study the issues of medical care insurance and report to the House of Delegates from time to time. The apparent purpose was not to advocate any compulsory insurance, but, according to I. M. Rubinow who became the executive secretary of the committee, "to bring about friendly understanding between all parties concerned and to protect the legitimate economic interests of the profession."

A few months before Rubinow's statement, the *Journal of the American Medical Association* ran an editorial regarding the model bill of the AALL: "It is hoped that physicians will take advantage of this opportunity [of studying the AALL bill] and that it will be possible to avoid that lack of co-operation between physicians and legislators which, for a time, marred some of the foreign legislation."

By 1920 officials of state medical societies were reacting vehemently against any deliberation on compulsory medical care insurance, particularly in New York, Michigan, Illinois, and California. A powerful group of delegates assembled at the annual session of the AMA in New Orleans in 1920 "to get Lambert" as they put it, who was then president of the association.

At the same session, the House of Delegates established a basic policy which has not been revised to the present day, and expressed it in the following resolution:

> The American Medical Association declares its opposition to the institution of any plan embodying the system of compulsory contributory insurance against illness, or any other plan of compulsory insurance which provides for medical service to be rendered contributors or their dependents, provided, controlled, or regulated by any state or Federal government.

The end of the controversy over compulsory medical care insurance was just as abrupt as the foregoing resolution was final.

Second Period, 1921-33

AFTER THE EMPHATICALLY worded resolution in 1920, the American Medical Association at several annual meetings considered resolutions concerned with definitions of "state medicine" and similar forms of medical care organized and operated by government.

In 1921 the Sheppard-Towner bill to provide grants-in-aid to states for maternal and child health programs was up for consideration in Congress. The bill aroused bitter controversy at the hearings, and many physicians testified in opposition. Although the bill was not proposing a system of compulsory medical care insurance, physicians regarded it as an entering wedge for encroachment of government in private practice. Nevertheless, the Sheppard-Towner Act was passed in 1922 with active support from citizens' groups. The act was disapproved officially by the House of Delegates at the annual meeting of the AMA in 1922.

Problems regarding the economic and social aspects of medical care were discussed on several occasions in 1925 and 1926 at conferences attended by physicians, members of the public health profession, and economists. These conferences were called to formulate plans for a study of the structure of medical services of the country, especially the economic aspects. As a result of the deliberations of these conferences, the Committee on the Costs of Medical Care (CCMC) was established. Its work was financed by six foundations: Carnegie Corporation, Josiah Macy, Jr., Foundation, Milbank Memorial Fund, Julius Rosenwald Fund, Russell Sage Foundation, and Twentieth Century Fund.

The committee consisted of 42 persons—14 private practitioners of medicine, 6 from public health, 8 from institutions interested in medicine, 5 economists, and 9 persons representing the general public.

From 1928 to 1932 the CCMC released twenty-eight reports on the incidence of illness, the cost of medical care, and related aspects of health. The period of study seemed to be one of watchful waiting. The AMA editorialized: "Most physicians and most economists and most social workers are willing to wait until the Committee on the Costs of Medical Care, a group with which the medical profession is cooperating wholeheartedly, has brought into the situation, data on which to base reasonable action for the future."

The effect of the final report dealing with recommendations for action on the basis of findings was immediate. Majority and minority reports split the CCMC and supporters of its objectives into factions. The lead in opposition to the majority report was taken by the AMA and some of the physician members of the CCMC.

The majority of the members of the committee were of the opinion that "medical service, both preventive and therapeutic, should be furnished largely by organized groups of physicians, dentists, nurses, pharmacists, and other associated personnel" and that "the costs of medical care be placed on a group payment basis," through the use of insurance, taxation, or both.

The minority group, while agreeing with the majority report in many matters, objected to the proposal for group practice and the adoption of insurance plans unless sponsored and controlled by organized medicine.

The editorial response of the AMA to the majority report has become a classic, and was presumably directed at the aspects of the report dealing with group practice and areas of government responsibility, and not at voluntary insurance, as such, if sponsored and controlled by organized medicine. The editorial read:

The alinement is clear—on the one side the forces representing the great foundations, public health officialdom, social theory—even socialism and communism—inciting to revolution; on the other side, the organized medical profession of this country urging an orderly evolution guided by controlled experimentation which will observe the principles that have been found through the centuries to be necessary to the sound practice of medicine.[1]

Third Period, Beginning 1933

THE RECOMMENDATIONS of the Committee on the Costs of Medical Care and the reactions to them formed the base of the third period of the compulsory medical care insurance movement. The main issues and factions were brought to the surface as the movement gained momentum and breadth during the following years. It will be recalled that the American Association for Labor Legislation, an organization composed chiefly of professional people, was the group most instrumental in initiating interest in and action for some type of compulsory medical care insurance in the first period; but during the third period, beginning in 1933, which has not yet ended, the Federal Government, through official committees and legislative activity, and later state governments, have been the agencies which spearheaded the reopening of the issue of government-sponsored medical care insurance. What government has done during this period has conditioned the attitudes and actions of other groups which feel that they have a stake in the future of medical care. There has been general agreement that a problem exists, and the depression made it more acute; but there has been profound disagreement as to what should be the solution.

The depression and the deliberations over the nature and scope of the impending social security program provided the framework for discussions and action regarding compulsory medical care insurance. The precedent-setting Federal *Rules and Regulations No. 7* of 1933 defined policies and procedures under which medical care might be given to those receiving unemployment relief in the states. Representatives of the American Medical Association participated in the formulation of the rules and regulations and gave their sanction. Access to medical care was now recognized by government as a basic minimum right together with food, clothing, and shelter.

In 1934 the President appointed the Committee on Economic Security to make recommendations for a program "against misfortunes which cannot be wholly eliminated in this man-made world of ours." In addition there were numerous committees established as advisory to the Committee on Economic Security, with a very broad range of representation of fields of interests and organizations. The research duties of the committee were divided into several problem areas; among them, medical care.

Medical care insurance was given short shrift, however, inasmuch as Edwin E. Witte, executive director of the Committee on Economic Security, reported that medical care insurance could not even reach the research stage, not to mention its incorporation in the social security program. He wrote:

[1] *Journal of the American Medical Association*, Vol. 99 (Dec. 3, 1932), p. 1952.

When in 1934 the Committee on Economic Security announced that it was studying health insurance, it was at once subjected to misrepresentation and vilification. In the original social security bill there was one line to the effect that the Social Security Board should study the problem and make a report thereon to Congress. That little line was responsible for so many telegrams to the members of Congress that the entire social security program seemed endangered until the Ways and Means Committee unanimously struck it out of the bill.

As a corollary, the AMA was also the object of pressure. Its *Journal* editorialized, on November 24, 1934:

The headquarters office of the American Medical Association has been besieged with telephone calls, telegrams and letters on this subject. . . . Some physicians are apparently opposed to all change and feel that the American Medical Association should officially make itself felt in opposition to the entire program of the government.

Following the Social Security Act.—The Social Security Act was passed in 1935. Thereafter the Government sponsored a series of activities which either deliberately or coincidently resulted in the introduction of the first compulsory medical care insurance bill in Congress to attract any widespread attention, the so-called Wagner bill of 1939 (S. 1620).[2] The series of activities was as follows:

1. The National Health Survey was made in 1935-36—a large-scale study of the incidence of illness and the underlying social and economic factors.

2. In 1935 the President appointed the interdepartmental Committee to Co-ordinate Health and Welfare Activities, entrusted with the task of making sure that the provisions of the Social Security Act were being effectively applied, and suggesting improvements. One of the chief interests of the committee was the problem of medical care.

3. Out of the Interdepartmental Committee was created the Technical Committee on Medical Care in 1937, consisting chiefly of experts from the Federal agencies concerned in whole or in part with health.

4. Early in 1938 the Technical Committee recommended, among other things, that there was a need for a general program of medical care and insurance against loss of wages as a result of illness.

5. Thereupon, the Interdepartmental Committee called the National Health Conference held in Washington, D. C., in July 1938, to discuss the findings and recommendations submitted by the Technical Committee. Invitations were sent to a large representation of people from the medical profession, from agencies working in health, and from labor, industry, agriculture, and other groups of citizens. The purpose of the conference was to clarify issues and stimulate constructive criticisms. No specific recommendations were expected from the conferees.

Succession of Bills.—The Wagner bill of 1939 was followed by: the Capper bill in 1941 (S. 489); the Eliot bill in 1942 (H. R. 7354); the Wagner-Murray-

---

[2] Actually, the first medical care insurance bills in Congress were those introduced by Senator Capper of Kansas in July 1935 (S. 3253) and in January 1937 (S. 855); but they received little attention.

Dingell bill in 1943 (S. 1161); a reintroduction of S. 1161 by Representative Dingell, Michigan, early in 1945 (H. R. 395); and in November of the same year, a new Wagner-Murray-Dingell bill (S. 1606). In 1947 there appeared the first counter-proposal to compulsory medical care insurance in the bill (S. 545) sponsored by Senator Taft and others to assist states in providing medical care for the indigent. The opposite type of bill was introduced in the same year by Senators Murray, Wagner, and others (S. 1320).

In May 1948 another health conference, the National Health Assembly, was held in Washington, attended by 800 professional and community leaders. Again all phases of the problem of medical care were examined. The Medical Care Section of the assembly unanimously agreed that the *principle* of contributory insurance should be the basic method of financing medical care for the large majority of the American people, but differed in their views on the method of implementation. Independent of the National Health Assembly, the Federal Security Administrator, Oscar R. Ewing, recommended a compulsory system, and in the report to the President marshaled a great array of data in an attempt to justify his conclusions.[3]

In 1949 bills in Congress on medical care became so numerous that they were difficult to follow, but two bills emerged as the focus of the conflict over compulsory medical care insurance—the administration bill, S. 1679, and the opposition bill, S. 1970. The latter bill proposed a "voluntary" approach by providing for Federal grants to the states to assist co-operating voluntary prepayment plans to make their services generally available to those wishing to utilize them. The difference between the two bills reflects diverse philosophies.

Because of the intense and prominent activities on the Federal level, parallel actions on the state level have been overlooked or discussed as of little importance, except in California. However, since 1935 compulsory medical care insurance bills have been introduced in over a dozen states, and in some of them repeatedly. In California, by law of 1949, compulsory insurance against the cost of hospitalization was introduced for all persons covered by compulsory unemployment insurance.

As stated previously, it appears that government activity was the stimulus for counteractivity on the part of proponents of voluntary health insurance. Today these plans are widespread.

Development of Issues.—To close the discussion of the third period let us trace the development of issues to the present time, so that we can be assisted in delineating current issues. Not until the National Health Conference held in Washington in 1938 did the issue of compulsory medical care insurance become a national issue in the sense that a great variety of groups throughout the country became aware of the problem and acted accordingly.

The shifts in issues since 1933 may be broadly indicated as follows:

1. In 1933 medical care insurance, regardless of type of sponsorship, was an issue.

[3] Oscar R. Ewing, *The Nation's Health, A Ten Year Program: A Report to the President,* Washington, D. C.: Federal Security Agency, 1948, 186 pp.

2. By 1939 insurance as a device to spread the economic risk of illness ceased to be an issue. The hospitals had for several years supported insurance plans pertaining to hospitalization, and the AMA recognized them and began to direct attention to medical plans along similar lines.

3. Also by 1939 an insurance system covering the Nation regardless of type of sponsorship was an issue.

4. By 1946 both the American Hospital Association and the AMA subscribed to a nation-wide system sponsored and operated by themselves.

5. The remaining basic issue has become a national compulsory medical care insurance system or a national voluntary system. There are important sub-issues, such as the questions of scope of service, extent of coverage of population, and pace of development.

Basically the AMA is in the forefront of the chief opposition group, and organized labor—the CIO and the AFL— is spearhead for some form of compulsory insurance. It will be recalled that the collapse of the movement for compulsory medical care insurance in the first period was partly due to the lack of effective support from organized labor; but the reverse is true today.

Bases of Agreement.—So much attention is being paid to disagreements between opposing factions that bases of agreement are ignored. The bases of agreement holding all parties and individuals within sparring distance of one another is the consensus that all should have access to medical care irrespective of income. Given this consensus, the next step is the struggle over means. The means is insurance, but there is disagreement as to sponsorship and control.

Another common orientation is that groups on both sides of the question of compulsory medical care insurance have a basic faith in the present political and economic institutions. The individuals and organizations supporting compulsory medical care insurance are not necessarily revolutionary; nor are those opposing such a system necessarily reactionary. As specific objects of a reform movement, physicians are naturally very much affected, and to them it seems a revolutionary step; but in the perspective of a deep-seated and world-wide movement gaining momentum in the United States with the Social Security Act in 1935, compulsory medical care insurance is a rounding out of a broad social program.

The exact form a national medical care insurance program might take would probably depend on the ability of the Blue Cross and Blue Shield plans to modify and deflect an all-out Federal-state compulsory medical care insurance system, and on the as yet unclear trends of the burgeoning union health and welfare plans. In other words, the third period of the medical care insurance movement in the United States is by no means over. Events are moving so rapidly that the last part of this article will become out of date in a year.

89. National Health Insurance: A Suggested Plan

A. THE PLAN IN OUTLINE *

EVERYONE SHOULD have ready access to all necessary medical, hospital, and related services.

I recommend solving the basic problem by distributing the costs through expansion of our existing compulsory social insurance system. This is not socialized medicine.

Everyone who carries fire insurance knows how the law of averages is made to work so as to spread the risk and to benefit the insured who actually suffers the loss. If, instead of the costs of sickness being paid only by those who get sick, all the people, sick and well, were required to pay premiums into an insurance fund, the pool of funds thus created would enable all who do fall sick to be adequately served without overburdening anyone. That is the principle upon which all forms of insurance are based.

During the past 15 years, hospital insurance plans have taught many Americans this magic of averages. Voluntary health insurance plans have been expanding during recent years; but their rate of growth does not justify the belief that they will meet more than a fraction of our people's needs. Only about 3 or 4 percent of our population now have insurance providing comprehensive medical care.

A system of required prepayment would not only spread the costs of medical care, it would also prevent much serious disease. Since medical bills would be paid by the insurance fund, doctors would more often be consulted when the first signs of disease occur instead of when the disease has become serious. Modern hospital, specialist, and laboratory services, as needed, would also become available to all and would improve the quality and adequacy of care. Prepayment of medical care would go a long way toward furnishing insurance against disease itself, as well as against medical bills.

Such a system of prepayment should cover medical, hospital, nursing, and laboratory services. It should also cover dental care—as fully and for as many of the population as the available professional personnel and the financial resources of the system permit.

The ability of our people to pay for adequate medical care will be increased if, while they are well, they pay regularly into a common health fund instead of paying sporadically and unevenly when they are sick. This health fund should be built up nationally in order to establish the broadest and most stable basis for spreading the costs of illness and to assure adequate financial support for doctors and hospitals

* From: *Message from the President of the United States, Transmitting His Request for Legislation for Adoption of a National Health Program,* by Harry S. Truman; Document No. 380, House of Representatives, 79th Cong., 1st Sess., Washington: U.S. Government Printing Office, 1945 (pp. 8-10). Reprinted with omissions, including initial paragraphs.

everywhere. If we were to rely on State-by-State action only, many years would elapse before we had any general coverage. Meanwhile health service would continue to be grossly uneven, and disease would continue to cross State boundary lines.

Medical services are personal. Therefore, the Nation-wide system must be highly decentralized in administration. The local administrative unit must be the keystone of the system so as to provide for local services and adaptation to local needs and conditions. Locally as well as nationally, policy and administration should be guided by advisory committees in which the public and the medical professions are represented.

Subject to national standards, methods and rates of paying doctors and hospitals should be adjusted locally. All such rates for doctors should be adequate and should be appropriately adjusted upward for those who are qualified specialists.

People should remain free to choose their own physicians and hospitals. The removal of financial barriers between patient and doctor would enlarge the present freedom of choice. The legal requirement on the population to contribute involves no compulsion over the doctor's freedom to decide what services his patient needs. People will remain free to obtain and pay for medical services outside of the health-insurance system if they desire, even though they are members of the system; just as they are free to send their children to private instead of to public schools, although they must pay taxes for public schools.

Likewise physicians should remain free to accept or reject patients. They must be allowed to decide for themselves whether they wish to participate in the health-insurance system full time, part time, or not at all. A physician may have some patients who are in the system and some who are not. Physicians must be permitted to be represented through organizations of their own choosing, and to decide whether to carry on in individual practice or to join with other doctors in group practice in hospitals or in clinics.

Our voluntary hospitals and our city, county, and State general hospitals, in the same way, must be free to participate in the system to whatever extent they wish. In any case they must continue to retain their administrative independence.

Voluntary organizations which provide health services that meet reasonable standards of quality should be entitled to furnish services under the insurance system and to be reimbursed for them. Voluntary cooperative organizations concerned with paying doctors, hospitals, or others for health services but not providing services directly, should be entitled to participate if they can contribute to the efficiency and economy of the system.

None of this is really new. The American people are the most insurance-minded people in the world. They will not be frightened off from health insurance because some people have misnamed it "socialized medicine."

I repeat—what I am recommending is not socialized medicine.

Socialized medicine means that all doctors work as employees of government. The American people want no such system. No such system is here proposed.

Under the plan I suggest, our people would continue to get medical and hospital services just as they do now—on the basis of their own voluntary decisions and choices. Our doctors and hospitals would continue to deal with disease with the same professional freedom as now. There would, however, be this all-important difference: whether or not patients get the services they need would not depend on how much they can afford to pay at the time.

I am in favor of the broadest possible coverage for this insurance system. I believe that all persons who work for a living and their dependents should be covered under such an insurance plan. This would include wage and salary earners, those in business for themselves, professional persons, farmers, agricultural labor, domestic employees, Government employees, and employees of nonprofit institutions and their families.

In addition, needy persons and other groups should be covered through appropriate premiums paid for them by public agencies. Increased Federal funds should also be made available by the Congress under the public-assistance programs to reimburse the States for part of such premiums, as well as for direct expenditures made by the States in paying for medical services provided by doctors, hospitals, and other agencies to needy persons.

Premiums for present social-insurance benefits are calculated on the first $3,000 of earnings in a year. It might be well to have all such premiums, including those for health, calculated on a somewhat higher amount such as $3,600.

A broad program of prepayment for medical care would need total amounts approximately equal to 4 per cent of such earnings. The people of the United States have been spending, on the average, nearly this percentage of their incomes for sickness care. How much of the total fund should come from the insurance premiums and how much from general revenues is a matter for the Congress to decide.

The plan which I have suggested would be sufficient to pay most doctors more than the best they have received in peacetime years. The payments of the doctors' bills would be guaranteed, and the doctors would be spared the annoyance and uncertainty of collecting fees from individual patients. The same assurance would apply to hospitals, dentists, and nurses for the services they render.

Federal aid in the construction of hospitals will be futile unless there is current purchasing power so that people can use these hospitals. Doctors cannot be drawn to sections which need them without some assurance that they can make a living. Only a Nation-wide spreading of sickness costs can supply such sections with sure and sufficient purchasing power to maintain enough physicians and hospitals.

We are a rich Nation and can afford many things. But ill health which can be prevented or cured is one thing we cannot afford. . . .

B. THE PLAN IN OPERATION: A PREVIEW *

Health Insurance as Seen by the Insured Person and His Family.—For the worker and his family, health insurance is primarily a method of prepaying the costs of

* From: *Medical Care Insurance,* by the Committee on Education and Labor, United States Senate; Committee Print No. 5, 79th Cong., 2nd Sess., Washington, U.S. Government Printing Office, 1946 (Part II, pp. 11-19). Reprinted with omissions, including initial paragraphs.

medical care. The worker will therefore have his first direct contact with the system when he pays his social insurance premium. The premium for health insurance, it may be assumed, will be part of the worker's total social insurance contribution, but a designated part. The worker and his family will know just how much of its income is being budgeted for prepayment of medical costs. If the worker is an employee, the employer will deduct the amount of the premium from his pay check, and forward the earnings record and premium to the Government agency, presumably at the same time and in the same clerical operation as that already practiced for old-age and survivors insurance. If the worker is in business or farming for himself (self-employed), he may report his earnings and pay his premium in a supplement to his income-tax return. If self-employed persons with income below the income-tax reporting limit are covered, they might make a simple declaration of income and annual, quarterly or other periodic installment payment of the premium.

A worker who has sufficient credited earnings to meet the eligibility test will have "insured status," that is paid-up rights to the medical care benefits for a year. In some social insurance programs, insured status and the individual's benefit year is determined at the time the risk occurs, as when a worker becomes unemployed, or disabled, or retires or dies. For medical care benefits, however, it would seem preferable to have a uniform benefit year for all beneficiaries. The establishment and continued maintenance of relations between the insured person and the doctor, dentist, or hospital, will be much simpler and easier if the eligibility determination has been made in advance of the time when medical care is needed, so that there is no reason for the insured person to have to deal with the insurance system or its offices at that time. Furthermore, since medical care benefits would be available to the worker's family as well as to the worker himself, the simplest and most understandable arrangement would be to have a uniform period, such as a year, within which the family has paid-up insured status and is entitled to the insurance benefits without having to take any further steps except to arrange with the doctor or hospital for the medical care that is needed and wanted.

The benefit year might be the calendar year; or it might be the 12 months from July 1 through June 30. If the benefit year begins on July 1, eligibility for the current benefit year will presumably be determined, for most workers, by their earnings and contributions in the previous calendar year, the period generally used for income-tax purposes. The interval between the end of the calendar year and the beginning of the benefit year would give the insurance agency time to obtain all the earnings records and to make a predetermination of insured status. After the insurance system has been started, each new benefit year would start at the end of the preceding one; there would be no gap between successive benefit years.

Somewhat in advance of the beginning of a benefit year, the insurance agency might issue a card to each insured worker, indicating that he and his qualified dependents had paid-up rights to medical care for the coming benefit year. In order to get his card, the worker would merely need to furnish the insurance office his current address, so that the insurance card could be mailed to him. Application blanks for this purpose would be available at local post offices, health agency offices, unions, work places, and elsewhere. The worker would presumably record on his application and his insurance card the names of his dependents, and possibly the signatures of his adult dependents, who would qualify for medical care benefits. A worker who failed to meet the eligibility test at the beginning of a benefit year might send in a new application and become eligible at the beginning of any subsequent calendar-quarter during the benefit year (when additional earnings credits had been acquired), and receive an insurance card entitling him and his family to benefits for the remainder of the benefit year. A family which acquired a new dependent during the course of a benefit year, could arrange to have the individual's name added to the card. Ordinarily, the entire family would probably find it easier to use one card, but separate cards could be provided for members of the family temporarily away from home or who for other reasons find this arrangement more convenient.

Insurance cards evidencing the right to medical care benefits for the current benefit year would also be issued to individuals brought under coverage through supplementary contractual arrangements between the insurance system and other public agencies. Whether in such cases the cards would be distributed by the insurance agency or by the public agency making the arrangements with the insurance system might be determined by mutual agreement between the two agencies. Whatever the method of distribution, the insurance cards issued to persons covered by contract would presumably be indistinguishable from the cards issued to insured workers.

At or shortly before the beginning of a benefit year, then, each insured person will presumably have a card evidencing right to medical care benefits for the coming year. What each family does from then on in selecting a doctor or dentist and obtaining needed services will depend largely on its own habits and preferences. A family which already has an established relationship with a family doctor, who is participating in the insurance system, will let him know—perhaps on the next call or visit—that they are insured for the coming year. Other families may be stimulated, by the receipt of the insurance card, to select a doctor and to make some contact with him in advance of illness. Many will no doubt wait until someone in the family is ill before making their selection.

Choice of doctor (or dentist) has always depended on many factors. And, as is the case today, previous experience, advice from friends and neighbors, convenience and personal compatibility may be expected to play important roles in determining a family's choice of doctor under the insurance system. The local administrative agency will see to it that lists of the names of all participating physicians are published locally and placed where the lists can easily be consulted by insured persons who do not already have a family doctor. The free choice of doctor by the insured person is limited, of course, by the right of the doctor to accept or reject anyone who chooses him. The continuity and duration of the relationship, once established between doctor and insured persons, depends upon them.

If the doctors in the community have chosen to receive their payments from the health insurance system on a fee-for-service basis, there will be no special reason for the insured individual to select a physician in advance of the time he needs service. The same holds true if the local doctors have chosen to be paid on a salary basis. The insured person will be able to go to one general practitioner or another, at will, among those who are participating in the insurance system, subject to the professional restraints on such "shopping-around" which operate today and would presumably continue to be imposed by the medical profession itself. Unless he establishes a continuing relationship with the doctor, he will have to present his insurance card each time he sees a new doctor, in order that the doctor may have the necessary information indicating the patient's insurance right and, where doctors are paid by fee-for-service, for billing the insurance system for the service rendered.

If the doctors in the community have chosen to be paid on the capitation basis —that is, according to a fixed amount of money per year or per month for each insured person who has chosen the doctor—insured persons will be encouraged to select a doctor in advance of actual illness, in order that the doctor and the insurance system may know how many persons are relying on a particular physician for care in case of illness or need for preventive service or advice. A person who failed to make an advance selection could, of course, still request the doctor's services when the need arises. An insured person could change doctors if he wished, but where the insurance system pays the doctor by the capitation method, he would be required to notify the local administrative agency or the doctor to transfer his name from one doctor's list to another—in order that only one doctor may receive the capitation payment for him. Unless he make such a change, he will not need to show his insurance card to his family doctor more than once in each benefit year.

If there are in the community physicians practicing together as an organized group, insured persons will be free to receive their medical care from such a group if they so choose. The groups themselves, like individual practitioners, may set up certain conditions as to whom they will accept for care.

Once an insured family has decided it wants a particular physician as its family doctor (or for any member of the family) and has been accepted by him, it will obtain his services just as it would today—according to prevailing practices in the community and the decisions and judgment of the individual doctor (or the medical group if such has been chosen). The doctor will see patients in his office, at their homes or in the hospital, as he does now. Decisions as to the course of treatment will rest entirely with the doctor. Because of the availability of laboratory and related services as insurance benefits, the doctor will be much freer to prescribe laboratory tests or treatments than he is in many cases today, where the family income and ability to pay for such supplementary services has to be taken into account. The general practitioner will also be able to call on specialist and consultant services whenever in his judgment they are needed. He will also be able to prescribe—at the cost of the insurance system rather than of the patient—such special medicines, appliances, etc., as are provided as benefit. Referral to specialists will ordinarily occur through the general practitioner or family doctor, or through a specialist who is already attending the patient; but in case an insured person (or the family of the sick person) is refused a referral which he thinks desirable, he would be able to ask for it through the medical officer of the local insurance office.

Whether or not a patient should be hospitalized and for how long will ordinarily be decided by the attending physician, as it is today. While the insured person will have the right to go to any participating hospital in the community or in the hospital-service area, his actual choice will no doubt be determined, as it is today, primarily by the advice of his doctor and the availability of space. When he goes to a participating hospital, the insured person may be required to present his insurance card as evidence of his right to hospitalization benefit. If the hospital has a service contract with the insurance agency, and he receives no services other than those to which he is entitled as insurance benefit, he will have no further financial obligation to the hospital. If the hospital does not have such a contract, he will have to pay his bill himself, and turn a receipt over to the local office to serve as a basis for paying him an indemnity (reimbursement) amount. If the hospital has a contract covering a limited credit, the insured person would have to pay the amount by which his total bill exceeds the amount payable to the hospital by the insurance system.

So far as the insured person is concerned, then, health insurance will mean advance payment of premiums, and the assurance that he and his family are entitled to all needed care provided as insurance benefits. The kind of care the insured person obtains will still be the responsibility of the doctor of his choice, and the methods by which be obtains it will be mainly those which the medical profession and the hospitals sanction and encourage.

Health Insurance as Seen by the Doctor.—For most doctors, also, prepayment will be the most important feature of health insurance. From the doctor's point of view, prepayment means guaranteed payment from the insurance fund—instead of individual payment by the patient—for services rendered.

It is suggested that all doctors licensed under State law should be guaranteed the right to participate as general practitioners or family physicians under the insurance system. A doctor who wishes to engage in insurance practice will signify his intent to the local administrative office and will have his name included on the list of participating physicians. A doctor who wishes to receive the higher rates of payment for specialist services will need to satisfy the requirements that will have been established to show that he is a qualified specialist for such services. Many will presumably qualify automatically on the basis of having been accredited by the existing professional specialty boards.

When the system first goes into operation, and periodically thereafter, all of the participating doctors in the community will be given the opportunity of selecting the method by which they wish to be paid, from among the several methods available. Individual doctors or groups of doctors who wish to be paid by a method different from that selected by the majority may be permitted to make appropriate special arrangements with the administrative agency.

Each participating doctor will decide for himself whether he wishes to restrict his practice to insured persons or whether he will accept noninsured patients as well; in other words, whether he will devote all or only part of his working time to insurance practice. For those services which he provides to insured persons as insurance benefits, he will be paid by the insurance system; he will not, therefore,

be free to charge such a patient or family any supplementary fee for such services.[1]
If he furnishes care to noninsured persons, or to insured persons who choose to
disregard their insurance rights and to consult him under a private arrangement,
or if he furnishes services which are not insurance benefits, he will be entirely free
to charge what he wishes and collect from them for such services, but of course
he will not bill the insurance system for these services.

A doctor who has chosen to receive payment on a fee-for-service basis, will
need to keep records of services provided to insured persons. Periodically, probably
once a month, the doctor will submit to the local insurance agency an accounting—
in effect, a consolidated bill—for insurance services rendered during that period,
possibly including identification of the insured persons served. Payments to the
doctor will be according to the bills submitted, except that if the aggregate of such
bills from all doctors in the community exceeds the funds available for all payments
to doctors on a fee-for-service basis, the bills will have to be prorated down. If
the aggregate bills are substantially less than the total funds available for these payments, the surplus would need to be held—for a while—as a contingency reserve
against subsequent periods when the aggregate bills may be in excess of the funds;
if a surplus persists, either too much money was allocated for the services or the fee
schedule needs to be reinspected for upward revision.

A doctor who is receiving payment on a capitation basis will need only to keep
a file of the names of those insured persons who are currently on his list as having
chosen him as their physician and whom he has accepted. Periodically, presumably
once a month, he will receive from the insurance system the agreed-upon per capita
payment for each person on his list. In addition, if the capitation amount has been
calculated on the basis of all the insured and not merely those who have chosen
their doctors, he will receive a prorata share of payments for those insured persons
who are not on any doctors' lists. Since it will be his responsibility to furnish all
needed services—that may be expected from a general practitioner or family
physician—to those persons, and since he will be paid the same amount per person,
regardless of how many services he has furnished any particular person on his list,
there will be no need for him to provide the insurance system with a detailed
accounting or bill for particular services rendered. The individual physician will
decide for himself the maximum number of insured persons whom he is willing to
accept on his list [2] (assuming that number choose him) and therefore how much
time, if any, he will reserve for noninsurance practice.

Some doctors will prefer to be paid on a salary basis for their insurance practice.
The amount of the salary will be a matter for negotiation between the doctor and
the insurance agency, on the basis of general salary scales (national, State, or local),
and in view of the experience and acquired skill of the particular doctor. A doctor
on full-time salary will be expected to devote his full time to serving insured persons
(except in emergency situations, of course). He will need, therefore, to make sure

[1] Except where supplementary charges have been temporarily authorized by the insurance
agency to prevent abuse.

[2] Except that the insurance system might not permit him to be paid for any length of time
for more than a specified maximum number.

that persons who come to him for service are insured, but will not need to give the insurance agency an accounting—for payment purposes—of the individual services he renders. A doctor on part-time salary will devote the appropriate portion of his time to insurance practice. Part-time salary agreements might provide that the doctor is available a specified number of hours a week or month, or on each of a specified number of days, for insurance patients, or might provide other similar arrangements.

Doctors who prefer to practice in groups will, of course, be free to do so. If such a group enters into an agreement with the insurance agency to furnish services as insurance benefits, it may distribute the payments it receives from the insurance system among the several doctors in the group in any way it pleases. How detailed an accounting of services rendered to insured persons the group would need to make to receive payment from the insurance system would depend largely on the scope and character of the services it provided and its choice of the method to be used in calculating the amount of the payment.

Individual doctors or groups of doctors who provide laboratory services more extensive than those usually furnished by doctors as an integral part of the physician's service may bill the insurance system separately for such services. In rural areas the payments to some or all doctors may also include mileage allowances and supplementary payments for medicines or other supplies dispensed to patients who do not have ready access to a pharmacy.

Whatever the method of payment, the content of services he provides will remain the responsibility of the individual doctor and of the medical profession. Except in the case of the salaried doctor, the amount of income an individual doctor earns will still depend on the number of patients he can attract and hold or on the number of services furnished insured persons.

The assurance of higher rates of payment for specialist than for general practitioner services should furnish an incentive to many doctors to become and remain proficient in some specialty, even though they intend to devote part or most of their time to general practice. The grants-in-aid for education and training provided by the insurance system would open increased opportunities for specialized training and for attendance on periodic "refresher" courses. The availability of specialist and consultant services, paid for as insurance benefits, will make it easier than at present for the family doctor to call on such services when they are needed. The insurance arrangements would thus afford individual doctors, those practicing in organized groups, and the medical profession as a whole new opportunities for service. What they will make of those opportunities, the doctors themselves will largely determine.

Health Insurance as Seen by the Hospital Administrator.—For the hospital administrator, inauguration of health insurance will mean primarily an assured source of income and an orderly basis of financing the hospital. The stabilization of income which the voluntary hospital insurance plans have accomplished for some hospitals with respect to some of their patients will be extended to most hospitals and to services for most of the population, the extent depending on the coverage of the insurance system.

A hospital which is to receive payments from the insurance system for its services to insured persons will have to be on the list of participating hospitals. For nearly all hospitals throughout the country—those which are now registered, certified, approved, and so forth, by the American Medical Association, the American College of Surgeons, the American Hospital Association, and so forth—acceptance as a participating hospital may be substantially automatic. Some of the few hospitals which fail to meet the national standards of professional associations may be able to meet standards which will be established by the central administration, after consultation with its advisory council, for particular localities or for institutions providing limited classes of services as insurance benefits. Apart from assuring that the institution meets the general standards for participation, the health insurance agency would presumably have no authority with regard to intramural management or administration of the hospital. Admission procedures, methods of selecting or paying its staff, intramural management, the scope of service provided, and so forth, will be determined by the hospital itself.

The payment arrangements between the insurance system and the hospital will depend upon what is finally provided in the health insurance law and upon decisions to be made by the hospital.

A hospital which chooses to receive payments directly from the insurance agency for all services furnished as insurance benefits, will negotiate an agreement with the agency for reimbursement for the costs of such services. The cost accounting necessary to determine a fair basis for reimbursement can be comparatively simple; many hospitals will already have had experience with such cost-accounting procedures in connection with other Government programs. Once a per diem charge has been agreed upon, the hospital will need only to submit accounts of the patient-days of service furnished to insured persons and be reimbursed for those services at the agreed per-diem rate by the insurance fund. Insofar as the hospital provides insured persons with additional services or more expensive facilities than those available as insurance benefits, it will collect the charges for such services directly from the patient or his family. If the insurance benefit is only a limited payment (so many dollars toward each day of hospital care) and the hospitals have only a limited-credit contract with the insurance system, the hospital would need to submit a bill for the patient-days furnished.

A hospital which does not wish to enter into a service contract with the insurance agency may agree to accept the assignment by an insured person of his right to a cash benefit, in complete or partial payment for hospital services. In this case, the hospital will need only to bill the insurance system for the assigned amounts, and collect the remainder from the patient. A hospital which does not wish to enter into any arrangement with the insurance system, will only need to continue giving patients or their families receipted bills for payments.

Hospitals having out-patient clinics and an associated staff of physicians and technicians will in many cases want to enter into agreements with the insurance agency to be reimbursed not only for hospital care but also for general and special medical services, laboratory services, and possibly dental and nursing services furnished to nonhospitalized persons, or for some of these classes of service. If they have such arrangements with the insurance system, they will bill it according to the terms of the agreements.

In communities with several or many hospitals, each hospital may prefer to deal with the local insurance office directly; in others, some or all of the hospitals may prefer to deal indirectly through the medium of a common representative, a local hospital council, a Blue Cross plan, or a hospital association.

Health Insurance as Seen by Other Practitioners.—The preceding pages have dealt primarily with physicians and hospitals. This course was followed only for the sake of simplicity. With variations in detail, according to the nature of the service or commodity provided, dentists, nurses, laboratories, pharmacists, optometrists, or others furnishing services or commodities as insurance benefits would establish relations with the insurance system similar to those described for doctors and hospitals.

Individuals and groups who wish to participate in providing services or commodities under the program will, like physicians and hospitals, have opportunity to make their interest known to the insurance agency and to give evidence of their ability to meet the standards applicable to their field. The contact between the insured person and the practitioner providing service will follow accepted professional patterns. In the case of dentists furnishing general dental services, access would be direct as in the case of the physician. The dentist will presumably have the same choices as to methods of payment as are open to the physician. Home-nursing services and laboratory services would ordinarily be available only when requested by an attending physician. Nurses will, for the most part, continue to be on the salaried staffs of nursing organizations and the insurance fund will ordinarily pay for nursing services through such organizations; some nurses, however, may be on independent contractual arrangements.

Health Insurance as Seen by the Community.—The health insurance system has special importance both for those receiving and for those providing medical care. If it is to be fully successful, the system must therefore live and grow as a community undertaking.

One of the first steps the local administrative agency will need to take in getting health insurance into operation will be to create a local community advisory council. The members of this council should, of course, include representatives of the insured persons and representatives of the medical, dental and nursing professions, of the hospitals, etc. It should also have among its members community leaders concerned with general or special local health programs or informed as to methods of providing adequate health services. This council would confer with and advise the local administrator on all important policies and problems relating to the operation of the program. It would also serve as the focus for community interest in high standards of medical care, and as the interpreter to the community of the objectives and procedures of the health insurance agency. The council may well provide the leadership necessary to fuse into a coordinated program the activities of the health insurance agency and of other agencies, public and private, having an active interest in health matters....

90. FEDERAL AID TO VOLUNTARY INSURANCE

A. THE SUBSIDY METHOD *

IT IS NOW CERTAIN that one of the big questions before the American people during the next few years will be public health.... Prospective candidates are sizing up the question and feeling for their positions. All signs point to a good, old-fashioned political debate.

The issues involved in the debate are momentous. There is first of all the issue of whether a nation whose health and health services rank among the best in the world needs any major legislation at all. But secondly, even if it is granted that major legislation is needed, the controversial question arises of the *kind* of legislation desired. Here the inquiring citizen runs straight into the so-called "welfare" issue, but on a scale larger than anything he is likely to have encountered thus far. The attempt to solve the problem of health by government initiative—as the [Truman] Administration proposes—would constitute a more advanced step in the direction of state socialism than the American people have yet been willing to take.

Now of all the proposals made thus far, only two approach this issue in a thoroughgoing manner on a national scale. One is the Administration proposal (S. 1679 and H.R. 4312 and 4313), which has as its keystone the principle of compulsory insurance administered through governmental agencies. The other is the remarkable proposal (S. 1970 and H.R. 4919) of a group of progressive Republican Senators and Congressmen, based upon the voluntary principle. This principle, of course, has been used in many plans, notably in the Hunt bill, which is comprehensive in scope, but vague as to its provisions and costs. More typically, however, as in the Taft bill and the Hill bill, voluntary plans are *partial* plans, aimed at alleviating some portion of the medical problem. But the progressive Republican plan defines a method of implementation (which the Hunt bill lacks) whereby the voluntary principle can be applied effectively on a national scale. This bill, therefore, which has had remarkably little publicity, ought to be better known, inasmuch as it seeks the achievement of an important social goal in a uniquely American manner....

It is true that millions of Americans desperately need medical care. It is true

* From: "Health Insurance Is Next," by Russell W. Davenport; reprinted by special permission from the March 1950 issue of *Fortune Magazine* (pp. 63-67, 142-52); copyright 1950 by Time, Inc. (Omissions include some author's italics.) The author was, until shortly before his death in 1954, an editor of *Life*.

also that for these people care of some sort, even if the standard is lower, would be better than nothing. Still, the Administration bill is in danger of promising the American people something that it cannot deliver. Should the bill succeed in its stated objective of reaching 80 per cent of the people, within (let us say) five years, not only would the care of the lower income groups be second rate, but a medical inflation would result, complete with black-market fees. People who could afford to do so would pay private fees for special attention. The inequitable distribution of good medical care would thus become even more pronounced. And the experience of our time teaches us what the remedy for this scarcity situation would surely be: more government controls.

The Administration plan, in short, can *succeed* only in so far as it *fails,* within the first several years, to reach its objective of service to 80 per cent of the people. A promise of medical care commensurate with American medical standards can only be honestly fulfilled if time is provided for orderly growth.

[The progressive Republican] bill starts from the proposition that any group of Americans can set up an insurance plan adapted to their needs. Such groups might include those already in existence, such as Blue Shield and Blue Cross, employer plans, union plans, benefit-association plans, or entirely new plans worked out by responsible citizens. State and regional boards must approve the plans, but they would not initiate them.

The major requirements laid upon the voluntary programs, if they are to participate in government aid, are (1) that they be non-profit; (2) that their governing boards shall be composed of a majority of laymen; and (3) that their subscriptions shall be determined as a percentage of the subscriber's income (up to incomes of $5,000 a year and with a minimum charge of $6 a year). This latter feature is unique. Almost all the voluntary plans now in existence charge flat rates, whatever the subscriber's income, and they are therefore usually beyond the reach of lower income groups. This fact should be remembered when it is claimed that, according to past experience, voluntary insurance provides insufficient coverage. By requiring that rates be based upon a percentage of income the Republican proposal makes such plans more available than they have ever been.

Thus in a 3 per cent plan, a family with an income of $5,000 a year would pay $150 a year, or $12.50 a month; one with $3,800 would pay $114 a year, or $9.50 a month; one with $1,500 a year would pay $45 a year, or $3.75 a month. They would all get the same services. It is estimated that the $3,800 family would just about pay its way on an actuarial basis. Smaller incomes would be subsidized, mostly by public funds, but partly also by the higher-income people in the plan. It is worth noting that this partial subsidization of the lower income groups by the higher ones is just what happens now, in a rough and unsatisfactory way, through the scaling of charges by the doctors and the hospitals. Persons with incomes over $5,000 could join a plan, and would undoubtedly choose to do so; but in most plans they would probably be paid fixed sums (called "indemnity benefits") rather than the complete costs of their care (called "service benefits").

The amount of government aid that any particular plan would receive would be determined by a formula that sounds rather complicated but is mathematically simple. To begin with, there is set up in the bill itself a "yardstick" plan, based on a charge of 3 per cent of a subscriber's income, and providing certain specified benefits (doctors, both general and specialist; visiting nurses; hospitalization for thirty days; ambulance service; and rehabilitation). A regional board estimates the cost of providing these benefits in its region, and this estimate (if accepted by the state) is called the "cost norm" for that region. Let us suppose it to be $50 per capita. Each plan in the region is then assigned an "allowed cost," depending on the number of services it offers. Manifestly, if it offers the "yardstick" services its "allowed cost" will be the "cost norm" of its region. If it covers lower income groups, however, its charge of 3 per cent of subscribers' incomes will result in something less than this allowed cost—let us say $37.50 per subscriber. The amount of government aid owing to a plan will be the difference between actual subscribers' payments and the allowed cost—in this case, the difference between $37.50 and $50, or $12.50 per subscriber.

An interesting feature of this formula is that if a plan is heavily loaded with lower income groups, and has consequently a lower gross income, government aid will be greater. Conversely, if the income groups served by the plan are relatively high, government aid will be less. It is estimated that on the average the government's contribution (state and federal) will be about a quarter of the allowed cost.

A plan does not have to adhere to the yardstick, however. It may provide fewer services, in which case its allowed cost will be correspondingly less than the cost norm and it will charge less to its subscribers (say 2 per cent). It will still get government aid to cover the difference between the allowed cost of its services and the payments from subscribers. Or it may (with state approval) offer more than the yardstick and charge more than 3 per cent.

By the use of this formula a maximum of freedom is assured for all concerned. Not only may patients, doctors, and hospitals stay out of all plans, but, if they want to come in, they will have a variety of plans to choose from. In fact, it is anticipated that the system will lead to a good deal of healthy competition. Some plans may devise means (for instance, by the installation of a first-rate system of group insurance) to provide more service than the yardstick, though charging only 3 per cent. They would not get more government aid than other 3 per cent plans, but their popularity with subscribers would exert a competitive pressure upon less efficient plans.

It is exceedingly difficult to estimate the cost of this proposal because it is not known how fast the plans would grow. The framers of the bill have made the assumption for working purposes that in four years the voluntary plans could build up to a volume of about $3 billion, to which the government contribution (part state, part federal) would be an additional $1 billion. This bill, then, contemplates a somewhat smaller expenditure than the Administration bill, although the two plans are set up so differently that an exact comparison is almost impossible. Since the long-range objective of both is complete national coverage, it may be assumed that their ultimate costs will be of the same order.

Since only one day's hearings have been held on the Republican bill, it has not yet received much criticism. One objection is that it subsidizes the high costs of voluntary plans, which, besides ordinary administrative expenses, include substantial items for collection and sales promotion. Yet this objection fails to take account of a number of factors. In the first place, government bureaus themselves are not ordinarily conspicuous for economical operation. The FSA * has given a good account of itself administratively, but the administration of the health bill would be infinitely more complex than that, say, of OASI.† It would involve not merely the administration of funds but the administration of services. Secondly, competition between the voluntary plans should foster economical operation. And finally, while sales promotion would still be necessary, this would constitute a form of medical education—which is very much needed if any kind of national insurance is to be a success. In such matters the cheapest way is not always the best. Americans encourage small enterprises, for example, even though in innumerable instances these are demonstrably less efficient than very big ones. As a supporter of the Republican bill has remarked, "The additional cost of voluntary programs, if any, represents the cost of free choice."

Some people object to the plan's complexity. It is admittedly difficult to understand at first, but this is partly because it embodies some really original thinking. So far as the yardstick formula is concerned, it entails very little actuarial work that is not already done to set up any voluntary medical plan. This work will be done by actuaries and statisticians, not by the subscriber. From the latter's point of view the proposal is simple enough: government aid to voluntary plans will enable you to insure yourself medically at a great bargain. Your concern, therefore, is to choose that plan which will give you the best service for your money.

Another and more serious objection concerns the states. The Republican plan makes federal aid contingent on state aid, according to a formula that gives the poorer states an advantage. Thus, in order for the plans to start, states must undertake to make substantial outlays. In addition, a great many states will have to change their laws (*a*) to allow consumer-sponsored plans and (*b*) to provide for the fixing of charges on the basis of a percentage of income. These difficulties are real, but surely not insuperable. They arise partly from the fact that the states are given a real choice, whereas by the Administration plan they are compelled.

The fundamental objection to the Republican proposal has to do with voluntary plans in general. Administration proponents assert that their growth has been inadequate, their costs high, and their coverage scanty. They declare flatly that the lower income groups will never subscribe to such plans. Moreover, how is the necessary capital for starting a plan to be raised? Private funds for such purposes are becoming increasingly difficult to get. In short, many an Administration advocate will declare that he would prefer the voluntary system in principle; but he will add, flatly, that it won't work.

In answer to the objection about the difficulty of raising the original capital funds, the advocates of the Republican bill admit that this exists. Nevertheless, they think that the Administration people exaggerate it. . . . The Republican bill,

* Federal Security Agency, now the Department of Health, Education and Welfare.

† Old Age and Survivors' Insurance system, administered by the Department of Health, Education and Welfare.

moreover, provides that the federal government may advance non-interest-bearing loans to an approved plan up to 50 per cent of the total of the starting capital.

The answer of the Republicans to the categorical objection to voluntary plans in general is made difficult by the fact that their bill is in effect proposing something entirely new. It is the contention of its sponsors *that a voluntary system has never really been tried.* It is true that many voluntary plans exist. But a concerted effort —promoted, possibly, by communities and civic organizations—has never been made to educate the people to the virtue of such plans, offered at below cost through government aid. The Republicans point out that the American people have been able to educate themselves on many other matters (life insurance, for example); that vast facilities exist for the purpose; and that if community leadership were aroused throughout the country, with the help of the right kind of legislation, an entirely different atmosphere could be created that would make past experience obsolete. . . .

The advocates of the Republican bill believe that if universal health insurance is ever to be achieved in this country, without sacrificing the qualitative excellence of American medicine, a fairly long evolution lies ahead. The compulsory system advocated by the Administration contemplates forcing this evolution. A voluntary system would stimulate it as much as possible, but never in excess of the ability of the medical profession to grow in an orderly way. The Republican plan contemplates starting with a nucleus of about 65 million people who are already educated, through voluntary plans, to the idea of *some* medical insurance. It would not be too difficult, the Republicans think, to educate these people to the idea of complete medical insurance. From this nucleus it is no far cry to the coverage of everyone on a payroll, where the device can conveniently be used of periodical deductions— undoubtedly with the employer sharing in the contributions. And at the same time, everyone on relief would be joining the plans, for the simple reason that most states would subscribe for them.

Such a growth of demand, the Republicans believe, would develop great pressures, not only for more medical services, but for better ones. The necessary expansion has already started in the Hospital Construction Act, and would be carried further by various provisions for direct aid to medical schools, backward areas, etc., proposed in their bill. At the end of five or six years some of this expansion would have taken place, and it would then be possible to push on toward complete national coverage. If special legislation is needed for this final step, we would then know what kind of legislation it ought to be. But to attempt to take the final step before the necessary preliminaries have been achieved seems to the Republicans both foolhardy and unnecessary.

Underlying all the arguments regarding these plans there are a number of important intangibles, not the least of which is the question of how far the power of government is to be extended.

The framers of the Administration bill have made a sincere effort to reduce federal powers to a minimum. The functions of the National Health Board, the top medical authority for the plan, would be essentially threefold: (1) to account for the funds; (2) to distribute the funds; and (3) to set standards. All other administrative tasks would be passed down to the states, and thence to regional boards. These powers sound innocent enough. Yet they are, after all, the *ultimate* powers so far as the plan is concerned; and since the whole plan is by federal law compulsory, the board is bound to prevail wherever its duties lead it into conflict with local interests.

But even assuming that the states would have a good deal of working power under the Administration bill, we should not forget that a state is also a government. And the question is whether any government, federal or state, ought to be drawn into such decisions as the Administration bill requires some government to make. . . .

. . . If you start with an entity called government and work downward, there is no real way to limit its power, because nobody has more power. *True limitation of government power can come only by working from the people upward.* This is perhaps the most basic concept of American politics, and we shall overlook it at our peril.

The chief virtue of the progressive Republican plan is that it proceeds in exactly that manner. It is true that in order to provide for full national coverage, and especially for the lower income groups, the Republican bill gives the federal government a lot of power. It has the power, that is, to approve a state's plans, and above all, to pass upon the propriety and accuracy of a state's claims for federal aid with reference to the yardstick. Even at that, the Republican proposal gives the federal government far less direct power than the Administration plan does: government has nothing whatever to say, for example, about medical fees, which are wholly determined by the doctors in their contracts with the voluntary plans. Yet all that is really secondary. The great advantage of the Republican proposal lies in the fact that the initiative must come from the people and not from any government, whether federal or state. The people and the local communities retain the power, because theirs is the decision whether to act and how to act. If the government yardstick is not realistic they will refuse to act. The power of government is thereby checked and balanced by the people themselves.

The ultimate question, therefore, is whether the American people have got the initiative and the intelligence to subscribe to voluntary health plans. The Administration supporters do not think so. The Republicans, on the other hand, do not declare flatly that they have. They merely say that nobody knows—because nobody has really tried. . . .

B. THE REINSURANCE APPROACH *

As a NATION, we are doing less than now lies within our power to reduce the impact of disease. Many of our fellow Americans cannot afford to pay the costs of medical care when it is needed, and they are not protected by adequate health insurance.

* From: *Message from the President of the United States, Transmitting Recommendations Relative to a National Health Program,* by Dwight D. Eisenhower; Document No. 81, House of Representatives, 84th Cong., 1st Sess., Washington: U.S. Government Printing Office, 1955 (pp. 2-3). Reprinted with omissions, including initial paragraphs.

Too frequently the local hospitals, clinics, or nursing homes required for the prevention, diagnosis, and treatment of disease either do not exist or are badly out of date. Finally, there are critical shortages of the trained personnel required to study, prevent, treat, and control disease.

The specific recommendations that follow are designed to meet this threefold deficiency.

Meeting the Costs of Medical Care.—For most Americans, insurance—private, voluntary insurance—provides a sound and effective method of meeting unexpected hazards which may be beyond the capacity of the individual to bear. Risk sharing through group action is in the best tradition of vigorous and imaginative American enterprise.

The Government should cooperate with, and encourage, private carriers in the improvement of health insurance. Moreover, a great many people who are not now covered can be given its protection, particularly in rural areas where group enrollment is at present difficult.

Existing health insurance can also be improved by expanding the scope of the benefits provided. Not all private expenditures for medical care can or should be covered by insurance; nevertheless, many policies offered today are too limited in scope. They are principally for hospitalized illness and for relatively short periods of time.

I recommend, consequently, the establishment of a Federal health reinsurance service to encourage private health insurance organizations in offering broader benefits to insured individuals and families and coverage to more people. . . .

The purpose of the reinsurance proposal is to furnish a system for broad sharing among health insurance organizations of the risks of experimentation. A system of this sort will give an incentive to the improvement of existing health insurance plans. It will encourage private, voluntary health insurance organizations to provide better protection—particularly against expensive illness—for those who now are insured against some of the financial hazards of illness. Reinsurance will also help to stimulate extension of private voluntary health insurance plans to millions of additional people who do not now have, but who could afford to purchase, health insurance.

The Department of Health, Education, and Welfare has been working with specialists from the insurance industry, with experts from the health professions, and with many other interested citizens, in its effort to perfect a sound reinsurance program—a program which involves no Government subsidy and no Government competition with private insurance carriers. The time has come to put such a program to work for the American people.

I urge the Congress to launch the reinsurance service this year by authorizing a reasonable capital fund and by providing for its use as necessary to reinsure three broad areas for expansion in private voluntary health insurance:

1. Health insurance plans providing protection against the high costs of severe or prolonged illness;

2. Health insurance plans providing coverage for individuals and families in predominantly rural areas;

3. Health insurance plans designed primarily for coverage of individuals and families of average or lower income against medical care costs in the home and physician's office as well as in the hospital. . . .

C. *Medical Care for the Nation: Two Views*

91. FOR THE VOLUNTARY PRINCIPLE *

MR. OSCAR R. EWING, Federal Security Administrator, in his report to the President urges compulsory Government health insurance as an essential part of a long-range program to improve the health of the nation. He points out that the 5,000,000 men rejected by the draft as unfit for the armed forces, the 4,300,000 man years of work lost through bad health and the national loss of $27,000,000 in national wealth through sickness and partial and total disability are evidences of the bad state of the national health, and that at least 70,000,000 people in this country will have difficulty in providing adequate minimal medical care for themselves and their families.

How do these more prominent reasons for the establishment of a federal insurance program stand up under factual analysis? Is there a real need for such a program? If not, what are the more important reasons for opposing it at this time?

Will Compulsory Health Insurance Improve the Nation's Health?

WE, AS PHYSICIANS, recognize the need for continually improving the many factors that contribute to better health. But are we, and is the public, properly informed when we are told that the way to better health is through compulsory health insurance? The following quotation from Simons and Sinai [1] is most instructive:

> When insurance systems are being urged upon governments, one of the strongest arguments offered is that improvement in general health will follow prompt, universal medical care. After the system has been adopted, one of the most amazing things to the outside observer is the almost complete absence in the vast amount of discussion

* From: "Medical Care for the American People: Is Compulsory Health Insurance the Solution?" by Leland S. McKittrick, M.D.; *New England Journal of Medicine* 240:998-1,002, June 23, 1949 (No. 25). Reprinted (with omissions) by permission of the author and publishers. The author is clinical professor of surgery at Harvard University Medical School, Boston.

[1] Simons, A. M., and Sinai, N. *The Way of Health Insurance*. Chicago: Univ. of Chicago Press, 1932, p. 156.

of any reference to public health in relation to insurance. Moreover, not even the most intense partisan of insurance has ever attempted to present any statistical proof that insurance has any effect upon the general death- and sickness-rate. No sort of statistical manipulation has ever been able to show any correlation between the movements of death-rate in insurance and non-insurance countries. They have declined in both at about equal rate, according to sanitary and health measures and other influences; but no difference in any way traceable to insurance can be discovered.

This is the more remarkable since water protection, better housing, tuberculosis care, isolation, immunization, and numerous other health measures do show such traceable results. At no point has a disappointment been greater than in the failure of insurance as a preventive measure.

Contrary to all prediction, the most startling fact about the vital statistics of insurance countries is the steady and fairly rapid rate of increase in the number of days the average person is sick annually and the continuously increasing duration of such sickness.

The average recorded sickness for each person per year practically doubled in Great Britain and Germany after the installation of Government insurance. What evidence does Mr. Ewing have to suggest that the effect of Government insurance upon work days lost through sickness will be any different in this country than in others?

We still read that the high percentage of rejections in the military recruitment program has provided striking evidence of the unsatisfactory state of the nation's health and that for this reason a national health insurance program is essential. We, as physicians, know that there are millions of men in this country in good health who will not meet the rigid requirements for combat duty in the armed forces. We know that at least 80 per cent of those rejected could not have been rehabilitated by any medical care known at this time, and we know that of the approximately 20 per cent who might have been influenced by medical care, it would have been necessary for them to have consulted the doctor, to have accepted his recommendation and for the treatment to have been completely successful.

We, as a profession, are the first to recognize the importance of improved sanitation and other public-health measures. They are fundamental to any program to improve the nation's health, but provision of these is in no way dependent upon or to be confused with a compulsory health insurance program.

Is Compulsory Health Insurance Necessary to Provide Medical Care to Half the Population?

WHAT ARE THE facts concerning the "70,000,000 people" who "will have difficulty in providing adequate minimal care for themselves and their families"?

About 28 per cent of the families of this country had incomes under $2000 in 1946. Many of these can pay nothing or only a portion of the cost of a serious illness. The indigent are provided for in the present [Truman] Administration bill (S. 5) only when "equitable reimbursements to the account on behalf of such needy or other individuals have been made, or for which reasonable assurance of such reimbursements has been given, by public agencies of the United States, the several states" and so forth. The same agencies could readily purchase such care from medical care programs already in existence or in process of formation. There is, then, no need for a compulsory Government health insurance agency to assure proper care for this group.

Approximately 50 per cent of our families are now earning between $2,000 and $5,000 a year. Good medical care is and will remain costly. The total expenses associated with a serious illness are too high for most of these families to meet without difficulty at the time of the sickness. However, many own automobiles, television sets and electric refrigerators, and, as a group, they spend a large amount on alcoholic beverages and other things. These are accepted as a part of the American life. But, at the same time, if these families had to pay cash for their automobiles, for their electric refrigerators or for their television or radio sets, many would not be in a position to buy them. Is it fair to say that because they cannot pay cash for these items, they cannot afford them? Because this same group cannot pay for a major illness at the time it occurs, is it just to assume that they cannot afford to pay for it? Because a mechanism to spread the costs of serious illness must be made available to these families, why must it be done under the costly, inflexible and inefficient machinery of federal Government before thorough exploration of reasonable alternatives?

We need have no great concern for those with incomes over $5,000, although we must also accept the fact that it is customary for most of us to adjust our standards of living pretty well to our incomes, to the end that many families with annual incomes between $5,000 and $10,000 will have difficulty in paying large medical bills at the time at which they are incurred. Many of these recognize the importance of spreading the cost of illness, and for them such a mechanism would be a convenience though not a necessity.

We have now in this country the highest quality of medical care, the best teaching and the most productive research of any country anywhere. As the science of medicine has improved to make this possible, the costs have increased. We have not developed a satisfactory means of paying these increased costs. Industry was faced with, and successfully met, a similar problem in selling its technical products. Because we as a profession have failed to lead the way, we as a nation are now being urged to make a complete change from a system of medical practice that places emphasis on quality of service and direct responsibility to the individual and his family, to a system that had its concept in the Bismarckian philosophy, which puts emphasis on quantity rather than quality, and which fixes the ultimate responsibility of the physician to the central Government rather than to the patient.

We are unable to find any factual evidence to support the contention that compulsory health insurance will improve the health of the nation. A sound program to afford medical care to the needy is not dependent upon a Government insurance system. There is urgent need for developing a method of paying for the medical care of the large segment of our population who cannot, or would prefer not to, meet the payment for serious illness when it comes. Does our failure to have provided a mechanism for doing this justify a complete change from any possible solution of this problem on a voluntary basis to a system of compulsion that has been tried in so many foreign countries and has as yet provided no country with the quality of medical care equal to ours?

Does Compulsory Health Insurance Meet the Qualifications of a Good Medical Care Plan?

WITHOUT careful analysis it might seem very reasonable for all of us to pay a tax to the federal Government, which, in turn, takes the responsibility of supplying us with and paying for our medical care whenever we need it. It is a very easy matter, in writing, from the platform or over the air, to develop a logical and apparently practical program. It must be remembered, however, that a successful program to provide prepaid medical care is dependent upon certain fundamental principles. The more important of these are: free choice of physician; mutual co-operation of the public, those rendering professional services and the administrative agencies; continuing improvement in the quality of care given, the teaching in medical schools and research; and a total cost of the program in keeping with the general economy of the community.

Free Choice of Physician.—Only a short time ago Mr. Ewing assured the public that from the patient's point of view there was absolutely no difference between the present system and that which the Administration was proposing (compulsory health insurance) except that the Government would pay the bill. If this is true it means that you as a patient can go to any physician you wish at any time, provided he is available and is willing to accept you. At present he is limited in the number of patients he can care for only by the number who seek his services or by the number of working hours in his week. Since those who can are expected to pay for his services, he is spared a multitude of demands upon his time for minor, insignificant complaints. The fact that longer hours mean greater income is an incentive for him to be available to prospective patients throughout most of each twenty-four hours. Mr. Ewing knows and his advisers know that a medical care plan of the magnitude proposed cannot remain solvent if the physician is paid each time he sees a patient. They know that removal of any financial responsibility from the patient will greatly increase the demands upon the physician's time for unimportant complaints. They know that the number of patients a physician will be permitted to care for must be limited. Every prospective patient in a community must register and have his name on some doctor's panel. The best known doctor in each community will be in the greatest demand, and in fairness to all, those first applying must be accepted until the panel is filled. When his panel is filled, all others desirous of being under his care must select another doctor or will be assigned to one by those responsible for carrying out the plan. Moreover, there will undoubtedly be a certain number of the most successful and older physicians in each area who may well prefer not to become part of such a program.

Under compulsory health insurance the free choice of physician cannot be assured to anywhere near the degree that it is available at the present time.

Co-operation.—Co-operation between those giving, those receiving and those administering any plan is essential. Co-operation means mutual confidence and mutual respect.

We hear Mr. Ewing over the public radio say that there will be absolutely no change in the relationship between the patient and the doctor, except that the Government pays the bill, and that the maximum payment that anyone will have to meet is $1.40 per week. We know that it will be absolutely impossible to maintain, under a Government program, the private practice of medicine as it now exists. We know, and Mr. Ewing should know, that a maximum of $1.40 per week on the part of the worker, in addition to a like amount from the employer, cannot possibly support the comprehensive program outlined. Such statements are misleading and do not inspire the confidence of an enlightened public or of the medical profession.

Mr. Ewing states that there are 325,000 lives lost in this country each year that we have the knowledge to save. We are not told the basis for these figures, but we read that 117,000 of these lives are lost through heart disease and cancer. We know that the death rate for heart disease among the physicians of the country is higher than it is in the population at large. We do not believe that lack of medical care is responsible for the greater number of our profession who die each year of this condition, and therefore we fail to understand how a compulsory health insurance program will help save the lives of others who have heart disease. We know that in the state of Massachusetts only 0.3 per cent of those coming to our cancer clinics have delayed in coming because of economic reasons. We do not know how to make an earlier diagnosis of cancer of the internal organs, many of which give symptoms too late for cure. We do not know how to remove from the patient the fear of reality, dread of an operation and other factors that postpone early diagnosis and treatment of cancer. We are certain that the introduction of a compulsory health insurance program will not alter these factors and therefore will have little effect upon the death rate from this disease.

We are, therefore, at a loss to understand the basis for Mr. Ewing's figures or how we, as a medical profession, can have confidence in an agency and its administrator that are responsible for giving to the public this kind of information. Nor do we understand how Mr. Ewing can have confidence in and co-operate with a profession of which he says, "Which is the more important? The personal, selfish business and professional values of 180,000 practicing physicians in this country, or the health and well-being of some 68,000,000 of our population?" [2]

Surely there is nothing in the material discussed above to assure the type of mutual confidence and respect that is essential to the smooth running of so important a program.

---

[2] Ewing, Oscar R. *Boston American,* December 21, 1948.

Quality of Care.—Whenever compulsory health coverage has been adopted, the emphasis has been on quantity and not on quality of care. This was so in Germany, was and is so in England, is so in New Zealand, and, if adopted, it will be so here. Unethical though it may be, it is common practice to get everything possible from anything as remote from the individual and as wealthy as a government. Seeing too many people with minor transient complaints and nothing wrong dulls the doctor's perception for the early signs of serious disease. History taking and examinations become superficial and a matter of routine.

Good medical care cannot be assured by legislation or by any mechanism of payment. It is personal, individual and intangible, and it depends not only on the training and experience of the physician, upon his scientific accomplishments and facilities but, more than anything else, upon the intensity and thoughtfulness with which he applies these to the individual patient who is sick. A feeling of responsibility directly to the patient and to his family, as well as ethical competition between physicians for the confidence of the public, is the more important factor in assuring each patient the personal care that he wants from his doctor. Any third party coming between the patient and his physician may interfere with this relationship, but when Government assumes complete responsibility for paying the physician and for providing medical care to the patient, such a relationship cannot survive.

It is difficult to foresee just how far-reaching the effect of compulsory health insurance might be upon the actual care of the more complicated illnesses. What, if any, effect might it have upon the training of young men in preparation for the actual care of the sick? To those of us who are actively interested in preparing young men for the specialties, it is disturbing to learn that in New Zealand many desirable young doctors are not being attracted to the ranks of the future specialists and teachers because the "unnaturally swollen rewards of general practice" [3] can be enjoyed after a much shorter and less arduous period of training than that necessary to qualify them for the all-important responsibilities of the specialists and of teaching.

The Cost.—Compulsory health insurance, as now advocated, is not insurance. There is no calculated risk, no payment of a premium to cover the cost of specific benefits and no contract. It is a form of taxation and should be recognized as such.

Comprehensive medical care is not an insurable risk. The demands upon such a program will be unlimited, indeterminate and uncontrollable. Abuse of the privileges is easy and attractive and therefore likely. The cost will be unpredictable and inordinately high. . . .

In England, three months after the beginning of the present health program, Mr. Bevan * made the following statement:

> Because things are free is no reason why people should abuse these opportunities. This is a great test of the maturity of the British people in so far as they have all the

---

[3] Robb, G. D. Health Reform in New Zealand. Auckland: Whitcombe and Tombs, Ltd., 1947, p. 35.

    * Minister of Health in the Labor Government that held power in Great Britain in 1945-51.

resources of the medical profession at their disposal without charge. If any individual abuses the opportunity, he must reckon with a sum total which might add up to one too grievous to carry and for which it would be very difficult to continue to provide.[4]

Two months before the end of the fiscal year the Ministry of Health asked for $233,820,000 in addition to the original estimate of $598,700,000 to meet the expenses of the program for the first nine months.

We find little to comfort us in the [1948] report of the subcommittee of the Hoover Commission, which studied the medical care program for which the Government is now responsible. The many evidences of extravagance and waste in money and in manpower are forcefully presented—for example, the Government pays $20,000 to $51,000 per bed for construction of hospitals in areas where voluntary hospitals are doing this for $16,000 per bed. . . . Evidence of the effect of the "free" hospital care of a Government-controlled program upon its cost is found in a comparison of the length of stay of patients after similar operations in voluntary and in Government hospitals (table 49).

TABLE 49. *Average hospital stay in voluntary and government hospitals*

Operative Procedure	Average Hospital Stay	
	Voluntary General Hospitals	Veterans Administration Hospitals
	days	*days*
Appendectomy	7.8	14.3
Tonsillectomy	1.4	15.1
Hemorrhoidectomy	6.9	34.3
Herniotomy (inguinal)	10.3	27.0

Not only is the actual cost for the care of each illness much greater in the Veterans Administration than in voluntary hospitals, but also the longer stay means that more beds are necessary to take care of the same number of patients. More beds means more construction, more personnel, more cost.

The people of this country must realize that there is no such thing as mass production of medical services. Each examination, whether x-ray or clinical study of the patient, is a personal service and one that takes time, and will remain costly if well done, even under the most efficient type of program. Such a program as advocated by Mr. Ewing cannot possibly be paid for by payroll deduction but may necessitate a bottomless pit with limitless money. This can only mean a tax burden out of all proportion to the benefits received.

Free choice of physician, co-operation, continuing improvement in the quality of care given and a total cost in keeping with the local and national economy cannot be expected if compulsory health insurance is adopted. Because we believe these to be essential to a succssful medical care plan, we are opposed to compulsory health insurance until sincere and co-ordinated efforts to attain these objectives by other means are made and found wanting.

[4] Bevan, A. *London Times,* October 8, 1948.

There are many who are very close to the problem of bringing good medical care to the American people who believe that a country so large and so diversified as ours may not lend itself to any single over-all plan, that our objective should be to provide the most widespread distribution of the best available medical care at the lowest cost possible, that our planning should be concentrated upon the end rather than the means, and that only through programs carefully planned and efficiently administered will we later have the experience and background necessary to put into effect that program which most nearly meets these objectives. The adoption of compulsory health insurance would eliminate any possibility of experimentation outside the structure of the compulsory, centrally controlled plan. "Once the whole employed population, wives and children included, is brought within the scope of compulsory sickness insurance, the great majority of doctors, dentists, nurses, and hospitals find themselves engaged in the insurance medical service which squeezes out most of the private practice on the one hand, and most of the medical care heretofore given by public authorities on the other. The next step to a single national medical service is a short one." [5] Are we ready to discard completely the tremendous advances made by non-profit and commercial agencies during the past ten years, or should our efforts be intensified to eliminate the many defects now recognized in present plans with the expectation that from these experiences will evolve a program that will be practical, effective, efficient and available to all who desire it?

Who Shall Be Our Keeper?

WHEN WE AS a nation become dependent upon the Government for our medical care we come to think of the Government as a paternal agency to which we turn and upon which we become increasingly dependent. Bismarck recognized the importance of this when he put a compulsory health insurance program into effect in 1883. Since that time the adoption of a compulsory, Government-controlled medical care program has been one of the most important early steps in the more complete socialization of a country. This was so in Germany, and it is so in England and in New Zealand. If this is the will of the American people, it should be so here, but we should be remiss if we did not point out the implications of making the Government rather than ourselves responsible for anything so personal and so essential as medical care. We are told that this is not socialized medicine, that it is no different from "buying fire insurance" (Ewing). But when the Government takes complete responsibility for providing a service, when we are compelled to pay a tax to the Government for that service, and when the Government in turn regulates and pays those who provide it, that service is socialized and is subject to the evils of political control.

There is little evidence that compulsory health insurance will improve the health of the nation or that it is necessary to assure adequate medical care to the

[5] International Labor Office. *Approaches to Social Security: An International Survey.* Montreal, Canada: International Labor Office, 1942, p. 50.

American people. There is much to suggest that such a program would gradually lower rather than continue to improve the quality of care received and that its cost would be inordinately high. We therefore oppose its adoption.

We believe that provision of adequate medical care for those unable to obtain it by voluntary prepayment plans or by direct payment is the responsibility of local or state government aided by charitable agencies and, if necessary, by federal grants-in-aid to state programs. Such a program is in no way dependent on compulsory health insurance.

We recognize the necessity of spreading the cost of serious illness by the development of more effective voluntary plans than those available today. We believe that the medical care of those able to purchase it through such plans or by direct payment is the responsibility of the individual, not of the Government.

The development and perfection of a complete medical care program presents many problems the solution of which is not yet at hand. However, the rapid advances in medical care during the past decade suggest that, given further opportunity and with the complete co-operation of all concerned—the public, those furnishing the services and the various private and Government agencies—this country can develop a most effective and efficient medical-care program and still retain the initiative and individual freedom that have made it so great.

92. For a Governmental System *

I

THE PAST DECADES have witnessed a ferment of ideas in the field of medicine and medical care. Physicians, typifying a segregated class, are satisfied for the most part with things as they are, or at most see the need for minor changes. But the people at large have become aware of grave deficiencies in medical care and have a dawning vision that better things are possible. The most articulate expression of this viewpoint is found in Franklin D. Roosevelt's new Bill of Rights. In January 1944 he said:

"We have accepted, so to speak, a second Bill of Rights, under which a new basis of security and prosperity can be established for all—regardless of station, race or creed." Among these, he said, is:

"The right to adequate medical care and the opportunity to achieve and enjoy good health; the right to adequate protection from the economic fears of old age, sickness, accident and unemployment."

* From: *Why Do We Need National Health Insurance?* by Ernst P. Boas, M.D.; New York: Society for Ethical Culture, 1945. Reprinted (with omissions, including initial paragraph) by permission of the author and publishers, from a revised edition (undated). The author was, at the time of his death in 1955, a consultant in internal medicine in New York.

Medical care is not a luxury whose availability should depend on the patient's ability to buy it. The sick person should not have to undergo a means test to determine whether or not he is eligible for treatment. Medical care should be regarded as a right to which all citizens are entitled, as they are to education.

If we accept this point of view we are faced with a serious dilemma. Medical care is a commodity that must be bought. Its distribution and availability depend on the incomes of the people in the community. Hence doctors and hospitals are plentiful in large cities and in wealthy industrial centers, for here there is money to pay for them.

But we are confronted with the basic fact that a large proportion of our population have not the money to buy decent medical care. In poorer communities, in the South, in farming areas, and in small towns the available medical resources are scanty or lacking. The National Health Survey and subsequent studies give ample evidence, but few realize the tremendous discrepancies that have developed.

II

Expenditures for medical care are consistently correlated with income. The lowest income group spends least, and the amount spent steadily increases as income increases. . . . So we find the higher income group spending over three times as much for medical care as do those with incomes of less than $1,000. Yet illness is nearly three times as frequent among those in the lowest income groups.

The same relation between medical care and income observed among families is seen in whole communities, even in States. In New York City, for instance, there is one doctor to every 700 of the population, in Mississippi the ratio is one to 2,100; in New York there is one general hospital bed to every 196 of the population, in Mississippi one to 667. It is ability to pay, rather than medical need that determines the availability of medical resources. . . .

III

Developments within the field of medicine itself have made more difficult the adequate distribution of medical care. Medicine in the United States, at its best, is unsurpassed. The past decades have been years of tremendous medical discovery and progress, resulting in a sharp reduction in disease and in marked prolongation of the average life span. But knowledge how to prevent and cure disease has far outstripped the actual performance. The techniques of medical care have become more and more complex and specialized. Medicine as it is practiced by organized medical staffs of our university and large voluntary hospitals offers the best there is of medical care. No longer is the solitary medical practitioner able to give adequate service to his patients. The constant development of new laboratory techniques, the increasing tempo of specialization, with the complex and difficult technical procedures which this involves, have brought it about that frequently many doctors must cooperate to reach a diagnosis and carry out treatment for a single patient.

The idea of cooperative group medicine has not yet penetrated to the general practice of medicine. Indeed it is constantly being thwarted by the present economic set-up of medical practice. The patient pays a separate fee for each service rendered, and the doctor is compelled to send the patient from one specialist or one laboratory to another in order to obtain the data that he needs to reach a diagnosis or carry out treatment. The costs rapidly mount, so that often needed special examinations are postponed or omitted because the patient cannot afford to pay for them. Moreover, it is to the practitioner's interest to minimize the number of these special examinations because that will make less money available for the payment of his own bill. Medical care still centers around the individual practitioner who is a private entrepreneur, and who singlehanded, to the best of his ability, provides medical care for those who seek him out, and who at the same time is compelled to make a living from these activities.

Good medical care today is better than it has ever been, but it is also more expensive, so costly, in fact, that the majority of patients cannot afford to benefit from the present available medical knowledge. Furthermore it is an old story that exceptionally heavy medical expenses affect only a relatively small number of families every year, families in which there is some major or catastrophic illness. . . .

This generation is also witnessing a radical change in the nature of disease, and this in turn leads to new problems in medical care. . . . More and more people are living to more advanced ages at which they acquire one of the so-called degenerative diseases, such as a heart disease, high blood pressure, diabetes, cancer or chronic rheumatism. It is these diseases that today are the great hazard to health and life. Their diagnosis and treatment, and still more so their prevention, is more difficult and complex and as a rule more expensive than that of the infectious diseases. Well established methods of sanitation or of mass vaccination are of no value in preventing their onset. Their control and prevention depend on making available to all complete medical care, not alone when the disease has run its course and is in its last stages, but at the time of its earliest manifestations, when it still may be checked and arrested. Preventive medicine has largely become a personal type of medicine which concerns itself with maintaining the health of the individual. The distinction between preventive medicine and the practice of medicine is being broken down, and one of the important fields for the public health official concerns itself with the creation of opportunity for early and adequate diagnosis and treatment of disease.

In spite of minor changes that have been engrafted on medical practice here and there, medicine is still practiced in the way it was practiced a generation ago, and the philosophy that justifies these methods, the philosophy proclaimed by organized medicine, is based on social and economic conditions, and a scientific and technological status of previous generations. Yet medicine is a public service or a public utility and should adapt itself to the framework of the society within which it functions. New methods must be found to assure the best medical care to everyone.

Physicians have traditionally espoused the view that medicine is an esoteric science and art, and that only they, the initiates in the cult, have the knowledge to determine what is good for the public and for their patients. Accordingly, physicians as individuals, as well as through their organizations, have insisted that they alone can plan for the medical care of the country, that medical care is a matter that does not concern the public or the government. And since any and every group dislikes and resists changes that may impair their traditions and their vested interests, doctors have balked at any plans that would alter the status quo. They have not been disinterested pleaders.

Yet it is clear that the patient, that is, the recipient of medical care, working through governmental agencies or through consumer organizations, has both the right and duty to be heard. He pays the bills and is entitled to determine the kind of medical care that he wants. Of course in the strictly professional and technical aspects of the problem, he must yield to the knowledge of the physician as expert advisor, but the layman is quite competent to decide whether or not he wishes to correct the gross inequalities in the distribution of medical care that exist today. That is why it is so important for laymen and doctors to work together to this end.

IV

We have learned that very many people cannot buy good medical care because their incomes are too small. If we agree that medical care is a right to which all are entitled, it is clear that a large part of the money to pay for it must come from other sources. There is ample precedent to look to government to fill this gap, whether it be local, State or Federal government. For years government has provided medical care for the indigent, and it has borne almost the total cost of the medical care of the mentally ill and of the tuberculous, because families are unable to bear the drain of such long drawn out chronic illnesses. . . .

No one challenges the principle of the use of public funds for the *prevention* of disease. But the prevention of disease today involves much more than the old line activities of the public health officer—sanitation and vaccination. Today the chronic, so-called degenerative diseases are the great hazard to life and health. Their control and prevention involves the creation of complete facilities for early diagnosis and treatment, and for making them freely available to all. People must be encouraged to consult a physician at the first intimation of a bodily disorder, and not wait until the disease has progressed to an advanced stage at which damage may be irreparable. The financial barrier that keeps patients from seeking medical advice must be eliminated.

Today we can no longer say, "This is preventive medicine, a proper function of government; and this, on the other hand, is curative medicine, the function of the practitioner of medicine whose services must be bought in the open market." These two aspects of sickness control have become merged; preventive medicine begins with measures of personal hygiene and health examinations instituted by the medical practitioner. So it is a logical and natural step to turn to government for funds to extend adequate medical care to all citizens of this country.

Because of the uneven distribution of wealth in the United States the Federal government must assume responsibility. A state such as New York could finance its own system of medical care, but there are many states that are unable to do so. . . . The increasing mobility of our population also makes it necessary that health plans be national in scope, so that the worker will not lose his benefits when he moves from one state to another.

To spread good medical care to all, the Federal government will have to spend a very large sum of money. Will this lead to "socialized medicine," the great bugaboo that we have been taught to fear? What is "socialized medicine"? The term as used today has an emotional, not a factual connotation; it is a catchword employed to arouse emotional resistance to plans to improve or change the methods of distributing medical care. The term socialized medicine, correctly used, means state medicine, an arrangement under which all medical facilities are owned by the state, all doctors are salaried civil servants, and all citizens have the right to complete medical care without charge. Only the Soviet Union has true socialized medicine, and there have been no proposals to introduce such a system in the United States. Yet we have a good deal of state medicine in this country—hospitals erected by cities, counties, by the State or Federal government and manned by salaried physicians. The care of the mentally ill, the tuberculous, and of veterans is managed in this manner.

V

The proposals for improvement of medical care have concerned themselves principally with application of the insurance principle to the payment for medical care. Sickness insurance is set up to spread the cost of illness. Application of the insurance method makes it possible to meet the extraordinary costs of major illnesses out of a common fund to which all contribute.

Many have cherished the hope that voluntary sickness insurance might fill the need. Even the conservative organized medical profession has accepted the principle of voluntary health insurance, provided the organization furnishing such protection is governed and controlled by physicians.

During the past decade an increasing number of voluntary health insurance plans have been launched. Broadly speaking, they may be divided into two great classes: one which operates on a fee-for-service basis; i. e., the doctor is paid out of the insurance fund for every individual visit or service rendered; a second, which is a per capita prepayment of service plan where the physician receives a certain sum annually, for which he renders complete general practitioner service to the patient. Organized medicine has insisted on the fee-for-service method of paying doctors, and has supported a number of plans developed on this principle throughout the country. In most of these benefits are restricted to all or part of the doctor's fee for a surgical operation, or for obstetrical services.

These plans are essentially medical expense indemnity insurance, much like accident and sickness insurance one can buy from a commercial insurance company. They are schemes to reimburse the patient for the costs of medical care provided through physicians. They give the patient a certain protection against the cost of catastrophic illnesses, but do not assure him adequate medical care. They guarantee the physician payment of certain of his bills, but do not make it much easier for him to provide the best medical service to his patients.

The cash indemnity plans strike at only one of the several weaknesses in the current medico-economic set-up, the unpredictability of heavy medical expense. Experience has demonstrated that medical insurance, to be practical and to provide adequate medical service, must cover all elements of medical care, and must be of a service rather than of an indemnity character. It must be a prepayment plan for medical services. The patient pays a certain sum annually, and for this receives complete medical coverage, for general practitioner, specialist, laboratory, hospital and preventive services.

A few such voluntary health insurance plans are in successful operation. They can exist only under special favored circumstances, among employees of one large industry, and as a rule with a subsidy from the employer. Usually they cover the worker, but not his family. They succeed in times of plenty, but with curtailment of employment, at a time when they need it most, many workers lose their insurance.

In all such plans that are functioning efficiently—plans such as those of the Endicott Johnson Shoe Company, of the Stanacola Company, of the Henry Kaiser Permanente Foundation, and of the Ross-Loos Clinic—the physicians are salaried. They do not operate on the fee-for-service system. Experience has shown that a certain small percentage of both patients and doctors take advantage of the insurance fund if payment is made for each service rendered, instead of by straight salary, and run up unnecessary bills. So in order to protect the insurance funds, plans employing the fee-for-service method of payment compel the patient to pay for the first few calls of any illness, and set up a complicated and expensive system of checks to detect cheating. Such safeguards discourage the patient from calling the doctor at the first signs of illness, and impede preventive services, but are essential to protecting the insurance fund from bankruptcy.... Insurance guaranteeing complete medical coverage cannot be set up, except at a prohibitive cost, if the fee-for-service principle is retained.

But even when doctors are paid by salary or by a capitation scheme, i. e., a certain sum annually for each patient on their panel, voluntary insurance against sickness is not cheap; the charges must be from $25 to $30 per person per year. For a family of four this amounts to $120 a year. For low income families, for those with incomes below $2500, this is far too expensive. The other necessities of life at these income levels are too demanding; prepayment for illness is put off in the hope that illness will not strike.

Skimping of charges to make the insurance plan available to persons with lesser incomes leads to poor medical service and to exploitation of the physicians. Many voluntary insurance plans have this defect, particularly those set up by labor or fraternal organizations. The reason lies in the simple fact that the clients have incomes too low to allow payment for complete satisfactory medical services.

For all these reasons, protection offered by voluntary sickness insurance in this country is minute in comparison to the need. A mere handful have complete medical coverage.... In this the experience of the United States reflects the experience of other countries more advanced in the organization for the distribution of medical care; voluntary plans fall far short of meeting the needs of the country.

VI

National compulsory health insurance is the only practical method of spreading the benefits of good medical care to the whole population. People can budget and make regular payments when they are well that will pay for medical services when they are ill. Such insurance would be financed by payments from all workers, with equal payments from their employers, supplemented by funds from general taxation. Contributions would be collected by payroll deductions, like other social security payments. Only by supplementing the workers' contributions by contributions from their employers and from taxation can sufficient funds be raised to finance a satisfactory medical care program. Since payroll deductions are calculated at a certain per cent of the worker's wages, those with small incomes would pay less than those with larger incomes. . . .

There are definite advantages in financing a national health program by contributory insurance payments through payroll deductions under the social security laws. It is just and psychologically sound for the worker to contribute to the costs of his own medical care. Knowing that he has paid for medical service, he will regard this service as a right, he will demand that it be adequate; and every stigma of charity that in the past has been associated with medical services provided by government, will be eliminated.

Tax funds will have to be provided in addition to the social security payments. Medical care of the indigent, who are not covered by virtue of employment, should also be included in a national health program. Additional funds are needed for the construction of hospitals and health centers, especially in rural areas, for the extension of full-time public health departments, for research, and for medical and other professional education. Without the leaven of teaching and scientific investigation no national health plan will develop the highest type of medical care. . . .

VII

The [Wagner-Murray-Dingell] Bill * will remove the economic barrier that prevents so many of our people from receiving adequate medical care. Opponents of national health insurance claim that it will lower the quality of medical care, that it will lead to regimentation and political control of medicine; that Washington bureaucrats will dictate every detail of medical practice, will select physicians for patients, and completely destroy the doctor-patient relationship. These arguments have no foundation in fact and have a very familiar ring. One hundred years ago they were hurled at advocates of public education; more recently they were used to prevent the enactment of child labor legislation, of the income tax and of workmen's compensation insurance.

* Senate Bill 1606.

The function of the Federal administrator of national health insurance is primarily to collect the funds to operate the program. This activity must be centralized, as it is today for old age retirement insurance. The Federal authority will also set minimum standards of performance for hospitals and for doctors participating in the insurance program. The Wagner-Murray-Dingell Bill provides specifically for decentralization of administration by directing the Surgeon General, as administrator, to give priority and preference to existing State and local agencies, and to establish committees in each locality to assure that the program will be adapted to local needs. Such committees shall include representatives of the insured population, doctors, hospitals, other agencies furnishing service under the program, and other persons informed on the need for, or provision of health benefits. The patient is free to choose his own physician, and the physician is permitted to reject a patient as he can today. Encouragement is given to the development of group medical practice. There will be no interference with the internal organization of existing institutions, nor with the methods of practice of individual doctors.

Since practically every person in the United States will be covered by this insurance, and since funds are appropriated to construct hospitals and health centers in areas where they are lacking or insufficient, the financial and professional inequalities that have led to the unequal distribution of physicians will largely disappear. There will result a more equitable distribution of doctors to rural and impoverished areas.

VIII

Patients, that is, the public, have everything to gain from this measure. It is not so generally recognized that the average doctor, too, will profit by its passage. The physician today is a split personality. He is a combination of a professional man and a small business man. These dual activities often conflict with one another, to the doctor's distress and the patient's disadvantage. All too often the physician is prevented from giving his patient the benefit of the full resources of medicine because the patient cannot afford the expense of the procedures involved. The doctor is unable to practice medicine in the way he wishes to and in the way it should be practiced. At present, all doctors are very busy and very prosperous. They forget that only a few years ago 60,000 doctors who are now in the armed services were competing with them for patients, and that a large number of these patients had no money.... Compulsory health insurance will stabilize the income of doctors over the years, and in fact will increase the incomes of the majority. They will be paid for taking care of the many persons whom they have been taking care of free. It has been reliably estimated that the average income both of practitioner and specialist will increase rather than suffer under the provisions of the bill. Of course the high priced specialist and surgeon may suffer some curtailment of income, but for the patient this is not an unmitigated hardship. Today the doctor wastes many of his early years building up a practice, meanwhile living at a starvation level, and after he has reached the age of sixty he finds his practice and his income rapidly shrinking. By providing a stabilizing economic base, compulsory health insurance will do much to eliminate this waste of skilled manpower. And it will give security to the doctor in youth and in old age just as it will to his patients.

Our parents thought of a doctor as someone to be called in times of serious illness, after the usual home remedies had failed to cure. We are learning to think in terms of positive health. We want our doctors to keep us well, to guard us against the ravages of diseases such as cancer or diabetes, and we know that to enable them to do so we must be able to consult them freely, before the disease process has become irreparable. We must give them the opportunity to employ in our behalf the complete resources of scientific medicine. As a nation we have learned the importance of good health of all our citizens, and are realizing that we cannot afford to leave the health of our people to the chance that they may have sufficient income to command modern medical care; or to expose them to the disadvantages that their race, their color, their occupation or their residence in a less favored economic community may bring about.

It is for such a national health program that all of us, doctors and laymen, must work together. Our efforts are needed to give actuality to the plans that have been developed by competent experts. The time has come to marshal the complete resources of modern medicine, and place them at the service of all our people.

FURTHER READINGS

Voluntary Medical Care Insurance

American Hospital Association, Blue Cross Commission. *Blue Cross Guide.* Chicago: The Association. (Issued annually).

American Medical Association. *Voluntary Prepayment Medical Care Plans.* (Issued annually, 1946-1952). *Voluntary Prepayment Medical Benefit Plans.* (Issued annually since 1953). Chicago: The Association.

Anderson, Odin W. with Feldman, Jacob J. *Family Medical Costs and Voluntary Health Insurance: A Nationwide Survey.* New York: McGraw-Hill, 1956. 251 pages.

Chamber of Commerce of the United States. *A Look at Modern Health Insurance.* Washington: The Chamber, 1954. 176 pages.

Chamber of Commerce of the United States. *Major Medical Expense Insurance.* Washington: The Chamber, 1956. 33 pages.

Commission on Financing of Hospital Care. *Financing Hospital Care in the United States.* (3 vols.). Vol. 2: *Prepayment and the Community.* New York: McGraw-Hill, 1955. 356 pages.

Department of National Health and Welfare. *Voluntary Medical and Hospital Insurance in Canada.* Memorandum No. 9, General Series, Research Division. Ottawa, Canada: The Department, 1955. 61 pages (processed).

Goldmann, Franz. *Prepayment Plans for Medical Care.* New York: Twentieth Century Fund and Good Will Fund, 1941. 60 pages.

Health Insurance Council. *The Health Insurance Story.* New York: The Council, 1954. 63 pages.

Klem, Margaret C. *Prepayment Medical Care Organizations.* (3rd ed.). Memorandum 55, Bureau of Research and Statistics, Social Security Board. Washington: U. S. Government Printing Office, 1945. 148 pages.

Rothenberg, Robert E. and Pickard, Karl. *Group Medicine and Health Insurance in Action.* New York: Crown, 1949. 278 pages.

United States Department of Health, Education, and Welfare, Public Health Service. *Comprehensive Dental Care in a Group Practice.* Publication No. 395, Public Health Service. Washington: U. S. Government Printing Office, 1954. 48 pages.

United States Senate, 79th Congress, 2nd Session. *The Experimental Health Program of the United States Department of Agriculture.* Monograph No. 1, Subcommittee on Wartime Health and Education, Committee on Education and Labor. Washington: U. S. Government Printing Office, 1946. 166 pages.

Warbasse, James P. *Cooperative Medicine.* (5th ed.). Chicago: Cooperative League of the U. S. A., 1951, 77 pages. (Includes references).

The Role of Government

American Medical Association, Council on Medical Service. *Voluntary Health Insurance vs. Compulsory Sickness Insurance.* A compilation of articles from various sources. Chicago: The Association, 1946. 124 pages.

Bachmann, George W. and Meriam, Lewis. *The Issue of Compulsory Health Insurance.* Washington: The Brookings Institution, 1948. 271 pages.

Bauer, Louis H. *Private Enterprise or Government in Medicine.* Springfield, Ill.: C. C. Thomas, 1948. 201 pages.

Canadian Welfare Council. *Health Insurance—What Are the Issues?* Ottawa, Canada: The Council, 1956. 60 pages. (Includes references).

Davis, Michael M. and Anderson, Dewey. *Medical Care for the Individual and the Issue of Compulsory Health Insurance: A Review of the Report of the Brookings Institution.* Committee Print, Committee on Labor and Public Welfare, United States Senate. 80th Congress, 2nd Session. Washington: U. S. Government Printing Office, 1948. 17 pages.

Falk, I. S. *Security Against Sickness.* New York: Doubleday, Doran and Co., 1936. 423 pages. (Includes references).

Means, James Howard. *Doctors, People, and Government.* Boston: Little, Brown and Co., 1953. 206 pages.

CHAPTER XIII

Principles and Proposals

MODERN MEDICINE is a wondrous thing, still very much a dynamic and not quite balanced blend of art and science. We accept its usefulness and call it essential for the prevention of disease, disability and premature death. Medical care is assigned a role of growing significance in the promotion of health and in the restoration of the disabled. It is a social thing and yet highly individual in so many ways. It is compounded of personnel and facilities, both specially developed to serve its unique purposes; of funds and organizations; of fundamental and clinical research. It represents a tremendous store of scientific knowledge and technical skill. A picture of these many parts and how they fit together, some loosely and some well, and of their changing shape has been the content of the preceding chapters. This final chapter brings directly and by implication a restatement of the purpose of medical care, and a series of definitive proposals for the achievement of the broadly accepted objective—that every man and woman and child shall have available the medical care services required to reach and maintain his or her personal optimum of good health.

Clearly implied is recognition of the fact that the social organization of medical care has lagged behind the scientific progress of medicine. While the several public and professional bodies whose proposals are quoted in this chapter would appear to agree on the need for extension and improvement of medical care, there are major differences concerning the methods of organization. Chapter XII has already suggested some of these differences as they pertain to the insurance methods of organizing payment for medical care services.

The proposals considered in this chapter are concerned primarily with the organization of service, although they include proposals relating to the general problems of financing medical care, of personnel, of facilities, of public and professional education. They have been chosen as representative of the major approaches to solution of the current problems of medical care.

New suggestions are made almost daily in this era of ferment. Recom· mendations come from a wide variety of community organizations, professional bodies, from both elected and self-proclaimed representatives of the public. National, state and even local legislative bodies see countless bills pertaining to the organization and financing of medical care. Hopefully, the background of information and the stimulation of the ideas presented in these pages will help us to select the more meaningful of these many proposals, to evaluate them intelligently, and to act upon them as mature and understanding citizens.

93. SOCIAL ORGANIZATION OF MEDICAL CARE *

FROM THE MEDICINE man of old to the modern clinic is a long way. Again and again mystery after mystery has been probed; again and again the utterly impossible has won acceptance against ancient truth; again and again the reach of medicine has been enlarged. The doctor's craft, with triumph after triumph to its credit, is still on its way. Yet it is set within a larger problem of human well-being which up to now has hardly been explored. It will not be solved until we learn to make culture in all its color and drama an instrument of health.

Institutions of some sort must be set up to serve each of the great needs of life. A people must be fed, given laws, protected against the weather, held to a moral code, provided with escapes from the dullness of everyday existence, fitted out with the comforts and frivolities which make life worth living. As we jog down the centuries and over the globe the ways in which these great tasks are performed present a most kaleidoscopic picture. If the job be to appease the gods, educate the young, ward off plagues, each people has its own way of doing it. Nowhere is there a final answer; there is always bother and striving that it may be better done.

Now the health of the people is among the mightiest of these great tasks. Yet the problem of the adequacy of medical care is unusually baffling. For it is only the exceptional person who has experienced all the arts—technical, economic, cultural —which converge in it. A beginning of understanding lies in a recognition of a distinction between the technology of medicine and its organization. By technology

---

* From: "Justice and the Future of Medicine," by Wendell Berge; *Public Health Reports* 60:1-16, Jan. 15, 1945. Reprinted with omissions, including initial paragraphs. The author is a former assistant attorney general of the United States, and is now a member of a Washington, D.C., law firm.

I mean all of those arts of diagnosis, therapeutics, surgery, radiology, dentistry, and the like, which constitute the profession of medicine. By organization I mean all of the arrangements, social and economic, by which medical service is made available. It is idle to dispute as to which is the more important; for there must be a medicine to practice, and there must be arrangements for bringing physician and patient together. It is no veiled mystery as to which is the more backward. In the advance of the art of medicine, you * have done a brilliant job. In the face of this advance it is all the more tragic that progress in the organization of medicine has lagged and, because of this lag, the nation has not had the full benefit of your superlative performance.

For backwardness in organization I am not disposed to pass out blame. But we should be quite frank in looking into reasons. You must be able to state your problem before you can solve it; and I wonder if a primary cause of the backwardness is not a failure to put the question clearly. Is not confusion found in attitude, in approach, at the very beginning of inquiry? To be specific, I profess no knowledge of the practice of medicine, and should I attempt to "lay down the law" as to how to treat an ailment you could—and quite properly—laugh me down. Yet, as a group, physicians have been little exposed to the discipline of the social sciences, and social organization is as intricate and as full of mysteries as the art of medicine itself. So when I hear a physician speaking about the organization of medicine in a tone of doctrinaire finality, I cannot fail to remark the contrast with the courageous and humble search for truth displayed in his own work. And when I hear the question put as a choice between private practice and socialized medicine, I cannot escape noting a confusion and dogmatism strikingly different from the scientific approach. As for the "either or" of private practice and socialized medicine, there is no such question. There are a myriad of schemes under which the doctor and the patient may be brought together—not a choice between just two.

Here, then, is the main reason for the great lag of organization behind art. Organization must be shaped in the full knowledge of the economic and social arts, yet it also must be shaped to the art of medicine and the distinctive service it renders. Advance, then, depends upon a range of understanding which neither you and your kind, nor I and my kind, alone possess. It demands a cooperation of professions which is not yet an accomplished fact. As we now take counsel together we are not going to clear up the problem. But this is the kind of thing, multiplied a myriad of times over, out of which will some day emerge the answer to the question of justice and the future of medicine.

Down through the centuries the common law has recognized the maintenance of the common health as one of the great tasks of society. In Europe, and in America, there never was such a thing, strictly speaking, as the private practice of medicine. From the earliest days the common law has made this clear. It is true that from days of old the doctor held no public office, but his service was, as the judges put it, "clothed with a public interest." At a time when any man, butcher, mercer, wheelwright, baker, fishmonger, or candlestick maker, was free to enter

* Physicians as a group, *i.e.* This selection was written as a speech for presentation to the 14th annual meeting of the American Urological Association, in St. Louis, June 21, 1944.

the trade of his choice, a license was required of the doctor. To secure his right to practice the candidate had to prove his knowledge, his integrity, his skills. The physician was not free to select or to reject patients at will. As one who followed a common calling he held himself ready to serve all in need to the limit of his capacity. Nor was inability to pay a valid excuse for the refusal of his service. The law recognized him as a kind of unofficial servant of the community and exempted him from the ordinary rules of the market. It wisely refused to crowd the relation of doctor and patient into the elementary forms of trade. The doctor rendered a service, the patient, if he was able, paid a fee, but the courts refused to regard the matter as a business deal.

On the contrary the law judged the relation by reference to the norm of common health. It was recognized that the patient, unversed in the mystery, was unable to judge the quality of service. Hence the doctor, in taking a case, assumed a trust unknown in respect to trade at large. The courts steadfastly refused to bring the rights and duties of the parties involved under the ordinary law of contract. And even in days when any old bargain was held valid, I have yet to discover a case in which a bungling physician was allowed to get off with a plea of caveat emptor.

The law went to lengths unknown elsewhere to make certain that the common health was served. In respect to the wares of trade the law of single price usually holds; a commodity is available to all who wish to purchase on exactly the same terms. To insure adequacy of service, a special rule of law was decreed for the physician; he was permitted to charge different fees to patients differently situated. The sliding scale, as much later it came to be called, served a definite social end. It elevated medicine above commerce, broke the pecuniary connection between the doctor's service and his reward, and gave legal recognition to the principle that persons were to be served according to their needs, that charges were to be assessed in terms of ability to pay. . . .

Let us briefly survey the great trends which converge upon medicine, for they decree a revision of means if the great ends of the Hippocratic oath are to be served.

First, the art of medicine has refused to stand still. The family doctor, with his bedside manner, his nostrums, his ponderous vocabulary to conceal his perplexities, his downright devotion to duty and sacrifice of self, was once the very epitome of the art of healing. He has been succeeded by the general practitioner who is the focus of a group of specialists, of which there are now more than a score, each with what a lawyer would call its own jurisdiction. The doctor's office, filled with gadgets and contraptions, has become a combination of consulting room, laboratory, and miniature hospital. A number of separate shops for X-rays, chemical tests, and pathological checkups have become necessary adjuncts. Access to a hospital has become a requirement of the individual physician. Consultation with his fellows has grown into an essential of practice. And behind all this is medicine which, as science and art, is on the march. Behind medicine stand optics, physics, chemistry, biology, and bacteriology, and still medicine continues to capture provinces which until recently lay beyond its frontiers.

Second, the community which the physician must serve has changed with the times. In the good old days the parson, the squire, and the doctor each held sway over his flock. Allegiance to the family doctor was a tie so firmly rooted that it took a crisis to break it. But our world no longer invites so durable, so personal, so exclusive a relationship. The machine, the corporation, and the pecuniary calculus have made over our work, our lives, our personal relationships. Our society has become urban, industrial, gregarious. We have become a new sort of wanderers, a race of modern nomads operating a material culture.

For most of us a job has come to replace an equity in the old homestead. For most of us livings, no longer taken directly from the farm, are pent in between the wages we receive and the prices we must pay. As individuals we are as stubborn as ever our ancestors were. But we act far less on our own and far more as managers, agents, or employees. Our industry is operated by corporations, our farmers band themselves into cooperatives, our workers, skilled and unskilled, gather into unions, even the great mass of our scientists make their discoveries while working for others. In our culture the group has come to be the regular thing.

Against such forces our minds cannot stand firm. Profound changes in habit, interest, and value have come in their wake. The standard of living has moved to a place of primacy among our everyday concerns. It makes the costs of medical service an inescapable problem. The care of the sick no longer can be absorbed by the family; it becomes an item of expense in the budget. If it is a wage earner who is ill, there is a double cost; absence from work means loss of earnings and bills are there to be paid. So medical service becomes a sheer economic necessity, for unless a man's capacity to work is maintained, he ceases to earn. Health thus becomes an aspect of the operation of the national economy.

Within this urban, industrial, wage-earning society, men and women are becoming increasingly conscious of what they want. Our workers demand health as a condition of their livelihoods. They insist upon adequate medical service at a price they can afford to pay, and in their newly won self-respect they will refuse all charity.

Third, a changing medicine has not yet been adapted to its new world. The high objectives of the profession endure, for they are eternal. But they must be freshly applied. Our society cannot be served by an instrument designed to fit the family physician into the village community. Neither my time nor your patience will permit a prolonged analysis. Yet two or three soundings will reveal the nature and contours of a very insistent problem.

In the not so long ago the old-fashioned doctor could be depended upon to administer medicine for the community. He could see to it that needs were met, service was adequate, and costs were justly distributed. The physician of today is in no position to discharge this office. His practice comprehends, not the whole community, but a mere fraction of it. If he is a specialist, the fraction is highly selective. And the whole body of physicians, each operating by himself, has no collective instrument by which it can apportion the totality of service in accordance with general need. Nor can it any longer take the specific responsibility of graduated charges. The sliding scale survives as a legacy from a simpler society and it has not yet been shaped to the circumstances of modern life. In the larger cities and even in smaller places, there is something of a trend toward fashionable, middle-class, or industrial-worker practice. Here obviously the sliding scale no longer operates, for different physicians serve persons in different income groups.

It is far more serious that charges as a whole are quite out of accord with the ordinary standard of living. As medicine has advanced, its arts have become more intricate. Yet very little attention has been given toward making up-to-date facilities available at prices the common people can afford to pay. It is not that on the whole physicians are paid too much; the statistics I have seen lead me to believe that their remuneration is quite inadequate. It is rather that there is waste, a failure fully to use facilities, a lack in getting the most out of a trained personnel.

The result is a national tragedy. The rich, who do not have to consider price, are often pampered with medical care which they may not need. Paupers are often indulged with a service which rises far above their ordinary way of life. The great middle class finds charges on the whole quite above its ability to pay. As a result, a great part of our population tries to reduce its demand for medical service to the minimum. A great volume of cases reach the doctors in an aggravated condition which, in an early stage, could have been easily handled. Necessary service is often secured at the cost of a heavy debt—a fact which does not make for health. And a far larger part of the people than I like to admit never become your patients.

Here then is challenge. The arts of medicine have advanced; the importance of medicine has been enhanced; it has become a necessity to the people and an essential in the operation of the industrial system. It has outgrown the organization into which, in days of petty trade, it was cast. The demand is for a vaster, more comprehensive, more reliable medical service. If an instrument of the common health can be provided on terms the people can afford, the people will rejoice. If you do not help them to it, the people will seize upon whatever agencies are at hand as a help in time of need, for the universal demand that the common health be served cannot much longer be stayed.

A new medical order is inevitable. Whether we shall cling to the old order or create a new one is not the question. The swift course of events has decreed that there can be no turning back. The question is rather what sort of a medical order it is going to be and whether it is the best which wisdom and knowledge can contrive. Like every promising venture, it has its hazards. Is it to be shaped by the best understanding which law, medicine, and the social studies can bring to it? Or is it to be constructed by amateurs in ignorance but with good intentions?

I can understand how, in the face of a new venture, you wonder whether change may not fail to constitute progress. I am certain that there will be serious loss if you sit upon the side lines and allow whoever may come to power to shape this new medical order.

As medicine gropes for a new organization, we all hear much of the doubts and fears of the profession. Many doctors are fearful lest objectives which have been hard won and which they value highly be lost. Many do not see how things which to them are essential can be fitted into a new order. Let us consider a few of the current perplexities.

A great many physicians are justly fearful that the quality of service may be compromised. From the profession I have frequently heard the argument that, when the Government undertakes to look after the health of the people, the service rendered is invariably poor. With this insistence on quality I fully concur. Nor do I dispute the fact that the new venture may provide a service that fails to meet the standards of the profession. But I cannot follow that argument that a causal relation exists between Government auspices and poor medicine. The truth is that the new system will bring medical care to hosts of people who before have had no access to it. For them there can be no falling off in quality: there has been no service to fall off in quality. Under a new system the provision of doctors and facilities almost always falls short of the new and enlarged demand. As a result, doctors with exacting notions discover much with which they can find fault.

But let us be fair and place the blame where it belongs. The shortcomings are not necessarily due to the new system. They are probably due to the shortage of personnel and equipment with which to work. It is hardly wise to blame untried arrangements, when there is a scarcity of doctors, nurses, clinical facilities, and drugs. No system can discharge its obligations if it lacks the men and materials with which to carry on.

Much is said, too, about the maintenance of a "personal relation" between doctor and patient. Like the law, medicine is practiced by persons and is practiced upon persons. The patient may be served by one or a number of physicians; the contact may endure for a single call, over a stretch of time, or for a long period of years. But in the practice of the profession, there is no escape from a personal relationship. The law has made this clear beyond a reasonable doubt. . . .

An oft-repeated variant of the same theme is the insistence upon the right of the patient freely to choose his physician. As a patient I am quite willing to have this right qualified for my own good. A well-recognized principle of economics has it that freedom of choice should be limited where the consumer is not a proper judge of the quality of the ware. If there is one field where freedom of choice should be qualified, it is medicine. For medicine is not one thing but many things. Its services are of a highly technical character. If we are downright honest, you and I know that the layman possesses neither the facts about the distinctive competence of particular physicians nor trustworthy norms to guide his judgment. In a matter of medicine, I am not foolish enough to trust my own choice, and a check with some of my lawyer colleagues indicates that they agree with me. I have over the years, through the devious ways by which a layman gets a little practical knowledge, discovered a physician or two whose judgment I have reason to trust. And with me it is their choice, not mine, which goes.

How many patients have walked into your office whose ailments have been aggravated by an amateur's choice of a physician? If for a moment I can be quite rash, I venture to say that in medicine competence does not wholly accord with ability to attract patients, as in law it does not always rest on ability to attract clients. List, if you will, the six physicians in your city in which you repose the greatest confidence. Let me, from the records of the Bureau of Internal Revenue, list the six who have the highest incomes. It's dollars to doughnuts, isn't it, that the lists do not match? People go to Johns Hopkins or the Mayo Clinic not to be treated by a particular doctor, but to secure skillful service. A personal choice, for that matter, can be secured even under State medicine. But far more important to the patient is the assurance of a high standard of competence.

Nor is wide-open freedom fair to the physician. He should on sheer merit advance in his profession. In all justice his work should be judged, not by the laity, to whom medicine is still a mystery, but by men of his craft who can distinguish brilliant from routine work. "The free choice of a physician," I fear, has become a shibboleth which will not stand analysis.

Candor compels me to say that I feel much the same about the argument that group practice robs the physician of his incentive. In its usual form it runs that if a man is on his own, he will give his best; if he works for a salary, he will put in his hours and let it go at that. The age-old traditions of your honorable profession deny the truth of such an argument. Your code of medical ethics has always elevated the relief of suffering above the pursuit of gain. Its purpose has always been to save the physician from avarice, one of the seven deadly sins. It has long been a canon of yours that service is to be given to rich and poor alike, that quality is not to be tempered to the ability of the patient to pay. My limited experience indicates —and a number of colleagues to whom I have put the question concur—that the mightiest urge to which the physician responds is the pride, the drive, the keeping faith with his calling. A doctor cares, and cares mightily, about the respect of his fellows. . . . You know better than I that a conscientious and resourceful physician is not, if he can help it, going to allow a case to lick him, and if the case is tough and he loses, it hurts.

Now I do not say that material things are to the doctor of no account. Like the judge, the lawyer, the engineer, the university professor, he has a right to demand advancement, security, an income adequate to his standard of life. For the professional man such things are necessities. Without them the physician is not in a position to give his best.

But such values depend upon no one single way of organizing medicine. To say that a doctor will give his utmost if he acts as his own business agent, and that his incentive will be stifled if he receives a salary, is not borne out by experience. The time was when the great scientific advance was the work of the solo inventor. Today the most creative of all work, the progress of science and the useful arts, is the product of men on salary. In the larger offices the great mass of lawyers now work on salary and work as hard and as heroically as the youngster who used to flaunt his own shingle in the breeze. It is true that the chance to become a partner is an incentive, but I would not rank it overly high, for work equally as good is done by the lawyers in the Government, where no such opportunity exists. In our institutions of higher learning, research as well as teaching falls to salaried employees and there you will observe an interest, excitement, devotion to duty, an urge to be up and doing. To return to medicine, how many thousands of our best doctors are today giving their all without stint in the service of the Army and the Navy?

Ambition, security, income are necessary things. They have in every age and among the most varied conditions of society driven men to accomplishment. If I were a youngster, I would rather leave the series of judgments which shape my career to men of my own profession than attempt to get ahead by translating my skills into the art of winning and holding patients. Most important of all, why is it that doctors are troubled by this doubt when university professors, lawyers in public service, officials who make of government a lifework, never even raise the question. And why is it that, when the Government of England first undertook to offer medical service, there was quite a chorus which viewed with alarm the loss of incentive, while today such a doubt remains unvoiced? It is easy enough to answer the argument that a salary will kill the urge to serve; it is hard to understand why the question is ever asked.

It is too late to turn away from that fearful subject of the State as employer, for I am already discussing it. As for myself I have no more fear of a venture of the State into medicine than I have of a venture of the State into law. The venture into law is old—judges, public counsel, prosecuting attorneys, are examples. The venture into medicine, the pauper and the criminal aside, is new, but the traditions and high standards which have long operated in one realm can be established in the other. Our Federal Government, in most of its activities, has adhered to a very high standard of professional competence. If for a moment I may be personal, I have experienced the practice of law in a large private New York office and in the Department of Justice. The Government has never imposed upon me restrictions which I have felt to be a burden. If anything, I have enjoyed a greater freedom than I could have had in a private law office. It is true that frequently my own judgment is tempered by the opinions of my colleagues. But usually a consultation, as you call it, leads to a sounder decision than any one of us alone would make.

You are right in insisting that high standards of medical care must not be compromised. But standards are a professional matter. Their chief dependence is upon adequacy of resources. They are not inherent in any type of organization. Your current way, as well as State medicine, has its insidious dangers, and, since comparative merits are at issue, I am not content with any argument which points out vices in the one without looking at the faults of the other. As it is now practiced, medicine is exposed to the corroding ways of business. Witness the recent exposure of fee-splitting in the city of New York. Under another dispensation, medicine may be exposed to the strange ways of politics. Which is the greater temptation, I am not able to say. But politics is a thing from which no activity of man is free. It can be employed to achieve holy as well as unholy results. And the State is not, as some of my physician friends seem to fear, a ward heeler telling the doctor how to practice.

I am not, mind you, presenting a case for or against the prevailing system, State medicine, or any particular medical order. There is, as I said at the beginning, no such question as private practice versus socialized medicine. For practice is never private and all medicine has a social function. The question to be faced is harder, more intricate, far more detailed than any such antithesis suggests. First of all you must ask what you want medicine to do. That is easy, to furnish to the whole population an adequate service of quality upon terms it can afford. Next, you must contrive ways and means of seeing to it that the great variety of services we call medicine are called into play to serve the common health. Next, you must set up protections against the hazards you and I see so clearly. And finally, all of these arrangements must be brought together into a going organization. Such a result is not to be attained by an act of faith or a single trial. The conditions of health vary from city to country, from section to section. The needs of the people as locally felt must me met, and this means variety, flexibility, and capacity for adaptation. It means, seek—honestly, objectively, courageously—and ye shall find; knock at many doors until the right ones shall be opened to you.

There is no royal road to a modern medical order. Thus the system we seek is not a choice between private practice and socialized medicine. In following his private calling the physician is fulfilling a social service; in medicine "private" and "social" always have been and always will be associated. These terms, so frequently set down as opposites, have only the most evasive content. Private practice has no stabilized form; the private practice of the country doctor who rode his horse, made his rounds, and was monarch of all he surveyed is not the private practice of a modern urologist. And "socialized medicine" embraces systems as distinct as the charity of the medieval church, the Royal College of Physicians, the clinic of a modern university, the bureau of public health, and the Russian way. You can no more get anywhere with such terms than you can practice your profession with a general concept of disease as your stock in trade.

The question demands, not an easy answer, but painful, constructive, detailed thought. It demands, too, an indulgence in downright trial and error without which nothing worthwhile emerges. A few experiments—far fewer than the length and breadth and depth of the subject demands—have been blazing fresh trails. Increasing numbers of physicians have enjoyed practice on their own and on salary, and are prepared, from experience rather than in speculative terms, to assess debits and credits. . . .

Last but most important of all, the war has accelerated a trend long in the making. A host of physicians now in service are conscious of the shortcomings of "military medicine" and have scores of suggestions as to how it can be improved. But they have become aware of the tremendous possibilities which inhere in a medicine directly organized to perform its function. Millions of soldiers, returned from the front, are going to demand for themselves and for their families the instruments of health to which they are entitled.

The course of events moves fast and a new medical order seems inevitable. My fear is not that we will not get it; an awakened public, sparked by our veterans, will see to that. My fear is that we will not bring to its creation all the knowledge, wisdom, and understanding we possess. A reference to the Wagner-Murray-Dingell bill will make my point. About its intent and objectives for me there can be no dispute. The detail of its provisions, however, may or may not fall short of its purpose—I do not know. On ways and means I am open to argument in behalf of something which is better. Of the necessity for distributing the cost of protection against illness I am wholly convinced, and I think the American people are adamant.

The medical order our stalwarts defend has already ceased to exist. A new medical order will come into being even though we do not will it, even, in fact, if we stubbornly resist it. For the medical order, like other institutions, cannot insulate itself against the impinging culture. It must make its response to the great pulsing tides which everywhere else enter our national life. The wiser physicians know that sheer opposition is not going to hold back the tide. They are putting forward—it seems to me a little timidly—proposals of their own. The other day the medical society right here in St. Louis voted approval of a plan for prepaid medical care, and the papers stated that a minority of doctors thought it did not go far enough. Timidity must be replaced by high resolve, and I am afraid that a very old adage which goes back at least as far as ancient Egypt applies here: "If you can't stop a movement, join it."

Seriously, support of the doctors is essential to the salvation of the movement. The organization of medicine is an affair of a couple of shops. It is a job for the craftsman in social order, but it must be shaped to the very life of the medical service it has to offer. If doctors oppose, or stand on the side lines, the layman will create a medical order which may prove to be indifferent or even blind to the values doctors prize most. If the doctors assume a role in its creation, they can see to it that no compromise is made with the standards of the profession.

The problem thus becomes one of creation. In respect to the selection of personnel, the standards of care, the carrying of risks, the methods of payment, the ways of remuneration, a score of ways are open. The form of organization may follow an agency of the State, the university pattern, the hospital set-up, or a combination of devices from all these. The Government may dominate the system, become one of a number of parties to its management, or be excluded from it altogether. The venture may fall into the legal form of a public health authority, a nonprofit-making corporation, a series of independent or interlocking corporations, a group of consumers' cooperatives, a mutual association of the profession and the laity, or something else. Its direction may be lodged with a tripartite board, representing the Government, the public, and the profession, or the public and the profession, free from Government interference, may assume joint responsibility. It may or may not be State medicine; it cannot escape being social medicine.

It is man for whom medicine exists. Its function must be to keep a whole people in health. The doctor must be the focus, but upon his office a host of unlike services must converge. The physician must not stop with asking, "Of what is this man ill and what can I do about it?" He must also inquire, "Why and how did this man become ill in the way he did?" The quest leads beyond cure to all the conditions upon which personal well-being depends. Food, clothing, housing, recreation, family, occupation, social life are all terms in the equation of health. Nor must man's habitat be forgotten, for adaptation is a requisite of the life process. Many arts must converge into the new medicine; prevention, sanitation, the public health must become a part of it. At its hub must stand the doctor; it is he who must direct this vast apparatus of skills, specialized personnel, facilities to the service of the human being. The medical order I suggest, and which the American people are going to have, will be vaster and mightier than anything we now know.

Such a medical order, it seems to me, should be hailed enthusiastically by the physician. In respect to professional matters his word will prevail. His opportunities for service will be greatly enlarged. He will have access to facilities which only the exceptional physician can now afford. A shift in work now and then will keep him alive in his profession. He can get away occasionally for further training. And above all, he ought to be better able to turn his clinical work to permanent account.

In an abstract way I recognize the value of ivory-tower research. But, after all, the heat of the daily round has its own contribution to make.... To me it seems that one of the great shortcomings of the prevailing medical system is that the practitioner is kept so busy with his patients that he cannot translate his work into medical discovery.

Thus, in the end, I return to my beginning. I can hand you no ready-made medical order on a silver platter. If I could, it would do you no good. I can only suggest to you, whose minds have long been busied with the subject, some reflections of a man of another profession. And I am positive that a service adequate to the times cannot be brought into being without the doctors' creative participation. As doctors and patients we face a crisis, and my appeal is to the ancient wisdom of the profession. The ends of medicine remain unchanged; ways and means must be found to adapt its practice to the conditions of present-day society. A new organization must be created that an ancient mission be not lost, that once again medicine shall be available to all in need and charges shall be graduated in accordance with ability to pay....

94. VARYING APPROACHES

A. AMERICAN MEDICAL ASSOCIATION *

A Federal Department of Health.—Creation of a Federal Department of Health of cabinet status with a Secretary who is a Doctor of Medicine, and the coordination and integration of all Federal health activities under this Department, except for the military activities of the medical services of the armed forces.

Medical Research.—Promotion of medical research through a National Science Foundation with grants to private institutions which have facilities and personnel sufficient to carry on qualified research.

Voluntary Insurance.—Further development and wider coverage by voluntary hospital and medical care plans to meet the costs of illness, with extension as rapidly as possible into rural areas. Aid through the states to the indigent and medically indigent by the utilization of voluntary hospital and medical care plans with local administration and local determination of needs.

* From: "Program of the American Medical Association for the Advancement of Medicine and Public Health," *Journal of the American Medical Association* 139:529, Feb. 19, 1949 (No. 8). Reprinted by permission of the publishers.

Medical Care Authority with Consumer Representation.—Establishment in each state of a medical care authority to receive and administer funds with proper representation of medical and consumer interest.

New Facilities.—Encouragement of prompt development of diagnostic facilities, health centers and hospital services, locally originated, for rural and other areas in which the need can be shown and with local administration and control as provided by the National Hospital Survey and Construction Act or by suitable private agencies.

Public Health.—Establishment of local public health units and services and incorporation in health centers and local public health units of such services as communicable disease control, vital statistics, environmental sanitation, control of venereal diseases, maternal and child hygiene and public health laboratory services. Remuneration of health officials commensurate with their responsibility.

Mental Hygiene.—The development of a program of mental hygiene with aid to mental hygiene clinics in suitable areas.

Health Education.—Health education programs administered through suitable state and local health and medical agencies to inform the people of the available facilities and of their own responsibilities in health care.

Chronic Diseases and the Aged.—Provision of facilities for care and rehabilitation of the aged and those with chronic disease and various other groups not covered by existing proposals.

Veterans' Medical Care.—Integration of veterans' medical care and hospital facilities with other medical care and hospital programs and with the maintenance of high standards of medical care, including care of the veteran in his own community by a physician of his own choice.

Industrial Medicine.—Greater emphasis on the program of industrial medicine, with increased safeguards against industrial hazards and prevention of accidents occurring on the highway, home and on the farm.

Medical Education and Personnel.—Adequate support with funds free from political control, domination and regulation of the medical, dental and nursing schools and other institutions necessary for the training of specialized personnel required in the provision and distribution of medical care.

B. AMERICAN PUBLIC HEALTH ASSOCIATION *

THE RECOMMENDATIONS presented in this report represent guides to the formulation of a policy for action. It is believed that study of these recommendations by the

* From: "Medical Care in a National Health Program," by the American Public Health Association; *American Journal of Public Health* 34:1,252-56, Dec. 1944 (No. 12). Reprinted (with omission of initial paragraphs) by permission of the publishers.

professions and others concerned in the states and localities will produce new and more specific recommendations for the attainment of the objectives of a national health program.

Recommendation I. The Services.—a. A national plan should aim to provide comprehensive services for all the people in all areas of the country. In light of present-day knowledge, the services should include hospital care, the services of physicians (general practitioners and specialists), supplementary laboratory and diagnostic services, nursing care, essential dental services, and prescribed medicines and appliances. These details of content must remain subject to alteration according to changes in knowledge, practices, and organization of services.

Because of inadequacies in personnel and facilities, this goal cannot be attained at once; but it should be attained within ten years. At the outset, as many of the services as possible should be provided for the nation as a whole, having regard for resources in personnel and facilities in local areas. The scope of service should then be extended as rapidly as possible, accelerated by provisions to insure the training of needed personnel, and the development of facilities and organization.

b. It is imperative that the plan include and emphasize the provision of preventive services for the whole population. Such services include maternity and child hygiene, school health services, control of communicable diseases, special provisions for tuberculosis, venereal diseases, and other preventable diseases, laboratory diagnosis, nutrition, health education, vital records, and other accepted functions of public health agencies, which are now provided for a part of the population.

c. In so far as may be consistent with the requirements of a national plan, states and communities should have wide latitude in adapting their services and methods of administration to local needs and conditions.

Recommendation II. Financing the Services.—a. Services should be adequately and securely financed through social insurance supplemented by general taxation, or by general taxation alone. Financing through social insurance alone would result in the exclusion of certain economic groups and might possibly exclude certain occupational segments of the population.

b. The services should be financed on a nation-wide basis, in accordance with ability to pay, with federal and state participation, and under conditions which will permit the federal government to equalize the burdens of cost among the states.

Recommendation III.   Organization and Administration of Services.—a. A single responsible agency is a fundamental requisite to effective administration at all levels —federal, state, and local. The public health agencies—federal, state, and local— should carry major responsibilities in administering the health services of the future. Because of administrative experience, and accustomed responsibility for a public trust, they are uniquely fitted among public agencies to assume larger responsibilities and to discharge their duties to the public with integrity and skill. The existing public health agencies, as now constituted, may not be ready and may not be suitably constituted and organized, in all cases, to assume all of the administrative tasks implicit in an expanded national health service. Public health officials, however, should be planning to discharge these larger responsibilities, and should be training themselves and their staffs. This preparation should be undertaken now because, when the public comes to consider where administrative responsibilities shall be lodged, it will be influenced in large measure by the readiness for such duties displayed by public health officers and by the initiative they have taken in fitting themselves for the task.

b. The agency authorized to administer such a program should have the advice and counsel of a body representing the professions, other sources of services, and the recipients of services.

c. Private practitioners in each local administrative area should be paid according to the method they prefer, *i.e.,* fee-for-service, capitation, salary, or any combination of these. None of the methods is perfect; but attention is called to the fact that fee-for-service alone is not well adapted to a system of wide coverage.

d. The principle of free choice should be preserved to the population and the professions.

e. State departments of health and other health agencies are urged to initiate studies to determine the logical and practical administrative areas for a national medical care plan.

Recommendation IV. Physical Facilities.—a. Preceding, or accompanying, the development of a plan to finance and administer services, a program should be developed for the construction of needed hospitals, health centers, and related facilities, including modernization and expansion of existing structures. This program should be based on federal aid to the states and allow for participation by voluntary as well as public agencies, with suitable controls to insure the economical and community-wide use of public funds. The desirability of combining hospital facilities with the housing of physicians' offices, clinics, and health departments should be stressed.

b. Federal aid to the states should be given on a variable matching basis in accordance with the economic status of each state.

c. Because of its record of experience and accomplishment in this field, the U. S. Public Health Service should administer the construction program at the federal level, in coöperation with the federal agencies responsible for health services and construction.

d. Funds available under this program should be granted only if:

(1) The state administrative agency has surveyed the needs of the state for hospitals, health centers, and related facilities, and has drawn up a master plan for the development of the needed facilities (taking account of facilities in adjacent states); or, in the absence of a state plan, the project is consistent with surveys of construction needs made by the U. S. Public Health Service;

(2) The proposed individual project is consistent with the master plan for the state; its architectural and engineering plans and specifications have been approved by the state agency and/or the U. S. Public Health Service; and there

is reasonable assurance of support and maintenance of the project in accordance with adequate standards.

e. State health departments are urged to conduct studies to develop state plans for the construction of needed hospitals, health centers, and related facilities. Such studies should be made in coöperation with official health agencies, with state hospital associations, and other groups having special knowledge or interests.

Recommendation V. Coördination and Organization of Official Health Agencies. —a. The activities of the multiple national, state, and local health agencies should be coördinated with the services provided by a national program. There is no functional or administrative justification for dividing human beings or illnesses into many categories to be dealt with by numerous independent administrations. It is difficult to reorganize agencies or to combine activities, and this cannot be accomplished hurriedly. Therefore studies and conferences should be undertaken without delay at the federal level, and in those states and communities where the health structure is already unnecessarily complex.

b. The federal and state governments should provide increased grants for the extension of adequate public health organization to all areas in all states. Increased federal grants should be made conditional upon the requirement that public health services of at least a specified minimum content shall be available in all areas of the state.

Recommendation VI. Training and Distribution of Service Personnel.—a. Within the resources of the program, financial provisions should be made to assist qualified professional and technical personnel in obtaining postgraduate education and training.

b. The plan should provide for the study of more effective use of auxiliary personnel (such as dental hygienists, nursing aides, and technicians), and should furnish financial assistance for their training and utilization.

c. Professional and financial stimuli should be devised to encourage physicians, dentists, nurses, and others to practice in rural areas. Plans to encourage the rational distribution of personnel, especially physicians, should be developed as quickly as possible, in view of the coming demobilization of the armed forces. Such plans should be integrated with the whole scheme of services and the establishment of more adequate physical facilities.

Recommendation VII. Education and Training of Administrative Personnel.— a. Education and training of administrative personnel should be encouraged financially and technically, especially for those who may serve as administrators of the medical care program, for hospital and health center administrators, and for nursing supervisors.

b. State health departments should utilize those funds that may be available to train personnel in such technics as administration of health and medical services, and hospitals. Such a training program may contribute more than any other single activity to the future rôle of the official public health agency. As a corollary, the attention of schools of public health is directed to the importance of establishing the necessary training courses.

Recommendation VIII. Expansion of Research.—a. Increased funds should be made available to the U. S. Public Health Service and to other agencies of government (federal, state, and local), and for grants-in-aid to non-profit institutions for basic laboratory and clinical research and for administrative studies and demonstrations designed to improve the quality and lessen the cost of services.

b. The research agencies and those responsible for making grants-in-aid should be assisted by competent professional advisory bodies to insure the wise and efficient use of public funds.

1950 Association Resolution on Medical Care.*—RESOLVED: † 1. That with respect to that segment of the public health field having to do with medical care, the Association reaffirms its position that its primary interest is with the ready availability of a high quality and adequate quantity of medical care for the people;

2. That the Association recognizes the intricacy of the problem of financing a high quality and adequate quantity of medical care and has not advocated and does not now advocate any one method of financing;

3. That no method of financing yet proposed by the Congress [of the United States] or elsewhere will *per se* assure a high quality and adequate quantity of medical care;

4. That regardless of the methods of payment, medical services must be adequately and securely financed, with due regard to ethical, professional, and administrative requirements;

5. That the Association continue its objective studies of medical care programs of all kinds, revising its statements of policy from time to time as sound information and experience accumulate;

6. That the Association urges all agencies, organizations, and individuals concerned with medical care problems to exchange views and experiences and to pool their knowledge, their resources and their efforts to the end that the best possible medical care for all the people may ultimately be developed under the conditions that prevail in the United States.

* From: "Policy on Medical Care in a National Health Program," by the American Public Health Association (Association Resolution No. 19, passed Nov. 1, 1950); *American Journal of Public Health* 40:1,592, Dec. 1950 (No. 12). Reprinted by permission of the publishers.

† This resolution concerning Association policy on medical care in a national health program was adopted by the membership of the American Public Health Association at its annual meeting in 1950. The purpose of the resolution, according to the Association, was to "reaffirm and clarify the purpose and meaning" of the organization's 1944 policy statement (reprinted immediately above) on the same subject, as well as to "clarify its present [1950] position."

C. NEW YORK ACADEMY OF MEDICINE *

THERE IS CONSENSUS concerning several important fundamentals. All are agreed that medical service should eventually provide everything that science can offer toward the preservation of health and the cure of disease, and that it should make available these benefits to the entire population. There is agreement that medical service is not now optimally organized, supervised, or distributed, but also that the development of plans for its improvement should be preceded by inclusive study of the many complex factors involved and should not be directed toward the support of any preconceived scheme which has not been based upon such study. It is apparent to all members of the Committee [on Medicine and the Changing Order] that in a country as vast as ours no one plan can be applicable to all parts and that many and various experiments for extending and improving medical care in conformity with local conditions are urgently needed. It is the belief of the Committee that the general public, as the intended beneficiary of plans for change, have such a vital interest in them that they should be adequately represented in their formulation, but that physicians, who in the last analysis must render medical care, should have a dominant role in the preparation of plans they will be called upon to carry out. The Committee agrees that gradual extension and improvement of medical service is preferable to revolutionary change and that, while government has a direct responsibility for the health of its citizens, rapid and sweeping changes accomplished by legislative action would defeat their own purposes by impairing the spirit and quality of a service which is essentially individualistic and personal.

As a result of its study the Committee is prepared to formulate several conditions which it believes are necessary for satisfactory improvement of medical service:

In extending medical service and perfecting its organization, quality must be preserved. Eventually only the best of medical care should be perpetuated. Extension of inferior service will at best be of limited value and under certain circumstances may be actually dangerous. It must be recognized, however, that during the past decade remarkable improvement has been evident and that any plans for future betterment should not impede the progress already made. Changes should be accomplished as far as possible without dismemberment, disorganization, or serious dislocation of any major section of the medical and allied professions or of established public and official institutions.

Provision of public health services is a prime essential. Great areas of rural America as well as many of its smaller cities are still without good or even adequate public health services. The Committee believes that correction of this condition is an essential first step in the evolution of good medical care. Its achievement,

* From: *Medicine in the Changing Order*, by the Committee on Medicine and the Changing Order, New York Academy of Medicine; New York: Commonwealth Fund, 1947 (Chap. XII, "The Method and the Goal"). Reprinted (with omissions, including initial paragraph) by permission of the publishers.

however, will require not only the establishment of well-equipped health centers but also the training of many more health officers than are now available. The Committee urges that this step be regarded as a local responsibility to be shared with state and federal agencies only where and when local resources in knowledge, funds, and personnel are inadequate.

Improvement in medical service requires effective use of hospitals with adequate facilities. If the aim of providing all that medical science can offer is to be achieved, the extensive facilities of a well-equipped hospital are essential. Conformity to this requirement, however, implies delay in many rural communities where hospitals are non-existent or of an inferior quality. The situation is not much better in many of the smaller communities. Even in larger urban centers where there are many hospitals, the facilities are less than optimal.

In a study of the situation it becomes apparent not only that there must be more hospitals but also that those which exist must be more effectively utilized. Among other things this implies development of better outpatient department clinics and the use of hospital facilities by groups of physicians to reduce the actual and relative costs of medical service. By such arrangements large items of capital investment and the failure to use in full the facilities available, now implicit in the office practice of individual physicians, may be eliminated. Under these circumstances the Committee favors the experimental development of diagnostic consultation services at a minimum flat fee, the services to be provided by teaching and other competently equipped hospitals.

Success will require trained professional and non-professional personnel. The provision of a hospital, of operating rooms, of x-ray equipment, of urological and orthopedic devices, will not serve an optimal purpose unless highly trained physicians, surgeons, radiologists, and orthopedists are available to utilize them. There must be well-trained nurses and social workers available both for the operation of the hospital and for visiting in the home. Highly skilled technical assistants must also be available to perform laboratory services. These requirements imply that in some situations progress in improving medical care will be slow until the requisite professional skill has been attained by training or importation. The difficulties of rapid progress are evident in all areas but are particularly apparent in rural communities. For reasons which the Committee has found to be numerous, the younger and better-trained physicians have in the main tended to settle and to practice in large cities. Correction of the deficit will depend in part upon better financial rewards, but perhaps more upon the provision in the district of resources essential to effective medical practice and upon education of the community in the desirability and the meaning of adequate medical care. There are several ways in which it might be possible to provide assurance of more adequate income, ranging from participation in a group serving a voluntary prepayment plan to partial subvention in the form of a salary for part-time service to the medically indigent provided by the local community, the state, the Federal Government, or by their combined participation. Distance in sparsely settled regions also enters into consideration since it implies social as well as physical limitations. This is a serious problem and becomes greater the worse the roads and the more irregular the terrain. For rapid progress, the physical phase of population dispersion must be dealt with effectively, and on this score the Committee recommends a variety of experiments such as local health centers with emergency bed facilities, mobile clinics, mobile laboratory facilities, and airplane ambulance services. It is also the belief of the Committee that substantial progress in improving service in rural districts may be made by experiments in exposing medical students during their clinical years to rural and small-town practice, this to be achieved through an association between the medical schools and the rural hospitals.

It is not to be expected that many rural communities will of and by themselves take up their health problems and resolve them. The Committee therefore recommends that surveys be initiated at the state level to define the local and other community health needs and that plans be thereafter formulated to provide for the necessary additions and changes in service.

For optimal results, organization and cooperation of physicians are required. The idea of the medical group now well established in this country offers advantages which cannot be attained by the individuals of the group acting separately. Cooperative enterprise between physicians working in a health center with facilities for curative and preventive medicine seems at the present time to offer an appropriate formula for rapid progress. For its accomplishment, however, organization is required and with it some sacrifice of the individual prerogatives and rights of each of the cooperating physicians. For successful operation there must also be strict standards of performance to be followed by all the individuals engaged in the enterprise. To enforce the standards and to achieve optimal results, supervision will be necessary.

In the improvement of medical services, voluntary prepayment plans are needed. While lower costs are not the prime requisite, the absolute and relative reduction in the cost of medical services is strongly urged by the Committee to meet the needs of those who under the existing fee-for-service system are medically indigent. The Committee recommends the extension of voluntary prepayment plans which, by spreading the risk, can make this group competent to provide for its medical needs. To assure the stability and solvency of such prepayment plans, the Committee urges that they should provide easy admission to the economically higher groups, the latter being generally better insurance risks. The Committee also recommends that those in a dependency condition should likewise be covered by the insurance of prepayment plans, the community paying the premium.

Voluntary prepayment plans, the Committee feels, leave free to physicians the play of initiative, of resourcefulness, and of individual responsibility. Voluntary prepayment plans can be developed when and where conditions are propitious and ready, and can be adapted in a variety of ways to local needs and circumstances. Being limited in scope, they are susceptible to easy change and modification, and being voluntary, they do not threaten disruptive effects on the medical and related professions or on medical institutions. The Committee therefore advocates grants, subsidies, employers' contributions, and other aids which may hasten the growth and extension of voluntary medical insurance.

The Committee believes that voluntary prepayment plans are much safer and more adaptable than compulsory insurance, the consequences of which are at best uncertain and are in any event irrevocable. It is convinced that if a program of voluntary insurance can obtain the understanding and cooperation of the public, the profession, and the government alike, it will more surely lead to the desired goal. It is on a voluntary basis that the great progress in medicine has been achieved in the past, and it is thus that continuance of progress can best be assured for the future.

The goal should be comprehensive medical service. If activities are to be undertaken to guide future trends in the practice of medicine as well as to meet current popular demands, they should be so arranged as to offer comprehensive care including health supervision and preventive as well as curative treatment. Segmental care as represented by diagnostic clinics or clinics for case-finding in a special disease will not suffice. The discontinuous care and patchwork now represented by hospitalization without adequate follow-up will furnish only partial solution. Examinations should not depend solely upon the accident of illness. They should be undertaken when no fault is apparent and should be sufficiently searching to permit early recognition of cancer and important infectious diseases such as tuberculosis and syphilis, as well as emotional abnormalities. Routine care should include procedures for immunization. The treatment should be focused not only on the care of the acutely ill or injured person but should also include management of convalescence and rehabilitation. The interest of physicians in such developments should also extend into the community and should include correlation of recreational and intellectual resources with medical needs.

Extensive education for both physicians and the public will be required. Few physicians are now equipped to practice both preventive and curative medicine or to conduct routine health surveys in a spirit which should make them effective. In order to make comprehensive health care on a large scale a reality, medical schools will be required to give the physician in training a new orientation. Progress will depend upon changes and improvements in the curricula of medical schools to meet the present-day needs in medical service, the recruitment of a competent and representative medical student body, and the continuing education of the physician.

There must also be education of the public. It is the opinion of the Committee that most patients at present are by no means ready to take advantage of comprehensive medical service and that much information will be required before people in general realize the advantages of hygiene, proper nutrition, and constant medical supervision in health as well as in illness. Success in the extension of the best medical service will demand physicians with more than ordinary interest in both preventive and curative measures, as well as an extensive and long-continued educational program for the community to be served.

Progress in the extension of medical service must be varied and adapted in each instance to the needs of the community.... In the [Committee's] report the medical care problems of urban and suburban dwellers, of the rural population, and of the distinct and particular groups to be found in each, have been defined and described in terms of their known social, economic, and educational circumstances. Out of these considerations has come the compelling realization of the multiplicity of problems involved in providing more and better care for the American people. There has come, too, the inescapable conviction that these various problems cannot be solved by any one single line of action. Experiments should be numerous and varied and should be undertaken with the idea that prolonged study may permit selection of the best and most appropriate.

Government aid will be required. It is unlikely that rapid progress can be made either in the establishment of adequate hospital and health facilities or in the provision of sufficiently skilled personnel without aid from government sources. While need of such aid is more apparent throughout rural America, it is also evident in many urban and suburban communities. In each case government aid should be applied with special attention to local requirements. This should include critical choice of location for new hospitals with an eye to greater utility for both the public and the local medical profession, and arrangements to facilitate coordination of other existing hospital facilities within ambulance range. It implies further an association between the hospital so established and some larger, preferably teaching, hospital proximate to the community. Promising efforts in these directions . . . are those of the Bingham Associates, the Kellogg Foundation, and the studies and experience of the Commonwealth Fund.

For the establishment of voluntary prepayment plans and for their support during the formative period, the Committee favors, where and when necessary, government support, the government being local, state, or federal, or a combination. The Committee is cognizant of the disadvantages and risks involved in every form of payment to the physician made from an insurance or prepayment fund, and has deliberately refrained from recommending any one form of payment, advising instead experimentation with the various possible forms of payment until time and experience prove which are the best.

In general the system of government grants-in-aid for the promotion of better medical care has been successful and provides a precedent for future developments along similar lines. It has the impressive advantage of allowing for local administration and experimentation to meet special conditions and also for the rectification of omissions or mistakes. It is applicable to the establishment of hospitals and health centers, to the support of group practice, especially in hospitals, and also to the support of voluntary plans for prepayment medical insurance. In general the Committee supports the grants-in-aid method of government contribution to the solution of many of the problems of medical care as a sound alternative to legislation for an over-all program of compulsory health insurance.

In acknowledging government participation as a reality which will probably be greatly expanded, the Committee strongly recommends a general method of grants-in-aids as the one that has stood the test of American experience in the past, presents the least difficulty and disadvantage for the present, and holds the brightest promise for the future.

The foregoing statement of the Committee's major working principles and recommendations should suffice to render clear the philosophy that has animated and directed its studies and report. The Committee began its labors in the full conviction that there is need and a real opportunity to extend the benefits of modern medicine to more of the people of this country. The crucial question to which the Committee devoted itself was how best the need is to be met. . . .

It is against the background of its historical studies that the Committee has dealt with the economic and legislative aspects of the problem.

Over and above the specific conclusions which the Committee derives from its studies and upon which it based its numerous particular recommendations, the Committee stands confirmed in the conviction that providing more and better care for the people is a task that will require many years for its achievement; that it can be accomplished only step by step and in a cumulative and accelerating fashion. Those who believe it can be accomplished quickly, and chiefly through legislative enactments, are, in the Committee's conviction, grossly in error and their proposals place in jeopardy the very aims they have in mind. The Committee has, therefore, felt justified not only in offering a series of recommendations applicable now and in the immediate future, but also in charting such developments in the provision of more and better medical care as may require a generation or more to achieve. Toward this end it is hoped that some permanent agency may come into being which will carry into the future the continued study of the problems of medical care, destined to change in the future as they have in the past. The Committee hopes that this report may serve as a preliminary introduction to such a continuing study.

D. NATIONAL HEALTH ASSEMBLY *

1. ADEQUATE MEDICAL care [1] for the prevention of illness, the care and relief of sickness, and the promotion of a high level of physical, mental, and social health should be available to all without regard to race, color, creed, residence, or economic status.

2. The principle of contributory health insurance should be the basic method of financing medical care for a large majority of the American people, in order to remove the burden of unpredictable sickness costs, abolish the economic barrier to adequate medical services, and avoid the indignities of a "means test."

3. Health insurance should be accompanied by such use of tax resources as may be necessary to provide additional

* From: *America's Health: A Report to the Nation by the National Health Assembly;* New York: Harper, 1949 (Chap. VIII, "What Is the Nation's Need for Medical Care?" pp. 221-22). Reprinted (with omissions, including initial paragraphs) by permission of the publishers.

1. Medical care, as used here, aims at the organization of all the facilities and personal services necessary to attain the highest level of health, prevent disease, cure or mitigate illness, and reduce if not prevent disability, economic insecurity, and dependency associated with illness.

   (a) Services to persons or groups for whom special public responsibility is acknowledged; and

   (b) Services not available under prepayment or insurance.

   4. Voluntary prepayment group health plans, embodying group practice and providing comprehensive service, offer to their members the best of modern medical care. Such plans furthermore are the best available means at this time of bringing about improved distribution of medical care, particularly in rural areas. Hence such plans should be encouraged by every means.

   5. The people have the right to establish voluntary insurance plans on a cooperative basis, and legal restrictions upon such right (other than those necessary to assure proper standards and qualifications), now existing in a number of states, should be removed.

   6. High standards of service, efficient administration, and reasonable costs require:

   (a) Coordination of the services of physicians, hospitals, and other health agencies in all phases of prevention, diagnosis and treatment; and

   (b) Effective cooperation between the providers and the consumers of such services.

   7. A medical care program by itself will not solve the health problems of the nation. It must be coordinated with all efforts directed toward providing the people with adequate housing, a living wage, continuous productive and creative employment under safe working conditions, satisfying recreation, and such other measures as will correct conditions that adversely affect the physical, mental, and social health of the people.

   8. There are areas on which the planning committee of the Medical Care Section * is not yet prepared to report. In the Section's meetings differing views were expressed as to the method of effectuating the principle of prepayment or insurance. Some believe it can be achieved through voluntary plans. Others believe that a national health insurance plan is necessary. . . .

E. COMMISSION ON HEALTH NEEDS OF THE NATION †

THE PHYSICIAN no longer makes his sole contribution to the health of individuals and the Nation by treating disease. Now, a broader view of health service is being developed—one that takes into account more than what a physician does in

---

   * The term "medical care section" here denotes that panel of the National Health Assembly (one of fourteen into which the Assembly was divided) which discussed questions relating to the financing of medical care, and whose "planning committee" (comprising a small executive group of panel delegates) was responsible for formulating the report of the panel's deliberations; the eight points listed, which were called "Main Principles" in the official Assembly report, formed part of the "Conclusions" section of the medical care panel's discussions.

   † From: *Building America's Health,* by the President's Commission on the Health Needs of the Nation; Washington: U.S. Government Printing Office, 1953 (Vol. 1, "Introduction," p. 3, and Section VII, "Financing Personal Health Services," pp. 47-48). Reprinted with omissions, including initial paragraphs. (Note: Four of the volumes comprising the Report of the President's Commission on the Health Needs of the Nation were published in 1953; Vol. 1, "Findings and Recommendations," was actually issued in 1952).

the diagnosis and treatment of disease. It includes things that are done in the absence of disease, namely, the promotion of health and prevention of disease; and what is done beyond the ordinary treatment of disease, namely, rehabilitation. This view, a spectrum of comprehensive health services, specifically includes the contribution of a variety of personnel and of community services. The physician leads the over-all effort, but as one member of a well-trained team comprised of dentists, nurses, technicians, and many other professional health workers. Only through such joint endeavor can the whole range of services be delivered.

To be most effective the health team, with community and national support, must achieve a smooth continuum of care—embracing promotion of health, prevention of diseases, diagnosis and treatment, and rehabilitation—all of which is constantly improved through education and research.

Health Principles.—From such considerations the Commission has formulated these principles to be used as a guide in approaching our health problem.

WE BELIEVE THAT:

1. Access to the means for the attainment and preservation of health is a basic human right.

2. Effort of the individual himself is a vitally important factor in attaining and maintaining health.

3. The physician-patient relationship is so fundamental to health that everyone should have a personal physician.

4. The physician should have access to proper facilities and equipment, affiliation on some basis with a hospital, and the help of trained personnel in order to fulfill his part in providing comprehensive health services.

5. Comprehensive health service includes the positive promotion of health, the prevention of disease, the diagnosis and treatment of disease, the rehabilitation of the disabled—all supported by constantly improving education of personnel and a continuous program of research.

6. Comprehensive health service is the concern of society and is best insured when all elements of society participate in providing it.

7. Responsibility for health is a joint one, with the individual citizen and local, State, Federal governments each having major contributions to make toward its fuller realization.

8. The American people desire and deserve comprehensive health service of the highest quality and in our dynamic expanding economy the means can be found to provide it.

9. The same high quality of health services should be available to all people equally.

10. A health program must take into account the progress and experience of the past, the realities of the present, and must be flexible enough to cope with future changes.

We set as a goal for this Nation a situation in which adequate health personnel, facilities, and organization make comprehensive health services available for all, with a method of financing to make this care universally accessible. . . .

Recommendations.—In order to move toward the goal of comprehensive personal health services for all people in this country,

WE, THEREFORE, RECOMMEND THAT: *

1. The principle of prepared health services be accepted as the most feasible method of financing the costs of medical care.

2. The present prepayment plans be expanded to provide as much health service to as many people as they can; be judged by the criteria mentioned earlier in this chapter; and be aided by government through allowing payroll deductions

---

* Dissenting opinions, or supplementary statements clarifying their individual positions, were recorded here by several Commission members, as follows:

1. Dissenting opinion signed jointly by A. J. Hayes [President, International Association of Machinists], Elizabeth S. Magee [General Secretary, National Consumers League], and Walter P. Reuther [President, United Automobile Workers, CIO]:

"... The majority recommendations [regarding the financing of personal health services] will not accomplish the objectives of the Commission as stated throughout the report ... 'that all persons in the country should have ready access to high quality comprehensive personal health service.'

"Any legislation which would leave participation in a health or health insurance program to the option of each State, or which would be dependent upon special kinds of organizations of medical personnel, could not possibly accomplish the objective ... In fact, such legislation would discriminate against those persons whose States chose for any reason not to participate.

"If the basic recommendations in [this section] of the Commission's Report are to be considered as a means of achieving the objectives set forth throughout the report, then the participation of every State must be assured by Federal statute, or the Federal government must make such health services available in those States which for any reasons do not participate. In the event this cannot be accomplished for any reasons, then [these] objectives ... should be accomplished through a National Health Insurance Act supported by joint employer-employee contributions and tax revenues."

2. Supplementary statement by Clarence Poe [President and Editor, The Progressive Farmer]:

"I heartily agree with the Commission's endorsement of (a) the prepayment principle as the only foundation on which we can build and (b) Federal matching grants to States (upon the basis of relative wealth and needs) as the only effective way of insuring medical care for all people.

"[In rural areas], however, [there is] a sense of urgency and a desperate need for prompt action. Among our rural people, we have neither the wealth nor the insurance needed. Every day men, women, and children are dying needlessly for lack of proper medical and health facilities. ...

"I hope that our report will lead more and more people to accept the principle ... that our democracy will never be complete until every person, rich or poor, high or low, urban or rural, white or black, has an equal right to adequate hospital and medical care whenever and wherever he [requires such care]. And as for the method by which this equal right should be achieved we need to use the prepayment mechanism and add these three basic principles:

"(a) The family that can pay its way should do so.

"(b) The family that can partly pay its way should pay this part, government and philanthropy providing the remainder.

"(c) Whatever family poverty, illness, or misfortune has left honestly incapable of paying anything will nevertheless be helped by government and philanthropy to an equal chance with the rest of us."

3. Supplementary statement by Joseph C. Hinsey [Dean, Cornell College of Medicine]:

"I concur in these recommendations only if comprehensive personal health services are developed so as to maintain free choice of health personnel, freedom of type of practice, and a system of remuneration that is mutually satisfactory to the members of the health professions and the consuming public."

for government employees, removing the restrictions on organization of prepayment plans, and promoting research on health service administration.

3. A cooperative Federal-State program be established to assist in the financing of personal health services. Under this program, a single State health authority would be set up in each participating State. Each State would draw up an over-all State plan for assisting the development and distribution of personal health service for all persons. It would use public or private agencies and resources, or a combination of them. State plans would be developed in cooperation with local or regional authorities and would be linked with the planned expansion of health resources so as to provide ultimately more comprehensive, more efficient, and more economical services. State plans would be expected to conform to certain Federal minimum standards and would be submitted to the Federal health agency for approval. Federal funds for the program might be derived from several different sources as recommended below.

4. Funds collected through the Old Age and Survivors Insurance mechanism be utilized to purchase personal health service benefits on a prepayment basis for beneficiaries of that insurance program, under a plan which meets Federal standards and which does not involve a means test.

5. Federal grants-in-aid be made from general tax revenues for the purpose of assisting the States in making personal health services available to public assistance recipients. This should be done under a prepayment plan which is established in consultation with a State advisory council, which is approved by a Federal health agency in accordance with Federal standards, and which specifies:

a. A State-wide program administered by a single State agency, with an advisory council representing the public interest.

b. Services to all persons who are declared eligible, with no discrimination as to age, race, citizenship, or place or duration of residence, and with no means test at the time care is needed.

c. As comprehensive personal health services as local resources will permit, with maximum utilization of all available health personnel and facilities.

d. Administration on a local or regional basis.

6. Federal grants-in-aid be made from general tax revenues for the purpose of assisting the States in making personal health services available to the general population, under a plan meeting the same criteria as above.

7. Federal grants-in-aid be made to the States to assist them and local governments in operating facilities for tuberculosis and mental disease and developing similar facilities for other long-term illness. These institutions should be available to all persons in the population without the application of a means test.

8. The Federal government continue to meet through use of its own facilities its obligations for providing personal health services to military personnel, veterans with service-connected disabilities requiring long-term care, and merchant seamen —with no expansion of federally operated facilities except when needed for the Armed Forces. It should also continue to meet its present commitments to veterans for service-connected disabilities requiring short-term care and to the Indians, through direct operation of health services—until such time as the administration of

these services can be transferred to the States and localities in accordance with approved local and State plans which guarantee a proper standard of care. . . .

F. AMERICAN DENTAL ASSOCIATION *

THE AMERICAN DENTAL Association believes that the following elements are essential for the success of a national program for the promotion of dental health.

Federal Department of Health.—A federal department of health, with cabinet status, should be established independently of welfare and educational agencies and should be administered by persons trained in the health sciences and qualified to coordinate all federal health activities except those of the military services.

Dental Research.—Dental research should be promoted through the National Institute of Dental Research and through grants to public and private agencies and individuals qualified to carry on significant research. New resources for dental research should be sought continuously from private agencies.

Dental Health Education.—Dental health education should be carried on through appropriate state and community agencies to provide authentic information on health practices, to motivate people to assume personal responsibility for health and to inform them of the facilities available for dental health care.

Dental Care.—Dental care should be available to all regardless of income or geographic location as rapidly as resources will permit. Private and community programs should provide for priority treatment, prevention and control of dental disease in children, and for the elimination of pain and infection in adults. The community in all cases shall determine its methods for providing services.

Program Planning.—In all major conferences that may lead to the formation of a national dental health program, authorized representatives of the American Dental Association should participate. Similarly, in all major conferences that may lead to the formation of a community or state dental health program, authorized representatives appointed by constituent or component dental societies should participate that public health and welfare may be best protected.

Councils on Dental Health.—The establishment of councils on dental health at state and local levels should be completed as rapidly as possible in order to provide a mechanism through which the development of dental health programs can be facilitated. Such councils should have lay and consumer consultants.

General Health Plans and Programs.—It should be the consistent policy of all dental groups to cooperate as fully as possible with other health groups in the development of programs designed to promote the total health of the patient.

* From: *Official Policies of the American Dental Association on Dental Health Programs*, by the Council on Dental Health, American Dental Association; Chicago: The Association, 1954 ("The National Program," pp. 7-9). Reprinted by permission of the publishers.

Public Health Dentistry.—Each of the states should be urged to establish a division of dental health within the department of health and the administration of the dental program should be in the hands of a qualified dental officer who is directly responsible to the state health officer.

Veterans' Dental Care.—The dental care of veterans should be maintained at a high standard and should be provided under a state program in which the veteran has free choice of practitioners in private practice.

Hospitals and Health Centers.—The construction or addition of adequate dental facilities should be undertaken in all hospital and health centers. Such dental facilities should be operated and maintained in accord with standards established by the American Dental Association and administered by a qualified dentist.

Methods of Payment.—Voluntary prepayment and postpayment plans consistent with sound experience should be developed as rapidly as possible. A federal compulsory health insurance program should be opposed on the ground that it is not in the interest of the public or of the profession.

Dental Education and Personnel.—Facilities for the training of dental personnel should be expanded. Such expansion should be consistent with local and regional needs. Improved support for dental education should be sought provided that such support does not entail a loss of independence on the part of the educational institutions.

Dentistry in Military Services.—Dental programs in the military services should provide high quality care for the military patient. All policies dealing with dentistry should be developed, administered and controlled by the dental officer.

FURTHER READINGS

American Nurses Association and National Organization for Public Health Nursing. *Guide for the Inclusion of Nursing Services in Medical Care Plans.* New York: The Association, 1950. 31 pages.

American Public Health Association, Subcommittee on Medical Care. *The Quality of Medical Care in a National Health Program.* New York: The Association, 1949. 27 pages. (Includes references).

American Public Health Association, Committee on Child Health. *Services for Handicapped Children.* New York: The Association, 1955. 150 pages. (Includes references).

American Public Health Association and American Public Welfare Association, Joint Committee on Medical Care. *Tax-Supported Medical Care for the Needy.* New York: American Public Health Association, 1952. 18 pages. (Includes references).

Burns, Eveline M. *Social Security and Public Policy.* New York: McGraw-Hill, 1956. 291 pages. (Includes references).

Commission on Financing of Hospital Care. *Financing Hospital Care in the United States.* (3 vols.). New York: McGraw-Hill, 1954-55.

Committee on the Costs of Medical Care. *Medical Care for the American People.* Publication No. 28 (Final Report) of the Committee. Chicago: University of Chicago Press, 1932. 213 pages.

Davis, Michael M. *Medical Care for Tomorrow.* New York: Harper and Bros., 1955. 497 pages. (Includes references).

Dickinson, Frank G. *Analysis of a Statement on Medical Care.* Bulletin 77, Bureau of Medical Economic Research, American Medical Association. Chicago: The Association, 1950. 6 pages.

Massachusetts Memorial Hospitals. *Health for the American People: A Symposium.* Boston: Little, Brown and Co., 1956. 105 pages.

INDEX

Index *

* Prepared by George A. Chaffee

697

Group practice, and GP's, 206-7, 224; and specialists, 228-9; hospital data, 271-2; in clinics, 326, 328; patterns and problems, 331-9; advantages, 339-43; disadvantages, 344-6; and free choice, 346-7; in operation, 347-50; and prevention, 356-8; and rural problems, 428, 439, 443; and HIP (N.Y.), 580-4; and compulsory health insurance, 634, 637; slow development of, 656
Guidance for handicapped, 479-80
Guilds, medieval, medical care in, 10
Guy's Hospital (London, England), 259

Hamilton, C. Horace, 178
Hammurabi, code of medical practice, 4
Handicapped persons, VA care, 464-5, 468; crippled children, 469-75; disabled adults, 475-81. *See also* Rehabilitation
Hanes, Fred, 204
Harvard Medical School, history, 23
Hawley, General Paul R., 458-9
Health, new and positive concept, 30-1; a definition of, 31-2; status of U.S., 34-6; means to improvement, 36; trends in children, 40-4; among Negroes, 44-7; in the aged, 47-54; the nation's medical bill, 121-5; consumer spending trends, 126-44; ability to pay for, 144-8
Health, Education and Welfare, Department of (U.S.), reinsurance approach, 646
Health center, concept of hospital as, 255, 268; regional concept, 352-6; role in integration of prevention and cure, 362-5; and group practice, 580-4; proposals, 693
Health departments. *See* Public health departments
Health education, proposals, 677, 685, 692
Health examinations, and prevention of chronic disease, 380
Health Information Foundation, 3
Health insurance. *See* Commercial insurance companies, Compulsory health insurance, *and* Voluntary prepayment health insurance
Health Insurance Council, 3
Health Insurance Plan of Greater New York (HIP), 51-2; utilization of physicians' services, 84-6; on utilization of nursing services, 89; payment of physicians, 198; on GP's, 213, 216; organization of, 334; comprehensive service benefits, 579-84
Health services, utilization of, 83-90, 99-100
Hill bill, 640
Hill-Burton Act. *See* Hospital Survey and Construction Act

Hippocratic oath, 199, 206, 668
Hitchcock Memorial Hospital (Hanover, N.H.), 333
Holmes, Dr. Oliver Wendell, 23
Home care, and hospitals, 272, 287; maternity cases, 372; and chronic illness, 382-3, 408-12; VA, 467; HIP (N.Y.), 584
Hospital care, standards of, 302-7
Hospital Council of Greater New York, on bed-death ratio, 297-8
Hospital services, utilization of, 86-8
Hospital Survey and Construction Act (Hill-Burton Act), program of, 268-9, 273-8, 283-4, 300-1; and bed needs, 299; and regionalization of hospitals, 354; and state responsibility, 372; facilities for chronic illness, 384; and rural needs, 426, 427, 428, 436, 442; and public medical care, 447
Hospitalism (cross-infection), banishment by Lister, 261
Hospitalization, needs of individual for, 105-6
Hospitalization insurance, 292-5. *See also* Voluntary prepayment health insurance
Hospitals, history and development, 24, 257-65; bed shortages, 26-7, 76-7, 269-70, 271-8, 295-9, 461-3; increase in utilization, 86-7, 90-2, 98, 116, 129-43, 298; and discriminatory patterns, 180-2; and GP's, 202, 204, 211-2, 223-4; as health centers, 206, 255, 268; and development of modern nursing, 231-2, 235-7; dental programs, 241; and medical social worker, 247-8; as medical institutions, 256-67; status of present system, 267-72; construction needs, 272-8; program for service improvement, 279-84; administrative and financial problems, 284-92; and hospitalization insurance, 292-5; standards of care, 302-7; and the physician, 307-28; definition, 315-6; medical practice *in never by*, 316-20; out-patient services, 320-8; and group practice, 337; and regionalization, 351-6; role in integration of prevention and cure, 358-62, 365-72; and chronic illness, 383-407; and home care, 408-12; and rural problem, 423-5, 427, 435-6, 442-3; and public medical care, 448, 453, 455; and VA program, 457-8, 461-3, 466, 468; and crippled children, 470-5; and disabled adults, 477; and mentally ill, 482-5, 490; and industrial medical care, 501, 514-5, 523-4; and voluntary health insurance, 559-608 *passim*, 653; and compulsory health insurance, 630, 631, 637-9, 653; proposals, 683, 693

Private ambulatory service, as a form of group practice, 335
Private group clinics, 332-3
Professional associations, hospital standards of, 302-7
Prosthetic progress, VA, 465
Provident Medical Associates, on discriminatory patterns, 180, 181
Psychiatry, need for training in by GP's, 207; and VA program, 465, 466; and public medical care of mentally ill, 484-91
Public health departments (and services), and the regional concept, 355; coordination with hospitals in prevention and cure, 362-3, 365-72; advantages of joint housing with hospitals, 366-8; and rural medical care, 440, 443; and public medical care, 446-93 *passim;* and individual medical care, 496, 550-1; proposals concerning, 677-83, 693
Public health education, and hospitals, 281
Public health nurses, in out-patient clinics, 327
Public Health Service (U.S.), on shortage of physicians, 158, 171; methods of payment of physicians, 198; dental service, 239; on mental hospitals, 271; direction of Hill-Burton Act, 273; hospital operation, 274; on extent of disability, 418; aid to rural areas, 437; and industrial medical care, 502; proposals concerning, 679, 681

Quality of medical care, basic principles, 100-9; concept of adequacy, 110-1; criteria for assessment of, 111-4

Reciprocity, in Blue Cross plans, 566-7
Referrals, and group practice, 331-9, 341-8
Regionalization, 350-6; as aid to rural problem, 439
Rehabilitation, and hospitals, 272; for chronic illness, 374, 387-8, 416-21; and the VA, 468; federal vocational program, 470-81; under workmen's compensation, 535-6, 540-8
Reinsurance, for voluntary health insurance, 645-7
Relief status, and illness rates, 55-60
Replacement needs, hospitals, 299-302
Research, in hospitals, 280, 286; and integration of prevention and cure, 360; on chronic illness, 380-1; VA program, 465-6; proposals, 676, 681, 692
Residencies, standards, 303, 306; duties, 310; VA program, 465

Robinson, G. Canby, 207
Rochester (N.Y.), plan of regionalization, 355-6
Rockefeller Sanitary Commission, on rural needs, 425
Rome (Italy), history of medical care, 4, 8-9
Roosevelt, Franklin Delano, on medical care, 655
Ross-Loos Clinic (Los Angeles, Calif.), 333, 660
Rotating internships, to encourage GP's, 203, 208
Rubinow, I. M., 622-3
Rural areas, decline in medical services, 155-7, 168, 174-9, 422-6; hospital needs, 283; integration of prevention and cure, 363, 364, 368; joint housing of health departments and hospitals, 366; effect of population shift, 423; health status, 425; medical care programs, 432-41; suggested programs for, 441-5; public medical care for the mentally ill, 489; and Blue Cross plans, 563; and voluntary health plans, 595
Rural families, utilization of physicians' services, 85, 86; of hospital services, 92; of care for children, 94-8
Rural general practitioners, encouragement for, 205; distribution pattern of, 211-2; functions, 217-8
"Rush medicine," 196
Rusk, Howard, 378, 542-3
Russia, history of medical care, 13

Saint Bartholomew's Hospital (London, England), 258-9
St. Thomas's Hospital (London, England), 232, 258-9
Salary basis, of payment for physicians, 189-90, 193, 196-8, 660; under compulsory health insurance, 634, 636-7
Saskatchewan (Canada) Hospital Services Plan, 51-3, 84, 295
Screening, for chronic illness, 390; definition, 396-7; principles, 397-8; multiple, 398-402
Semi-private patients, increase under Blue Cross plans, 294-5
Serbein, Oscar N., 138
Service benefits, under voluntary health plans, 560-74, 612-3
Service facilities, availability under voluntary health plans, 607-8
Service plans, voluntary health insurance, 559, 560-74, 612

www.ingramcontent.com/pod-product-compliance
Lightning Source LLC
Chambersburg PA
CBHW021022210326
41598CB00016B/883

* 9 780807 879511 *